Essential Revision Notes in Paediatrics for the MRCPCH

Second edition

Edited by

Dr R M Beattie BSc MBBS MRCP FRCPCH
Consultant Paediatric Gastroenterologist
Paediatric Medical Unit
Southampton General Hospital
Southampton

Dr M P Champion BSc MBBS MRCP FRCPCH
Consultant in Paediatric Metabolic Medicine
Department of Paediatric Metabolic Medicine
Evelina Children's Hospital
London

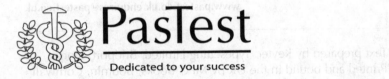

PasTest
Dedicated to your success

Second edition published 2006

First edition published 2002

ISBN: 1 904627 62 5
9781904627623

A catalogue record for this book is available from the British Library.

The information contained within this book was obtained by the author from reliable sources. However, while every effort has been made to ensure its accuracy, no responsibility for loss, damage or injury occasioned to any person acting or refraining from action as a result of information contained herein can be accepted by the publishers or author.

Every effort has been made to contact holders of copyright to obtain permission to reproduce copyright material. However, if any have been inadvertently overlooked, the publisher will be pleased to make the necessary arrangements at the first opportunity.

PasTest Revision Books and Intensive Courses

PasTest has been established in the field of postgraduate medical education since 1972, providing revision books and intensive study courses for doctors preparing for their professional examinations.

Books and courses are available for the following specialties:

MRCGP, MRCP Parts 1 and 2, MRCPCH Parts 1 and 2, MRCPsych, MRCS, MRCOG Parts 1 and 2, DRCOG, DCH, FRCA, PLAB Parts 1 and 2.

For further details contact:

PasTest, Freepost, Knutsford, Cheshire WA16 7BR

Tel: 01565 752000   **Fax: 01565 650264**
www.pastest.co.uk enquires@pastest.co.uk

Text prepared by Keytec Typesetting Limited, Bridport, Dorset
Printed and bound in the UK by MPG Books, Bodmin, Cornwall

Contents

v

Contents

Karyn Moschal MBChB MRCP (UK) MRCPCH DTM+H
Consultant in Paediatric Infectious Diseases
Great Ormond Street Hospital for Children
London

Vasanta R Nanduri MBBS DCH MRCP MD FRCPCH
Consultant Paediatrician
Watford General Hospital
Watford

Mr Ken Nischal FRCOphth
Consultant Ophthalmic Surgeon and Fellowship Director
Great Ormond Street Hospital for Children
London

Joanne Philpot BA MBBS MD DCH MRCPCH
Consultant Paediatrician
Wrexham Park Hospital
Slough

Waseem Qasim BMedSci MB BS MRCP MRCPCH PhD
Clinical Lecturer
Molecular Immunology Unit
Institute of Child Health
London

Christopher J D Reid MB ChB MRCP(UK) FRCPCH
Consultant Paediatric Nephrologist
Evelina Children's Hospital
London

Vel K Sakthivel FRCS(Ed), FRCS(Tr&Orth)
Specialist Registrar in Trauma and Orthopaedics
Southampton General Hospital
Southampton

Neil H Thomas MA MB BChir FRCP FRCPCH DCH
Consultant Paediatric Neurologist
Southampton General Hospital
Southampton

Stephen R Tomlin MRPharmS
Principal Paediatric Pharmacist
Evelina Children's Hospital
London

Robert M R Tulloh BA BM BCh MA DM FRCP FRCPCH
Consultant Paediatric Cardiologist
Bristol Royal Hospital for Children
Bristol

Angie M Wade MSc PhD CSTAT ILTM
Senior Lecturer in Medical Statistics
Centre for Paediatric Epidemiology and Biostatistics
Institute of Child Health
London

Robert A Wheeler
Consultant Neonatal and Paediatric Surgeon, Consultant in Medical Law
Wessex Regional Paediatric Surgical Centre
Southampton General Hospital
Southampton

Louise C Wilson BSc MBChB FRCP
Consultant in Clinical Genetics
Clinical and Molecular Genetics Unit
Great Ormond Street Hospital for Children NHS Trust and Institute of Child Health
Department of Genetics
London

The Publisher and Editors would also like to thank the following contributors to the 1ˢᵗ edition for their contribution:

Katy Fidler BSc MBBS MRCPCH
Clinical Research Fellow in Paediatric Infectious Diseases
Institute of Child Health
London

Bobby Gaspar BSc MBBS MRCO PhD MRCPCH
Senior Lecturer and Consultant in Paediatric Immunology
Molecular Immunology Unit
Institute of Child Health
University College London
London

Nigel Klein BSc MBBS MRCP FRCPCH PhD
Reader/Honorary Consultant in Paediatric ID and Immunology
Department of Infectious Diseases and Microbiology
Institute of Child Health
London

Preface to the Second Edition

The first edition of *Essential Revision Notes in Paediatrics for the MRCPCH* was the response to an often expressed desire by candidates for a revision book covering all the essential information required for the Paediatric Membership in an accessible and concise way. Contributors were then sought who were both experts in their chosen field, but also experienced teachers. The resultant text was somewhat larger than first envisaged, but has also found a place on many a bookshelf as a reference source long after the MRCPCH is passed.

This second edition has been thoroughly updated and revised, with the addition of 5 new chapters: ethics and law, emergency paediatrics, hepatology, orthopaedics and surgery. Once more we hope that the book will prove useful to GP trainees preparing for the DCH and to our allied health care professionals who want a concise General Paediatric reference.

We remain indebted to the individual contributors of the various chapters who are the key to the success of this book and to Pastest for their expertise and support in its production.

To all the candidates we wish you every success in the exam and your future career and hope that this book will contribute in some way to your success.

Mark Beattie
Mike Champion

Preface to the First Edition

There are numerous question books useful in the preparation for the paediatric membership. The feedback is that it is often the concise and focused summary notes that are the most helpful. This book attempts to bring all that together in one text. We hope prospective candidates will find it useful in the preparation for the exam and subsequently as a reference text.

We have tried to emphasise topics which are of particular relevance to the exam and therefore future practice.

We hope that book will also be useful for GP trainees studying for the DCH and the allied health care professionals who want to broaden their general paediatric knowledge base.

We are indebted to PasTest for their considerable expertise and support, our impressive list of contributors all of whom are experts in their fields and experienced teachers, and the candidates who on many MRCPCH courses by the commitment and enthusiasm for the specialty have provided the inspiration for the book.

Mark Beattie
Mike Champion

Chapter 1

Cardiology

Robert Tulloh

CONTENTS

Cardiology

1. DIAGNOSIS OF CONGENITAL HEART DISEASE

1.1 Fetal cardiology

Diagnosis

In the south of England, most children (> 70%) who require infant surgery for congenital heart disease (CHD) are diagnosed during pregnancy at 16–20 weeks' gestation. This gives a significant advantage to the parents who are counselled by specialists who can give a realistic guide to the prognosis and treatment options. A few undergo termination of pregnancy (depending on the diagnosis). Most continue with the pregnancy and can be offered delivery within the cardiac centre if there could be neonatal complications or if treatment is likely to be needed within the first 2 days of life. Surgical intervention during fetal life is not yet routinely available.

Screening (by a fetal cardiologist) is offered to those with:

- Abnormal four-chamber view on routine-booking, antenatal-anomaly ultrasound scan
- Increased nuchal translucency (thickness at back of the neck), which also increases the risk of Down syndrome
- Previous child with or other family history of CHD
- Maternal risk factors, such as phenylketonuria or diabetes
- Suspected Down, or other, syndrome

Important normal findings on fetal echocardiography include echodensities:

- Used to be called 'Golf-balls'
- Found on anterior mitral valve papillary muscle
- Thought to be calcification during development
- No importance for CHD
- Positive association with Down syndrome
- Do not need echocardiogram after delivery

Arrhythmias

- Diagnosed at any time during pregnancy: an echocardiogram is required to confirm normal anatomy and to confirm type of arrhythmia. Fetal electrocardiogram (ECG) is not yet a routine investigation
- Multiple atrial ectopics are usually not treated
- Supraventricular tachycardia is usually treated with maternal digoxin or flecainide

5

- Heart block may be treated with maternal isoprenaline or salbutamol
- Presence of hydrops is a poor prognostic sign

1.2   Epidemiology of congenital heart disease

Eight per 1,000 live births have CHD, of which the commonest are:

- Ventricular septal defect   30%
- Persistent arterial duct   12%
- Atrial septal defect   7%
- Pulmonary stenosis   7%
- Aortic stenosis   5%
- Coarctation of the aorta   5%
- Tetralogy of Fallot   5%
- Transposition of the great arteries   5%
- Atrioventricular septal defect   2%

Incidence is increased by a positive family history, so the proportion of live births with CHD will be:

- Previous sibling with CHD   2%
- Two siblings with CHD   4%
- Father with CHD   3%
- Mother with CHD   6%

Incidence also increased by

- Presence of other anomaly or syndrome
- Parents with an abnormal genotype
- Maternal ingestion of lithium (Ebstein anomaly)
- Third-trimester enterovirus or coxsackievirus infection (myocarditis, dilated cardiomyopathy)
- Maternal systemic lupus erythematosus (anti-ro, anti-la antibodies leading to congenital heart block)

1.3   Cardiac anatomy

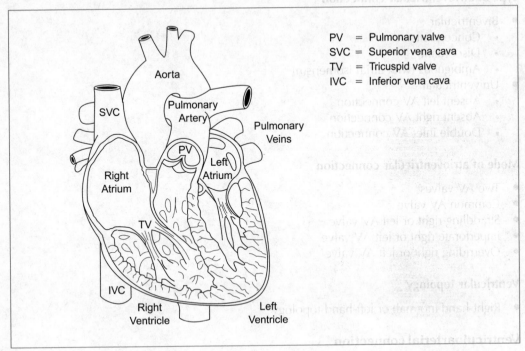

PV = Pulmonary valve
SVC = Superior vena cava
TV = Tricuspid valve
IVC = Inferior vena cava

Normal heart

1.4   Nomenclature for sequential segmental arrangement

The European (as opposed to American) system for complete heart diagnosis is referred to as 'sequential segmental arrangement'. The advantage is that it is no longer necessary to remember the pattern of an eponymous syndrome. The disadvantage is that it is quite long-winded. The idea is that each component is described in turn:

Atrial arrangement (atrial situs)

- Usual (solitus)
- Mirror image (inversus)
- Right isomerism (asplenia syndrome)
- Left isomerism (polysplenia syndrome)

Atrioventricular (AV) connection

Type of atrioventricular connection

- Biventricular
  - Concordant
  - Discordant
  - Ambiguous (with atrial isomerism)
- Univentricular
  - Absent left AV connection
  - Absent right AV connection
  - Double inlet AV connection

Mode of atrioventricular connection

- Two AV valves
- Common AV valve
- Straddling right or left AV valve
- Imperforate right or left AV valve
- Overriding right or left AV valve

Ventricular topology

- Right-hand (normal) or left-hand topology

Ventriculoarterial connection

Type of ventriculoarterial connection

- Concordant
- Discordant
- Double outlet
- Single outlet:
  - Common arterial trunk
  - Solitary arterial trunk
  - With pulmonary atresia
  - With aortic atresia

Mode of ventriculoarterial connection

- Two perforate valves
- Left or right imperforate valve

Infundibular morphology

Arterial relationships

Associated malformations

- Position of heart in the chest — left, right or middle
- Systemic and pulmonary veins

- Atrial septum
- Atrioventricular valves
- Ventricular septum
- Semilunar valves
- Anomalies of great arteries (e.g. double aortic arch)

Surgical or interventional procedures

Acquired or iatrogenic lesions

1.5   Examination technique

To many candidates the diagnosis of congenital heart disease is daunting. Certainly, if the candidate examines the child, listens to the heart and then tries to make a diagnosis, this will prove difficult. The following system should be used instead.

History

The history-taking is short and to the point. The candidate needs to know:

- Was the child born preterm?
- Are there any cardiac symptoms of:
  - Heart failure (breathlessness, poor feeding, faltering growth, cold hands and feet)
  - Cyanosis
  - Neonatal collapse
- Is it an asymptomatic heart murmur found on routine examination?
- Is there a syndrome such as Down syndrome?
- Is there any family history of congenital heart disease?
- Did the mother have any illnesses or take any medication during pregnancy?

Examination

- Introduce yourself to mother and patient. Ask if you can examine the child.
- Position child according to age:
  - For a 6-year-old — at an angle of 45 degrees
  - For a toddler — upright on mother's knee
  - For a baby — flat on the bed
- Remove clothes from chest
- Stand back and look for:
  - Dysmorphism
  - Intravenous infusion cannula
  - Obvious cyanosis or scars

The following examinations should be performed.

Heart failure

The delivery of oxygen to the peripheral vascular bed is insufficient to meet the metabolic demands of the child. Usually because of left to right shunt with good heart pump function.

- A thin, malnourished child (Faltering growth)
- Excessive sweating around the forehead
- Tachycardia
- Breathlessness +/– subcostal or intercostal recession
- Poor peripheral perfusion with cold hands and feet
- A large liver
- Never found with ventricular septal defect (VSD) or other left to right shunt in first week of life
- An emergency if found up to 7 days of age. Implies a duct-dependent lesion, e.g. hypoplastic left heart syndrome or coarctation

Cyanosis

- Mild cyanosis is not visible — use the pulse oximeter

Clubbing

- Visible after 6 months old
- First apparent in the thumbs or toes
- Best demonstrated by holding thumbs together, back to back to demonstrate loss of normal nail-bed curvature
- Disappears a few years after corrective surgery

Pulse

- Rate (count for 6 seconds × 10)
- Rhythm (only 'regular' or 'irregular', need ECG for 'sinus rhythm')
- Character at the antecubital fossa with the elbows straight, using the thumbs — on both arms together

Head and neck

- Anaemia — for older children only — ask the patient to look up and examine the conjunctivae (not appropriate in a baby)
- Cyanosis — the tongue should be examined for central cyanosis. If in doubt ask the child to stick out their tongue and ask the mother to do the same. This will detect oxygen saturations of < 85%
- Jugular venous pressure — the head is turned towards the candidate so that the other side of the neck (the left side) can be seen with the jugular venous pressure visible, outlined against the pillows. In a child who is under 4 years, the jugular venous pressure should not be assessed
- Carotid thrill — essential part of the examination, midway up the left side of the neck, felt with the thumb, proof of the presence of aortic stenosis

Precordium

Inspection

- Respiratory rate
- Median sternotomy scar (= open heart surgery — see Section 9)
- Lateral thoracotomy scar (Blalock–Taussig (BT) shunt, patent ductus arteriosus (PDA) ligation, pulmonary artery (PA) band, coarctation repair)
- Additional scars, e.g. on the abdomen

Palpation

- Apex beat 'the most inferior and lateral position where the index finger is lifted by the impulse of the heart'. Place fingers along the fifth intercostal space of both sides of chest (for dextrocardia) and count down apex position only if patient is lying at 45 degrees
- Left ventricular heave
- Right ventricular heave at the left parasternal border
- Thrills at upper or lower left sternal edge

Auscultation

- Heart sounds and their character
- Additional sounds
- Murmurs, their character, intensity and where they are best heard

Heart sounds

First heart sound is created by closure of the mitral and then tricuspid valves. It is not important for the candidate to comment on the nature of the first heart sound.

Second heart sound, however, is more important, created by closure of first the aortic and then the pulmonary valves.

- Loud pulmonary sound — pulmonary hypertension
- Fixed splitting of second sound (usually with inspiration the sounds separate and then come together during expiration). Listen when patient is sitting up, at the mid-left sternal edge in expiration
  - Atrial septal defect
  - Right bundle-branch block
- Single second sound in transposition of great arteries (TGA), pulmonary atresia, or hypoplastic left heart syndrome
- Quiet second sound may occur in pulmonary valve stenosis or pulmonary artery band

Additional sounds

Added sounds present may be a normal third or fourth heart sound heard in the neonate or these sounds can be pathological, for example in a 4-year-old with a dilated cardiomyopathy and heart failure. An ejection click is heard at aortic valve opening, after the first heart sound, and is caused by a bicuspid aortic valve in most cases.

Murmurs

Before listening for any murmurs, the candidate should have a good idea of the type of congenital heart disease, which is being dealt with. The candidate should know whether the child is blue (and therefore likely to have tetralogy of Fallot) or is breathless (likely to have a left to right shunt) or has no positive physical findings before auscultation of the murmurs (and therefore more likely to either be normal, have a small left to right shunt or mild obstruction). By the time the murmurs are auscultated, there should only be two or three diseases to choose between, with the stethoscope being used to perform the fine tuning. It is best to start at the apex with the bell, and move to the lower left sternal edge with the diaphragm. Then on to the upper left sternal edge and upper right sternal edge both with the diaphragm. Additional areas can be auscultated, but provide little additional information. Murmurs are graded out of 6 for systolic, 1 = very soft, 2 = soft, 3 = moderate, 4 = loud with a thrill, 5 = heard with a stethoscope off the chest, 6 = heard as you enter the room. Murmurs are out of 4 for diastolic, again 2, 3 and 4.

Ejection systolic murmur

Upper sternal edge — implies outflow tract obstruction. Right or left ventricular outflow tract obstruction can occur at valvar (+ ejection click), subvalvar or supravalvar level.

- Upper right sternal edge (carotid thrill)   = Aortic stenosis
- Upper left sternal edge (no carotid thrill)   = Pulmonary stenosis or atrial septal defect (ASD)
- Mid/lower left sternal edge   = Innocent murmur (see below)
- Long harsh systolic murmur + cyanosis   = Tetralogy of Fallot

Pansystolic murmur

- Left lower sternal edge (+/− thrill)   = VSD
- Apex (much less common)   = Mitral regurgitation
- Rare at left lower sternal edge (+/− cyanosis)   = Tricuspid regurgitation (Ebstein anomaly)

Continuous murmur

- Left infraclavicular (+/− collapsing pulse)   = Persistent arterial duct
- Infraclavicular (+ cyanosis + lateral thoracotomy)   = BT shunt
- Any site (lungs, shoulder, head, hind-quarter)   = Arteriovenous fistula

Diastolic murmurs

- Unusual in childhood
- Left sternal edge/apex (+/− carotid thrill or VSD)   = Aortic regurgitation
- Median sternotomy (+/− PS (pulmonary stenosis) murmur)
    = Tetralogy of Fallot, repaired
- Apical (+/− VSD)   = Mitral flow/(rarely stenosis)

NB Listening to the back gives little diagnostic information, but is useful thinking time.

Presentation of findings

Few candidates pay enough attention to the case presentation. This should be done after the examination is complete. The candidate should stand, look the examiner in the eye, put hands behind his/her back and present. The important positives and negatives should be stated quickly and succinctly with no 'umms' or 'errrs'. It is important to judge the mood of the examiner, if he/she is looking bored, then go faster. Practise with a tape recorder or video-recording.

To complete the examination you would:

- Measure the blood pressure
- Measure the oxygen saturation
- Feel the femoral pulses
- Feel the liver edge

The presentation should be rounded off with the phrase 'the findings are consistent with the diagnosis of . . .'.

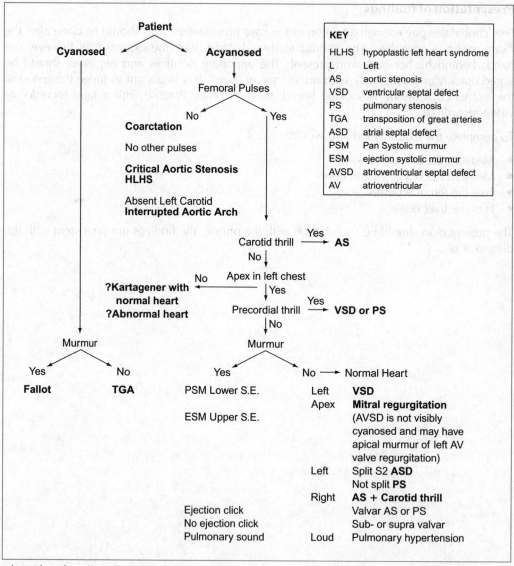

Algorithm for clinical examination

The patient with surgical scars:

- Left lateral thoracotomy
  - PA band   Thrill + ejection systolic murmur at upper left sternal edge
  - Coarctation   +/– left brachial pulse
  - Shunt   Blue + continuous murmur
  - PDA No signs

- Right lateral thoracotomy
  - Shunt   Blue + continuous murmur
- Median sternotomy
  - Any intracardiac operation

1.6   Innocent murmurs

The commonest murmur heard in children is the functional, innocent or physiological heart murmur (40% of all children). They are often discovered in children with an intercurrent infection or with anaemia. These all relate to a structurally normal heart but can cause great concern within the family. There are several different types depending on the possible site of their origin. It is clearly important to make a positive diagnosis of a normal heart. The murmur should be:

- **S**oft (no thrill)
- **S**ystolic
- **S**hort, never pansystolic
- **AS**ymptomatic
- Left **S**ternal edge

It may change with posture.

Innocent murmurs do not require antibiotic prophylaxis.

Diastolic murmurs are not innocent.

An innocent murmur is not associated with abnormal or added heart sounds.

Types of innocent murmur include:

- Increased flow across branch pulmonary artery — this is frequently seen in preterm neonates, is a physiological finding and resolves as the pulmonary arteries grow. The murmur disappears after a few weeks of age, and never causes symptoms
- Still's murmur — this is vibratory in nature and is found at the mid-left sternal edge. It may be caused by turbulence around a muscle band in the left ventricle
- Venous hum — it may be easy to hear the venous blood flow returning to the heart, especially at the upper sternal edge. This characteristically occurs in both systole and diastole and disappears on lying the child flat

2.   BASIC CARDIAC PHYSIOLOGY

2.1   Physiology of adaptation to extrauterine life

During the adaptation from fetal life there are a number of changes in the normal child:

- A fall in the pulmonary vascular resistance, rapidly in the first few breaths, but this continues until 3 months of age
- A resultant fall in the pulmonary arterial pressure
- Loss of the placenta from the circulation

- Closure of the ductus venosus
- Closure of the ductus arteriosus
- Closure of the foramen ovale

The arterial duct is kept patent with prostaglandins E_1 or E_2 infusion in children with duct-dependent circulation such as transposition of the great arteries, or pulmonary atresia.

2.2 Physiology of congenital heart disease

The main principles of congenital heart disease are

- The pressure on the left side of the heart is usually higher than that on the right
- Any communication between atria, ventricles or great arteries leads to a left to right shunt
- Pulmonary vascular resistance falls over the first 12 weeks of life, increasing the shunt
- There will only be cyanosis if the desaturated blood shunts from the right to left side
- Common mixing leads to cyanosis and breathlessness
- Duct-dependent conditions usually present at 2 days of life
- Prostaglandin E_2 or E_1 can be used to reopen the duct up to about 2 weeks of life

2.3 Physiology of heart muscle and heart rate

Arterial pulse volume depends on stroke volume and arterial compliance.

- Small pulse volume in
  - Cardiac failure
  - Hypovolaemia
  - Vasoconstriction
- Large pulse volume in
  - Vasodilatation
  - Pyrexia
  - Anaemia
  - Aortic regurgitation
  - Hyperthyroid
  - CO_2 retention
- Pulsus paradoxus
  - Exaggeration of normal rise and fall of blood pressure with respiration, seen in airways obstruction, such as asthma
- Sinus arrhythmia
  - Variation of the normal heart rate with respiration. Faster in inspiration and slower in expiration. Can be very marked in children

Cardiac output is increased by
- Adrenergic stimulus
- Increased stretch (Starling's curve)
- Increased preload
- Reduced afterload

3. LEFT TO RIGHT SHUNT

(Pink +/– breathless)

General principles

No signs or symptoms on first day of life because of the high pulmonary vascular resistance. Later, at 1 week, infant can develop symptoms and signs of heart failure.

Symptoms of heart failure

- Tachypnoea
- Poor feeding, Faltering growth
- Cold hands and feet
- Sweating
- Vomiting

Signs of heart failure

- Thin
- Tachypnoea
- Displaced apex
- Dynamic precordium
- Apical diastolic murmur
- Hepatomegaly

3.1 Atrial septal defect (ASD)

Types of defect

- Secundum ASD
- Primum ASD (partial atrioventricular septal defect)
- Sinus venosus ASD
- Other

Secundum ASD

A defect in the centre of the atrial septum involving the fossa ovalis.

Clinical features

- Asymptomatic
- 80% of ASDs
- Soft systolic murmur at upper left sternal edge
- Fixed split S2 (difficult to hear)

ECG

- Partial right bundle-branch block (90%)
- Right ventricle hypertrophy

Chest X-ray

- Increased pulmonary vascular markings

Management

- Closure at 3–5 years (ideally)
- 90% undergo device closure in catheter laboratory
- 10% undergo surgical closure (too large or personal preference)

Partial atrioventricular septal defect (Primum ASD)

A defect in the lower atrial septum, involving the left atrioventricular valve which has three leaflets and tends to leak.

Clinical features

- Asymptomatic
- 10% of ASDs
- Soft systolic murmur at upper left sternal edge
- Apical pansystolic murmur (atrioventricular valve regurgitation)
- Fixed split S2 (difficult to hear)

ECG

- Partial right bundle-branch block (90%)
- Right ventricle hypertrophy
- Superior axis

Chest X-ray

- Increased pulmonary vascular markings

Management

- Closure at 3–5 years
- All require surgical closure (because of the need to repair valve)

Sinus venosus ASD

A defect at the upper end of the atrial septum, such that the superior vena cava (SVC) overrides the atrial septum. The right pulmonary veins are usually anomalous and drain directly into the SVC or right atrium adding to the left to right shunt.

Clinical features

- Asymptomatic or heart failure
- 5% of ASDs
- Soft systolic murmur at upper left sternal edge
- Fixed split S2 (easily heard)

ECG

- Partial right bundle-branch block
- Right ventricle hypertrophy

Chest X-ray

- Increased pulmonary vascular markings
- Cardiomegaly

Management

- Closure at 1–5 years
- All require surgical closure and repair to the anomalous pulmonary veins

There are other rare types of ASD, which are similarly treated.

3.2 Ventricular septal defect (VSD)

Small defect

A defect anywhere in the ventricular septum (perimembranous or muscular, can be inlet or outlet). Restrictive defects are smaller than the aortic valve. There is no pulmonary hypertension.

Clinical features

- Asymptomatic (80–90%)
- May have a thrill at left lower sternal edge
- Loud pansystolic murmur at lower left sternal edge (the louder the murmur, the smaller the hole)
- Quiet P2

ECG

- Normal

Chest X-ray

- Normal

Management

- Review with echocardiography
- Spontaneous closure, but may persist to adult life

Large defect

Defects anywhere in the septum. Large defects tend to be the same size or larger than the aortic valve. There is always pulmonary hypertension.

Clinical features

- Symptomatic with heart failure after age 1 week
- 10–20% of VSDs
- Right ventricular heave
- Soft or no systolic murmur
- Apical mid-diastolic heart murmur
- Loud P2

ECG

- Biventricular hypertrophy by 2 months (see Section 15 — ECG)

Chest X-ray

- Increased pulmonary vascular markings
- Cardiomegaly

Management

- Initial medical therapy, diuretics +/– captopril + added calories
- Surgical closure at 3–5 months

3.3 Persistent ductus arteriosus (PDA)

There is persistence of the duct beyond 1 month after the date the baby should have been born.

Clinical features

- Asymptomatic usually, rarely have heart failure
- Continuous or systolic murmur at left infraclavicular area

ECG

- Usually normal
- If large, have left ventricle volume loading (see Section 15 — ECG)

Chest X-ray

- Usually normal
- If large, have increased pulmonary vascular markings

Management

- Closure in cardiac catheter laboratory with coil or plug at 1 year
- If large, surgical ligation age 1–3 months

NB The presence of an arterial duct in a preterm baby is not congenital heart disease. If there is a clinical problem, with difficulty getting off the ventilator, or signs of heart failure with bounding pulses, the problem is usually treated with indomethacin or ibuprofen (< 34 weeks). If medical management fails, surgical ligation is undertaken.

3.4 Aortopulmonary window

A defect in the wall between the aorta and pulmonary artery.

Clinical features

- Rare
- Usually develop heart failure
- Continuous murmur as for PDA

ECG

- If large, have left ventricle volume loading (see Section 15 — ECG)

Chest X-ray

- If large, have increased pulmonary vascular markings

Management

- If large, surgical ligation age 1–3 months

3.5 Others

There are other rare causes of significant left to right shunt, such as arteriovenous malformation. These are all individually rare. Medical and surgical treatment is similar to that for large ducts or VSDs.

Summary

Disease	Symptoms	Treatment
ASD	Minimal	Surgery/catheter device at 3–5 years
VSD	None	None (in 80–90% of cases)
	Moderate	Diuretics/captopril/added calories then review early
	Severe	Surgery at 3–5 months (10–20% cases)
PDA	None	Coil occlusion at cardiac catheter (at 1 year old)
	Mod/severe	Surgery, especially in preterm babies
Others rare (A-P window, etc.)		Surgery at 3–4 months

4. RIGHT TO LEFT SHUNT

(Cyanosed)

General principles

Cyanosis in a newborn can be caused by:

- Cardiac problems (cyanotic heart disease)
- Respiratory problems (diaphragmatic hernia, etc.)
- Metabolic problems (lactic acidosis, etc.)
- Infections (pneumonia, etc.)

Cardiac cases which present on day 1–3 are usually duct-dependent:

- Transposition of great arteries (common)
- Tetralogy of Fallot with pulmonary atresia (less common)
- Pulmonary atresia with intact ventricular septum (PA/IVS) (rare)
- Tricuspid atresia or other complex hearts (rare)
- Ebstein anomaly (rare)

Investigations

- Chest X-ray (to exclude lung pathology and large 'wall to wall' heart in Ebstein anomaly)
- Blood culture (to exclude infection)
- ECG (superior axis in tricuspid atresia)
- Hyperoxia test, 10 min in 100% O_2 + blood gas from right radial arterial line. If $pO_2 > 20$ kPa then it is not cyanotic heart disease — **you must not use a saturation monitor, because this is notoriously inaccurate in the presence of acidosis**
- Echocardiogram is not first line but should be considered early on

Management

- Resuscitate first
- Ventilate early
- Prostaglandin E_1 or E_2 infusion (5–20 ng/kg per min) (may cause apnoeas)
- Transfer to cardiac centre
- Treat as for specific condition

4.1 Tetralogy of Fallot

Ventricular septal defect + subpulmonary stenosis + overriding aorta + right ventricular hypertrophy (RVH)

Clinical features

- Asymptomatic usually, rarely have severe cyanosis at birth, worsens as they get older
- Loud, harsh murmur at upper sternal edge day 1
- Do not usually develop heart failure

ECG

- Normal at birth
- RVH when older

Chest X-ray

- Usually normal
- If older have upturned apex (boot shaped) + reduced vascular markings

Management

- 10% require BT shunt in newborn if severely cyanosed
- Most have elective repair at 6–9 months

4.2 Transposition of the great arteries

Aorta is connected to the right ventricle, and pulmonary artery is connected to the left ventricle. The blue blood is therefore returned to the body and the pink blood is returned to the lungs. These children have high pulmonary blood flow and are severely cyanosed, unless there is an ASD, PDA or VSD to allow mixing.

Clinical features

- Cyanosed when duct closes
- No murmur usually
- Can be very sick, unless diagnosed antenatally
- May be associated with VSD, coarctation or pulmonary stenosis (PS)

ECG

- Normal

Chest X-ray

- Normal (unusual to detect 'egg-on-side' appearance)
- May have increased pulmonary vascular markings

Management

- Resuscitate as above
- 20% require balloon atrial septostomy at a cardiac centre (usually via umbilical vein — see Section 17 — Cardiac catheterization)
- Arterial switch operation usually before 2 weeks

4.3 Pulmonary atresia

Duct-dependent pulmonary atresia

Clinical features

- Cyanosed when duct closes
- No murmur usually
- Can be very sick, unless diagnosed antenatally
- May have IVS or VSD

ECG

- Normal

Chest X-ray

- Normal at birth (unusual to diagnose 'boot-shaped' heart, until much older)
- Decreased pulmonary vascular markings

Management

- Resuscitate as above
- BT shunt inserted surgically
- Radiofrequency perforation of atretic valve — if appropriate

Pulmonary atresia with VSD and collaterals

Collaterals are abnormal arterial connections direct from the aorta to the lung substance.

Clinical features

- Not usually duct-dependent
- No murmur usually
- Usually present with heart failure at 1 month but may present with cyanosis at any age if collaterals are small

ECG

- Bi-ventricular hypertrophy

Chest X-ray

- Boot-shaped heart
- Cardiomegaly
- Increased pulmonary vascular markings if in heart failure, or reduced vascular marking if severely cyanosed

Management

- Diuretics, if in failure
- Further imaging with cardiac catheter or magnetic resonance imaging (MRI)
- Staged surgical repair

4.4   Ebstein anomaly

The tricuspid valve is malformed such that it leaks, and is set further into the right ventricle than normal.

Clinical features

- Cyanosed at birth
- Loud murmur of tricuspid regurgitation
- Can be very sick
- May be associated with maternal lithium ingestion ✗

ECG

- May have a superior axis

Chest X-ray

- Massive cardiomegaly (wall to wall heart)
- Reduced pulmonary vascular markings

Management

- Resuscitate as above
- Pulmonary vasodilator therapy (ventilation, oxygen, etc., see Section 12)
- Try to avoid surgical shunt insertion, in which case prognosis is poor

4.5   Eisenmenger

This is secondary to a large left to right shunt (usually VSD or AVSD (atrioventricular septal defect)) where the pulmonary hypertension leads to pulmonary vascular disease (increased resistance) over many years. Eventually the flow through the defect is reversed (right to left) so the child becomes blue, typically at 15–20 years of age.

Clinical features

- Cyanosed in teenage life
- Uncommon
- Usually secondary to untreated VSD or AVSD
- No murmur usually
- Develop right heart failure eventually

ECG

- Severe RVH + strain

Chest X-ray

- Decreased pulmonary vascular markings

Management

- Supportive
- May need diuretic and anticoagulant therapy
- Oxygen at night, consider other therapy (see *Pulmonary hypertension*, Section 10)
- Consider heart/lung transplantation

Summary of right to left shunts

Disease	Symptoms	Treatment
Fallot	Loud murmur	Surgery at 6–9 months
TGA (transposition	No murmur	Septostomy at diagnosis (20%)
of great arteries)	Neonatal cyanosis	Arterial switch at < 2 weeks
Pulmonary atresia	No murmur	BT shunt
(duct-dependent)	Neonatal cyanosis	or radiofrequency perforation
Pulmonary atresia	No murmur	Staged surgical repair
(VSD + collaterals)	Heart failure/cyanosis	
Ebstein anomaly	Loud murmur of	Pulmonary vasodilation (O_2, NO, etc.)
	tricuspid regurgitation	
	Cardiomegaly	
Eisenmenger	Severe cyanosis	Pulmonary vasodilators
	No murmur, loud P2	Diuretics
		Transplantation

5. MIXED SHUNT

(Blue and breathless)

General principles

- Tend to present either antenatally (most often) or at 2–3 weeks. Symptoms are that of mild cyanosis and heart failure
- Includes most of the complex congenital heart diseases

5.1   Complete atrioventricular septal defects

There is an atrial and ventricular component to the defect, so there is pulmonary hypertension as with a large VSD. There is a common atrioventricular valve with five leaflets, not a separate mitral and tricuspid valve.

Clinical features

- May be cyanosed at birth
- No murmur usually at birth, may develop in first few weeks
- Often present on routine echo screening (neonatal Down syndrome)
- May present with heart failure at 1–2 months

ECG

- Superior axis
- Bi-ventricular hypertrophy at 2 months old
- Right atrial hypertrophy (tall P-wave)

Chest X-ray

- Normal at birth
- Increased pulmonary vascular markings and cardiomegaly after 1 month

Management

- Treat increased pulmonary vascular resistance at birth if blue
- Treat as for large VSD if in failure (diuretics, captopril, added calories)
- Surgical repair at 3–5 months

5.2   Tricuspid atresia

There is no tricuspid valve and usually the right ventricle is very small.

Clinical features

- Cyanosed when duct closes if duct-dependent
- No murmur usually
- Can be very well at birth

ECG

- Superior axis
- Absent right ventricular voltages
- Large P-wave

Chest X-ray

- May have decreased or increased pulmonary vascular markings

Management

- BT shunt inserted surgically if very blue
- PA band if in heart failure
- Hemi-Fontan after 6 months old (see Section 9.2 — Fontan)
- Fontan at 3–5 years old

5.3   Others

There are many other types of complex congenital heart disease.

- Common arterial trunk
- Double inlet left ventricle
- Total or partial anomalous pulmonary venous connection (unobstructed)
- Right or left atrial isomerism +/– dextrocardia

Individually, these are quite rare and their management is variable, depending on the pulmonary blood flow, the sizes of the two ventricles, etc. For further information a larger textbook of congenital heart disease should be consulted.

6.   OBSTRUCTION IN THE WELL CHILD

(Neither blue nor breathless)

General principles

- Often present to general practitioner with murmur
- Asymptomatic

6.1   Aortic stenosis

The aortic valve leaflets are fused together, giving a restrictive exit from the left ventricle. There may be two or three aortic leaflets.

Clinical features

- Asymptomatic
- Always have a carotid thrill
- Ejection systolic murmur at upper sternal edge
- May be supravalvar, valvar (and ejection click) or subvalvar
- Quiet A2 (second heart sound aortic component)

ECG

- Left ventricular hypertrophy

Chest X-ray

- Normal

Management

- Review with echocardiography
- Balloon-dilate when gradient reaches 64 mmHg across the valve

6.2 Pulmonary stenosis

The pulmonary valve leaflets are fused together, giving a restrictive exit from the right ventricle.

Clinical features

- Asymptomatic (not cyanosed)
- May have a thrill at upper left sternal edge
- Ejection systolic murmur at upper sternal edge from day 1
- May be supravalvar, valvar (ejection click) or subvalvar
- Quiet P2

ECG

- Right ventricular hypertrophy

Chest X-ray

- Normal

Management

- Review with echocardiography
- Balloon-dilate when gradient reaches 64 mmHg across the valve

6.3 Adult-type coarctation of the aorta

Not duct-dependent, this gradually becomes more severe over many years.

Clinical features

- Rare
- Asymptomatic
- Always have systemic hypertension in the right arm
- Ejection systolic murmur at upper sternal edge
- Collaterals at the back
- Radiofemoral delay

ECG

- Left ventricular hypertrophy

Chest X-ray

- Rib-notching
- '3' sign, with a visible notch on the chest X-ray in the descending aorta, where the coarctation is

Management

- Review with echocardiography
- Stent insertion at cardiac catheter when gradient reaches 64 mmHg, or surgery via a lateral thoracotomy

6.4   Vascular rings and slings

Embryological remnant of aortic arch and pulmonary artery development.

Clinical features

- Often present with stridor
- May have no cardiac signs or symptoms

ECG

- Normal

Chest X-ray

- May have lobar emphysema as a result of bronchial compression

Management

- Diagnose with barium/gastrografin swallow
- Review with echocardiography
- Additional imaging often required (computerized tomography, magnetic resonance imaging, angiogram)
- Surgical treatment

7.   OBSTRUCTION IN THE SICK NEWBORN

General principles

- Present when duct closes or antenatally
- Often have normal ECG and chest X-ray when first present
- Must feel pulses!!

7.1 Coarctation of the aorta

Duct-dependent narrowing, the ductal tissue encircles the aorta and causes an obstruction when the duct closes.

Clinical features

- Very common diagnosis
- Often diagnosed antenatally
- Absent femoral pulses
- Should be born in a cardiac centre
- If not detected antenatally, presents as sick infant with absent femoral pulses
- No murmur, usually
- Signs of right heart failure (large liver, low cardiac output)
- May be breathless and severely acidotic
- Associated with VSD and bicuspid aortic valve

ECG

- Normal

Chest X-ray

- Normal, or cardiomegaly with heart failure

Management

- Resuscitate
- Commence prostaglandin E_1 or E_2 (5–20 ng/kg per min)
- Ventilate early (before transfer to cardiac centre)
- Surgery 24 hours later, usually through a left lateral thoracotomy, to resect the narrow segment, unless the whole aortic arch is small, in which case the surgery is performed via a median sternotomy on bypass.

7.2 Hypoplastic left heart syndrome

A spectrum of disorders where the mitral valve, left ventricle and/or the aortic valve are too small to sustain the systemic output.

Clinical features

- Common diagnosis (200–400 born annually in UK)
- Usually diagnosed antenatally
- Should be born in a cardiac centre
- If sick, presents with absent femoral + brachial pulses
- No murmur
- Signs of right heart failure (large liver, low cardiac output)
- May be breathless and severely acidotic
- Anatomy varies from mitral stenosis to mitral and aortic atresia

ECG

- Absent left ventricular forces

Chest X-ray

- Normal, or cardiomegaly with heart failure

Management

- Resuscitate
- Commence prostaglandin E_1 or E_2 (5–20 ng/kg per min)
- Ventilate early (before transfer to cardiac centre)
- Surgery (see Section 9.3 — Norwood) 3–5 days later

7.3 Critical aortic stenosis

Critical means duct-dependent, i.e. there is not enough flow across the stenotic valve to sustain the cardiac output.

Clinical features

- Rare diagnosis
- Usually diagnosed antenatally
- Should be born in a cardiac centre
- If sick, presents with absent femoral + brachial pulses
- No murmur
- Signs of right heart failure (large liver, low cardiac output)
- May be breathless and severely acidotic
- Poor prognosis

ECG

- Left ventricular hypertrophy

Chest X-ray

- Normal, or cardiomegaly with heart failure

Management

- Resuscitate
- Commence prostaglandin E_1 or E_2 (5–20 ng/kg per min)
- Ventilate early (before transfer to cardiac centre)
- Balloon dilation 24 hours later, may require cardiac surgery

7.4   Interruption of the aortic arch

A gap in the aortic arch, which may occur at any site from the innominate artery around to the left subclavian artery. It is always duct-dependent.

Clinical features

- Rare diagnosis
- Presents with absent left brachial + femoral pulses
- No murmur
- Heart failure (large liver, low cardiac output)
- Breathless and severely acidotic
- Associated with VSD and bicuspid aortic valve
- Associated with 22q11.2 deletion and Di George syndrome (see Section 10.5)

ECG

- Normal

Chest X-ray

- Normal, or cardiomegaly with heart failure

Management

- Resuscitate
- Commence prostaglandin E_1 or E_2 (5–20 ng/kg per min)
- Ventilate early (before transfer to cardiac centre)
- Surgery 24 hours later

7.5   Total anomalous pulmonary venous connection

The pulmonary veins have not made the normal connection to the left atrium. Instead they can drain up to the innominate vein (supracardiac), to the liver (infracardiac) or to the coronary sinus (intracardiac).

Clinical features

- Uncommon diagnosis
- Not a duct-dependent lesion
- If obstructed, presents day 1–7 with cyanosis and collapse
- No murmur
- Signs of right heart failure (large liver, low cardiac output)
- May be breathless and severely acidotic
- May, however, present later up to 6 months of age if unobstructed, with murmur or heart failure

ECG

- Normal in neonate
- RVH in older child

Chest X-ray

- Normal, or small heart
- 'Snowman in a snowstorm' or 'cottage loaf' because of visible ascending vein and pulmonary venous congestion. Appearance usually develops over a few months

Management

- Resuscitate (ABC)
- Ventilate early (before transfer to cardiac centre)
- Prostaglandin not effective if obstructed pulmonary veins
- Emergency surgery if obstructed

Summary of obstructed hearts

Disease	Symptoms	Treatment
Coarctation	Absent femoral pulses	Surgery at 24 hours
Hypoplastic left heart	+Absent brachial pulses	Norwood 3–5 days
Interrupted aortic arch	+Absent left brachial	Surgery >24 hours
Critical aortic stenosis	+Absent brachial pulses	Balloon >24 hours
Total anomalous pulmonary venous connection	Cyanosed, sick if obstructed	Emergency surgery

Overview

Left to right shunt	Right to left shunt	Mixed	Well obstructions	Sick obstructions
VSD	Fallot	AVSD	AS	TAPVC
ASD	TGA		PS	HLHS
PDA	Eisenmenger			AS
				CoA
				Int Ao Arch

There are other causes in each column, but these are less common and are unlikely to appear in examinations.

VSD	Pansystolic murmur at LLSE
ASD	Ejection systolic murmur at ULSE + fixed split S2
Partial AVSD	ASD + apical pansystolic murmur of mitral regurgitation.
PDA	Continuous murmur under left clavicle +/– collapsing pulses

Tetralogy of Fallot	Blue + harsh long systolic murmur at ULSE
TGA	No murmur. Two-thirds have no other abnormality, never in examinations
Eisenmenger	10 years old +/– Down syndrome, often no murmurs, loud P2
Complete AVSD	Never in examinations
AS	Ejection systolic murmur at URSE + carotid thrill
PS	Ejection systolic murmur at ULSE +/– thrill at ULSE
TAPVC/HLHS/AS/CoA/ Interrupted aortic arch	Never in clinical exam, but common in vivas, grey cases, data; present in first few days of life. May see postoperative cases

Key: AS, aortic stenosis; ASD, atrial septal defect; AVSD, atrioventricular septal defect; CoA, coarctation; HLHS, hypoplastic left heart syndrome; Int Ao Arch, interrupted aortic arch; LL/LRSE, lower left/right sternal edge; PDA, persistent ductus arteriosus; PS, pulmonary stenosis; TAPVC, total anomalous pulmonary venous connection; TGA, transposition of great arteries; UL/RSE, upper left/right sternal edge; VSD, ventricular septal defect

8. NON-BYPASS SURGERY FOR CONGENITAL HEART DISEASE

Non-bypass surgery is performed by means of a lateral thoracotomy, right or left. The scar is found underneath the right or left arm, the anterior border of the scar tends to end under the axilla and may not be seen from the front of the chest. It is imperative that the arms are lifted and the back inspected as a routine during clinical examination otherwise the scars will be missed.

8.1 Shunt operation

- Right or left modified BT shunt
- Modified shunts will mean an intact brachial pulse on that side
- Most likely to be for tetralogy of Fallot with pulmonary atresia
- If there is no median sternotomy, the infant will still be cyanosed
- Definitive repair will be performed usually by age 18 months

8.2 Coarctation of the aorta repair

- May have absent left brachial pulse (subclavian flap technique) or a normal left brachial pulse
- May have no murmur and normal femoral pulses

8.3 Pulmonary artery band

- Uncommon operation these days
- Usually for complex anatomy which may be palliated in the neonatal period
- There may be a thrill at the upper left sternal edge

- When present, the child is cyanosed
- The band is usually removed at 1–2 years old as part of the next procedure

8.4 Arterial duct ligation

- Rare except for the ex-preterm neonate
- No murmurs and no abnormal pulses
- Usually not associated with other defects

9. BYPASS SURGERY FOR CONGENITAL HEART DISEASE

Any child who undergoes open cardiac surgery, cardiopulmonary bypass, placement of a central shunt or repair of the proximal aortic arch will need a median sternotomy. Therefore any repair of intracardiac pathology will need to be performed via a midline incision.

9.1 Switch operation

- Performed for transposition of the great arteries
- Undertaken before 2 weeks of age (if no VSD present)
- Involves cutting aorta and pulmonary artery and changing them round
- Have to relocate coronary arteries as well
- Mortality is low now, around 5%
- Outcome is affected by presence of associated defects, such as VSD, coarctation, abnormal coronary artery patterns

9.2 Fontan

- Any child with a complex heart arrangement which is not suitable for a repair with two separate ventricles will end up with a Fontan operation. If the pulmonary blood flow is too low at birth (cyanosis), they will have a BT shunt. If the pulmonary blood is too high (heart failure) they will have a PA band. If physiology is balanced, then conservative treatment will be undertaken until the Hemi-Fontan is performed
- At about 6–8 months, the venous return from the head and neck is routed directly to the lungs. A connection is therefore made between the superior vena cava and the right pulmonary artery. The Hemi-Fontan (or a Glenn or Cavopulmonary shunt) is performed on bypass, via a median sternotomy. Following the operation, the oxygen saturations will typically be 80–85%
- At 3–5 years, there will be insufficient blood returning from the head to keep the child well. Hence a Fontan operation will be performed, where a channel is inserted to drain blood from the inferior vena cava up to the right pulmonary artery. This means that the child will be almost pink, saturations around 90–95%
- When completely palliated, the ventricle pumps pink oxygenated blood to the body, whereas the blue deoxygenated blood flows direct to the lungs

9.3   Norwood

- Used to palliate hypoplastic left heart syndrome
- Stage I at 3–5 days of age
  - Pulmonary artery sewn to aorta so that right ventricle pumps blood to body, branch pulmonary arteries are isolated.
  - Atrial septectomy so that pulmonary venous blood returns to right ventricle
  - BT shunt from innominate artery or a conduit from right ventricle to pulmonary arteries
- Stage II (Hemi-Fontan) at 5–6 months old
- Stage III (Fontan) at 3–5 years old
- Results of survival to 5 years are approximately 70–80%
- Unknown long-term results

9.4   Rastelli

- Used for TGA/VSD/PS
- Left ventricle is channelled through VSD to aorta
- VSD is closed with a patch of Gortex material
- Right ventricle is connected to pulmonary artery with a homograft (donor artery)
- Homograft is replaced every 20 years

9.5   Other operations

- A child with median sternotomy scar and lateral thoracotomy scar with a systolic and diastolic murmur at the left sternal edge
  - This is typical of a child who has undergone insertion of a BT shunt, and then had complete repair for tetralogy of Fallot
- The child with Down syndrome who has a murmur at the left lower sternal edge and a median sternotomy scar
  - Atrioventricular septal defect or ventricular septal defect, who has undergone repair and who has a residual ventricular septal defect — the child may also have residual left atrioventricular valve (i.e. mitral) regurgitation with systolic murmur at the apex
- Bikini incision — in girls, for cosmetic reasons who have undergone closure of atrial septal defect
- Groin puncture site — it may be worth inspecting the area of the right and left femoral vein to look for the small puncture scar of previous cardiac catheterization, for example for balloon dilatation of pulmonary stenosis

For further information, consult a larger textbook (see Section 19 — Further reading).

10. SYNDROMES IN CONGENITAL HEART DISEASE

General principles

- Septal defects are the most common
- Anomalies of kidneys, vertebra or limbs are often connected with cardiac disorders
- Genetic causes of many syndromes now known

10.1 Isomerism

- Genetic defect — multifactorial, several candidates isolated

Right atrial isomerism

Heart defects

- Both atria are morphological right atria
- May have apex to right (dextrocardia)
- Must have anomalous pulmonary venous connection (no left atrium to connect to)
- May have complex anatomy, with AVSD, pulmonary atresia, etc.

Associated defects

- Asplenia (penicillin prophylaxis)
- Midline liver
- Malrotation of small bowel
- Two functional right lungs

Left atrial isomerism

Heart defects

- Both atria are morphological left atria
- May have anomalous pulmonary venous connection
- May have complex with AVSD, etc.

Associated defects

- Polysplenia (usually functional)
- Malrotation (less often than in right isomerism)
- Two functional left lungs

10.2 Trisomy

Down syndrome

- Genetic defect — trisomy 21

Heart defects

- 30% have CHD
- Usually VSD and AVSD
- All offered surgery with low risk

Associated defects

- Diagnosed antenatally — increased nuchal translucency

Edward syndrome

- Genetic defect — trisomy 18

Heart defects

- VSD
- Double outlet right ventricle

Associated defects

- Rocker bottom feet
- Crossed index finger
- Developmental delay

Patau syndrome

- Genetic defect — trisomy 15 or 13

Heart defects

- VSD
- Double outlet right ventricle

Associated defects

- Holoprosencephaly
- Midline facial cleft
- Renal anomalies

10.3 William syndrome

- Genetic defect — 7q11.23 deletion including elastin gene *ELN*

Heart defects

- Supravalve aortic stenosis
- Peripheral pulmonary artery stenosis

Associated defects

- Gene abnormality on long arm of chromosome 7
- Hypercalcaemia
- Serrated teeth
- Carp-shaped mouth
- Hypertelorism
- Cocktail party chatter

10.4   Noonan syndrome

- Genetic defect — 12q locus

Heart defects

- Hypertrophic cardiomyopathy
- Pulmonary valve stenosis
- ASD

Associated defects

- Almond-shaped eyes and shallow orbits
- Shield-shaped chest, widely spaced nipples
- Short
- Not 'male Turner', can be girls

10.5   Di George syndrome

- Genetic defect — 22q11.2 deletion

It is increasingly recognized that Di George syndrome may not always occur with the classical form of hypocalcaemia, absent thymus, lymphopenia, cardiac defect and characteristic facies (CATCH 22). Chromosomal abnormalities have been recognized in partial cases, or even in those with familial VSD or tertalogy of Fallot (22q11.2 deletion). Deletions of the chromosome are detected using fluorescent *in situ* hybridization (FISH) probes.

Heart defects

- Conotruncal anomalies
- Common arterial trunk
- Interrupted aortic arch
- Tetralogy of Fallot
- Familial VSD

Associated defects

- 22q11.2 deletion
- Only have full Di George if there is deletion + heart + two out of three of:
  - Cleft palate
  - Absent thymus (T cells low)
  - Absent parathyroids, hypocalcaemia
- Small jaw, small head, pinched nose, hypertelorism
- Small baby, slow development
- Renal anomalies (20%)

Physical examination

Features to describe or exclude in this syndrome are as follows:

- Dysmorphic features of face, skull or pelvis
- Exclude cleft palate
- Check spine for scoliosis
- Check males for hypospadias

Investigations

- Full blood count and film (ask for haematologist's report)
- Calcium and magnesium levels
- Thyroid function tests
- Check total CD4 count
- Measure total immunoglobulin E levels
- Chest X-ray
- Thymic ultrasound
- If abnormal: T-cell precursors and response to tetanus, *Haemophilus influenzae* type B (HIB) and pneumococcus vaccination

Medical treatment (if T-cell-deficient)

- Maintenance co-trimoxazole (if lymphocyte count $< 1.5 \times 10^9/l$)
- Regular intravenous immunoglobulin infusions
- Cytomegalovirus-negative, irradiated blood until immunological status is known
- No live vaccines, but with component or fixed vaccines

10.6   Alagille syndrome

- Genetic defect — Jagged 1 gene (*JAG1*) mutations in 70%

Heart defects

- Peripheral pulmonary artery stenosis

Associated defects

- Prominent forehead; wide-apart, deep-set eyes
- Small, pointed chin
- Butterfly vertebra
- Intrahepatic biliary hypoplasia — jaundice
- Embryotoxon (slit lamp for cornea)
- Kidney, growth, abnormalities of development, high-pitched voice

10.7 Turner syndrome

- Genetic defect — XO

Heart defects

- Coarctation of the aorta

Associated defects

- Webbed neck
- Short stature
- Shield-shaped chest, wide-spaced nipples
- Infertility

10.8 VACTERL

Heart defects

- VSD
- Tetralogy of Fallot
- Coarctation
- PDA

Associated defects

- **V**ertebral
- **A**norectal
- **C**ardiac
- **T**racheo-o**E**sophageal fistula
- **R**enal/Retardation
- **L**imb

10.9 Holt–Oram/TAR (Thrombocytopenia and Absent Radius) (TAR)/Fanconi syndromes

- Genetic defect for Holt–Oram — 12q2 mutations

Heart defects

- ASD

Associated defects

- Radial aplasia
- Limb abnormalities

10.10 CHARGE

Heart defects

- VSD
- Tetralogy of Fallot

Associated defects

- **C**oloboma
- **H**eart
- **A**tresiae choanae
- **R**enal/retardation
- **G**enital/growth
- **E**ar

10.11 Pentalogy of Cantrell

Heart defects

- Tetralogy of Fallot

Associated defects

- Absent sternum
- Absent pericardium
- Absent diaphragm
- Absent heart (ectopic, on the front of the chest)
- Absence of normal heart (tetralogy of Fallot)

10.12 Dextrocardia

A clinical diagnosis with the apex beat in the right chest. It is dangerous to use in cardiology because it gives no information about the connections or orientation of the heart. For example, if the right lung was collapsed and there was a tension pneumothorax on the left, it would be possible to find the apex beat in the right chest. However, the child would not suddenly have developed a cardiac anomaly. We use the term 'apex to right' to imply the orientation of the heart and then talk about the connections such as situs inversus (right atrium is on the left and left atrium is on the right) or some other situs.

In practice, most children with dextrocardia have a normal heart. This is most often the case when the liver is on the left. It may be part of Kartagener syndrome (primary ciliary dyskinesia) where the organs failed to rotate properly during embryological development. It is easily diagnosed by performing nasal brushings to look at the dynein arms of the cilia on electron microscopy. Associated with bronchiectasis, sinus occlusion and infertility.

If the child is blue with dextrocardia, there is almost always complex heart disease with right atrial isomerism (see above).

10.13   Other syndromes

Cri du chat

- Genetic defect — 5p–
- Heart defects — VSD, ASD

Tuberous sclerosis

- Genetic defect — *TSC1* and *TSC2* genes
- Heart defects — cardiac rhabdomyoma which reduce in size with age

Hypertrophic obstructive cardiomyopathy

- Genetic defect — multiple genes
- Heart defects — obstruction in left ventricle may be associated with Noonan syndrome and many more. In general, cardiac defects may be associated with other defects. The commonest cardiac defect is a septal defect (ASD or VSD).

11.   SYNCOPE IN CHILDHOOD

Syncope in childhood is very common. Most episodes are benign, not dangerous and are the result of neurocardiogenic syncope. Most of the investigations are of limited use and most often, it is reassurance that is needed. A suggested protocol follows for the paediatrician.

- Careful history — is syncope associated with a drop in blood pressure on standing
- Known groups of causes are:
  - Neurally mediated syncope, including postural hypotension, is commonest. Tend to have prodrome with dizziness on standing, or sitting upright. Nausea, vomiting and pallor before loss of tone and consciousness
  - Cardiovascular causes, including arrhythmia, structural and vascular
  - Non-cardiovascular pseudo-syncope, including psychogenic
- Investigations
  - ECG, 12-lead. Exclude long Q-T interval, pre-excitation or heart block
- If there is a good history of neurally mediated syncope, then no further tests are required, but if very frequent or severe attacks, then refer to a cardiologist for Tilt testing

- If there are some warning bells, such as exercise-related symptoms, then:
  - Exercise ECG if the symptoms relate to exercise
  - Cardiac event monitoring (longer than 24-hour) or Reveal implantation
  - Electroencephalogram is rarely helpful
- Management, in increasing complexity:
  - Reassurance, advice to stand slowly and sit down if dizzy
  - Encourage to drink more water and take more salt
  - Fludrocortisone 50–100 µg per day
  - β-blocker

12. PULMONARY HYPERTENSION

For children, pulmonary hypertension is when the systolic pulmonary artery pressure is higher than 50% systemic systolic pressure. Needless to say this is normal in the 1-day-old baby, but is abnormal after that time.

Classification of pulmonary hypertension

1. Pulmonary arterial hypertension
   1.1 Idiopathic pulmonary hypertension
      (a) Sporadic
      (b) Familial
   1.2 Related to:
      (a) Collagen vascular disease
      (b) Congenital systemic to pulmonary shunts
      (c) Portal hypertension
      (d) HIV infection
      (e) Drugs/toxins
         (i) Anorexigens
         (ii) Other
      (f) Persistent pulmonary hypertension of the newborn
      (g) Other

2. Pulmonary venous hypertension
   2.1 Left-sided atrial or ventricular heart disease
   2.2 Left-sided valvar heart disease
   2.3 Extrinsic compression of central pulmonary veins
      (a) Fibrosing mediastinitis
      (b) Adenopathy/tumours
   2.4 Pulmonary veno-occlusive disease
   2.5 Other

3. **Pulmonary hypertension associated with disorders of the respiratory system and/or hypoxemia**
   3.1 Chronic obstructive pulmonary disease
   3.2 Interstitial lung disease
   3.3 Sleep-disordered breathing
   3.4 Alveolar hypoventilation disorders
   3.5 Chronic exposure to high altitude
   3.6 Neonatal lung disease
   3.7 Alveolar-capillary dysplasia
   3.8 Other

4. **Pulmonary hypertension caused by chronic thrombotic and/or embolic disease**
   4.1 Thromboembolic obstruction of proximal pulmonary arteries
   4.2 Obstruction of distal pulmonary arteries
      (a) Pulmonary embolism (thrombus, tumour, ova and/or parasites, foreign material)
      (b) In situ thrombosis
      (c) Sickle cell disease

5. **Pulmonary hypertension caused by disorders directly affecting the pulmonary vasculature**
   5.1 Inflammatory
      (a) Schistosomiasis
      (b) Sarcoidosis
      (c) Other
   5.2 Pulmonary capillary haemangiomatosis

12.1 Persistent pulmonary hypertension of the newborn

Aetiology

A relatively uncommon scenario, there are numerous causes, most commonly:

- Structural lung disease (e.g. congenital diaphragmatic hernia)
- Respiratory distress syndrome (hyaline membrane disease)
- Group B streptococcal infection
- Idiopathic

Diagnosis

- Persistent hypoxia
- Low cardiac output
- Loud P2 on examination
- Oligaemic lung fields

- Hepatomegaly
- Episodic desaturation, preceding a fall in blood pressure
- Echocardiographic appearance of pulmonary hypertension
  - High-velocity tricuspid regurgitation jet
  - Dilated right ventricle
  - Right to left shunt via atrial septum
  - Long right ventricle ejection time
  - High-velocity pulmonary regurgitation jet
  - Right to left shunt via arterial duct

Treatment

- Good ventilation (High O_2, low CO_2)
- Use oscillation ventilation if necessary
- Sedation with morphine or fentanyl
- Paralysis
- Good chest physiotherapy
- Restricted fluids
- Pharmacology
  - Nitric oxide (5–20 ppm, inhaled)
  - Prostacyclin (50 ng/kg, nebulized each 15 minutes)
  - Magnesium sulphate (200 mg/kg intravenous)
- Extracorporeal membrane oxygenation (ECMO) as last resort

12.2 Increased pulmonary blood flow

Post-tricuspid shunts

- Ventricular septal defect
- Arterial duct
- Common arterial trunk
- Aortopulmonary window

Treatment

- Repair defect by 3 months of age to avoid irreversible pulmonary vascular disease

12.3 Chronic hypoxia

Aetiology

- Bronchopulmonary dysplasia
- High altitude
- Cystic fibrosis
- Upper airway obstruction
- Chronic bronchiectasis

Investigation

- Sleep studies
- ECG (right ventricular hypertrophy)
- Ear/nose/throat opinion (upper airway obstruction)
- Chest X-ray
- Echocardiogram
- Cardiac catheterization with pulmonary vascular resistance study

Treatment

- Ensure good airway mechanics
- Treat underlying cardiac condition if appropriate
- Added O_2 to keep O_2 saturations > 94%
- Maintain low CO_2 (consider night-time ventilation)
- If responsive to vasodilators:
  - Nifedipine (0.1 mg/kg three times per day)
  - Dipyridamole (2.5 mg/kg/12 hourly)
  - Nebulized or intravenous prostacyclin
- Consider heart/lung transplantation if appropriate

12.4 Pulmonary venous hypertension

Aetiology

- Uncommon
- Mitral valve stenosis (rare in children)
- Total anomalous pulmonary venous connection
- Pulmonary vein stenosis
- Hypoplastic left heart syndrome

Investigation and treatment are determined by aetiology.

13. DRUG THERAPY FOR CONGENITAL HEART DISEASE

13.1 Heart failure

- Diuretics (furosemide (frusemide) and spironolactone or amiloride)
- Captopril
- Added calories
- **NB** Digoxin not routinely used now in left to right shunt

13.2 Anticoagulation

- Aspirin — for arterial platelet aggregation prevention orally (5 mg/kg per day)
- Heparin — for arterial anticoagulation, intravenous

- Warfarin — for venous or arterial thrombus prevention
- Streptokinase — for thrombolysis
- Tissue plasminogen activator — for thrombolysis

13.3 Pulmonary hypertension

- Oxygen — therapeutic vasodilation
- Low CO_2 — good ventilation
- Alkalosis — bicarbonate if needed
- Dipyridamole — increases cyclic guanosine monophosphate (cGMP) levels
- Nifedipine — only if proven to tolerate it
- Nitric oxide — 2–20 parts per million
- Prostacyclin — nebulized (Iloprost) or intravenous
- Bosentan — endothelin (ET_A and ET_B) antagonist
- Sildenafil — increases cGMP levels

13.4 Antiarrhythmia

Supraventricular tachycardia (SVT)

- Vagal manoeuvres first
- Adenosine intravenous 50–250 µg/kg
- DC synchronized cardioversion 0.5–2 J/kg

Ventricular tachycardia (VT)

- Cardioversion if pulse present — synchronized 0.5–2 J/kg
- Defibrillation if no pulse — 2–4 J/kg

Prophylaxis for arrhythmias

This tends to be very variable from unit to unit. Suggestions are:

- SVT — flecainide, sotalol, digoxin or propranolol
- VT — flecainide, sotalol, amiodarone (toxic side-effects on thyroid, skin and lungs)

14. ACQUIRED HEART DISEASE

14.1 Kawasaki disease

Clinical features

- Fever > 5 days
- Plus at least four of:
  - Rash
  - Lymphadenopathy
  - Mucositis (sore mouth, strawberry tongue)

- Conjunctivitis
- Extremity involvement (red fingers/toes)
- +/– coronary artery aneurysms (25% of untreated cases, 4.6% of treated cases)
- +/– abdominal pain, diarrhoea, vomiting, irritable, mood change, hydrops of gallbladder, peeling extremities, thrombocytosis

Pathology

- Marked similarity to toxic shock syndrome
- Perhaps immune response to disease or toxin

Investigation

Erythrocyte sedimentation rate (ESR), C-reactive protein (CRP), white blood count (WBC), blood culture, antistreptolysin-O test (ASOT), viral, throat swab, ECG

Heart

- Pericardial effusion
- Myocardial disease (poor contractility)
- Endocardial disease (valve regurgitation)
- Coronary disease
  - Ectasia, dilatation
  - Small, 3–5 mm, aneurysms — resolve
  - Medium, 5–8 mm, aneurysms — usually resolve
  - Giant, > 8 mm, aneurysms — ischaemia later

Greatest risk if male, < 1 year, fever > 16 days, ESR > 100, WBC > 30,000

Echocardiogram at 10–14 days, 6 weeks, 6 months or longer if abnormal.

Treatment

- Immunoglobulin 2 g/kg over 12 hours
- Aspirin 30 mg/kg per day (four times per day dosage) reduce to 5 mg/kg per day when fever resolves
- Continue aspirin until 6 weeks or longer if abnormal echocardiogram

14.2   Dilated cardiomyopathy

History

- Multiple transfusions, recent viral illness, family history of myopathy or autoimmune diseases. Consider nutritional deficiencies (e.g. selenium, thiamine, etc.)

Examination

- Full cardiovascular examination
- Exclude myopathy

ECG

- Evidence of ischaemia
- Arrhythmias — unrecognized tachycardia

Echocardiogram

- Exclude anomalous coronary artery

X-ray

- Look for arterial calcification

Blood

- Metabolic
  - Carnitine (and acylcarnitine) profile
  - Amino acids, organic acids, lactate
  - Creatinine and electrolytes (including phosphate)
  - Liver function tests and lactate dehydrogenase, creatine kinase-membrane-bound
  - Selenium and thiamine
- Autoimmune
  - Antinuclear, anti-DNA antibodies; immune complexes
- Virology
  - Full blood count, ESR, CRP,
  - Polymerase chain reaction for Epstein–Barr virus, coxsackievirus, adenoviruses, echoviruses
  - Stools for viral culture

Other investigations include abdominal ultrasound for arterial calcification, electromyography and muscle biopsy if there is myopathy. Rare causes include endomyocardial fibrosis, tropical diseases, amyloid.

14.3 Hypertrophic cardiomyopathy

History

Family history of sudden unexplained death, cardiomyopathy, or myopathy. If a neonate, check if an infant of diabetic mother, or if mother was given ritodrine. Hypertrophy is more suggestive of metabolic cause compared to dilated cardiomyopathy. Consider inherited causes.

Examination

- Exclude syndromes, Noonan, Leopard, Friedreich ataxia, neurofibromatosis, lipodystrophy
- Exclude endocrine disease, thyroid (hyper- and hypo-), acromegaly
- Exclude hypertension; check for gross hepatomegaly
- Check for cataracts, ophthalmoplegia, ataxia, deafness, myopathy

* Look for signs of mucopolysaccharidoses

Echocardiogram

* Exclude tumours, amyloid, endocardial infiltration

ECG

* Look for short PR + giant complexes (Pompe syndrome)
* Look for QRS–T axis dissociation (Friedreich ataxia)

Blood tests

* Carnitine (decreased) + acylcarnitine profile
* Creatine phosphokinase (increased = glycogen storage disease type III)
* Blood film for vacuolated lymphocytes, if positive check white cell enzymes (suggesting storage disorders)
* Calcium (hyperparathyroidism)
* Thyroid function tests, fasting blood sugar
* Lactate, amino acids

Urine

* Glycosaminoglycans (for mucopolysaccharidosis)
* Organic acids
* Vanillylmandelic acid

If no cause is found, screen family for hypertrophic obstructive cardiomyopathy (HOCM) and consider a gene probe for HOCM

14.4 Suspected bacterial endocarditis

All children and adults with congenital, and many with acquired, heart disease need antibiotic prophylaxis before dental extraction and potentially septic procedures. Only those with secundum ASD do not. After surgery, prophylaxis is required for 1 year — if no residual defect — or until the residual defect closes.

History

* If a child is admitted with an unexplained fever, has or might have congenital heart disease, has murmurs (? changing), suspect bacterial endocarditis
* Ask for history of recent boils, sepsis, dental extraction, etc.
* Suspected bacterial endocarditis may be found postoperatively following insertion of prosthetic material such as homograft or prosthetic valve

Examination

- Full cardiovascular examination
- Hepatosplenomegaly, fever, heart sounds and signs of infected emboli: Osler's nodes, Roth's spots, septic arthritis, splinter haemorrhages, haematuria, nephrosis

Investigations

- Six blood cultures from different sites at different times over 2 days, using the most sterile technique possible, but do not clean blood culture bottles with alcohol (or else the organisms will be killed off)
- Full blood count, ESR, CRP, ASOT throat swab
- Echocardiogram and ECG
- Consider V/Q scan, white cell differential
- Urine test for blood
- Dental opinion

Treatment

- If proven, treatment is for 6 weeks, predominantly intravenous
- Blood antibiotic levels may be taken for back titration after stabilization on antibiotic regimen — this will be used to assess that there is sufficient antibiotic present to have a bactericidal effect
- Antibiotics chosen should be those with a good record of deep-tissue penetration, e.g. fusidic acid, gentamicin

14.5 Rheumatic fever

- Uncommon in UK
- Increasing incidence with reduced use of antibiotics to treat sore throats
- Diagnosed by modified Duckett–Jones criteria (two major or one major + two minor criteria):
- Major criteria
    - Carditis
    - Polyarthritis
    - Chorea
    - Erythema marginatum
    - Subcutaneous nodules
- Minor criteria
    - Fever
    - Arthralgia
    - Previous rheumatic fever or carditis
    - Positive acute-phase reactants (ESR, CRP)
    - Leukocytosis
    - Prolonged P–R interval

Investigations

- ASOT
- Throat swab for streptococcus A
- ECG
- Echocardiogram (mitral regurgitation, myocarditis, pericarditis)

Treatment

- Penicillin or cefuroxime (if sensitive)
- Prophylactic penicillin V orally for 25 years

14.6   Pericarditis

Aetiology

- Coxsackieviruses
- Enteroviruses
- *Staphylococcus*
- Tuberculosis
- Oncological
- Rheumatic fever

Presentation

- Chest pain (inspiratory)
- Acute collapse (effusion)
- Soft, muffled heart sounds

Examination

- Pericardial friction rub
- Fever

ECG

- ST elevation, convex upwards
- T-wave inversion

Treatment

- Anti-inflammatory drugs (ibuprofen)
- Drain large pericardial effusion

15. ECG

15.1 The ECG and how to read it

Before interpreting a paediatric ECG it is essential to know the following:

- How old is the child?
- Is the ECG recorded at a normal rate (25 mm/s) and voltage (10 mm/mV)?

Rate

When measuring the heart rate on the ECG, the number of large squares is counted between the R-waves. The rate is calculated as 300/number of squares.

Rhythm

Sinus rhythm can only be inferred if there is one P-wave before each QRS and if the P-wave axis is between 0 and 90 degrees.

Axis

QRS axis

This is calculated by adding the total positive deflection (R-wave) and subtracting the negative deflection (Q+S-wave). The resulting vector is plotted for lead I and AVF:

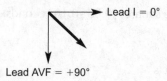

The P-wave and T-wave axes should be plotted similarly. This is important. For example, if there is left atrial isomerism, there is no sinoatrial node (a right atrial structure). This means that the P-wave axis is abnormal (superior) and can lead to the diagnosis. Similarly, in cardiomyopathies, such as Friedreich ataxia, there is a difference in the axis between QRS and T of more than 75 degrees. This can help to make the diagnosis (see below).

Normal QRS axis for

- newborn — 90–180 degrees
- 2–5 years — 45–135 degrees
- > 5 years — 10–100 degrees

Causes of a superior axis (> 180 degrees)

- Atrioventricular septal defect
- Tricuspid atresia
- Ebstein anomaly
- Noonan syndrome

- Wolff–Parkinson–White syndrome
- < 1% of normals

NB AVSD will have right ventricular hypertrophy, whereas tricuspid atresia usually has no right ventricular forces. Either can have large P-waves.

P-wave

The axis should be from 0 to 90 degrees. The normal size is 2×2 little squares (0.08 seconds, 0.2 mV). If there are not regular P-waves before each QRS consider the following:

- Complete heart block — there is complete dissociation between the QRS and P-waves, i.e. with no fixed relationship; see below for list of causes
- Atrial flutter — usually with 2 : 1 block, there is a typical saw-tooth baseline
- Inverted P-waves — these are typically seen with:
  - Left atrial isomerism (no RA → no sinus node)
  - Postoperatively
  - Occasionally in normals (coronary sinus rhythm).
- Peaked P-waves — seen in right atrial hypertrophy:
  - Tricuspid regurgitation (e.g. Ebstein anomaly)
  - Atrioventricular septal defect
  - Pulmonary hypertension
  - Cardiomyopathy

P–R interval

Normal in children is 2–4 little squares (0.08–0.16 seconds).

Causes of a long P–R interval

- Atrioventricular septal defects
- Myocarditis
- Digoxin toxicity
- Hyperkalaemia
- Duchenne muscular dystrophy
- Hypothermia
- Diphtheria

Causes of a short P–R interval

- Wolff–Parkinson–White syndrome
- Pompe disease (wide QRS)
- Lown–Ganong–Levine syndrome (normal QRS)

Q-wave

Not often seen in paediatrics. Rare to see signs of infarct. Normal Q-waves are seen in V1,V2 in young children and are allowed in other leads if small <0.2 mV.

Causes of Q waves

- Dextrocardia
- Left ventricular volume overload V5,V6 (e.g. large PDA or VSD)
- Congenitally corrected transposition
- Ischaemia (Kawasaki, anomalous left coronary artery from pulmonary artery)
- Ischaemia postoperatively

QRS-wave

Normal duration is 0.08 seconds. Prolonged in right bundle-branch block, e.g. after repair of tetralogy of Fallot.

- Delta (δ) wave — seen in Wolff–Parkinson–White syndrome, the slurred upstroke to R-wave, represents depolarization via the accessory pathway, with a short P–R interval. There will be a wide QRS and the QRS axis will be unusual, even superior. Likely to have supraventricular tachycardias (re-entry).
- R–S progression — the best way to assess ventricular hypertrophy. The following pattern should be seen:

	Lead V1	**Lead V6**
Newborn (0–1 month)	Dominant R ∧	Dominant S ∨
Infant (1–18 months)	Dominant R ∧	Dominant R ∧
Adult (> 18 months)	Dominant S ∨	Dominant R ∧

Therefore, if there is persistence of the newborn pattern in an infant then right ventricular hypertrophy is suggested. Other features of hypertrophy are:

- Right ventricular hypertrophy
  - Upright T-waves V1 (from 1 week to 16 years is abnormal)
  - Q-wave in V1
  - R-waves > 20 mm in V1
- Left ventricular hypertrophy
  - Inverted T-waves in V6
  - Q-waves in V6
  - Left axis deviation for age
  - R-waves > 20 mm in V6
- Biventricular hypertrophy
  - Total voltage (R+S) in V3 or V4 of > 60 mm only sign of large VSD

Q–T interval

Measured from the start of the Q-wave to the end of the T-wave (U-wave if present). This represents the total time taken for depolarization and repolarization. Normal is < 0.44 seconds for a heart rate of 60/min. To correct for the heart rate use the Bazett formula:

$$QTc = QT/\sqrt{(RR)}$$

i.e. QT (corrected) = QT measured/(square root of time from R to R).

for example: if QT measured = 0.30 s at a rate of 120

then QTc = $0.3/\sqrt{(0.5)}$ = 0.4 (normal)

If Q–T interval is long then abnormal T-waves and a slow heart rate may result. The cause of long Q–T is thought to be differential sympathetic drive to the two sides of the ventricle, allowing one side to repolarize before the other, hence prolonging the total time of repolarization. This also explains why the T-waves are abnormal.

Causes of long Q–T interval

- Genetic causes of long Q–T syndrome (LQT1, LQT2, LQT3, LQT4, formerly Roman–Ward syndrome and Jervell–Lange–Nielsen syndrome and may be associated with sensori-neural deafness)
- Hypocalcaemia
- Hypokalaemia
- Hypomagnesaemia
- Head injury
- Hypothermia
- Drug administration such as cisapride or erythromycin

S–T segment

Unusual to get marked changes in S–T segments. May represent ischaemia in Kawasaki disease, anomalous left coronary artery from pulmonary artery and postoperative cardiac surgery.

T waves

Normally T-waves are downward in V1 from 1 week to 16 years of age.

T-wave axis should be within 75 degrees of QRS. If not think of:

- Friedreich ataxia
- Dilated cardiomyopathy
- Noonan syndrome
- Long Q–T syndrome

Peaked T waves seen in hypokalaemia and digoxin toxicity.

15.2 Tachycardias

Supraventricular tachycardia (SVT)

- Likely if the heart rate is > 240/min
- Tend to be faster rates ~ 300/min
- Tend to be narrow complex (< 0.08 s, unless aberrant conduction)

- Often caused by Wolff–Parkinson–White syndrome
- Respond to adenosine (intravenous rapid bolus) or vagal manoeuvres such as immersion in ice-cold water, carotid sinus massage or valsalva in older children

Can use flecainide, propranolol, sotalol, esmolol, amiodarone for treatment/prophylaxis.

Do NOT use eyeball pressure, or intravenous verapamil.

For atrial flutter, adenosine challenge brings out flutter waves. Standard treatment is then to use synchronized DC cardioversion (0.5 J/kg)

Ventricular tachycardia (VT)

- Tend to be slower rates ~ 200/min
- Tend to be wide complex (> 0.08 s)
- There is P-wave dissociation
- Can have torsade de points, which can degenerate to ventricular fibrillation
- Treatment is usually amiodarone (can use flecainide, etc.)

15.3 Bradycardias

Complete heart block

Often present at birth but may be diagnosed antenally. Baby is born (sometimes following emergency Caesarean section) with heart rate ~ 70/min but is perfectly well. Usually needs no treatment for several years. Intervene if Faltering growth, collapses, heart failure, Stokes–Adams attacks or resting heart rate < 40/min. These would be indications for pacemaker insertion.

Causes

- Maternal systemic lupus erythematosus
- Congenitally corrected transposition of the great arteries
- Post-operative
- Myocarditis
- Rheumatic fever

Sick sinus syndrome

- Tachy/brady syndrome
- May be seen after heart surgery
- Caused by scar formation over sinus node
- To be differentiated from sinus arrhythmia which is normal variation in heart rate caused by the effects of respiration

If symptomatic needs pacemaker insertion.

16. CHEST X-RAYS

16.1 Cardiac outlines

Neonatal

- 'Egg-on-Side'
  - Transposition of great arteries
  - Narrow vascular pedicle (aorta in front of pulmonary artery)
- Boot-shaped
  - Tetralogy of Fallot with pulmonary atresia
  - Pulmonary artery bay because of absent pulmonary artery
- 'Snowman in a snowstorm'
  - Obstructed total anomalous pulmonary venous connection
  - Small heart with pulmonary venous congestion
- Wall-to-wall heart
  - Ebstein anomaly
  - Massive cardiomegaly with right atrial dilation

Infantile

- Cottage loaf
  - Total anomalous pulmonary venous connection
  - Visible ascending vein on upper left border

The older child

- Cardiomegaly with increased pulmonary vascular markings
  - Atrial septal defect
- Small heart with pulmonary oligaemia
  - Eisenmenger syndrome
  - Probably secondary to VSD or AVSD

Globular heart

Usually associated with pericardial effusions, perhaps secondary to pericarditis or dilated cardiomyopathy.

Situs

Check the heart is on the left along with the stomach bubble, and that the liver is on the right. This may be helpful in diagnosing right atrial isomerism, etc., as above.

Oligaemic lung fields

Reduced pulmonary blood flow such as tetralogy of Fallot, Ebstein anomaly, persistent pulmonary hypertension.

Plethoric lung fields

Left to right shunts, especially VSD and AVSD. Useful in transposition of the great arteries.

Normal lung fields

Those lesions with no shunt, such as pulmonary stenosis and aortic stenosis.

17. CARDIAC CATHETERIZATION

17.1 Diagnostic cardiac catheterization

Normal	Right atrium $SaO_2 = 65\%$ Press = 4 mmHg	Left atrium $SaO_2 = 99\%$ Press = 6 mmHg
	Right Ventricle $SaO_2 = 65\%$ Press = 25/4	Left Ventricle $SaO_2 = 98\%$ Press = 75/6 (age-dependent)
	Pulmonary artery $SaO_2 = 65\%$ Press = 25/15	Aorta $SaO_2 = 97\%$ Press = 75/50 (age-dependent)

To analyse cardiac catheter data, it is important to start with the aortic saturations. Follow the algorithm below.

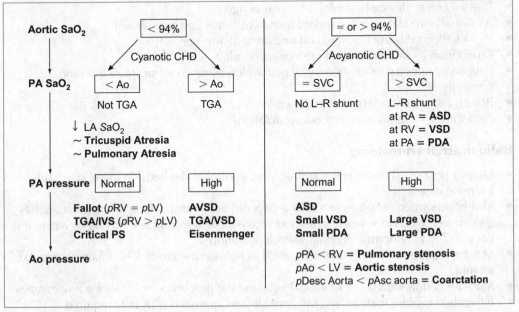

Algorithm for cardiac catheter data

- If pink (aortic SaO$_2$ ≥ 94%) check pulmonary artery SaO$_2$. If this is greater than systemic venous SaO$_2$, then there is a left to right shunt. If it is the same as venous SaO$_2$ then look for a pressure drop (AS/CoA).
- If blue (aortic SaO$_2$ < 94%) check pulmonary artery SaO$_2$. If this is greater than aortic SaO$_2$, then the diagnosis is transposition of the great arteries. If it is less than aortic SaO$_2$ then the problem is not TGA. Check pulmonary artery pressure. If less than right ventricular pressure then there is right ventricular outflow obstruction, probably tetralogy of Fallot.
- True diagnostic catheterization is rarely performed, use echocardiography instead
- Usually for assessment between staged surgical operations
- Pulmonary vascular resistance assessments for left to right shunts to determine operability
  - Measure pulmonary artery pressure and resistance (PVR) at baseline
  - Measure oxygen consumption for accurate determination
  - Repeat measurement in nitric oxide at two different doses
  - Repeat measurement in oxygen or prostacyclin
  - If PVR > 7 Wood units × m^2, then inoperable
  - If PVR falls by more than 20% then is partly reversible

17.2   Interventional cardiac catheterization

Interventional cardiac catheters

80% of cardiac catheters are used for interventional treatment

- ASD — septal occlusion device in 90% of secundum ASD after 3 years old
- VSD — not usually used, but may be appropriate in apical muscular VSDs
- PDA — coil or device occlusion at 1 year of age
- AS — balloon dilatation is standard treatment at any age (see above)
- PS — balloon dilatation is standard treatment at any age
- Coarctation — stent insertion in teenagers or adults
- Pulmonary atresia — radiofrequency perforation as newborn or shunt insertion surgically
- Branch PS — stent insertion in older children
- Arrhythmias — radiofrequency or cryoablation

Balloon atrial septostomy

- Usually performed under echocardiographic control at the bedside in the paediatric intensive care unit
- Mostly performed in babies less than 2 days old with transposition of the great arteries (see above), who are severely cyanosed where there is insufficient mixing or where it is not possible to perform a neonatal switch operation
- May be required in other conditions, such as pulmonary atresia with intact ventricular septum
- Most are performed via the umbilical vein and the procedure only takes a few minutes
- If the child is older than 3 days, the femoral vein approach is usually required

- A catheter is passed via the vein into the right atrium and hence into the left atrium across the foramen ovale. The balloon on the end of the catheter is inflated and the balloon is withdrawn rapidly into the right atrium. This tears a hole in the atrial septum allowing blood to pass freely from right to left and vice versa.

18. IMAGING

18.1 Echocardiography

- Mainstay of diagnostic tools
- Doppler to assess velocity (and hence pressure gradient) across valves or VSD
- Colour-flow to highlight small defects or turbulent blood flow
- Transoesophageal echo for posterior heart structures or during interventional cardiac catheterization, especially in adults with congenital heart disease
- Future uses for intravascular ultrasound, three-dimensional ultrasound and contrast echocardiography

18.2 Magnetic resonance imaging

- Standard diagnostic imaging for complex diseases where echocardiogram is insufficient
- Spin-echo for routine imaging
- Contract-enhanced for blood flow
- Three-dimensional magnetic resonance imaging for reconstruction

18.3 Positron emission tomography

- Uses ammonium ion to give blood-pool images
- Best for myocardial perfusion imaging

18.4 Radionuclear angiography

- For quantifying left to right shunt (e.g. ASD)
- For determining right or left ventricle function and ejection fraction

19. FURTHER READING

Anderson RH, Baker EJ, Macartney FJ, Rigby ML, Shinbourne EA, Tynan M (Eds). 2002. *Paediatric Cardiology*, 2nd edn. London: Churchill Livingstone.

Andrews RE, Tulloh RMR. 2002. Hypoplastic left heart syndrome: diagnosis and management. *Hospital Medicine* 63:1, 24–7.

Brogan PA, Bose A, Burgner D, Shingadia D, Tulloh R, Michie C, Klein N, Booy R, Levin M, Dillon MJ. 2002. Kawasaki disease: an evidence-based approach to diagnosis, treatment, and proposals for future research. *Archives of Diseases in Childhood* 86:4, 286–90.

Park MK, Guntheroth WG. 1987. *How to Read Pediatric ECGs*. Chicago: Year Book Medical Publishers (still the best ECG book).

Tulloh RMR. 2005. Congenital heart disease in relation to pulmonary hypertension in paediatric practice. *Paediatric Respiratory Reviews* 63:3, 174–80.

Chapter 2

Child Development, Child Psychiatry and Community Paediatrics

Joanne Philpot and Ruth Charlton

CONTENTS

Child Development

Child Development

1. DEVELOPMENTAL ASSESSMENT

This is a key part of the assessment of any child. It is important to learn the common milestones.

1.1 Milestones

It is important to consider the four areas:

- Gross motor
- Fine motor and vision
- Speech and hearing (language)
- Social

Milestones in child development

Age	Gross motor	Fine motor and vision	Language	Social
6 weeks	Head lag still present on pulling from a supine to sitting position When held in ventral suspension, head can be held in the same plane as the body	Maintains fixation and follows an object through 90° in the horizontal plane	Makes throaty noises	Smiles in response to appropriate stimuli
3 months	Able to raise head and chest on forearms in the prone position Head steady when pulled to sit	Will fix and follow an object through 180° in the horizontal plane Hands beginning to be brought to the mid-line Attempts to make contact with offered object	Vowel sounds and noises uttered on social contact Turns head to sound, level to the ear	Social smile (infant has awareness that smile attracts attention) May show displeasure on interruption of social contact
6 months	Can roll over Sits briefly or with some support	Transfers Reaches out for objects Mouthing objects	Unintelligible babble Will turn when name is called	Plays with feet Holds onto bottle when fed

Age	Gross motor	Fine motor and vision	Language	Social
9 months	Sits steadily Pivots to reach objects Stands holding onto objects	Looks for toy fallen from view Pokes objects with index finger	Shouts to gain attention Understands 'no' Two-syllable babble	Finger feeds Resists when objects removed
12 months	Crawling Pulls to stand Cruising	Pincer grip Banging bricks together	Two words with meaning Responds to 'give it to me' Shows recognition of objects by using them, e.g. brush	Waves bye bye Claps hands Empties cupboards
15 months	Walking well	Pincer grip refined, tiny objects can be picked up delicately Casting	Expression several words Understands words such as cup, names of brothers and sisters Jargon and jabbering Echolalia (repetition of words spoken to the child)	Drinks from a cup Indicates wants without crying, i.e. pointing, pulling, asking
18 months	Stoops and retrieves objects Carries toys while walking	Delicate pincer grasp Scribbles	Points to parts of body Understands up to 50 words Knows common objects by name, e.g. cat Follows one-step command, e.g. 'give me a doll' Expression 25 to 50 words	Holds spoon and gets food to mouth Into everything Takes shoes and socks off Indicates toilet needs
2 years to 2.5 years	Climbs and descends stairs one step at a time Kicks a ball Climbs furniture	Copies vertical line Tower of eight bricks	Uses plurals Follows two-step request, eg 'get the ball and put it in the box' Identifies objects from hearing their use Selects toy from others, i.e. 'Give me the sheep, brush'	Plays alone Eats with spoon and fork

continues

Age	Gross motor	Fine motor and vision	Language	Social
3 years	Pedals tricycle Jumps well Momentarily balancing on one foot	Copies a circle Matches two colours	Knows some colours Three- to four-word sentences Name, age and sex on request Pronouns and plurals Knows more about time, today and not today Starts to tell stories	Out of nappies during the day Separates from mother easily (less apprehensive about you the candidate) Eats with knife and fork Dresses with supervision
4 years	Stands on one foot well Hops	Copies a cross and square Draws man with three parts	Count to 10 Identifies several colours 100s of questions Understands numbers Past tense Increasing concentration	Shares toys Out of nappies by night Brushes teeth Toilet alone
5 years	Walks down stairs one foot per step Bounces and catches ball	Copies triangle Draws man with six parts Writes name Do up buttons	Comprehension: 'what do you do if you are hungry, cold, tired?' Comprehension of prepositions: 'put brick on, under, in front of'; opposites: hot, cold; if elephant is big, a mouse is small definition of words, e.g. ball, banana	Chooses friends Comforts in distress Acts out role play

Primitive reflexes

- Sucking and rooting present from 0–6 months
- Palmar grasp present from 0–3 months
- Stepping present from 0–6 weeks
- Asymmetrical tonic neck reflex (ATNR) present from 1–6 months — with the child supine, the head is rotated to one side leading to extension of the arm and leg on the side towards which the head is turned and flexion of the arm and leg on the opposite side. A good way to remember this is the 'Archer's reflex, like firing a bow and arrow. A strong ATNR is usually abnormal and a sign of cerebral palsy
- Moro present from 0–4 months
- Head-righting present from 6 months and persists
- Parachute reflex present from 9 months and persists

1.2 Developmental examination for the Short Case examination

It is important when assessing development to make comments under the four main headings (see above).

Inspect

- Look for clues. Remember the families will have come equipped for the day. Look for feeding equipment, nappy bag, the toys they have brought
- Is the child well?
- Does the child look dysmorphic?
- Are there any obvious neurological abnormalities?

Assessment

- Pitch in at around the age you think the child is, i.e. if they look around 18 months do not start asking them to copy circles, etc
- Assess each of the four developmental categories. Once you have demonstrated they can do one level push up to the next level until they are not able to perform the task. For example: if you have demonstrated the child can copy a square do not ask them to copy a circle as you have already demonstrated the child is past this level, instead see if they can copy a triangle
- Keep control of the situation. If the child is playing already, WATCH. You may be able to complete the whole assessment by observation alone
- If the child is already sitting use the opportunity to assess language, social and fine-motor development. Do not disrupt the child to do gross-motor tests — you may well have difficulty settling him again and in the older child gross motor gives you the least additional information. Leave it to the end
- Use the parents if the child is shy or apprehensive, e.g. ask the parents to draw a circle for the child to copy or test the child about colours, numbers, stories, etc.
- If the child does not co-operate do not panic. You can still get clues from observing. Remember stranger awareness and non-compliance are developmental milestones in themselves

Presentation

- Summarize any relevant clinical findings, e.g. this girl looks ill, has a drip in, a Hickman line, etc, which may be affecting your assessment. If the child looks dysmorphic then say so
- This child has a developmental age of X because:
  - Gross motor — I have demonstrated that they can do this but not that
  - Fine motor — I have demonstrated, etc

'Demonstrated' is better than 'can' or 'cannot'. It means that the parents cannot correct you by saying 'yes he can'! Remember you are only assessing the child over a few minutes.

If you have a developmental discrepancy between the four areas then present this, e.g. this child has a developmental age of 4 in gross- and fine-motor skills but a developmental level of 2 years in speech and language and social skills. Follow this by saying what you would like to do next, e.g. I would like to formally test his hearing to exclude a hearing problem.

Children likely to be seen

- Dysmorphic, e.g. Down syndrome. Just keep to the same format and in each of the four sections demonstrate what they can and cannot do to determine their developmental level
- Global developmental delay
- Gross-motor delay (cerebral palsy)
- Delay in specific areas

1.3   Management of the child with global developmental delay

Developmental delay can result from many causes:

- 40% have chromosomal abnormalities
- 5–10% have developmental malformations
- 4% have metabolic disorders

Causes of developmental delay

Static causes
Prenatal
   Chromosomal abnormalities
   Intrauterine infections
   Teratogens
   Congenital brain malformations, e.g. neuronal migration defects
   Specific syndromes
Perinatal
   Prematurity
   Ischaemic hypoxic encephalopathy
   Birth trauma
   Meningitis
Postnatal
   Trauma
   Intracranial infections

Progressive causes
Endocrine
   Hypothyroidism
Metabolic
   Aminoacidurias
   Galactosaemia
   Mucopolysaccharidoses
   Lesch–Nyhan

Degeneration of the cerebral grey matter

- Tay–Sachs disease
- Gaucher disease
- Niemann–Pick disease
- Batten disease
- Leigh disease
- Menkes disease

Degeneration of the cerebral white matter

- Krabbe disease
- Metachromatic leucodystrophy
- Canavan disease

Peroxisomal disorders

- Zellweger syndrome

Infection
- Subacute sclerosing panencephalitis (SSPE)

History

A good history is essential to help determine the cause and appropriate investigations. Information is required on prenatal history, perinatal history and postnatal development. Are there any associated symptoms such as seizures? General health is important when considering metabolic disorders. Family history may give the strongest clue to a chromosomal disorder. Enquire about previous pregnancy losses.

Examination

A thorough examination is essential.

Neurodegenerative conditions affecting the grey matter tend to present with dementia and seizures. Conditions affecting the white matter tend to present with spasticity, cortical deafness and blindness.

Inspect for:

- Sex of child — X-linked conditions such as fragile X, Menkes, Hunter, Lesch–Nyhan syndromes
- Age of the child:
  - First 6 months — Tay–Sachs disease, Leigh disease, infantile spasms, tuberose sclerosis
  - Toddlers — infantile metachromatic leukodystrophy, mucopolysaccharidoses, infantile Gaucher, Krabbe disease
  - Older children — juvenile Batten disease, SSPE, Wilson disease, Huntington chorea

- Dysmorphic features — Down syndrome, mucopolysaccharidoses
- Neurocutaneous signs — ataxia telangiectasia, Sturge–Weber syndrome, incontinentia pigmenti, tuberose sclerosis
- Extrapyramidal movements — cerebral palsy, Wilson disease, Huntington chorea
- Tremor — Wilson disease, Friedreich's ataxia, metachromatic leukodystrophy

Note growth of child

- Large head — Alexander, Canavan, Tay–Sachs syndromes, mucopolysaccharidoses
- Small head — cerebral palsy, autosomal recessive microcephaly, Rubinstein–Taybi, Smith–Lemli–Opitz, Cornelia de Lange syndromes
- Growth pattern (e.g. faltering growth with metabolic disease, gigantism with Soto syndrome)

Systematic examination

- Eyes — corneal clouding, cataract, cherry-red spot, optic atrophy
- Neurological examination including gait, scoliosis, tremor, extrapyramidal movements, tone, power and reflexes of limbs
- Associated system involvement (e.g. cardiac abnormalities, organomegaly in metabolic disease)
- Genitalia
- Hearing and vision should be checked

Further assessment often involves input from other professionals of the child development team, e.g. speech and language therapists and physiotherapist.

Investigations

A thorough history and examination may lead to targeted investigations, e.g. a specific genetic test or metabolic test. For approximately 40% of cases no cause is found. The two most useful investigations are genetic studies and brain imaging.

If no specific diagnosis is suggested then consider:

Blood tests

- Chromosomal analysis
- Thyroid function tests
- TORCH serology in infants (TORCH, **t**oxoplasmosis, **o**ther (congenital syphilis and viruses), **r**ubella, **c**ytomegalovirus and **h**erpes simplex virus)
- Plasma amino acids
- Ammonia
- Lactate
- White cell enzymes

Urine tests

- Urinary organic acids
- Urinary amino acids
- Urinary mucopolysaccharidoses

Brain imaging

This will identify congenital brain abnormalities and diagnose degenerative conditions such as the leukodystrophies and grey matter abnormalities.

EEG

This will identify SSPE, Batten disease

Management

This is multidisciplinary. The precise make-up of the team depends on local resources. It can include:

- Community paediatrician
- Speech and language therapist
- Physiotherapist
- Occupational therapist
- Child psychologist/psychiatrist
- Play therapist
- Pre-school therapist, e.g. portage
- Nursery teachers
- Health visitors
- Social workers

2. VISION

Each year around 500 children are registered blind or partially sighted. Early diagnosis is important because:

- Appropriate treatment may reduce the severity of the disability or stop progression
- Other medical conditions associated with visual problems can be diagnosed
- Genetic counselling can be offered
- Pre-school learning support can be started

Causes of visual impairment in childhood

- Cataract
- Glaucoma
- Optic nerve
  - Leber's optic atrophy
  - Septo-optic dysplasia
  - Raised intracranial pressure, e.g. hydrocephalus
- Retinal
  - Retinopathy of prematurity
  - Hereditary Leber's amaurosis
  - Retinoblastoma
- Amblyopia as a result of squint, refractive error, ptosis

2.1 Assessment of visual acuity

There is no national policy on visual screening or who should do it (primary care or orthoptists) in the UK. At present there are different screening policies in different health authorities. Visual screening is under review in conjunction with the results from trials on treatment of amblyopia.

Current recommendations

- Newborn screening inspecting the eyes for anomalies
- Repeat eye examination at the 6-week check
- Orthoptist's assessment of all children in the 4- to 5-year age group. This is to assess acuity and to detect squints. The advantage of screening at this age is easier testing of visual acuity compared to younger children. Parents will usually recognize a squint but amblyopia as a result of refractive error will only be detected when the child's vision is assessed monocularly
- Screening very low birth-weight babies to detect retinopathy of prematurity
- Visual screening in children with other major disabilities

Between the ages of 6 weeks and 4 years identification of visual defects will rely on concern being raised by the parents or other professionals.

Methods of testing visual acuity

Newborn — inspection of the eye for cataract and other abnormalities — including red reflex.

6 weeks — inspection of the eye. The child should also be able to fix and follow an object held at arms' length through 90° in the horizontal plane.

12 weeks — the child should be able to fix and follow an object 180° in the horizontal and vertical planes.

10 months — an infant can pick up a raisin. By one year they can pick up individual '100 and 1000s' sweets. If possible try to test the acuity of both eyes.

2 to 3 years — test each eye individually. Various tests for visual acuity are available.

- Preferential looking test — this can be used in a child too young to identify objects. Large cards with pictures on in different positions, i.e. top right-hand corner, bottom left-hand corner, are shown to the child and the eye movements are observed as the child focuses on the picture as it moves around the card
- Picture cards — children asked to identify picture cards at a set distance. Picture size varies to determine the acuity

3 years — visual acuity should be assessed in each eye. By this age the Sheridan–Gardner test can usually be used. The child has a card with five letters on, the Key card. The examiner stands 6 m away and holds up a letter which the child has to identify on his card.

4 years and upwards — by this age the child can usually verbally identify letters and therefore a Snellen chart can be used.

2.2   Squints

Squints are common, occurring in approximately 4% of children. There is a strong familial incidence. A squint is usually noticed by the parents first and parental report of squint should be taken seriously.

A squint is a misalignment of the visual axis of one eye.

It is either:

- Latent — i.e. only there at certain times (such as fatigue, illness, stress)
- Manifest — i.e. present all the time

It is either:

- Alternating — the patient uses either eye for fixation while the other eye deviates. As each eye is being used in turn, vision develops more or less equally in both
- Monocular — only one eye is used for fixation and the other eye consistently deviates. The child is more prone to develop amblyopia as the deviated eye is consistently not being used

It is either:

- Convergent — i.e. turns in
- Divergent — i.e. turns out

It is either:

- Non-paralytic
- Paralytic

Non-paralytic squint

This is the more common type of squint and includes the following:

- Comprises the majority of the congenital and infantile convergent squints
- The accommodative convergent squint. In some infants accommodation results in over-convergence or crossing of the eyes. This type of deviation most commonly occurs around 18 months to 2 years of age. The child is also usually long-sighted. In most cases the eye crossing can be controlled with glasses that correct for the long-sightedness
- In a few cases a non-paralytic squint is the result of an underlying ocular or visual defect, e.g. cataract, high refractive errors, retinopathy of prematurity, retinoblastoma

Paralytic squints

These are the result of weakness or paralysis of one or more of the extraocular muscles. They are less common.

- The deviation worsens on gaze into the direction of action of the affected muscle.
- Congenital paralytic squints are more commonly the result of developmental defects of the cranial nerves, muscle disease, or congenital infection
- Acquired paralytic squints usually signify a serious pathological process, e.g. brain tumour, central nervous system infection, neurodegenerative disease

Assessment of squint

- Ocular movements assessed to exclude paralytic squint
- Corneal reflex examined, looking for symmetry of the light reflex
- Cover/uncover test. The child sits comfortably on a parent's lap. Their attention is attracted and while they are looking at an object one of the eyes is covered. If the uncovered eye moves to fix on the object there is a squint present, a manifest squint. This may be a:
  - Unilateral squint — the squinting eye takes up fixation of the object when the other eye is covered. When the cover is removed the squinting eye returns to its original squinting position
  - Alternating squint — the squinting eye takes up fixation of the object when the other eye is covered. When the cover is removed the squinting eye maintains fixation and the previously fixing eye remains in a deviated position, i.e. the squint alternates from one eye to the other
- Rapid cover/uncover test. Sometimes a squint is not present all the time but only when tired or stressed. In the rapid cover test the occluder is moved quickly between the eyes. If the eye that has been uncovered moves to take up fixation there is a latent squint

Principles of treatment for a squint

- Develop best possible vision for each eye:
  - Correct any underlying defect, e.g. cataract
  - Correct refractive errors with glasses
  - Treat any amblyopia with occlusion therapy
- Achieve best ocular alignment:
  - In accommodative squints correction of long-sightedness by glasses usually controls the excessive convergence.
  - For other types of squints surgery is required. This is particularly important for congenital squints. The longer the defect persists untreated the less chance there is for development of good visual function

2.3 Examination of the eyes for the Short Case

- Observe for obvious eye abnormalities, e.g. coloboma, ptosis, squint
- Assess visual acuity of both eyes separately
- Assess visual fields
- Test eye movements
- Cover test for squint
- Direct and consensual light reflex
- Examination of the fundi

Order of examination may be influenced by your findings along the way, e.g. if you find an abnormality such as a squint you may focus on the assessment of that.

3. HEARING

Between 1 and 2 children per 1,000 population have permanent childhood deafness, 84% congenital and 16% acquired. Early detection of hearing problems and treatment have permanent beneficial effects.

Possible interventions

- Hearing aids
- Cochlear implant — will allow more deaf children to develop spoken language
- Involvement of Speech and Language therapy services
- Pre-school/in-school learning support, e.g. signing

Routine hearing screening programme

Neonatal screening
There is a move towards universal neonatal screening to allow early detection of deafness. At present in many areas only high-risk infants are screened.

- Low birth weight
- Jaundice at the exchange level
- Anomalies of the ears, preauricular pits, tags
- Special Care Baby Unit (SCBU) admission for more than 72 hours
- Family history of deafness
- Gentamicin treatment

The screening test used: otoacoustic emissions test or auditory brainstem response testing.

At 8 months
Testing of all children by the health visitor. Screening test used is the hearing distraction test.

At pre-school entry
At 4–5 years, testing for all children by school nurse. Screening test used is the sweep audiogram.

If the screening test is positive the child is referred to an audiologist for further assessment. Referrals to audiology can also be made at any time if concerns are raised about hearing or speech and language development, e.g. by the parents.

3.1 Assessment of auditory function

- Babies
  - Diagnostic auditory brainstem response testing
  - Otoacoustic emissions test

- **8 months**
  - Hearing distraction test
- **2 years**
  - Visual reinforcement audiometry
  - Performance games
  - Speech discrimination test
  - Free-field audiometry
- **3 years and over**
  - Pure-tone audiometry

It is important to consider both the developmental and the chronological age when deciding which test to use.

Otoacoustic emissions test

Otoacoustic emissions are thought to arise from the cochlear sensory mechanism and are only present if the cochlear is functioning. This test does not test the whole of the hearing pathway, but pure problems distal to the cochlear are very rare and this test detects most causes of deafness. For measuring emissions a soft-tip probe is placed into the ear. The test is easy, quick and requires minimum preparation. This test is now widely used to screen infants in the neonatal period for sensorineural deafness.

Auditory brainstem response

This test measures sound-induced electrical activity in the brain using scalp electrodes. It tests the whole hearing system but takes longer to perform, more equipment is needed and baby needs to stay calm. It is time-consuming, but it is very useful for babies and children who are difficult to test by behavioural means because they have developmental difficulties.

Distraction test

This test is performed routinely by health visitors on all infants at 8 months. The child sits on the mother's lap with a distracter sitting in front of them and the noise stimulus presenter remaining behind the child (out of sight). The test relies on the normal child's response to turn to locate the source of the sound and on the fact that they have not yet developed permanence of objects, so that once they have been distracted again by the person in the front they forget about the tester behind them. A series of sounds at different frequencies are presented at a level of about 40 dB at a set distance of 1 m behind the child at ear level. There are standardized sounds and test materials — Manchester rattle, warbler, Nuffield rattle, voice.

Visual reinforced audiometry

Sounds are presented to the child via a loudspeaker arrangement that enables the sound to be presented precisely at different decibels for each frequency tested. If the head turns to the sound the child is rewarded by a visual stimulus, e.g. a toy lighting up in a box. Headphones can be used in a compliant child so allowing individual ears to be tested.

Performance test or Go games

These tests are useful for children with an actual or developmental level of 2–4 years. They require some understanding and co-operation. The child is asked to perform a task when they hear a noise, i.e. put man in boat. It can be performed by health visitors.

Speech discrimination test

This test is useful for children with a 2.5 years plus actual or developmental level. An example is the McCormick Toy Test. Toys are laid out in front of the child on the table and the examiner asks the child to identify the toy called. The examiner must test voice level against a sound meter. The mouth is covered to prevent lip reading and the tester has to be careful not to give visual clues. The toys are in pairs to test for consonants, e.g. duck/cup.

Free-field testing

Suitable for children aged 2 years and over. It does not require understanding or co-operation so is useful for children with developmental delay or behavioural problems. Sounds are produced within a free field at different frequencies. The child's reaction to sound is observed and assessed if satisfactory.

Pure-tone audiometry

By 4 years of age a child should be able to co-operate with this test. Both ears can be tested separately. The audiometer delivers sounds at different frequencies and intensities. It is possible to determine the child's threshold at each sound frequency. It takes at least 10 minutes to perform.

The audiogram

Key to symbols used:

x-axis = frequency (Hz)
y-axis = hearing level (dBHL)
O = air conduction right ear
X = air conduction left ear
△ = bone conduction unmasked — vibrator vibrates whole skull no matter which mastoid it is placed on. Assesses both cochleas unless one ear is masked.
[= masked bone conduction right
] = masked bone conduction left
↓ = off scale (no response)

Air conduction assesses the whole auditory system, bone conduction assesses the auditory pathway from the cochlea and beyond. A difference between the two suggests a conductive loss (middle or outer ear). Equal impairment suggests a sensorineural loss. Impairment greater in air than bone suggests a mixed loss.

Normal range	−10 to +20 dBHL
Moderate hearing loss	20–40 dBHL
Profound hearing loss	90–120 dBHL

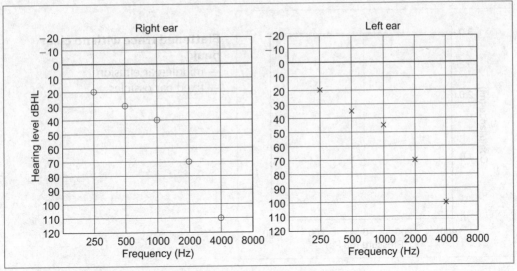

High-frequency hearing loss in a child with speech delay

Sweep audiometry

Same principle as above but quicker to perform because various sound frequencies are tested at only one intensity (around 25 dB). It is used as a screening test at the pre-school entry. If the child fails at any frequency then full audiometry is performed.

Tympanometry

The compliance of the tympanic membrane and ear ossicles is assessed by a probe that fits snugly in the external auditory canal and which is able to generate positive and negative pressures while recording the sound reflected back from a small microphone within the probe. Suitable for any age child. Primarily used to check for 'glue ear'. In the normal ear, the peak is at 0 pressure, reflecting the equal pressures either side of the drum. The trace is flattened if a middle-ear effusion is present.

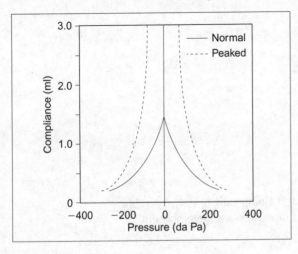

Normal trace
If compliance is much greater than normal (peaked) consider flaccid drum or disarticulation of the ossicles.

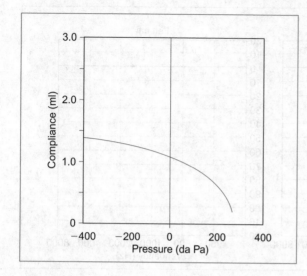

Flattened trace with no clear peak
— middle-ear effusion
— fixed ear ossicles

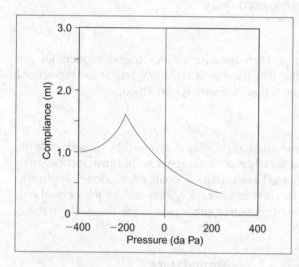

Peak at negative pressure (shift to left)
— eustachian tube dysfunction (retracted drum)

4. SPEECH AND LANGUAGE

4.1 Communication

Acquisition of communication involves:

Speech

- Expressive — production of speech
- Comprehension — understanding what is being said
- Comprehension development is ahead of expressive development

Non-verbal communication

- Eye contact, pointing, body gestures

Social communication

- Reciprocity and sharing of communication, insight into what is socially acceptable, sharing communication, listening skills

Problems in speech and language development are very common in pre-school children (5–10%) and more common in boys.

4.2 Differential diagnosis of speech and language problem

Problem with language input

- Hearing deficit
- Reduced exposure to spoken language, e.g. social circumstances, twins, poor parenting skills

Problems with language processing

- Specific speech and language delay
- Associated with general developmental delay
- Associated with reduced communicative intent and poor social skills, i.e. autistic spectrum disorder
- Associated with brain abnormalities, e.g. epilepsy, Llandau–Kleffner syndrome

Problems with language output

- Neurological or muscular problems, e.g. cerebral palsy

4.3 Specific speech and language delay

Problems in auditory/linguistic processing leading to difficulties with:

- Phonology — articulation and making the speech sounds
- Grammar — understanding the forms and structure of language

Problems in understanding the appropriate meaning and use of language

- Semantics — the meaning of words and sentences
- Pragmatics — the appropriate social use of language

Many children have a mixture of problems.

4.4   Clinical assessment

Clinical assessment determines:

- The nature of the speech and language problem
- If there are other problems such as general delay, autistic spectrum
- Any underlying cause, e.g. deafness

Investigations

- It is important to confirm that the hearing is normal (see earlier)
- EEG if there is a clear history of loss of language skills to exclude epilepsy syndromes
- Chromosomal studies if there are other associated difficulties

Management of speech and language problem

- If speech and language delay is the only problem it is usually managed by speech and language therapists alone without continuing paediatric input.
- If there are other additional problems, multidisciplinary assessment is usually necessary, involving some or all of the multidisciplinary team.
- It is also important that advice is given to education about the child's difficulties to enable them to access the national curriculum. Children with severe difficulties are sometimes placed in language units with access to on-site speech and language therapists. The majority, however, are managed in mainstream school with a speech and language programme incorporated into their individual education plans. Speech and language therapists then review the programme intermittently.

5.   AUTISTIC SPECTRUM DISORDER

Recent studies suggest that autism is becoming more common and the prevalence in industrialized countries may be as high as 1 per 1,000, not including Asperger's syndrome. Boys tend to outnumber girls by 3 to 1.

There is a wide variation in clinical presentation (autistic spectrum disorder). Three areas of development are affected:

Social skills

- Non-verbal behaviours, e.g. eye contact, body posture
- Failure to develop peer relationships
- Lack of social and emotional sharing

Verbal and non-verbal communication

- Delay in development of spoken language
- No attempt to communicate by other means
- Inability to initiate conversation
- Stereotyped and repetitive language, lack of imaginative play

Repetitive and stereotype patterns of behaviour

- Adherence to routines
- Lack of imaginative play and behaviour
- Restrictive patterns of interest
- Preoccupation with parts of objects
- Repetitive motor mannerisms, e.g. hand flapping, door closing

Other features

- The abnormal functioning is observed in one of these areas of development before the age of 3 years
- The behaviour is not accounted for by another diagnosis. A large number of children with syndromes and chromosomal abnormalities have autistic features
- Over 50% also have associated intellectual impairment that can affect the behaviours observed
- By middle age 30% have developed epilepsy
- Hearing and visual problems are common
- Dyspraxia is common

Asperger's syndrome

This is a condition at the mild end of the autistic spectrum. There is normal early language development and intellectual functioning. In early childhood it becomes apparent that the child has behavioural and social difficulties and some speech and language problems. The diagnosis can often be missed.

5.1 Assessment of children on the autistic spectrum

This is by multidisciplinary assessment. The format varies depending on local services but should include: a developmental paediatrician, a psychiatrist/psychologist and a speech and language therapy assessment.

- **History** — important to get thorough history including developmental milestones. Information about behaviour from other sources is helpful, e.g. nursery.
- **Examination** — to exclude any other diagnosis presenting with autistic features, e.g. fragile X syndrome. If possible, try to watch the child in different settings to observe the behavioural difficulties. A child in a one-to-one consultation situation may behave very differently when put into a group. Hearing and vision should also be checked.
- **Investigations** — there is no consensus regarding investigations. Some perform EEGs and chromosomal studies routinely. Others only perform the tests if there is a clinical indication, e.g. chromosomes if dysmorphic features are found, EEG if variation in symptoms or associated developmental regression.

Management

Each child needs to be assessed as an individual to determine the degree of difficulty in social and communication skills, and an individual management plan must be decided upon.

Health

Communication with parents about their concerns and difficulties with management of the child is essential. Access to more information should be provided, e.g. the National Autistic Society. Access to psychiatric/psychology services for the individual and the family are essential.

Education

Liaison with education is essential. Pre-school intervention within the home and nursery is possible with early diagnosis. Local outreach services may be available to go into the home to give management advice. Formal pre-school notification by health to education allows the child's needs to be assessed before school placement. School placement can vary from mainstream with support through to a special unit depending on the individual child. Children on the autistic spectrum often require a high teacher to pupil ratio in a highly structured environment to minimize disruptions. Speech and language input to help communication skills is also important.

Social services

Living with a child on the autistic spectrum affects all members of the family. Families often need respite care and support in the home.

6. DYSPRAXIA

Dyspraxia is a common type of sensory-processing problem that causes difficulty in performing co-ordinated actions. The child is often described as clumsy. There may be associated problems of language, perception and thought processing. Concern about dyspraxia is one of the commonest reasons for a referral to a paediatrician from education.

In the younger child symptoms include:

- Slow gross-motor development
- Poor motor skills, e.g. running, jumping, not able to catch a ball
- Difficulty dressing
- Poor pencil grip
- Difficulty with jigsaws
- Anxiety

In the older child symptoms include:

- Avoidance of physical education
- Slow school progress
- Reduced attention span
- Difficulty with maths, reading
- Trouble copying from blackboard
- Poor writing skills
- Inability to follow instructions
- Poor organizational skills

Differential diagnosis

- Learning disability
- Neuromuscular problem
- Attention-deficit hyperactivity disorder
- Specific speech and language delay
- Visual problem

Remember that a child can have more than one difficulty, e.g. dyspraxia and attention-deficit hyperactivity disorder.

Assessment

In the pre-school child initial assessment is usually by a paediatrician to exclude other pathologies, including general developmental delay. The school-age child is also often assessed by a paediatrician, but information should also be obtained from the school about the child's difficulties and overall progress. Often a speech and language assessment and occupational therapy assessment are also required.

The occupational therapist examines:

- Fine- and gross-motor developmental levels
- Visual motor integration (e.g. doing puzzles or copying shapes)
- Visual perception
- Balance and posture
- Responses to sensory stimulation
- Bilateral co-ordination
- Motor planning

Management

Dyspraxia is not curable but the child often improves in some areas with maturity. Liaison between education, health professionals and the child and parents is crucial to help the child within the classroom and the home environment. The school's special educational needs co-ordinator (SENCO) and school nurse can play an important role in the communication between health and education. Speech and language therapists and occupational therapists give advice to the school to help with difficulties in the classroom. Sometimes group and individual therapy can help, e.g. a phonology course for articulation difficulties. Advice for parents to help with home activities is also important.

7. SPECIAL EDUCATIONAL NEEDS AND THE EDUCATIONAL STATEMENT

Many children have special educational needs, but only a small percentage (approximately 2%) need statements because their difficulties are such that they require provision which is additional to or different from that normally available to children. In a statement the child's needs are clarified and a plan of how to meet these needs within the education setting is made. The statement is a legal contract and allows extra funding for the individual child to meet the special educational needs. Information from health is requested because:

- With the pre-school child it is often health that first becomes aware of the special educational needs, e.g. global developmental delay, Down syndrome, cerebral palsy
- Some medical conditions may have significant impact on the child's academic attainment and the ability to participate fully in the curriculum. Some of the commonest medical conditions are congenital heart disease, epilepsy, cystic fibrosis, haemophilia and childhood cancers

Pre-school children

- Health are required by law to notify the local education authority (LEA) of children over the age of 2 years who may have special educational needs
- The parents, nursery and social services are also able to notify education
- The LEA then collects information about the child, which is passed onto the educational psychologist who decides if a formal assessment for statementing is appropriate
- If formal assessment is requested health are asked to write a report on the child's needs, the 'E medical'. This report will give information about health, e.g. hearing, vision, epilepsy, physical problems, and a summary of the developmental problems. It also informs education of other therapists involved such as physiotherapy, speech and language. It also describes the practical needs of the child, e.g. toileting, feeding, dressing, what to do if the child has a fit. Other professionals also submit reports including the parents

Once the formal assessment is completed the LEA decides whether to statement the child or not. (The majority of children are issued a statement after formal assessment)

Schoolchildren

The process is the same, but the initial notification usually comes from the school or the parents rather than health, as the children are in school.

Child Psychiatry

8. ATTENTION-DEFICIT HYPERACTIVITY DISORDER (ADHD)

It is estimated that 1% of school-age children meet the diagnostic criteria for attention-deficit hyperactivity disorder (ADHD). Commoner in boys.

Diagnosis

Problems occur in three areas:

- Inattention
- Hyperactivity
- Impulsiveness

It is possible to have one of these features without the others, e.g. marked inattention without the hyperactivity or hyperactivity without inattention.

In addition:

- The behaviour should have persisted for at least 6 months
- The behaviour should be inconsistent with the child's developmental age
- There must be clinically significant impairment in social or academic development
- The symptoms should occur in more than one setting
- There should be no other explanation for the symptoms, e.g. psychiatric illness

Diagnosis requires detailed history and information gathering from parents, school and other professionals involved.

Children with ADHD develop emotional and social problems, poor school performance and problems within the home because of the difficult behaviour. Associated with unemployment, substance abuse and crime in adulthood.

Differential diagnosis

- Inappropriate expectations
- Language/communication disorder
- Social problem
- Specific learning difficulty
- Chronic illness, e.g. asthma
- Epilepsy
- Dyspraxia

Management

Management involves a comprehensive treatment programme. There needs to be multi-professional collaboration including the parents.

- **Psychological/behavioural interventions** — range of interventions from support groups through to psychotherapy
- **Educational support** — close communication with school is vital with the development of an individual education plan if necessary
- **Social services** — support if necessary
- **Drug treatment and dietary manipulation**

Dietary interventions are possibly useful. Some parents observe that certain foods aggravate the symptoms.

Methylphenidate (Ritalin) is used for the treatment of ADHD. It is a central nervous system stimulant and is usually given twice a day, morning and lunchtime. An evening dose is avoided because of difficulties with sleep. A drug holiday is recommended once a year. Side-effects include weight and growth retardation and hypertension. Treatment should be started and monitored by child psychiatrists or paediatricians with expertise in ADHD. Height, weight, pulse and blood pressure should be monitored at least 6-monthly. Drug treatment does not cure ADHD. It improves the symptoms to allow the other interventions an opportunity to take effect.

The National Institute for Clinical Excellence (NICE) has issued guidance on the use of methylphenidate. It has recommended:

- Methylphenidate can be used as part of a comprehensive treatment programme for children with severe ADHD
- Not licensed for those under 6 years
- Diagnosis should be made by a psychiatrist or paediatrician with expertise in ADHD
- The clinical expert should supervise the medication
- Treatment should be stopped if there is no effect
- Treatment should also include advice and support to parents and teachers
- Children should be regularly monitored

NICE is part of the National Health System (NHS). It provides guidance on medicines, medical equipment, diagnostic tests and clinical procedures and where they should be used.

9. SCHIZOPHRENIA WITH CHILDHOOD ONSET

Schizophrenia is rare in childhood and adolescence with an incidence of less than 3 in 10, 000. A genetic component can be implicated in at least 10% of cases, but other factors including perinatal difficulties, psychosocial factors and difficulties with premorbid personality are also important. Boys outnumber girls by approximately 2 : 1.

Presentation

May be acute or insidious (gradual withdrawal and failing schoolwork).

Major symptoms include:

- Delusions
- Hallucinations
- Distortions of thinking (thought insertion and withdrawal)
- Movement disorders, commonly catatonia

Differential diagnosis

It may be difficult to distinguish from major mood disturbance, e.g. manic depressive psychosis or organic causes of psychosis e.g. neurodegenerative or drug-induced episode, systemic lupus erythematosus, epilepsy, Wilson disease, thyrotoxicosis and vasculitis. (Any child presenting with psychotic symptoms should have an EEG and brain MRI scan).

Treatment

- Drugs — antipsychotics, e.g. clozapine (few extrapyramidal side-effects but risk of agranulocytosis), chlorpromazine, haloperidol
- Individual and family therapy
- Adequate educational provision essential

Prognosis

- Chronic or relapsing course is common
- Good prognostic factors include high intelligence, acute onset, precipitating factors, older age at onset and normal premorbid personality

10. DEPRESSION IN CHILDHOOD AND ADOLESCENCE

Depression affects around one in every 200 children under the age of 12 years and two to three in every 100 teenagers. The cause is usually multifactorial but recognized 'risk factors' include:

- Adverse personal experiences/life events such as family breakdown, death of friend/family member, neglect, abuse, bullying
- Physical illness including infectious mononucleosis (acute trigger) or chronic disease
- Stress — especially if unable to share concerns and/or lack of practical support
- Positive family history
- Female sex
- History of drug/alcohol problems

Symptoms

These include:

- Moodiness/irritability
- Withdrawal from friends, family, regular activities
- Self-critical/self-blaming
- Poor concentration

- Lack of care for personal appearance
- Changes in sleep pattern – may sleep too little or too much
- Tiredness
- Changes in appetite
- Frequent minor health problems particularly headaches/abdominal pain

Treatment

General advice should be given to all children and young people with mild, moderate or severe depression on:

- Self-help materials
- The benefits of regular exercise
- Sleep, hygiene and anxiety management
- Benefits of a balanced diet

Mild depression – if this persists for 4 weeks or more with no significant co-morbid problems or suicidal ideation offer one of the following psychological therapies for a limited period of 2–3 months:

- Individual non-directive supportive therapy
- Group cognitive behavioural therapy
- Guided self-help
- Antidepressant medication should not be used for the initial treatment of mild depression

Moderate/severe depression:

- First-line treatment is psychological therapy such as individual cognitive behavioural therapy or interpersonal therapy or family therapy
- If depression is unresponsive consider additional psychological therapies or medication (after multidisciplinary review)
- Fluoxetine is the most commonly prescribed but it is not licensed for under 18s and should be used extremely cautiously, especially in under 11s
- Second-line drug treatments unclude sertaline or citalopram

High-risk of suicide, serious harm and self-neglect:

- Consider inpatient treatment
- Use electroconvulsive therapy very rarely in 12–18 year olds

Do not use:

- Paroxetine, venlafaxine, tricyclic antidepressants, St John's wort

Consideration should be paid to the parent's mental health particularly the possibility of depression and substance abuse.

11. SUICIDE AND SUICIDAL BEHAVIOUR

Suicide is rare before puberty, yet it is the third leading cause of death for adolescents with rates in young men continuing to rise. Methods include drug overdose, hanging, inhalation of car exhaust fumes and shooting. It is by far the minority of adolescents who make suicide attempts who have either an underlying psychiatric disorder or serious suicidal intent. All individuals who attempt suicide must undergo psychiatric assessment. The use of violent methods, attempts which take place in isolated places and the writing of a suicide note should ring particular alarm bells.

Risk factors for suicide in adolescents

- Male sex
- Broken home, disturbed relationships with parents
- Living alone
- Immigrant status
- Family history of affective disorder, suicide or alcohol abuse
- Recent loss or stress
- Previous suicide attempt
- Drug or alcohol addiction

Characteristics of deliberate self-harm in adolescents

Self-poisoning

- Much more common in females
- Accounts for over 90% of cases of deliberate self-harm
- Overdose often taken in environment where patient is likely to be found
- Drugs most commonly taken include paracetamol, aspirin, benzodiazepines and antidepressants
- Multiple drug ingestion common (often with alcohol)
- Under 20% need intensive medical management but all should be admitted until assessed by child psychiatrist/social services as appropriate
- Mortality well below 1%
- Blood and urine toxicology screens are useful because there is often a poor correlation between the quantity of drugs taken and their clinical effect
- Paracetamol and aspirin levels should be taken routinely

Self-mutilation

- Includes scratching, cutting, cigarette burns, tattooing, bruising, biting and inserting needles
- Typically seen in teenage girls with personality problems, e.g. aggressive/impulsive behaviour, eating disorders, poor self-esteem
- Also occurs in those with schizophrenia/learning disability

Difficult to treat — need to address underlying personality/emotional problems.

Over 10% of adolescents who attempt suicide will repeat within 1 year.

12. EATING DISORDERS IN CHILDHOOD AND ADOLESCENCE

The eating disorders anorexia nervosa and bulimia nervosa have become increasingly recognized in paediatric practice over the last two decades. Both are rare in pre-pubertal children. Anorexia nervosa increases in incidence through mid- and late adolescence and is thought to affect around 1% of females aged between 15 and 25 years. Bulimia nervosa most commonly presents in the late teens or early 20s. Over 90% of those affected by eating disorders are female.

Many clinical features are common to both anorexia and bulimia nervosa and patients may satisfy criteria for anorexia or bulimia at different stages of their illness.

Diagnostic criteria for anorexia nervosa

- Self-induced weight loss of > 15% body weight (avoidance of 'fattening' foods aggravated by self-induced vomiting, purging or exercise)
- Intense fear of gaining weight or becoming fat, even though underweight
- Abnormal perception of body image
- Amenorrhoea in post-menarchal female (absence of at least three menstrual cycles)

Diagnostic criteria for bulimia nervosa

- Recurrent episodes of binge eating, characterized by consuming an excessive amount of food within a short, defined time span, with lack of control of eating during the episode
- Recurrent inappropriate compensatory behaviour to prevent weight gain, e.g. laxative abuse or self-induced vomiting
- Binges and compensatory behaviour occur at least twice per week for 3 months
- Self-evaluation unduly influenced by body shape and weight
- Disturbance does not occur exclusively during periods of anorexia nervosa

Aetiology

- **Familial factors** — concordance rate for anorexia nervosa in monozygotic twins is 50%, as compared to 10% for dizygotic twins. Other risk factors include family history of depression, alcoholism, obesity or eating disorder. Children with anorexia nervosa often come from overprotective and rigid families where there is a lack of conflict resolution
- **Individual factors** — e.g. previous obesity, fear of losing control, self-esteem dependent on the opinion of others and previous or ongoing abuse
- **Sociocultural factors** — there is a higher prevalence in high social classes and certain occupations, e.g. ballet dancers
- **Neurohumoral factors** — controversy remains over the exact role of substances such as serotonin in the pathogenesis of eating disorders

Clinical features

Anorexia nervosa
Usually this begins as a 'typical' adolescent diet to reduce stigmatization from obesity. Once weight begins to reduce, weight goals are constantly reset and compulsive weighing becomes a feature. Often physical activity is increased and social contacts diminish. Disordered thinking and poor concentration develop as the disease process progresses.

Bulimia nervosa
Bulimia is even more common than anorexia in those with a past history of obesity. Self-loathing and disgust with the body are also greater than in anorexia. Patients are more likely to seek medical help for their symptoms. Coexisting substance abuse is not uncommon. Both bulimia and anorexia are frequently associated with major depressive and anxiety disorders.

Medical complications of anorexia nervosa and bulimia

Central nervous system
- Reversible cortical atrophy
- Non-specific EEG abnormalities

Dental
- Caries
- Periodontitis

Pulmonary
- Aspiration pneumonia (rare)

Cardiovascular
- Bradycardia
- Hypotension
- Arrhythmias
- Cardiomyopathy (rare)

Gastrointestinal
- Parotitis
- Delayed gastric emptying
- Gastric dilation
- Constipation
- Raised amylase (bulimia)

Renal/electrolyte
- Hypokalaemia
- Hypochloraemic metabolic alkalosis
- Oedema
- Renal calculi (rare)

Neuroendocrine
- Amenorrhoea
- Oligomenorrhoea (bulimia)

Musculoskeletal
- Myopathy
- Osteoporosis and pathological fractures

Haematological
- Anaemia
- Thrombocytopenia
- Hypercholesterolaemia
- Hypercarotenaemia

Dermatological
- Dry, cracking skin
- Lanugo
- Callous on dorsum of hand (from vomiting)
- Perioral dermatitis

Treatment

Most patients with anorexia can be treated as outpatients, with hospital admission only if adequate weight gain at home is not possible or there are complications such as depression.

A combined multidisciplinary approach with monitoring of eating and weight, biochemical monitoring and ongoing psychotherapy is required. At present the psychotherapy usually involves behavioural, cognitive and psychodynamic components. Rarely medication such as antipsychotics or antidepressants may be required. Appetite stimulants are used even less often. Prokinetics such as cisapride and domperidone may be useful in patients with delayed gastric emptying. Adequate provision for education is essential. Feeding against the will of the patient can only be done in the context of the Mental Health Act 1983 or the Children Act 1989.

Young people with bulimia may be treated with cognitive behavioural therapy, adapted to suit their age and development. A trial of selective serotonin reuptake inhibitors (SSRIs) may be considered but no other drugs are recommended for the treatment of bulimia nervosa.

Course and prognosis

Five to 10 years after the diagnosis of anorexia nervosa around 50% will have recovered, 25% will have improved but still have some features of an eating disorder and the remainder will either not have improved or be dead. Mortality rates are between 5% and 20% with the most frequent causes of death being starvation, electrolyte imbalance, cardiac failure and suicide.

Good prognostic factors

- Younger age at onset
- Less denial
- Improved self-esteem

Poor prognostic factors

- Parental conflict
- Bulimia nervosa
- Coexisting behavioural disorders

The long-term outcome of bulimia nervosa is less clear.

13. COMMON BEHAVIOURAL PROBLEMS IN PRE-SCHOOL CHILDREN

13.1 Sleep disorders

Reluctance to settle at night and persistent waking during the night are common problems in young children, with one in five 2-year-olds waking at least five times per week.

Factors contributing to sleep difficulties

- Adverse temperamental characteristics in child
- Perinatal problems
- Maternal anxiety
- Poor accommodation
- Physical illness
- Medication, e.g. theophyllines
- Timing of feeds
- Co-sleeping with parents

Medication, such as sedating antihistamines, are usually unhelpful in this situation. A behavioural strategy is usually successful but often needs to be combined with some respite for the parents. Unlicenced melatonin, however, is sometimes used to reduce both the time to sleep onset and the number of episodes of night wakenings. Its use in children with co-existing neurodevelopmental pathology has been well described.

Nightmares are most common between the ages of 3 and 5 years with an incidence of between 25% and 50%. The child who awakens during them is usually alert and can recall the dream and frightening images. They are usually self-limiting and may be related to obvious frightening or stressful events. In severe cases the involvement of a psychologist or psychiatrist may be needed.

13.2   Feeding problems in infancy and childhood

Most children at some point will be 'picky eaters' — a phase which will usually pass spontaneously. Infants and children may also, however, refuse to feed if they find the experience painful or frightening. Reasons contributing to this may include:

- Unpleasant physical experiences associated with eating, e.g. gastro-oesophageal reflux, oral candidiasis, stricture post-oesophageal atresia repair
- Oral motor dysfunction
- Children who have required early nasogastric tube feeds
- Maternal depression
- Being forced to eat by caregiver
- Developmental conflict with caregiver
- Emotional and social deprivation

Non-organic faltering growth is a diagnosis of exclusion.

Evaluation of feeding disorders

- Complete history including detailed social history
- Complete physical examination — need to exclude physiological, anatomical and neurological abnormalities
- Assess emotional state and developmental level
- Observe feeding interaction
- Help parents to understand that infants and children may have different styles of eating and food preferences

Management of feeding disorders

- Eliminate and/or treat physical cause
- Multidisciplinary approach including paediatrician, GP, health visitor, speech therapist, dietician and/or psychologist
- Child's behaviour may need modification
- If there is also faltering growth, exclude medical disorders and maltreatment

Pica (the ingestion of inedible material such as dirt and rubbish) may be normal in toddlers but persistent ingestion is found in children with learning difficulties and in psychotic and socially deprived children. Lead poisoning is a theoretical risk from pica.

13.3   Temper tantrums

These are common in the pre-school child and generally occur when the child is angry or has hurt themselves. Usually they are typified by screaming and/or crying, often in association with collapsing to the floor. It is rare for the child to injure themselves during such episodes. If necessary the child should be restrained from behind by folding one's arms around the child's body. It is important to minimize any additional attention to the child and to respond and praise only when behaviour is back to normal.

13.4   Breath-holding attacks

These episodes typically occur after a frustrating or painful experience. The child cries inconsolably, holds his breath and then becomes pale or cyanosed. In the most serious cases loss of consciousness may ensue and there may be stiffening of the limbs or brief clonic movements. Clearly it may be difficult to distinguish from a generalized seizure; however, the fact that after a breath-holding attack the child will take a deep breath and immediately regain consciousness may facilitate differentiation. Typical onset is between 6 and 18 months. No specific treatment is needed and the episodes diminish with age.

14.   COMMON PROBLEMS IN THE SCHOOL-AGED CHILD

14.1   School refusal

This problem refers to the child's irrational fear about school attendance and most commonly is seen at the beginning of schooling or in association with a change of school or move to secondary school. Typically the child is reluctant to leave home in the morning and they may develop headache or abdominal pain.

Factors contributing to school refusal include:

- Separation anxiety
- Specific phobia about an aspect of school attendance, e.g. travelling to school, mixing with other children, games lessons, etc.

- A more generalized psychiatric disturbance such as depression or low self-esteem
- Bullying

Characteristics of school refusers

- Good academic achievements
- Conformist at school
- Oppositional at home

Treatment

- Avoid unnecessary investigation of minor somatic symptoms
- Early, if necessary graded, return to school
- Support for parents and child
- Close liaison with school

In chronic cases a gradual reintegration back into school is required, possibly with a concurrent specific behavioural programme and targeted family therapy.

Overall two-thirds of children will return to school regularly. Those who do badly are often adolescents from disturbed family backgrounds.

Truancy

In contrast to the above, truancy always reflects a lack of desire to go to school rather than anxiety re school attendance and as such may be part of a conduct disorder.

Bullying

Bullying may be defined as 'the intentional unprovoked abuse of power by one or more children to inflict pain or cause distress to another child on repeated occasions'. Estimates on the prevalence of bullying vary widely, but many studies report that between 20% and 50% of school-aged children have either participated in or been victims of bullying. Verbal harassment is the commonest form of bullying and is often not recognized as such.

Although it is important not to stereotype, certain characteristics are commonly exhibited by bullies:

- Poor psychosocial functioning
- Unhappiness in school
- Concurrent conduct disorders
- Emotional problems
- Social problems
- Alcohol and nicotine abuse

Children who suffer at the hands of bullies may consequently suffer from:

- Anxiety
- Insecurity
- Low self-esteem and self-worth
- Mental health problems

- Sleep difficulties
- Bed wetting
- Headaches
- Abdominal pain

Carefully planned programmes may reduce the incidence of bullying by 50% or more. Such strategies rely on teaching appropriate social skills to children who bully, developing clear rules which they are expected to adhere to, providing an increased level of supervision, particularly within the school environment, and facilitating access to other services they may require, e.g. child psychiatry, social services, etc.

14.2 Non-organic abdominal pain/headache/limb pains

Over 10% of children experience such symptoms. It is important to exclude organic pathology promptly and to search for any underlying stresses. Most run a short course but if symptoms are persistent and involve several systems the term 'somatization disorder' is used.

14.3 Sleep problems in the school-aged child

To understand sleep disorders a basic knowledge of the sleep cycle is necessary.

Sleep stages

Sleep consists of several stages that cycle throughout the night. One complete cycle lasts 90–100 minutes.

Sleep stage	Features
1 Slow wave sleep (SWS) or non-rapid eye movement (NREM)	Transition state between sleep and wakefulness Eyes begin to roll slightly Mostly high-amplitude, low-frequency theta waves Brief periods of alpha waves — similar to those when awake Lasts only a few minutes
2 SWS or NREM	Peak of brain waves higher and higher sleep spindles Lasts only few minutes
3 SWS or NREM	Also called delta sleep or deep sleep Very slow delta waves account for 20–50% of brain waves

Sleep stage	Features
4 SWS or NREM	Also called delta sleep or deep sleep Over 50% of brain waves are delta waves Last and deepest of sleep stages before REM sleep
5 REM	Frequent bursts of rapid eye movement and occasional muscular twitches Heart rate increases Rapid shallow respirations Most vivid dreaming during this phase

Night terrors

These are most commonly seen in children between the ages of 4 and 7 years. Typically the child wakes from deep or stage 4 sleep apparently terrified, hallucinating and unresponsive to those around them. Usually such episodes last less than 15 minutes and the child goes back to sleep, with no recollection of the events in the morning. It is unusual to find any underlying reason or stresses contributing to the problem.

Nightmares

These occur during REM sleep and the child remembers the dream either immediately or in the morning. Underlying anxieties should be sought.

Sleepwalking

This occurs during stages 3 or 4 of sleep and is most often seen in those between 8 and 14 years.

14.4   Tics

These occur transiently in 10% of children and are much more commonly seen in boys. Onset is usually around the age of 7 years and, while simple tics are seen most commonly. Gilles de la Tourette syndrome may occur in childhood. This phenomenon is characterized by complex tics occurring in association with coprolalia (obscene words and swearing) and echolalia (repetition of sounds or words).

Factors predisposing to tics

- Positive family history
- Stress (including parental)
- Neurodevelopmental delay

Treatment

- Most resolve spontaneously
- Reassure accordingly
- Behavioural or family therapy if appropriate
- Medication: haloperidol, pimozide, clonidine (in very severe cases only)

Outcome

- Simple tics — complete remission
- Tourette's syndrome — 50% have symptoms into adult life

15. ENURESIS

This is defined as the involuntary passage of urine in the absence of physical abnormality after the age of 5 years. Nocturnal enuresis is much more common than diurnal enuresis, affecting at least 10% of 5-year-olds. Although most children with nocturnal enuresis are not psychiatrically ill, up to 25% will have signs of psychiatric disturbance. Diurnal enuresis is much more common among girls and those who are psychiatrically disturbed.

Aetiology

- Positive family history in 70%
- Developmental delay
- Psychiatric disturbance
- Small bladder capacity
- Recent stressful life events
- Large family size
- Social disadvantage

Treatment

- Exclude physical basis (history, examination, urine culture, +/– imaging)
- Look for underlying stresses
- Reassure child and parents of benign course
- Star chart
- Enuresis alarm (7 years and older)
- Drugs (short-term control only) desmopressin, tricyclic antidepressants

It must be remembered that child sexual abuse may present with enuresis and/or encopresis.

16. ENCOPRESIS AND SOILING

This is defined as the inappropriate passage of formed faeces, usually onto the underwear, after the age of 4 years. It is uncommon, with a prevalence of 1.8% among 8-year-old boys and 0.7% for girls. Psychiatric disturbance is common and enuresis often coexists. Broadly speaking, children with encopresis may be divided into those who retain faeces and develop subsequent overflow incontinence (retentive encopresis) and those who deposit faeces inappropriately on a regular basis (non-retentive).

Type of encopresis and common family characteristics

- Retentive — obsessional toilet-training practices
- Non-retentive — continuous, disorganized, chaotic families

Other risk factors for encopresis

- Poor parent/child relationship
- Emotional stresses (including sexual abuse)
- Past history of constipation/anal fissure

Treatment

- Exclude physical problems, e.g. Hirschsprung's disease/hypothyroidism/hypercalcaemia
- Laxatives to clear bowel
- Education for parents and child
- Star chart
- Individual psychotherapy
- Family therapy

It is unusual for this problem to persist into adolescence

17.   CONDUCT DISORDERS

Persistent antisocial or socially disapproved of behaviour often involving damage to property and unresponsive to normal sanctions.

Prevalence

- Approximately 4%
- Strong male predominance

Clinical features

- Temper tantrums
- Oppositional behaviour (defiance of authority, fighting)
- Overactivity
- Irritability
- Aggression
- Stealing
- Lying
- Truancy

- Bullying
- Delinquency, e.g. stealing, vandalism, arson in older children/teenagers

'Oppositional defiant disorder' is a type of conduct disorder characteristically seen in children under 10 years. It is characterized by markedly defiant, disobedient, provocative behaviour and by the absence of more severe dissocial or aggressive acts that violate the law or the rights of others.

Aetiology

- Family factors: lack of affection, marital disharmony, poor discipline, parental violence/aggression
- Constitutional factors: low IQ, learning difficulties, adverse temperamental features
- Oppositional peer group values
- Urban deprivation/poor schooling

Differential diagnosis

Young people with conduct disorders have an increased incidence of neurological signs and symptoms, psychomotor seizures, psychotic symptoms, mood disorders, ADHD and learning difficulties.

Treatment

- Family/behavioural therapy
- Practical social support, e.g. rehousing

Prognosis

- Half have problems into adult life

Community Paediatrics

18. CHILD HEALTH SURVEILLANCE

The health authority is responsible for ensuring that an adequate surveillance programme is offered to all children and that it is monitored effectively. The programme should comprise:

- Oversight of health and physical growth of all children
- Monitoring developmental progress of all children
- Provision of adequate advice and support to parents
- Programme of infectious disease prophylaxis
- Participation in health education and training in parenthood
- Identification of 'children in need' in accordance with the Children Act
- Identification and notification of children with special educational needs in accordance with the 1981 Education Act

18.1 Pre-school children

At present in the UK, all children, at birth, are assigned a health visitor who has regular contact with the child and their family at home and at child health clinics. A parent-held child health record 'red book' is given at birth. All contact that professionals have with the child and family should be clearly documented. The current pre-school child health programme is:

- **Neonatal examination** — performed by hospital doctor, nurse practitioner or GP. Full physical examination including weight, head circumference, heart, eyes, hips, eyes for red reflexes, genitalia. Screening for phenylketonuria, hypothyroidism +/– haemoglobinopathy is performed by midwife around day 5. In some regions in the UK screening is also performed for cystic fibrosis and Duchenne muscular dystrophy. Universal neonatal hearing screening is currently being phased in.
- **6-week check** — physical examination by doctor and health visitor
- **7- to 9-month check** — physical examination, hearing distraction test, squint assessment, assessment of growth and development (doctor and health visitor)
- **18–24 months** — developmental assessment by health visitor (has been stopped in some areas)
- **36–54 months** — physical examination and identification of health problems that will either affect education or require medication in school

All these visits provide the opportunity for appropriate health promotion. The immunization schedule is discussed in detail below.

18.2   School-aged children

Programmes differ significantly between local authorities. A health questionnaire is completed on school entry and reviewed by the school nurse. Screening of hearing and vision is also undertaken. In most areas medical examination is carried out only on a selective basis.

Regular health interviews are subsequently carried out with intermittent screening of vision. Informal 'drop-in centres' run by the school nurse provide valuable support to the child and their family. A full medical may be requested if parents, teachers or school nurse have concerns.

19.   IMMUNIZATION IN CHILDHOOD

19.1   Immunization schedule

The current immunization schedule for infants and children in the UK

Age	Vaccine
Neonatal period	BCG if in high-risk category*
2 months	First diphtheria, tetanus, acellular pertussis, inactivated polio vaccine, *Haemophilus influenzae* type b (DTaP/IPV/Hib) — single vaccine
	+
	First pneumoccal vaccine
3 months	Second DTaP/IPV/Hib and first meningococcal group C (Men C)
4 months	Third DTaP/IPV/Hib and Men C + pneumococcal vaccine
12 months	Hib and Men C
13 months	Measles, mumps, rubella (MMR) + pneumococcal vaccine
3.5 years	MMR second dose
	DTaP/IPV
10–14 years	BCG (after skin test, if not given in infancy)
13–18 years	DTa and IPV booster

Notes on immunization schedule

*Bacillus Calmette–Guérin (BCG) vaccine

High-risk categories include:

- Infants born to immigrants from countries with high prevalence of tuberculosis
- Infants who are to travel abroad to high-prevalence areas
- Infants born in UK where high prevalence of tuberculosis

Rubella vaccine

Any girl who missed the MMR should be immunized between the ages of 10 and 14 years.

Hepatitis B vaccine

At present the vaccine is recommended only for:

- Babies born to mothers who are chronic carriers of hepatitis B virus or to mothers who have had acute hepatitis B during pregnancy
- Families adopting children from countries such as Southeast Asia, in whom hepatitis status is unknown

19.2   Contraindications to immunization

General considerations

- **Acute illness** — immunization should be deferred if the individual is acutely unwell but not if they have a minor infection without fever or systemic upset
- **Previous severe local or general reaction** — if there is a definite history of severe local or general reaction to a preceding dose, then subsequent immunization with that particular vaccine should not be performed
- **Local reactions** — extensive redness and swelling which becomes indurated and involves most of the anterolateral surface of the thigh or a major part of the circumference of the upper arm
- **General reactions** — this is defined as: fever over 39.5°C within 48 hours of vaccination; anaphylaxis; bronchospasm; laryngeal oedema; generalized collapse. In addition, prolonged unresponsiveness; prolonged inconsolable or high-pitched screaming for more than 4 hours; convulsions or encephalopathy within 72 hours

Live vaccines (e.g. BCG, MMR, polio)

Contraindications to live vaccine administration include:

- Prednisolone (orally or rectally) at a daily dose of 2 mg/kg per day for at least a week or 1 mg/kg per day for a month; corticosteroid use via other routes (e.g. intra-articular or inhaled) does not contraindicate live vaccine administration
- Children on lower doses of steroid also on cytotoxic drugs or with immunosuppression secondary to an underlying disease process
- Those with impaired cell-mediated immunity, e.g. Di George syndrome
- Children being treated for malignant disease with chemotherapy and/or radiotherapy, or those who have completed such treatment within the last 6 months
- Children who have had a bone marrow transplant within 6 months
- Immunoglobulin administration within previous 3 months

Myths surrounding contraindications

The following are **NOT** contraindications to immunization:

- Family history of adverse immunization reaction
- Stable neurological condition, e.g. Down syndrome or cerebral palsy
→• Egg allergy — hypersensitivity to egg contraindicates influenza vaccine and yellow fever vaccine, but there is good evidence that MMR can be safely given to children who have had previous anaphylaxis after egg
- Personal or family history of inflammatory bowel disease does not contraindicate MMR immunization
- Family history of convulsions
- Mother is pregnant

In addition, it should be noted that the Council of the Faculty of Homeopathy strongly supports the immunization programme.

19.3 Immunization in HIV-positive children

Current recommendations are that it is perfectly safe for HIV-infected children to receive:

- MMR (measles may be contraindicated if there is severe immunosupression)
- Inactivated polio
- Pertussis, diphtheria, tetanus, polio, typhoid, cholera, hepatitis B and Hib

They should not receive:

- BCG
- Yellow fever
- Oral typhoid

19.4 Additional information on vaccines

Vaccine type	Other specific contraindications*	Side-effects**	Comments
Diphtheria	Inactivated toxoid + adjuvant	As above	Swelling + redness common Malaise, fever, headache Severe anaphylaxis rare Neurological reactions very rare	
Tetanus	Inactivated toxoid + adjuvant NB *Bordetella pertussis* also acts as adjuvant	As above	Pain, redness, swelling common General reactions uncommon Malaise, myalgia, pyrexia Acute anaphylaxis and urticaria are common Peripheral neuropathy rare	

Vaccine type		Other specific contraindications*	Side-effects**	Comments
Pertussis	Killed *Bordetella pertussis* (as part of DTP) Acellular pertussis now used	As above + evolving neurological problem	Swelling and redness at injection site less common with acellular vaccine Crying, fever with DTP or DT Persistent screaming and collapse now rare with current vaccines Convulsions and encephalopathy vv rare and link with vaccine itself contentious Much more common after disease than vaccination	
Polio	Live, attenuated OPV *or* Enhanced potency inactivated polio vaccine (eIPV)	As above + OPV Vomiting or diarrhoea Not at same time as oral typhoid vaccine Not for siblings and household contacts of immunosuppressed children Not within 3 weeks of immunoglobulin injection Contraindications Inactivated polio vaccine (IPV) Acute or febrile illness Extreme polymyxin B and neomycin sensitivity	Vaccine-associated polio in recipients of OPV and in contacts of recipients at rate of one of each per 2 million oral doses	Faecal excretion of vaccine virus lasts up to 6 weeks Contacts of recently immunized baby should be advised re need for strict personal hygiene, e.g. after nappy changes Babies on Special Care Baby Unit (SCBU) should be given IPV Recently immun-ized children may go swimming
Hib	Conjugate	As above	Local swelling and redness 10% — rate declines with subsequent doses	Disease incidence has fallen dramatically since introduction in 1992

Vaccine type		Other specific contraindications*	Side–effects**	Comments
MMR	Live, attenuated	As above + allergy to neomycin or kanamycin	Malaise, fever, rash within 7 –10 days, Parotid swelling 1% Febrile convulsion 1/1,000 Arthropathy/thrombocytopenia rare Theoretical risk of encephalitis but causal evidence lacking Encephalitis much more likely secondary to measles in unimmunized child All side-effects less common after 2nd dose	Medical Research Council and CSM concluded no link between MMR and autism or bowel disease. Separate vaccines may be harmful. Adverse publicity led to a fall in uptake rates and consequent increased risk of measles outbreak
Men C	Conjugate (carrier proteins are diphtheria toxoid or tetanus toxoid derivatives)	As above + hypersensitivity to vaccine components incl. diphtheria toxoid or tetanus toxoid	Swelling at injection site common particularly in older children Systemic symptoms incl. irritability and fever much more common in infants Headaches, dizziness	Protects against *N. meningitides* group C only If travelling abroad, should still receive meningococcal polysaccharide
BCG	Live, attenuated A and C vaccines	As above + positive sensitivity skin test to tuberculin protein Generalized septic skin conditions	Vertigo and dizziness occasional Immediate allergy/anaphylaxis rare Severe injection site problems usually due to poor injection technique Adenitis Lupoid-type local reaction (rare) Widespread dissemination of organism (v. rare)	If child has eczema give at eczema-free site Tuberculin skin test must be done First in all children over 3 months Reaction to tuberculin protein may be suppressed by: infectious mononucleosis, other viral infection, live viral vaccines, Hodgkin's disease, sarcoid, corticosteroids, immunosuppressant treatment or diseases

* Please refer to notes above for general contraindications to immunizations.

** All immunizations may be complicated by local or general side-effects as discussed above.

DTP, diphtheria + tetanus + pertussis; DT, diphtheria + tetanus; OPV, oral polio vaccine; Hib, *Haemophilus influenzae* type b; MMR, measles, mumps, rubella; CSM, Committee on Safety of Medicines; Men C, meningitis C.

20. ADOPTION AND FOSTERING

20.1 Adoption

Adoption is about meeting the needs of a child and not those of the prospective parents. When a child is adopted full parental rights are taken on by the adopting parents and the child has all the rights of a natural child of those parents. Approximately 2,000 children per year are adopted in England, the majority of these being children over 4 years of age. Over half involve children being adopted by step-parents. Adoption of newborn babies is increasingly uncommon. Whilst infants and children from overseas are brought into the UK for adoption, it must be recognized that the legal complexities surrounding this area are immense.

In England and Wales social services and voluntary organizations act as adoption agencies. Before any child is adopted the following steps must occur:

- Freeing of child for adoption — baby/child's natural parents must give consent for adoption. Cannot be done until at least 6 weeks after birth for newborn infants. May not be required if parents are deemed incapable of decision-making (e.g. severe mental illness)
- Meticulous assessment of prospective adoptive parents — carried out by social services. There are very few absolute contraindications to adoption (certain criminal offences will exclude). Detailed medical history of prospective parents important to ensure they are physically able to look after child. Disabled adults are encouraged to adopt. Choice of family will ideally reflect birth heritage of child (i.e. ethnic origin)
- Application for adoption order — can be applied for as soon as the child starts living with prospective adoptive parents but it will not be heard for at least 3 months (for newborn infants the 3-month period begins at the age of 6 weeks)
- Adoption hearing — an Adoption Panel, including social workers and medical advisers, consider the both needs of the child and the prospective parents. May be contested. Decision on day as to whether Adoption Order to be granted

Medical services are involved at two levels:

- In an advisory capacity to the adoption agency, e.g. scrutinizing reports, collecting further medical information if needed
- Carrying out pre-adoption medicals — it is essential that prospective parents have all available information on, for example, the health of both natural parents, pregnancy, delivery, neonatal problems, development, etc. so that they can make a fully informed decision about adopting the child. Any special needs of the child should be identified at such an examination and additional reports by psychiatrists/psychologists may be needed. Children with special needs usually thrive in secure family environments, but full medical information must be made available to prospective adopters.

There are no medical conditions in the child which absolutely contraindicate adoption.

20.2 Fostering

Foster care offers a child care in a family setting but does not provide legal permanency as parental rights remain with the natural parents, local authority or courts, depending on the legal circumstances. Different types of foster care include:

- Care of babies awaiting adoption
- Young children in whom return to parents is anticipated

For some children with strong natural family ties long-term fostering is appropriate.

Foster parents are selected by a foster panel and, as with adoption, their health and that of the children awaiting fostering is considered.

21. DISABILITY LIVING ALLOWANCE

Disability Living Allowance (DLA) is a tax-free, social security benefit for people with an illness or disability who need:

- Help with getting around
- Help with personal care
- Help with both of the above

Obviously all children need some help and supervision. Families can make a claim if the child needs more help and supervision than another child of the same age. The claim is not affected by the money the child or family already have. Children can only receive DLA for help getting around if they are 5 years old or over. The rate they get depends on the type of help or supervision they need. Children can only receive DLA for help with personal care if they are 3 months or over. The rate again depends on the amount of help and supervision the child needs.

Additional support funds

There are other sources of financial support, e.g. The Family Fund Trust, to help families with severely disabled children. The Family Fund Trust is funded by the national government and family's financial circumstances are taken into consideration when deciding whether to give support.

22. THE CHILDREN ACT 1989 AND HUMAN RIGHTS ACT 1998

22.1 Aims of the Children Act

This Act introduced extensive changes to legislation affecting the welfare of children. Its main aims included:

- Restructuring custody and access in divorce

- Moving towards a 'family court' handling all public and private proceedings about children
- Creating a single statutory code for the protection of children through the courts
- Promoting interagency co-operation in the prevention, detection and treatment of child abuse and neglect
- Making legal remedies more accessible while also encouraging negotiation, partnership and agreed solutions which avoid the need to resort to court

In all of the above, the Act stresses that the child's welfare is the paramount consideration. It provides a checklist of welfare parameters aimed at ensuring that in planning for the child's protection and upbringing, full account is taken of his or her needs, wishes and characteristics.

Child protection issues contained in the Act

Social services have a duty to investigate if they have reasonable cause to suspect that a child has suffered, is suffering or is likely to suffer 'significant harm'. If investigation confirms the suspicion then the child may need to be accommodated by social services while matters are taken further. Parents of an accommodated child retain full parental responsibility, including the right to remove the child at any time. An emergency protection order may be available, enabling the child to be detained in hospital, if parents do not agree to voluntary admission.

Emergency Protection Order

This replaced the 'Place of Safety Order' and may be needed if, for example, non-accidental injury is suspected. The order lasts a maximum of 8 days with a possibility of extension for a further 7 days. It may be granted by the court if one of the following is satisfied:

- There is reasonable cause to believe that the child is likely to suffer appreciable harm if not removed from their present accommodation
- Inquiries by local authority or an 'authorized person' are being frustrated by lack of access

In addition, a child likely to suffer significant harm may also be taken into **police protection** for 72 hours. This involves a decision internal to the police force, and in cases of extreme emergency is likely to be quicker than applying for an Emergency Protection Order.

A Care Order

This order confers parental responsibility on the social services (in addition to that of the parents) and usually involves removal from home, at least temporarily. It may be applied for in cases of non-accidental injury, where inquiries will take some time and where the child is not regarded as being 'safe' at home.

A Supervision Order

This gives social services the power and duty to visit the family and also to impose conditions, such as attendance at clinic, nursery, school or outpatient visits.

Both care and supervision orders may be taken out by a court if that court is convinced that thresholds for appreciable harm to the child have been met. The court, however, is under duties to consider the full range of its power and not to make any order unless doing so would be better for the child than making no order. Whilst proceedings for either of these orders are pending, the court may make 8- and then 4-weekly cycles to allow time for the child's needs to be comprehensively assessed, and for parties to prepare their proposals for court.

Child Assessment Order (CAO)

This order may be used if there is a situation of persistent but non-urgent suspicion of risk. It is available if:

- Significant harm is suspected
- A necessary medical or other assessment would be unlikely or unsatisfactory without a court order

It therefore overrides the objections of a parent to whatever examination or assessment is needed to see whether the significant harm test is satisfied. In addition it may override the objection of a child who 'is of sufficient understanding to make an informed decision'. This order lasts up to 7 days.

Wardship

If insufficient powers are available via the Children Act then wardship via the High Court may be applied for. This gives the court almost limitless powers and is used in exceptional circumstances, such as when a family objects to surgery or medical treatment for religious reasons.

Despite all the above, the implementation of the Children Act has been associated with a significant reduction in the number of compulsory child protection interventions through the courts, in part because of greater social services' reliance on voluntary help and increased partnership with parents.

22.2 Human Rights Act 1998

This act requires that all UK law is interpreted in accordance with the European Convention of Human Rights so as to give effect to the requirements of the convention rights. The Act enables individuals to take action for breach of these rights which include:

- Article 2 — Right to life
- Article 3 — Prohibition of torture
- Article 6 — Right to a fair trial
- Article 8 — Right to respect for private and family life

During child protection investigations there is potential conflict between the right of the child's family (Article 8) and the duties of the child protection team as they relate to Articles 2 and 3. Legal advice will need to be sought in situations of doubt.

National Service Framework (NSF)

The NSF for children, young people and maternity services was published in September 2004. The entire document, which is divided into three parts, promotes the delivery of high quality, integrated, patient-focused health care. The standards comprise:

Part 1

- Promoting health and well being, identifying needs and intervening early
- Supporting parenting
- Child, young person and family-centred services
- Growing up into adulthood
- Safeguarding the welfare of children and young people

Part 2

- Children and young people who are ill
- Children and young people in hospital
- Disabled children and young people and those with complex health needs
- The mental health and psychological well-being of children and young people
- Medicines for children and young people

Part 3

- Maternity services

23. CHILD ABUSE

Epidemiology

In Britain up to 100 children per year die as a result of non-accidental injuries. The incidence of non-accidental physical injury is around 1 per 2,000 children per year. In addition some reports suggest that by the age of 16 years up to 1 in 4 girls and 1 in 5 boys will have been sexually assaulted. Many victims, particularly those of sexual abuse, do not come forward for many years. Sadly around 80% of these children are sexually abused by people they know.

The Victoria Climbié Inquiry

The death of Victoria Climbié in February 2000 exposed many deficiencies in the child protection system. Lord Laming conducted an inquiry into the circumstances leading to and surrounding the death of Victoria. As well as establishing the circumstances leading to and surrounding her death, his report scrutinized the working practices within social services, health bodies and the police. The degree of co-operative interagency working was also examined. The report's recommendations aim to minimize the chance of another such tragedy ever occurring. Individual recommendations were made for health services, social services and the police services. The major healthcare recommendations include recommendations on:

- Initial assessment/notekeeping — when deliberate harm of a child is identified as a possibility and the child is admitted:
  - Consider taking the history directly from the child even without the consent of the carer
  - Ensure nursing care plan takes full account of concerns
  - Record any differences of medical opinion
  - Ensure all notes are comprehensive/contemporaneous (include content of all telephone calls, handovers etc.)
  - Ask about previous admissions to other hospitals and obtain such information
  - Ensure full physical examination within 24 hours
  - Permission for any relevant investigations should be obtained by a doctor above the grade of senior house officer
  - The name of the consultant responsible for the child protection aspects of the child's care should be clear
  - Within a given location, work from one set of medical records
- Discharge arrangements
  - Permission must be obtained from consultant or middle-grade doctor
  - Follow-up arrangements must be documented
  - Must have a GP identified before discharge
- Training
  - National ongoing training programme for doctors should be set up and integrated within revalidation of doctors
  - Training should be available for all staff who have regular contact with children
- Interagency working
  - Liaison between hospitals and community health services is crucial

Types of abuse

- Physical injury may be inflicted deliberately or by failure to provide a safe environment
- Neglect, e.g. inadequate provision of food
- Emotional neglect
- Sexual abuse
- Potential abuse, e.g. if another child was previously harmed

Diagnosing child abuse

History
With any injury a careful history should be sought. The following should alert the clinician to the possibility of non-accidental injury:

- Discrepancy between history and injury seen
- Changing story with time or different people
- Delay in reporting
- Unusual reaction to injury
- Repeated injury
- History of non-accidental or suspicious injury in sibling
- Signs of neglect or faltering growth

Social and family indicators of abuse

Factors commonly associated with child abuse include:

- Young, immature, lonely and isolated parents
- Poor interparental relationship
- Substance abuse in parent
- Parents who had rejection, deprivation or abuse in their childhoods
- Parents with learning difficulties or difficult pregnancy
- Early illness in child
- Difficult behaviour in child

Examination

If non-accidental injury without sexual abuse is suspected the child should be fully undressed and examined in a warm, secure environment by an appropriately experienced doctor. Careful charting of injuries is imperative. The recommendations of Lord Laming's report should be adhered to.

Certain injuries are 'typical' in abuse:

- **Bruises** — bruises are uncommon in children under 1 year, especially if not mobile; bruises of different ages or finger-shaped bruises raise concerns, as do bruises on head, face and lumbar region (often finger marks), bruising around wrists and ankles (swinging), bruising inside and behind pinna (blow with hand), ring of bruises (bite mark)
- **Two black eyes**
- **Strap or lash marks**
- **Torn frenulum** — blow or force feeding
- **Perforated eardrum** — slap or blow to side of head
- **Small circular burns** — cigarette burn
- **Burns or scalds to both feet or buttocks**
- **Fractured ribs** — shaking
- **Epiphyses torn off** — swinging
- **Subdural haematoma** — shaking
- **Retinal haemorrhages** — shaking
- **Multiple injuries and injuries at different ages**

Potential pitfalls

Underdiagnosis is much more common than overdiagnosis but beware of:

- Mongolian spots — most common in those of Asian origin; look like bruises, seen most commonly over buttocks
- Bleeding disorders — need full blood count and clotting test to exclude these if there are multiple bruises
- Underlying bony disorder — e.g. osteogenesis imperfecta or copper deficiency; if fractures are present, a paediatric radiologist must be able to exclude the former

Rough estimates of ages of bruises and fractures

Accurate dating is not possible.

Age of bruise	Bruise appearance
< 24 hours	Red or red/purple, swollen
1–2 days	Purple, swollen
3–5 days	Starting to yellow
5–7 days	Yellow, fading
> 1 week	Yellow, brown, have faded

Healing of fractures

Fracture appearance	Average timing
Swelling of soft tissue resolves	2–10 days
Periosteal new bone	10+ days
Loss of fracture-line definition	14+ days
Soft callus	14+ days
Hard callus	21+ days
Remodelling	3+ months

It is not possible to date skull fractures.

Management of suspected non-accidental injuries

- Put the interests of the child first
- Local protocols will be in place and should be adhered to
- If suspicion of non-accidental injury, check local 'at risk' register
- History and examination should be performed by senior, experienced paediatrician and well documented
- Additional information from school, GP, health visitor may be extremely helpful
- Skeletal survey and clotting may be needed
- Final diagnosis of non-accidental injury requires piecing together of information gleaned from many sources
- If non-accidental injury is thought likely and the child is not ill enough to warrant hospital admission, close liaison with social services/child protection team is needed to discuss the most appropriate place for child to be discharged to (see Child Protection issues in Section 22.1 Aims of the Children Act)
- Social services will decide whether to call a case conference (see below), at which whether to place the child's name on the 'at-risk' register will be discussed

Case conference

This is a formal gathering of individuals with a legitimate interest in the child and family. It allows:

- Exchange of relevant information
- Decision as to whether abuse has taken place
- Decision on whether to place name on Child Protection Register
- Action plan for protecting child and helping family
- Identification of individuals to implement plan

Neglect

This may manifest as faltering growth, failure of normal development or growth, or lack of normal emotional responses. Other causes need to be excluded, but typically the child progresses better in a hospital environment than at home.

Poisoning

Rare but consider if symptoms and signs are difficult to explain. Blood and urine will need to be screened.

Munchausen's syndrome by proxy

In this condition a child receives medical attention for symptoms that have either been falsified or directly induced by their carer. Among the most common symptoms are bleeding, fever, vomiting, diarrhoea, seizures and apnoea. The doctor may be persuaded to order a range of increasingly complex investigations. Diagnosis is difficult and may involve inpatient observation. Once confirmed, social services and psychiatry services will need to be involved and a child protection conference should be convened.

Sexual abuse

Presentation
Sexual abuse presents in many ways:

- Allegations by child or adult (children rarely lie about this)
- Injuries to genitalia or anus (including bleeding or sexually transmitted disease)
- Suspicious features including unexplained recurrent urinary tract infection, sexual explicitness in play, drawing, language or behaviour, sudden or unexplained changes in behaviour, e.g. sleep disturbance and loss of trust in individuals close to them, taking an overdose, running away from home
- Psychosomatic indicators including recurrent headache, abdominal pain, enuresis, encopresis, eating disorders

Physical signs
The examination should take place in a quiet, child-centred room with appropriate facilities. Older children may prefer a doctor of the same gender. Consent is required before the examination and a forensic pack will be needed if the last assault was within 72 hours. The signs elicited must be taken in the context of the complete investigation. Careful documentation should be made in the form of sketches and sometimes photographs. As there is significant chance of coexisting physical abuse a full general examination should also be performed.

NB It must be remembered that up to 50% of children subject to sexual abuse will have no abnormal physical signs.

The following should be looked for in girls:

- Reddening, bruising, lacerations and swelling of labia, perineum and vulva
- Presence of vaginal discharge (+ comment on colour and amount) (NB on its own not strongly suggestive of sexual abuse)
- Hymenal opening — size (mm), margin, tears, scars (in prepubertal girl, hymenal opening > 0.5 cm suspicious of sexual abuse, > 1 cm even higher likelihood)
- Posterior fourchette — laceration/scars
- Vaginal examination ONLY in older girls if indicated

In boys, the following signs should be looked for:

- Penis — bruising, laceration, scars, burns
- Perineum — reddening, bruising
- Scrotum — bruising, reddening, burns

Anal examination

Examine young children on the carer's knee and older children in the left lateral position. Rectal examinations are rarely necessary and instead inspection should determine the presence or absence of acute signs such as:

- Swelling, reddening, bruising, haematoma, laceration or tears of anal margin
- Spasm, laxity and dilatation of anal sphincter
- Dilatation of perianal veins

Chronic signs should also be looked for including:

- Smooth thickened anal margin with shiny skin
- Chronic and acute fissures (single fissure unlikely to be significant)
- Spasm laxity and dilatation of anal sphincter
- Dilatation of perianal veins

Investigations

In certain cases it may be appropriate to send swabs for:

- Gonorrhoea
- Trichomonas
- Chlamydia
- Herpes

And forensic samples to look for:

- Spermatozoa
- Semen
- Grouping of semen
- Saliva, etc.

Management of sexual abuse

The child must be believed and handled in a skilled and sensitive fashion. After completion of history and examination the points outlined in 'Management of suspected non-accidental injury' should be followed.

Long-term legacy

The long-term problems associated with child sexual abuse include:

- Post-traumatic stress
- Suicidal behaviour
- Psychiatric illness
- Problems with relationships and sexual adjustment

24. SUDDEN INFANT DEATH SYNDROME (SIDS)

Definition

The definition of sudden infant death syndrome (SIDS) is 'the sudden death of an infant under 1 year of age which remains unexplained after the performance of a complete post-mortem examination and examination of the scene of death.'

Incidence

UK figures for 2004 — 0.4 per 1,000 live births

Many hypotheses have developed about the causes of SIDS. The search for an individual cause has shifted towards a more complex model. It seems likely that SIDS is the result of an interaction of risk factors — developmental stage, congenital and acquired risks and a final triggering event.

Established risk factors for SIDS

- Age 4–16 weeks
- Prone sleeping position and side sleeping position*
- Overheating/overwrapping
- Soft sleeping surfaces
- Fever/minor infection
- Bed sharing with parents (contraindicated if parent has had alcohol, smokes, has taken sedative medication, or feels very tired)
- Maternal smoking (ante- and postnatal)**
- Low maternal age
- High birth order
- Low birth weight
- Preterm delivery***
- Medical complications in the neonatal period
- Social deprivation
- Male sex
- Inborn errors of metabolism****

*The 'Back to Sleep' Campaign,** whereby parents are educated re the protective effect of supine infant sleeping, is well documented to have led to a very significant drop in the incidence of SIDS in the UK over the last decade. Similar campaigns have also been successful in other countries such as New Zealand, Scandinavia and the USA.

Smoking increases the risk of SIDS by up to threefold. There is an increase in risk with increased likelihood of spontaneous apnoea and decreased ability to compensate after such an episode. Such effects are likely to be enhanced by intercurrent illness.

***Relative risk of SIDS with preterm delivery**

Gestational age	Relative risk of SIDS
< 28/40	3.6
28–31 weeks	4
32–33 weeks	2.4
34–36 weeks	1.7

The period for which infants born preterm are at risk of SIDS is also longer than for term infants.

****Inborn errors of metabolism** — around 1% of cases of SIDS are likely to be the result of the enzyme deficiency: medium-chain acyl coenzyme A dehydrogenase deficiency (MCAD). It is likely that other enzyme deficiencies contribute to SIDS in a subset of patients, especially those cases of SIDS which occur at > 6 months. Appropriate investigations should be initiated.

Other potential risk factors implicated in aetiology of SIDS

- *Helicobacter pylori* (leads to increase in ammonia production)
- Prolonged QT interval
- Small pineal gland with altered melatonin production
- Gastro-oesophageal reflux
- Paternal cannabis use

There is **no** hard evidence that antimony (a substance present in some cot mattresses) is implicated in SIDS. Similarly, while there used to be a seasonal variation in SIDS, this is now no longer observed.

Protective factors for SIDS

- Supine sleeping position
- Appropriate environmental temperature
- ? Pacifier use (may prevent baby sleeping deeply)

Practical guidance on management of sudden unexpected deaths in infancy

Each hospital should have its own protocol for dealing with SIDS, which should be adhered to. Multiagency working is essential. The following are general guidelines:

- Contact consultant paediatrician immediately
- Ensure parents have a member of staff allocated to them and an appropriate room in which to wait
- Baby should be taken to appropriate area within A&E and **not** to the mortuary
- Initiate resuscitation unless it is evident baby has been dead for some time (e.g. rigor mortis or blood pooling)

- Parents should have option of being present during resuscitation with nurse supporting them throughout
- Take brief history of events preceding admission, including baby's past illnesses, recent health and any resuscitation already attempted; identify any predisposing factors for SIDS
- Consultant should decide, in consultation with parents, how long resuscitation should be continued for (it is usual to discontinue if there is no detectable cardiac output after 30 minutes)
- Once baby has been certified dead, consultant paediatrician should break news to parents, with support nurse present
- Explain to parents the need to inform the coroner and arrange a post-mortem

Physical examination

Carried out by most senior paediatrician present as soon as resuscitation has been completed/abandoned. Need to record:

- Baby's general appearance, state of nutrition and cleanliness
- Weight, and position on centile chart
- Rectal temperature
- Marks from invasive or vigorous procedures such as venepuncture, cardiac massage
- Any other marks on skin
- Appearance of retinae
- Lesions inside mouth
- Any signs of injury to genitalia/anus

Further action within A&E

- Keep all clothing removed from baby in labelled specimen bags as it may assist the pathologist and may be needed for forensic examination
- Inform coroner's office and discuss collection of further laboratory specimens, take photographs and mementoes such as lock of hair or hand and footprints
- Arrange for skeletal survey
- Contact Coroner's Office and request them to instruct a specialist paediatric pathologist for the post-mortem
- Check Child Protection Register
- If there are any concerns re suspicious death contact the police urgently (NB In some areas police may wish to be informed immediately of all unexpected infant deaths routinely)

Taking of samples

In some centres all samples are taken at post-mortem, however in others some or all of the following should be taken within the A&E department:

- Blood for urea and electrolytes, full blood count, blood culture, toxicology (clotted sample)
- Metabolic screen including amino and organic acids, oligosaccharides, blood spot on Guthrie card (for MCAD)
- Chromosomes (if dysmorphic)

- Nasopharyngeal aspirate, swabs (as appropriate) for bacteriology, suprapubic aspirate for urine microscopy, culture and sensitivity
- Consider skin and muscle biopsy

Support for family

- Ensure the family have Foundation for Study of Infant Death leaflet and helpline number and Department of Health leaflet on post-mortem
- Offer to put in touch with local support organizations
- If mother was breast-feeding discuss suppression of lactation
- If baby was a twin recommend admission/investigation of surviving twin
- Ensure family have telephone numbers of appropriate members of hospital team
- Offer to organize psychological support for older siblings
- Give details of counselling services
- Arrange transport home

Communication checklist
The following should be informed as soon as possible about the baby's death:

- Coroner
- Coroner's officer
- Police
- Family doctor
- Health visitor
- Social worker
- Medical records
- Other paediatric colleagues previously involved in care
- Immunization office

Follow-up arrangements
Ideally the paediatric consultant involved should organize to visit the family at home, as soon as is convenient for them. This allows more information on the family and baby to be obtained and also presents an opportunity for the parents to ask questions. Follow up information from such a visit should be included in a report done to assist the pathologist. A multidisciplinary discussion should be set up and should include all those who have been professionally involved with the family. Further follow-up visits should be organized, as necessary, and the post-mortem result should be discussed as soon as available.

25. ACCIDENT PREVENTION

Around 400 children per year die as a result of accidents in England and Wales and several thousand others suffer serious injuries.

Examples of how mortality and morbidity rates may be reduced include:

- Use of cycle helmets and car restraints (reduce severity of injury in road traffic accidents)

- Urban safety measures (e.g. crossing patrols, traffic redistribution schemes, improving safety on individual roads)
- Use of home safety devices (e.g. smoke detectors, stairgates, thermostat control of hot water)

Studies have established that educational programmes alone are not successful in preventing accidents and that to reduce accidents the educational material must be accompanied by:

- Targeting the families most at risk of accidents
- Home visits
- Free distribution of devices such as smoke alarms

26. CHRONIC FATIGUE SYNDROME

This remains an ill-understood condition which may present to either paediatricians or psychiatrists. The cardinal symptoms are severe and disabling physical and mental fatigue lasting for more than 3 months. Symptoms are usually continuous, their effects on the individual manifest to a pathological degree and are rarely objectively confirmed. The diagnosis excludes known causes of chronic fatigue such as chronic illness and also excludes known psychological disease.

Aetiology

Whilst viruses such as Epstein–Barr virus and the enteroviruses are often implicated in the disease process, direct evidence of this is often hard to find. Case clustering does occur and while anecdotal cases have suggested that immunization may be a trigger there is no direct evidence to support this theory. The aetiology is likely to be a combination of physical, psychological and behavioural factors. Often a trigger for the child's symptoms can be found.

Depression may be an associated feature, and the chronic course the disease takes makes psychological support and evaluation essential.

Epidemiology

The UK prevalence of chronic fatigue syndrome/myalgic encephalomyelitis (CFS/ME) in children and young people is 50–100 per 100,000 with the highest prevalence in adolescents. Where studies have reported a difference in gender, girls outnumber boys 3 : 1.

Clinical features

The onset may be gradual or sudden. In addition to fatigue other frequently reported symptoms are:

- Headaches
- Sleep disturbance
- Concentration difficulties
- Memory impairment

- Depressed mood
- Myalgia/musle pain
- Nausea
- Sore throat
- Tender lymph nodes
- Abdominal pain
- Arthralgia/joint pain

Less commonly there may be:

- Feeling too hot or too cold
- Dizziness
- Cough
- Eye pain
- Vision or hearing disturbance
- Weight gain or loss
- Muscle weakness
- Diarrhoea

Diagnostic criteria for CFS/ME

There are no accepted diagnostic criteria for CFS/ME in children and young people and the diagnosis should be based primarily on the impact of the condition and not require a specific illness duration.

Initial assessment

All patients referred for consideration of the diagnosis require a full and thorough assessment with an appreciation of the reality of the child's symptoms and acknowledgement of their validity. A thorough history and examination should be taken, exploring precise symptomatology. Organic and psychological disease should be looked for. Of particular importance is determining the effect of the child's symptoms on their normal daily routine including activities at home and attendance at school.

Investigation

Routine tests on all patients should include a blood test and a urine test for the following investigatons:

- Full blood count and film
- Erythrocyte sedimentation rate and C-reactive protein
- Blood glucose
- Blood biochemistry (to exclude renal insufficiency and Addison's)
- Creatine kinase
- Thyroid function
- Liver function
- Urine for protein/glucose and infection screen
- Viral titres Epstein–Barr virus IgM, IgG and EBNA

Other investigations may be required if there are specific disease pointers.

Investigations should be performed early on and, if possible, on one occasion only to prevent reliance on test results.

Management

Management is complex and requires the input of many professionals. It needs to be tailor-made to the individual child. Key points are:

- Facilitate the child and family to acknowledge the diagnosis, understand its implications and embark on a period of rehabilitation
- Assess current level of functioning by completing a daily programme to establish periods of eating, rest and activity
- Liaise closely with school/education authority
- Set goals:
  - Attendance at school is a key aim but gradual reintegration is usually required, with rest periods within school. Part days in school are preferable to exclusive home tuition
  - Aim to increase activity levels by around 5% each week
- Encourage child to keep a diary
- Advice re healthy balanced diet
- Help/support with sleeping difficulties
- Recognize early any predominant psychological symptoms including school phobia or depression and seek appropriate psychological or psychiatric help
- Appropriate pain management (may include psychological intervention and/or low-dose amitriptyline or nortriptyline)
- Pharmacological interventions such as corticosteroids, antidepressants (particularly SSRIs) and immunoglobulin have been used, but in a recent meta-analysis of treatments only physiotherapy (with a graded exercise programme) was shown to have a clearly beneficial effect
- There is no evidence to support the use of magnesium injections, essential fatty acids, high-dose vitamin B12 supplements, anticholinergic drugs, staphylococcus toxoid or antiviral therapies
- Cognitive techniques are used to assist patients to re-evaluate their understanding of the illness, combat depression and anxiety and look for underlying thoughts and assumptions that may contribute to disability
- Inpatient admission is rarely needed in the context of children with severe/very severe CFS/ME

Prognosis

The prognosis of chronic fatigue syndrome in children, in the absence of complications, is good. The onset of disease is more rapid and the response to therapy better than in adults, with a return to normal by 6–12 months after diagnosis in 80–90%.

Good prognostic factors in chronic fatigue syndrome are:

- Clearly defined trigger to illness
- Short duration of symptoms

- Supportive family with good interpersonal relationships
- Young age (adolescents overall do better than young or older adults)

27. FURTHER READING

Hall, D. Hill, P. Ellerman, D. 1994. *Child Surveillance Handbook*. Oxford: Radcliffe Med.

National Service Framework of Children Young People and Maternity Services, September 2004.

NICE. 2004. *Eating disorders: core interventions in the treatment and management of anoerexia nervosa, bulimia nervosa and related eating disorders*. National Institute for Clinical Excellence.

NICE. 2005. *Depression in children and young people. Identification and management in primary, community and secondary care*. National Institute for Health and Clinical Excellence.

RCPCH. 2005. *Evidence Based Guideline for the Management of CFS/ME in Children and Young People*. London: RCPCH.

Rutter, M. 2002. *Child and Adolescent Psychiatry — Modern Approaches*. Oxford: Blackwell Science.

HMSO 1996. *Immunisation against infant disease*.

The Baroness Kennedy QC. 2004. *Sudden unexpected death in infancy*. A report from the working group of the Royal College of Paediatrics and Child Health and the Royal College of Pathologists.

The Foundation for the Study of Infant Deaths 'Responding when a baby dies' campaign.

Sudden unexpected deaths in infancy: suggested guidelines for Accident and Emergency departments.

The Victoria Climbié Inquiry 2003 – Report of an Inquiry by Lord Laming.

Chapter 3

Clinical Governance

Robert Wheeler

CONTENTS

Clinical Governance

1. HISTORY

After the inception of the NHS in 1946 the practice of medicine was governed by professional judgement. Clinical decisions were made on the basis of knowledge accumulated during an apprenticeship, and this knowledge was validated by certification from the Royal Colleges. Compulsory registration with the General Medical Council was assumed to provide an assurance of fitness to practise and propriety, together with sanctions for transgressions.

Clinical practice itself, based on written and oral precedent, was seen as an evolving body of knowledge, against which new information could be evaluated.

These arrangements lasted, with varying degrees of satisfaction depending on the commentator, for more than 40 years. However, because of the inexorable rise of the cost of litigation,[1] the drug budget, and institutional catastrophes (such as those at the Bristol Royal Infirmary[2] and the Royal Liverpool Children's Hospital[3]), there has been a profound shift from the internal standard of medical self-regulation to an externally imposed regulatory apparatus, conforming to standards derived from state control.

It was with the advent of the hospital Trusts that politicians took renewed interest in quality issues. The Conservative administration had already coined the phrase 'Clinical Governance' by 1996; the advent of the new Labour government in 1997 confirmed Clinical Governance as the byword for quality assurance and enforcement.

A White Paper followed in 1997,[4] translating the concept into several national developments, with a mission to set or enforce standards. These included the National Institute for Clinical Excellence (NICE), the Commission for Health Improvement (CHI) and National Service frameworks, the latter to 'drive up' the quality of services for specific groups of patients, (e.g. cardiac, cancer) by setting national standards and describing service modules.

Into this initiative were drawn several other apparently disparate concepts: Appraisal/Assessment of Doctors, Integrated Care or Managed Pathways, and Evidence-Based Practice.

2. DEFINITIONS

It is fair to report that by late 1998, when interested parties had recovered from the onslaught of novel watchdogs, words and concepts, a steady stream of contradictory literature had begun to flow at national and local level, all trying to make sense of what 'Clinical Governance' actually meant.

133

The concept of governance was adapted from industry,[5] meaning 'to control and direct, with authority'.[6] It was conceived as being based upon seven central 'pillars' (Risk Management, Clinical Effectiveness, Education and Training, Patient and Public Involvement, Using Information, Research and Development, Management and Manpower). Organized within these broad categories, any aspect of clinical practice that could be regarded as pertaining to 'quality of care' could be subjected to intense scrutiny.

This arrangement has been rapidly incorporated into hospital practice, measured within the 'star rating' system. Although the pursuit of 'quality' seems uncontroversial, the reaction by doctors was not universally favourable;[7] many feeling that governance added no further value to their standard of care, which already exemplified many of the principles contained within the pillars. This conflict of understanding may have arisen from the necessity for clinical governance to be delivered by a team, rather than by an individual doctor. Consultants considered that they still retained 'ownership', the basis of continuity of care, which remained the their touchstone of 'quality'.

The widespread medical disaffection with clinical governance has continued, although there are high-profile exceptions. Adequate funding for clinical governance has not been forthcoming, resulting in a cutting-back in both central and local aspirations (i.e. the post of Commissioner for Patient and Public Involvement was abolished in the most recent review).

Shrinkage of the original seven-pillar plan has occurred, resulting in a largely risk-based agenda. This is reflected in the *Standards for Better Health*, where only Risk and Patient and Public Involvement survive as independent specified activities. The rest of the original agenda is subsumed into the 'core activities', although there is concern that the audit (clinical effectiveness) and educational elements are insufficiently established properly to service the *Standards* agenda.

3. EXTERNAL AGENCIES

Scrutiny of the management of illness nationally is institutionalized through the external agencies. As a starting point, NICE was responsible for setting uniform national standards on which to base clinical practice. (NICE was established in 1999 by the NICE (Establishment and Constitution) Order 1999 SI 1999 No. 220, www.nice.org.uk.) The agency provides guidance in three areas. Technology appraisals review the use of new and existing medicines and treatments. This gives an opportunity to control expenditure on high-cost drugs whose claims of efficacy failed to satisfy critical review, although as a government agency, there remains the concern that the need for financial saving may militate against the ratification of potentially effective (but expensive) treatments.[8]

Clinical guidelines are commissioned to designate the appropriate treatment and care of specific conditions and diseases. This should lead to clinical uniformity, and make a 'postcode lottery' less likely. At the same time, guidelines may lead to cost savings, at the price of reducing patient choice.[9] However, implicit in this is a reduction of clinical freedom, which has been demonstrated to disadvantage the sickest patients.[10]

Finally, reviews are commissioned by NICE into the safety and efficacy of new interventional procedures, in an effort to restrict the unregulated introduction of new technology.

This has led to a host of interventional guidelines, although little or no funding has yet been provided to establish the central registries that are required.

The resulting 'evidence base' is produced as a compilation.[11] Adherence to the advice may be seen as regulation by compliance, as opposed to deterrence.[12] Although clinicians are ready to adopt the advice providing the normal criteria apply,[13] there is considerable evidence that NICE guidance is not being followed.[14] There is also a growing recognition that the plethora of guidance has overloaded the system, and NICE is now calling for clinical advice on where to focus attention for future work.[15]

Scrutiny of the care that health organizations deliver to their patients was initially under-taken by the CHI (established by s19 of the Health Act 1999, and Commission for Health Improvement (Functions) Regulations 2000, S.I. 2000 No. 662, reg 3, transiently reconstituted as the Commission for Healthcare Audit and Improvement (CHAI) before being re-launched on 1 April 2004 as the Healthcare Commission (HC) — www.chai.org.uk). The Commission is an example of regulation by deterrence. Its remit was radical in comparison with the previous arrangements, which were described in the words of the Bristol inquiry as 'There was, in truth, no system'.[16] This abrupt shift to external regulation was recognized as a momentous event.[17] With a motto of 'Inspecting, Informing, Improving', the HC has an ever-increasing remit across public and private healthcare provision, including the value for money derived from healthcare expenditure, and aspects of the complaints procedure.[18] Amongst many other functions, the HC is responsible for issuing National Service Frame-works to promote uniformity and quality in areas of healthcare that are seen to be in need of support; the most recent was for the care of children.

4. STANDARDS FOR BETTER HEALTH

The 'core' activity until now has been clinical governance reviews, which are published regularly.[19] The HC has reconstituted the clinical governance agenda within the *Standards for Better Health*.[20] These are to be used to assess the performance of healthcare providers, and provide a banding system to replace the heavily criticized star ratings,[21] which initially emerged from the CHI. At the time of writing, the *Standards* are being employed for the first time, following a consultation process that ran until 21 February 2005 (feedback can be found at feedback@healthcarecommission.org.uk). The chairman of the HC has prefaced the consultation with the wish to employ a lighter touch in the process of assessment and audit.[22]

The *Standards* provide a highly prescriptive checklist for the Trust, enabling executives to judge how close their organization is to conforming to the required level of service. How do the concepts of Risk, Clinical Effectiveness, Patient and Public Involvement and Education fit into this exercise, and how do they interrelate?

5. IMPLEMENTATION

What follows is a recipe for establishing Clinical Governance.

5.1 Risk management

Risk describes anything that may put the patient, clinician, or parent in harm's way. This may be as specific as the risk of injecting the wrong chemotherapy into the spine, or as banal as ensuring that the doors to the outpatients department do not trap children's fingers.

Risks can thus come from the spectrum of practice, and the principle of management is to identify them before they cause damage.

A formal **Risk Assessment Exercise** can be run throughout the Unit, effectively taking a clipboard through the entire department, noting all possible potential problems. Since this is actually even more tedious than it sounds, Risk 'tools' have been developed; series of minutiae-type questions designed to ferret out any potential hazards, whether emanating from clinical practice or Health and Safety issues.

This is more exciting than it sounds. If, by use of the risk assessment it is possible to demonstrate that one's colleagues are overworked and overtired, then this is undoubtedly a significant risk. Bearing in mind that the chief executive bears ultimate responsibility for clinical governance matters; your use of the risk tool has promptly and legitimately transferred the burden of an 'hours' issue to the management.

A risk assessment performed carefully, accurately and on a yearly basis gives a good foundation of predicting (prospectively) the risks faced by a Unit. Equally, immediate retrospective data are acquired by **Critical Incident reporting**. In this way, any mishap that a member of staff subjectively considers a risk can be reported promptly. Examples of critical incidents include a staff nurse feeling the ward is unsafe; prescribing errors by undertrained or overtired doctors; or medical equipment malfunction.

Such reports are collated and reviewed on a monthly basis by senior medical, nursing and administrative staff. Some reports are dismissed as frankly trivial; for others a simple 'local' solution is obvious, while more fundamental flaws in the system may require such fundamental change as to merit consideration by the Trust Board.

The attraction of such reporting is that it encourages staff to be freely critical, which tends to expose weaknesses in practice, which would otherwise go unrecognized.

There are other sources of these risk data. Complaints from distressed or damaged patients, whether relating to domestic or clinical issues, serve to highlight hazards. Nationally recognized risks can also be contemplated: Do you have safeguards against imperfect consent for research procedures? Are your neonatal central venous catheter tips in a safe site?

Risk Management thus means identifying risks prospectively or retrospectively, then finding a solution for them. If the solution is not immediately available to the clinician, then the risk (and the liability) is passed to the executive body.

5.2 Education/appraisal

This element of clinical governance can be run in parallel with other activities. Continuing education for doctors is now mandatory, and in the future is likely to be reflected in demands for dedicated fixed consultant education sessions. Colleges have already recognized that education comes in various forms; formal teaching, courses, private reading, preparing lectures and research, among others.

Assessment and Appraisal are prominent on the political agenda, hence the anxiety of the General Medical Council to produce a workable formula in 2001, to facilitate revalidation of a doctor's original medical registration. It is a tribute to the difficulty of the task that by 2005, an adequate solution has yet to be found. To an extent, this has been delayed by the political reaction to the crimes of Dr Harold Shipman. Although apparently a convenient moment to incorporate a mechanism to identify potential mass murderers through the revalidation process, it is becoming clear that this is unworkable, and that cyclical revalidation of doctors will be largely based on local appraisal. The local appraisal process remains a matter for individual medical directors. It seems that reforms to the laws concerning the registration of death are more likely to reduce the risk of another similar tragedy.

Assessment (which is a mere observation; a measuring of attendance, workload, waiting times, educational target fulfilment) is a great deal easier to perform than **Appraisal** (a process of valuation, estimating the worth and quality of clinical activity).

This is because the individual can perform Assessment themselves; it may involve tedious and time-consuming data collection and form filling but it is an objective exercise. Appraisal, however, can only be performed by an outsider, who shares enough of the appraisee's training to allow pertinent questions to be asked, and relevant feedback to be given. This is equally time-consuming but is also potentially threatening and more subjective than Assessment.

5.3 Clinical effectiveness

The much-publicized medical errors of recent years, together with a logarithmic rise in medical negligence litigation, has led to calls for measurement of clinical performance. At its most simplistic, it has afforded the government an opportunity to publish 'league tables' for Trusts in such areas as cardiac mortality. Whilst recognized as a potential oversimplification, this has led to a call for individual practitioners to publish their results. Such data are now available via 'Dr Foster' (www.drfoster.co.uk).

The response has been to answer this call with **Audit**; i.e. establishing a gold standard, measuring whether the local Unit is at variance with the standard, modifying practice to improve results and then re-measuring (re-audit) to ensure that the modification has achieved the desired result.

Any conceivable clinical intervention has the potential for audit and audit has been a highly satisfactory tool as a measure of clinical performance, provided it is used appropriately and correctly.

Audit programmes can be integrated with other aspects of clinical governance. If a clinical intervention is identified as a risk either by a Risk Assessment, by Critical Incident reporting or as the result of a cluster of similar complaints, then this gives an ideal opportunity for audit.

At present, audit remains the single most effective method of performance measurement. Isolated specialities such as cardiac surgery have developed national databases of results, allowing comparison between units, but this obviously demands close integration and co-operation within a professional speciality. The advantage of audit is that it can be performed equally well in isolation, as long as a gold standard for comparison can be identified.

To maintain enthusiasm for audit within a department is quite a different matter, partly because some doctors see this as a merely self-fulfilling process. A pragmatic approach is a rolling audit, where a topic is chosen which continually poses a clinical challenge; the adherence to the Unit protocol for the management of bronchiolitis would be a recurring theme.

An audit can be set up along the usual lines, but then the re-audit phases, together with retrospective comparisons and prospective protocol adjustment, can be undertaken by successive generations of junior staff. In this way, audit becomes an integrated part of the working routine, not dependent on additional enthusiasm or drive by the medical team. Ideally, a combination of rolling 'routine' audit with additional audits reacting to risks should run simultaneously.

5.4 Patient and public involvement

Emerging with the initial tranche of clinical governance themes, Patient and Public Involvement has been elusive in definition. It is easy to identify what it represents, which is the laudable aim to tailor medical services to the requirements of the patient, rather than make the patient fit in with what proves convenient for the doctor. It also lends itself admirably to politicians, ever anxious to be seen to be listening to patients and to be affording them choice. The difficulty, of course, is to do either of these things in a meaningful way, leading to benefit. Furthermore, there appears to be little or no evidence that these efforts at patient participation create any measurable benefit to the patient.

Trusts have struggled to implement the political agenda of listening to patients. Considerable creativity has resulted in patient forums, surveys, focus groups, and a variety of methods by which patients feed their comments back to providers, ranging from the distribution of postcards to patients, or providing contact numbers for text messaging. One great difficulty is determining what to ask. Although the political demand for patient involvement can be met by simply asking 'how was your stay', the yield of useful information is low, once the problems surrounding car parking, decent food, clean wards and reliably communicative clinicians have been addressed. These are hardly revelations.

The choice element is being implemented at a national level, with the rapid enforcement of the patients' ability to choose where and by whom they should be treated. It remains to be seen whether this will result in improved patient satisfaction, or clinical outcome.

5.5   Interaction

The various elements of clinical governance interact, giving endless opportunities for flow diagrams and presentations.

If you start with a Risk topic, an audit will measure the Unit's performance. The audit will demand a gold standard for comparison, which can (possibly) be supplied from the available Evidence base. Obtaining this evidence or the consensus view may well be the appropriate use of a consultant's private study time, i.e. Continued Medical Education.

Once the gold standard has been determined, it can be incorporated as a module within the appropriate Integrated Care Pathway. This may then be subject to rolling audit, etc. The Patient and Public Involvement element can be involved, to either assess the patients' perception of the risk, or their reaction to the chosen remedy, or the priority that they feel should be given to implementing the remedy, given the obvious restrictions on resources.

6.   CONCLUSION

There is little doubt that hospital patients and clinicians should equally welcome additional supervision of clinical activities. Clinical 'freedom' may seem insufficiently controllable to guarantee adequate quality of care, and it is understandable that any government would wish to demonstrate an augmented quality of care, rather than merely reiterate a financial commitment to health. External regulation has become a cornerstone of the government's 'third way' in healthcare.[23] This has been achieved by asking doctors to comply with standards set by NICE, and deterring variance by the employment of agencies such as the Healthcare Commission. The product of this alliance is implemented by the clinical governance structure. There remains concern that the evidence base is unreliable, and that the individual patient's best clinical interest may not be best achieved by following a guideline produced from an averaged population. Effectively enforced 'bullet-point' medicine is likely to interfere significantly with the therapeutic relationship between patients and their doctors,[24] although from a utilitarian point of view, it may confer the least risk on the greatest number.

7.   ELECTRONIC SOURCES

www.chai.org.uk/assetRoot/04/01/00/32/04010032.pdf Most recent HC review: of Malden & South Chelmsford PCT

www.dh.gov.uk/publications

www.dh.gov.uk/publicationsandstatistics/bulletins/ChiefExecutiveBulletin

feedback@healthcarecommission.org.uk (*Standards for Health*)

www.healthcarecommission.org.uk/ContactUs/ComplainAboutNHS/fs/en

www.nice.org.uk

www.drfoster.co.uk

8. FURTHER READING

1. Harpwood V. 2001. *Negligence in Healthcare*, chapters 10, 11. London: Informa Publishing Group.

2. Department of Health. 2001. *Report of the Public Inquiry into Children's Heart Surgery at Bristol Royal Infirmary 1984–1995: Learning from Bristol*. London: DoH (Cm5207).

3. Department of Health. 2001. *The Royal Liverpool Children's Inquiry Report*. London: Stationery Office.

4. Department of Health. 1997. *The New NHS — Modern, Dependable*. London: Stationery Office.

5. Originally Sir Adrian Cadbury, referred to by Donaldson L. 2000. Clinical Governance. *Medico-Legal Journal* 68:3, 89–100.

6. *A First Class Service; Quality in the New NHS*. 1998. Government White Paper.

7. Klein R. 2000. *The New Politics of the NHS*, 4th edn. London: Prentice Hall.

8. Newdick C. 2002. NHS Governance after Bristol: holding on or letting go? *Medical Law Review* 10, 111–31.

9. NICE. 2004. NICE guidance issued on caesarean sections. *Medical Law Monitor* May 3–4.

10. Dranove D *et al.* 2002. Is more information better? The effects of 'Report Cards' on health care providers. *National Bureau of Economic Research* Paper 8697.

11. NICE. 2003. *Summary of Guidance issued to the NHS in England and Wales*, Issue 7 October 2003. London: NICE.

12. Reiss AJ. 1984. Selecting strategies of social control over organisational life. In Hawkins K, Thomas JM (Eds) *Enforcing Regulation*, Boston, MA, USA: Kluwert Nijhoff.

13. Editorial. 2004. If guidance is clear, based on an understanding of clinical practice, if the evidence is strong and relatively stable, if adequate funding is available and if guidance is supported and disseminated by professional bodies. *BMJ* 329, 999–1003.

14. Freemantle N. 2004. Is NICE delivering the goods? *BMJ* 329, 1003–1004.

15. NICE asks what not to assess. *Hospital Doctor*, 2004, 9 December, 4.

16. Department of Health. 2001. *Report of the Public Inquiry into Children's Heart Surgery at Bristol Royal Infirmary 1984–1995: Learning from Bristol*. London, DoH (Cm5207), chapter 6, para. 30; p.192 para. 21.

17. Smith R. 1998. All changed, changed utterly: British medicine will be transformed by the Bristol case. *BMJ* 316, 1917.

18. *Health and Social Care (Community Health and Standards) Act* 2003, explained at www.healthcarecommission.org.uk/ContactUs/ComplainAboutNHS/fs/en

19. Most recent reviews (e.g. of Maldon and South Chelmsford PCT) www.chai.org.uk/assetRoot/04/01/00/32/04010032.pdf

20. Department of Health. 2004. *National Standards, Local Action. Health and Social Care Standards and Planning Framework 2005/06-2007/08 Annex 1* Leeds, DoH www.dh.gov.uk/publications.

21. Editorial. 2004. Commission proposes end to star rating system for hospitals. *BMJ* 329, 1303.

22. Editorial. 2004. Commission plans to adopt 'a lighter touch' *BMJ* 329, 997.

23. Walshe K. 2002. The rise of regulation in the NHS. *BMJ* 324, 967.

24. Teff H. 2000. Clinical guidelines, negligence and medical practice. In Freeman M, Lewis A (Eds) *Law Medicine: Current Legal Problems*, vol. 3. Oxford: Oxford University Press.

Chapter 4

Clinical Pharmacology and Toxicology

Steve Tomlin and Michael Capra

CONTENTS

Clinical Pharmacology and Toxicology

1. PHARMACOKINETICS AND DYNAMICS

Pharmacokinetics is what the body does to a drug, pharmacodynamics is what the drug does to the body.

1.1 Absorption

- Liquid and intravenous forms of drugs (i.e. those already in solution) are readily absorbed into the body's systemic circulation
- Solid dosage forms (tablets and capsules) and suspensions must first be dissolved in the gastrointestinal tract (dissolution phase) before they can be absorbed, and so absorption is slower
- The term 'bioavailability' is applied to the rate and extent of drug absorption into the systemic circulation

First-order kinetics

Oral absorption of drugs is often considered as demonstrating first-order kinetics. This is especially true with oral solutions. 'First-order kinetics' implies that the fractional rate of absorption is constant, so absorption decreases the less there is left in the stomach. If a drug is absorbed at a constant rate independent of the amount left to absorb, then it is referred to as having 'zero-order kinetics'.

Ionization

Absorption of the majority of medicines is dependent on how ionized they are (their pK_a) and the acidity at the site of absorption. Drugs with acidic pK_as (for example: aspirin, phenoxymethylpenicillin (penicillin V)) will be mainly non-ionized in the acid stomach and so readily absorbed. Phenobarbital being a weaker acid is better absorbed in the more alkaline intestine.

Neonates

Neonates (especially those who are premature) have reduced gastric acid secretion, therefore the extent of drug absorption is altered and less predictable.

At birth, drugs with an acidic pK_a will have decreased absorption. Twenty-four hours after birth, acid is released into the stomach therefore increasing the absorption of acidic drugs. Normal adult gastric acid secretions are achieved by about 3 years of age.

Gastric motility is decreased during infancy, thus increasing the absorption of drugs that are absorbed in the stomach. However, drugs absorbed from the intestine will have a decreased or possibly delayed absorption.

Absorption and pK_a of some drugs in adults and neonates

Drug	Neonatal oral absorption compared to adult	pK_a
Ampicillin	Increased	2.7
Penicillin	Increased	2.8
Phenytoin	Decreased	8.3
Paracetamol	Decreased	9.9
Diazepam	Same	3.7

1.2 Distribution

The concentration of a drug at various sites of action depends on the drug's characteristics and those of the tissue. Most drugs are water-soluble and will naturally go to organs such as the kidneys, liver, heart and gastrointestinal tract.

At birth, the total body water and extracellular fluid volume are much increased, and thus larger doses of water-soluble drugs are required on a mg/kg basis to achieve equivalent concentrations to those seen in older children and adults. This has to be balanced against the diminished hepatic and renal function when considering dosing.

	Pre-term	Full-term	4–6 months	1 year	>1 year	Adult
Extracellular fluid volume (%)	50	45	40	30	25	25
Total body water (%)	85	75	60	60	60	60
Fat content (%)	3	12	25	30	variable	18

Distribution is also affected by a decreased protein-binding capacity in newborns, and particularly in pre-term newborns, therefore leading to increased levels of the active free drug for highly protein-bound drugs.

- For example, phenytoin is highly protein-bound but because there is less protein binding in neonates (lower plasma protein levels and lower binding capacity) there is more free phenytoin than in older children and adults. Thus the therapeutic range for phenytoin in neonates is lower than in the rest of the general population as it is the free phenytoin that has the therapeutic action and can cause toxicity.
  - Therapeutic range for neonates = 6–15 mg/l
  - Therapeutic range for children and adults = 10–20 mg/l

The reduced protein binding is the result of:

- Low levels of plasma protein, particularly albumin
- Qualitative differences in binding capacity
- Competition with endogenous substances, particularly increased bilirubin after birth

Volume of distribution

Distribution is measured by a theoretical volume in the body called the 'volume of distribution'. It is the volume that would be necessary to dilute the administered dose to obtain the actual plasma level within the body. The volume will be affected by the following characteristics (body size, body water composition, body fat composition, protein binding, haemodynamics and the drug characteristics). As a rule of thumb: drugs that are plasma protein-bound will mainly stay in the plasma and thus have a small volume of distribution; highly lipid-soluble drugs (especially in people with a high fat content) will have high volumes of distribution. Water-soluble drugs have increased volumes of distribution in neonates because of the increased total body water content of neonates.

The parameter can change significantly throughout childhood. Plasma albumin levels reach adult levels at approximately 1 year of age.

Blood–brain barrier

The blood–brain barrier in the newborn is functionally incomplete and hence there is an increased penetration of some drugs into the brain.

Transfer across the barrier is determined by:

- Lipid solubility
- Degree of ionization

Drugs that are predominantly un-ionized are more lipid-soluble and achieve higher concentrations in the cerebrospinal fluid. It is as a result of this increased uptake that neonates are generally more sensitive to the respiratory depressant effects of opiates than infants and older children.

Some drugs will displace bilirubin from albumin (for example: sulphonamides), so increasing the risk of kernicterus (encephalopathy due to increased bilirubin in the central nervous system — in at-risk neonates).

1.3   Half-life

Half-life is the time taken for the plasma concentration of a drug to decrease to half of its original value. Thus it follows that less drug will be eliminated in each successive half-life.

- For example, theophylline:
  - if there is initially 250 mg in the body, after one half-life (4 h) 125 mg will remain; after two half-lives (8 h) there will be 62.5 mg left; and so on

When a medicine is first given in a single dose, all the drug is at the absorption site and none is in the plasma. At this point, absorption is maximal and the rate of elimination is zero. As time goes on the rate of absorption decreases (first-order kinetics) and the rate of elimination increases. All the time that the absorption rate is higher than the elimination rate the plasma level will increase. When the two rates are equal, the concentration in the plasma will be at a maximum. After this point, the elimination rate will be higher and the levels will drop. A drug is said to be at 'steady state' after about four to five half-lives. So if multiple dosing is occurring the plasma levels at any particular point after a dose will always be the same.

1.4   Hepatic metabolism

Hepatic metabolism is generally slower at birth compared with adults. However, it increases rapidly during the first few weeks of life, so that in late infancy hepatic metabolism may be more effective than in adults.

The age at which the enzyme processes approach adult values varies with the drug and the metabolic pathway. For drugs such as diazepam, which are extensively metabolized by the liver, the decrease in half-life with age demonstrates this process.

	Pre–term babies	Full–term babies	Children
Diazepam half-life (h)	38–120	22–46	15–21

The hepatic metabolism process occurs either by sulphation, methylation, oxidation, hydroxylation or glucuronidation. Most hepatically metabolized drugs will undergo one or two of these processes.

Processes involving sulphation and methylation are not greatly impaired at birth, whereas those involving oxidation and glucuronidation are. It might be assumed that neonates would be at an increased risk of paracetamol toxicity; however, neonates use the sulphation pathway instead of glucuronidation and are able to deal with paracetamol as well as (if not more efficiently than) adults.

Hydroxylation of drugs is deficient in newborns, particularly in pre-term babies, and this is the process that accounts for the huge variation in diazepam half-life as shown in the table above.

Grey-baby syndrome is a rare, but potentially fatal, toxic effect of chloramphenicol in neonates. It is the result of the inability of the liver to glucuronidate the drug effectively in the first couple of weeks of life if correct doses are not given.

It is impossible to predict with any accuracy the possible toxic dose for a neonate and young infant even by applying all the above rules. For example, neonates unlike adults convert most theophylline to caffeine in the liver. Thus without dedicated studies we really are only guessing as to what toxic or non-toxic metabolites are being formed in this age group.

First-pass metabolism

Medication that is absorbed from the gastrointestinal tract goes straight to the liver before entering the systemic circulation. This is useful for some types of medication, which have to go to the liver to be activated (pro-drugs), e.g. enalapril. It is, however, limiting for medications that have to achieve good levels when given orally. Propranolol has a high first-pass metabolism, so quite large doses need to be given to achieve adequate systemic levels. Inhaled budesonide is often said to be relatively free of systemic side-effects because the steroid that is deposited in the throat and swallowed is almost entirely eliminated by first-pass metabolism.

1.5   Renal excretion

Drug excretion by the kidneys is mainly dependent on glomerular filtration and active renal tubule secretion. Pre-term infants have approximately 15% (or less) of the renal capacity of an adult, term babies have about 30% at birth, but this matures rapidly to about 50% of the adult capacity by the time they are 4–5 weeks old. At 9–12 months of age, the infant's renal capacity is equal to that of an adult.

1.6   Other clinical considerations

Many other factors influence drug handling and may alter an individual's response to a given dose.

Genetic considerations can lead to altered drug metabolism or altered responses, e.g. glucose 6-phosphate dehydrogenase (G6PD) deficiency; succinylcholine sensitivity; acetylation status.

G6PD deficiency

This is a commonly inherited enzyme abnormality. It is an X-linked recessive disorder. Male homozygotes show significant drug-related haemolysis, but females only have minor symptoms. Anaemia is the most common presentation.

Main drugs to avoid:

- dapsone, nitrofurantoin, quinolones (ciprofloxacin, nalidixic acid, ofloxacin, norfloxacin), sulphonamides (co-trimoxazole), quinine, quinidine, chloroquine

Succinylcholine sensitivity

Some people are extremely sensitive to the muscle relaxant succinylcholine. Serum pseudocholinesterase activity is reduced and the duration of action of the muscle relaxant (usually a few minutes) may be greatly increased, thus leading to apnoea (deaths have been reported). The incidence is about 1 in 2,500 of the population.

Acetylation status

Differences in the metabolism of isoniazid are seen in certain people and inherited as an autosomal recessive trait. People who are 'slow inactivators' have reduced activity of acetyltransferase, which is the hepatic enzyme responsible for the metabolism of isoniazid and sulphadimidine (and thus affects phenelzine and hydralazine metabolism). Toxic effects of such drugs may be seen in people who are 'slow acetylators'.

Slow acetylators are also predisposed to spontaneous and drug-induced systemic lupus erythematosus (SLE).

Examples of drugs that may induce SLE

Phenytoin	Isoniazid	Procainamide
Penicillin	Chlorpromazine	Tetracyclines
Hydralazine	Beta-blockers	Lithium
Sulphonamides	Clonidine	Methyldopa

Liver disease

Toxic substances normally cleared by the liver may accumulate in patients with liver impairment.

- Opioids and benzodiazepines may accumulate and cause central nervous system depression, thereby causing respiratory depression
- Diuretics (loop and thiazide) may cause hypokalaemia
- Rifampicin, which is excreted via the bile, will accumulate in patients with obstructive jaundice
- Cirrhosis may cause hypoproteinaemia and thus reduce the number of binding sites for highly protein-bound drugs (e.g. phenytoin)
- Clotting factors are reduced in liver impairment, thus increasing the chances of bleeding in patients on warfarin

Renal disease

- Nephrotoxic drugs will make any renal impairment worse by exacerbating the damage. Drugs that are renally excreted (most water-soluble drugs) will accumulate in renal impairment and the dosing intervals will need to be increased to avoid toxicity

Drugs that cause toxicity in severe renal impairment include:

- Digoxin — cardiac arrhythmias, heart block
- Penicillins/cephalosporins (high-dose) — encephalopathy
- Erythromycin — encephalopathy

Nephrotoxic drugs include:

- Aminoglycosides (gentamicin, amikacin)
- Amphotericin B
- Non-steroidal anti-inflammatory drugs (e.g. diclofenac, indomethacin)

2. FORMULATION

Medicinal preparations often contain ingredients (i.e. excipients) other than the medicine that is being prescribed. These adjuvants can have a pharmacological effect that needs to be taken into account when looking at medication consumption and assessing possible toxicity.

- Benzyl alcohol and methylparaben can displace bilirubin from albumin-binding sites, leading to exacerbation of jaundice. Benzyl alcohol may also cause a potentially fatal 'gasping syndrome'
- Propylene glycol is a common solubilizing agent. In excess, it may cause severe toxicity including hyperosmolarity, lactic acidosis, dysrhythmias and hypotension
- Polysorbate 20 and Polysorbate 80, which are used as emulsifying agents, have been associated with renal and hepatic dysfunction as well as hypotension (secondary to hypovolaemia), thrombocytopenia and metabolic acidosis
- Lactose is a common additive, but rarely associated with severe toxicity. It may, however, be important if a child has lactose intolerance
- Sugar and sorbitol are frequently added to liquid preparations for sweetness and occasionally cause problems. Sugar can cause dental caries and sorbitol may cause diarrhoea
- Alcohol is another common ingredient of many liquid pharmaceutical products and the quantity is often fairly significant. Products such as phenobarbital BP contains as much as 38% alcohol per 15 mg/5 ml. Equating this to a mg/kg quota, it would not be that unusual to subject a neonate to the equivalent of an adult swallowing one or two glasses of wine

Formulation issues are a fundamental problem in paediatric medicine management. Palatability causes many problems with compliance and it is well demonstrated that taste preferences change with age. Few medicines are made specifically for children and thus products needed in clinical use may not be available in a formulation that is appropriate for young children. This often leads to tablets being crushed and aliquots being given. If this is necessary the properties of the preparation may change significantly or the dose may be inaccurate depending on whether the tablet dissolves or disperses and on the release mechanisms built into the tablet originally (e.g. coating or matrix). A pharmacist should be consulted if there is any doubt.

3. PAEDIATRIC DOSING

Pharmacokinetic and pharmacodynamic data are seldom available for the paediatric population, this is because most medications are only licensed for adult use and have not undergone specific pre-marketing clinical studies in children. Data on therapeutic dosing for children are often anecdotal and based on case reports or very small population studies. New drugs are usually only studied in adult populations.

Some of the reasons for this are the stringent regulations put in place in 1962 following the thalidomide tragedy; these had the effect of discouraging research. The legislation surrounding drugs trials currently discourages trials in children, although in recent years there has been a call for more studies and European Legislation should be changing in 2006 to encourage more drug companies to seek paediatric licences.

The surface area and the weight are the only common methods currently available to predict paediatric therapeutic doses from those used for adults.

Surface area

The surface-area or percentage method for estimating doses is calculated as follows:

$$\frac{\text{Surface area of child } (m^2)}{1.76m^2} \times 100 = \text{percent of adult dose}$$

where 1.76 m^2 is the average adult surface area.

Children are often said to tolerate or require larger doses of drugs than adults based on a weight basis, and the percentage method helps to explain this phenomenon. Body water (total and extracellular) is known to equate better with surface area than body weight. It thus seems appropriate to prescribe drugs by surface area if they are distributed through the extracellular fluid volume in particular.

Weight

$$\frac{\text{Adult dose } (mg)}{70kg} = \text{mg/kg dose}$$

where 70 kg is the average adult weight.

This method will give lower doses than the surface-area method. It is far less accurate in clinical terms and is usually inappropriate for accurate therapeutic dosing. However, as it gives lower and thus safer estimates of what the toxic dose may be, it is a more practical and reasonably cautious method for extrapolating toxic doses.

Most paediatric doses given in textbooks are described in small age or weight groups on a mg/kg basis. However, these will often have been originally obtained from surface-area data and thus are larger than the adult dose divided by 70.

There are, however, many medications which can be used in children and accuracy of prescribing is essential because of the vast physical size differences in children (i.e. from

0.5 kg to 120 kg) let alone their changes in kinetics. Children should be regularly weighed so that up-to-date weights can be used for prescribing. However, remember the practicalities of what is to be given to the child. If a child is 6.5 kg and requires 2 mg/kg of ranitidine, it would seem wiser to prescribe 15 mg, which is 1 ml of the oral liquid, rather than 13 mg, which equates to 0.867 ml. Some knowledge of the therapeutic range of the drug is required to know when and by how much it is suitable to round doses, however, and sometimes awkward quantities are required.

4. PRESCRIBING OUTSIDE LICENCE

The unlicensed and off-label (licensed drugs being used outside their licence) use of medicines in children is widespread. It has been accepted by the Royal College of Paediatrics and Child Health (RCPCH) and the Neonatal and Paediatric Pharmacists Group (NPPG) that informed use of such medicines is necessary in paediatric practice when there is no suitable licensed alternative. Those who prescribe for a child should choose the medicine which offers the best prospect for that child, with due regard to cost. Legally, the prescriber is required to take full responsibility for such prescribing, which must be justifiable in accordance with a respectable, responsible body of professional opinion.

The choice of a medicine is not therefore necessarily determined by its licence status, although it should take into account information made available as a consequence of licensing and contained in the *Summary of Product Characteristics*. This can be of only limited help when the medicine chosen is unlicensed or off-label, and the necessary information to support safe and effective prescribing must be sought elsewhere.

The national paediatric formulary *Medicines for Children* written by the RCPCH and NPPG was produced to meet the need for accessible sound information. In September 2005 this production in partnership with the British National Formulary (BNF) produced the first *BNF for Children* distributed to all doctors and pharmacists by the Department of Health. This is a fundamental move forward in accepting that medicines need to be used outside their licence for children and to try to rationalize and standardize some paediatric medicine management using evidence-based data and expert peer review.

If prescribing outside the licence, remember that the medication supplied has to legally be given with the manufacturer's patient information sheet. This will probably not mention the use for which you are prescribing and may even suggest that it should be avoided in such a condition or age group. This has fundamental implications with compliance and concordance. Leaflets are available on the RCPCH website explaining to children and their carers why this situation may arise and decreasing the fears that this situation may cause.

5. DRUG MONITORING

Most drugs have wide therapeutic windows and thus toxicity is unlikely at 'normal doses'. It is usually easy to see a medication effect, e.g. analgesics take away pain. There are, however, certain circumstances when it is important to measure drug levels to ensure that there are adequate levels for effect and/or that the levels are unlikely to cause toxicity.

A drug with a narrow therapeutic window has a narrow range between the drug concentration exhibiting maximum efficacy and that producing minimum toxicity.

Medications that have narrow therapeutic windows are often monitored, as it is hard to predict whether a dose for an individual patient will be clinically effective or will cause toxicity.

Common drugs for therapeutic monitoring	
Phenytoin	Warfarin
Carbamazepine	Gentamicin
Phenobarbital	Vancomycin
Digoxin	Theophylline

Indications for monitoring:

- To confirm levels are not toxic and are at a level that is normally effective (usually checked once steady-state has been reached), e.g. gentamicin, vancomycin
- If toxicity is expected
- If external factors may have changed a level (change in renal/hepatic function, change in interacting concomitant medication)
- To check compliance

It is important to know that a drug was at a steady state when a level was measured and whether trough levels or peak levels are important.

6. INTERACTIONS

Many situations arise where interactions between different medications are important. Drugs may either inhibit or induce the liver enzyme systems as follows.

6.1 Drugs and the liver

Liver induction

- Will lead to treatment failure of:
  - Warfarin, phenytoin, theophylline, oral contraceptive pill
- Caused by:
  - Phenytoin, carbamazepine, barbiturates, rifampicin, chronic alcohol consumption, sulphonylureas

Liver inhibition

- Will lead to potentiation of:
  - Warfarin, phenytoin, carbamazepine, theophylline, cyclosporin
- Caused by:
  - Omeprazole, erythromycin, valproate, isoniazid, cimetidine, sulphonamides, acute alcohol consumption

Absorption interactions

Medication that changes the pH of the stomach or the motility of the stomach may vastly change the absorption of another medication (see Section 1.1).

Compatibility

When medications are administered, always be aware of their interactions before they enter the body. This is particularly important with parenteral medication. Many medications interact to produce non-effective products, toxic products or precipitates.

Examples of incompatible injections

- Amiodarone: precipitates in the presence of sodium ions
- Fat (in total parenteral nutrition):   emulsifies when mixed with heparin
- Erythromycin: is unstable in acidic medium (glucose), so must be made up in sodium chloride
- Gentamicin: is partly inactivated by penicillin, so lines must be flushed between administrations

6.2 Drugs in breast milk

There is now a great deal of evidence establishing the benefits of breast-feeding for both the mother and the baby. The ability of a drug to pass into the breast milk will depend on its partition coefficient, pK_a, its plasma and milk protein binding and selective transport mechanisms. Unfortunately, lack of knowledge about drug safety in breast-feeding often causes women to stop breast-feeding or never start in the first place because of their own anxiety or that of the health-care professionals involved in their care.

The lists in the BNF are mainly based on manufacturers' advice and this is usually far too conservative to be of real practical help in a majority of circumstances. The *BNF for Children* takes a far more pragmatic approach. A majority of medications do pass into the breast milk, but most will have little or no affect on an infant at normal therapeutic doses as the dose being delivered to them is subclinical.

It must always be remembered that even if drugs do enter the breast milk they must still go through the infant's gut to be absorbed and this offers another barrier to many drugs such as omeprazole. The infant's short gastric emptying time also reduces exposure to some drugs.

The frequency and volume of the feeding must also be considered as there will be less exposure to the drug if the infant is receiving supplementary feeds and/or other liquids. Further reassurance can be given to a parent if the medication that is being given has a long term history of safety in children at therapeutic levels.

Taking all this into consideration there are very few drugs that are contraindicated in breast-feeding women. The table lists the medicines which are usually seen as a contraindication to breast-feeding. The benefits of breast-feeding usually outweigh the small theoretical risk of harm to the neonate. This said we should never become complacent and should look for the evidence and approach newer drugs with more caution.

Drugs which are contraindicated in breast feeding

Amiodarone	Ergot alkaloids	Oestrogens (high dose)
Androgens	Iodine, Iodides	Radiopharmaceuticals
Antithyroid drugs	Indomethacin	Reserpine
Cancer chemotherapy	Lithium	Sulphonamide (in jaundiced
Chloramphenicol	Nalidixic acid	or G6PD-deficient infants)
Dapsone	Nitofurantoin (in	Tetracyclines
Doxepin	G6PD-deficient infants)	Vitamins A and D (high dose)

7. TOXICOLOGY

Each year 40,000 children attend A&E Departments with suspected poisonings/accidental ingestion. These incidents fall into three categories:

- Accidental — typically boys in the 1–4 years age group
- Intentional — usually teenage girls
- Deliberate — suspected if the signs cannot be explained in any other way

Principles of management include the following:

- Resuscitation if necessary
- Contact a national poisons unit for advice
- Induction of emesis (with ipecacuanha for example) is no longer indicated
- Consider limiting absorption of poison by:
  - Activated charcoal — if ingestion is within 1 hour
  - Gastric lavage — if a life-threatening quantity of poison is ingested
- Acid, alkali or corrosive substances should be treated with caution — do not intervene with the above before seeking advice from the poisons unit

7.1 Paracetamol

Levels of > 250 mg/kg are likely to lead to severe liver damage.

Clinical features

- Nausea and vomiting are the only early symptoms although the majority of patients are asymptomatic
- Right subcostal pain may indicate hepatic necrosis

Management

- Activated charcoal if ingestion < 4 hours earlier
- Measure plasma paracetamol level at 4 hours or as soon as possible thereafter
- Acetylcysteine, a glutathione donor, is nearly 100% effective if administered up to 24 hours post ingestion in preventing hepatotoxicity and nephrotoxicity
- Be aware of 'high-risk' factors that may require a lower threshold (total paracetamol ingestion as low as 75 mg/kg) for active management. These include conditions that decrease hepatic glutathione stores (e.g. anorexia nervosa, cystic fibrosis, malnourishment) and drugs that induce cytochrome p450 microenzymes (e.g. phenytoin, carbamazepine, rifampicin, phenobarbitone)

7.2 Iron

Severity of poisoning is related to the amount of elemental iron ingested.

- A 200 mg tablet of ferrous sulphate contains 65 mg elemental iron
- A 300 mg tablet of ferrous gluconate contains 35 mg elemental iron

< 20 mg/kg	toxicity unlikely
> 20 mg/kg	toxicity may occur
> 60 mg/kg	significant iron poisoning

Clinical features

1st stage

- Within a few hours
  - Nausea and vomiting
  - Abdominal pain
  - Haematemesis

2nd stage

- 8 to 16 hours
  - Apparent recovery

3rd stage

- 16 to 24 hours
  - Hypoglycaemia
  - Metabolic acidosis (due to lactic acid)

Late stage

- Hepatic failure — 2 to 4 days

Management

- Initial treatment depends on the likelihood of toxicity, i.e. was > 20 mg/kg ingested?
- Plasma iron level
- Abdominal X-ray
  - No iron visible but > 20 mg/kg ingested: give desferrioxamine orally
  - Iron in stomach: gastric lavage with desferrioxamine in the lavage fluid
  - Iron in intestine: desferrioxamine orally, picolax orally — a bowel stimulant
- If > 60 mg/kg ingested: administer parenteral desferrioxamine

7.3   Tricyclic antidepressants

Ingestion of > 10 mg/kg of a tricyclic antidepressant is likely to produce significant toxicity, with 20–30 mg/kg potentially being fatal, as a result of sodium-channel block leading to cardiac conduction abnormalities.

Clinical features

- Depressed level of consciousness
- Respiratory depression
- Convulsion
- Arrhythmia
- Hypotension
- Anticholinergic effects:
  - Pupillary dilatation
  - Urinary retention
  - Dry mouth

Management

- Resuscitation
- Activated charcoal
- ECG monitoring
- Sodium bicarbonate and systemic alkalinization
  - Monitor potassium as sodium bicarbonate can cause hypokalaemia
- All antiarrythmics should be avoided especially class Ia agents. Treat convulsions aggressively with benzodiazepines and sodium bicarbonate and if refractory, with general anaesthesia and supportive care

7.4 Aspirin overdose

Mild toxicity follows ingestion of more than 150 mg/kg with severe toxicity associated with doses greater than 500 mg/kg.

Clinical features

In young children dehydration and tachypnoea. In older children and adults tachypnoea and vomiting with progressive lethargy. Tinnitus and deafness. Hypoglycaemia or hyperglycaemia can occur.

Three phases

Phase One

- May last up to 12 hours
- Salicylates directly stimulate the respiratory centre resulting in a respiratory alkalosis with a compensatory alkaline urine with bicarbonate sodium and potassium loss

Phase Two

- May begin straight away, particularly in a young child, and last 12–24 hours
- Hypokalaemia with, as a consequence, a paradoxical aciduria despite the alkalosis

Phase Three

- After 6–24 hours
- Dehydration, hypokalaemia and progressive lactic acidosis. The acidosis now predominating
- Can progress to pulmonary oedema with respiratory failure, disorientation and coma

Management

- Gastric lavage up to 4 hours. Activated charcoal for sustained release preparations. Salicylate level at 6 hours plotted on a normogram and repeat every 3–4 hours until level has peaked. Levels between 200 and 450 mg/l can be treated by activated charcoal and oral or intravenous rehydration while levels greater than 450 mg/l require alkalinization
- Alkalinization of the urine to aid drug excretion, adequate fluids including bicarbonate sodium and potassium with close monitoring of acid–base and electrolytes
- Discuss care with National Poisons Centre

7.5 Lead poisoning

Lead poisoning is uncommon but potentially very serious. It often results from pica (persistent eating of non-nutritive substances, e.g. soil) and is therefore more common in pre-school-age children. Other causes include sucking/ingesting lead paint, lead pipes, discharge from lead batteries and substance abuse of leaded petrol.

Lead intoxication can be divided into acute and chronic effects, and results from its combination with and disruption of vital physiological enzymes.

Acute intoxication

- Reversible renal Fanconi-like syndrome

Chronic intoxication

- Failure to thrive
- Abdominal upset: pain/anorexia/vomiting/constipation
- Lead encephalopathy: behavioural and cognitive disturbance, drowsiness, seizures, neuropathies, coma
- Glomerulonephritis and renal failure
- Anaemia — microcytic/hypochromic, basophilic stippling of red cells

A co-existing iron deficiency is common which first, further exacerbates the anaemia and second, actually contributes to increased lead absorption. Basophilic stippling is the result of inhibition of pyrimidine 5′ nucleotidase and results in accumulation of denatured RNA.

Treatment involves

- Removing source
- Chelation:
  - Mild — oral D-penicillamine
  - Severe — intravenous sodium calcium edetate (EDTA)
  - Very severe — intramuscular injections of dimercaprol to increase effect of EDTA

Some US states implement universal screening for elevated lead levels in children.

7.6 Carbon monoxide

- Carbon monoxide is a tasteless, odourless, colourless and non-irritant gas
- Carbon monoxide binds to haemoglobin to form carboxyhaemoglobin which reduces the oxygen-carrying capacity of the blood and shifts the oxygen dissociation curve to the left. The affinity of haemoglobin for carbon monoxide is 250 times greater than that for oxygen
- Endogenous production occurs and maintains a resting carboxyhaemoglobin level of 1–3%
- Smoking increases carboxyhaemoglobin levels. Other sources of raised levels include car exhaust fumes, poorly maintained heating systems and smoke from fires
- Clinical features of carbon monoxide poisoning occur as a result of tissue hypoxia. PaO_2

is normal but the oxygen content of the blood is reduced. Toxicity relates loosely to the maximum carboxyhaemoglobin concentration. Other factors include duration of exposure and age of the patient

Maximum carboxyhaemoglobin concentration

10%	Not normally associated with symptoms
10–30%	Headache and dyspnoea
60%	Coma, convulsions and death

Neuropsychiatric problems can occur with chronic exposure.

- Treatment of carbon monoxide poisoning is with 100% oxygen which will reduce the carboxyhaemoglobin concentration. Hyperbaric oxygen is said to reduce the carboxyhaemoglobin level quicker

7.7 Button batteries

- Commonly ingested by children
- Systemic toxicity is rare while localized mucosal ulceration is common, possibly leading to gastrointestinal haemorrhage or perforation
- Batteries identified on plain film to be within the oesophagus are to be removed endoscopically
- Patients with batteries within the stomach are to be admitted and re-imaged within 24–48 hours. If battery is still in the stomach after 48 hours then it is to be removed endoscopically
- Batteries distal to the pylorus should not cause problems as long as there is no delay in transit time. It is recommended to monitor progress of the battery with plain films every 48 hours to ensure it remains intact and has been passed

8. FURTHER READING

Greene SL, Dargan PI, Jones AL. 2005. Acute poisoning: understanding 90% of cases in a nutshell. *Postgraduate Medical Journal* 81, 954, 204–16.

Young YL, Koda Kimble MA. 2001. *Applied Therapeutics: The Clinical Use of Drugs,* sixth edition. Chapters 95 and 96. Lippincott Williams & Wilkins.

Royal College of Child Health/Neonatal & Paediatric Pharmacists Group. 1999. *Medicines for Children.*

Maxwell GW. 1989. Paediatric drug dosing. *Drugs* 37, 113–15.

Rylance GM. 1988. Prescribing for infants and children. *British Medical Journal* 296, 984–6.

Watson D *et al.* 1993. Principles of drug prescribing in infants and children: a practical guide. *Drugs* 46:2, 281–8.

Chapter 5

Dermatology

Helen M Goodyear

CONTENTS

Dermatology

1. STRUCTURE AND FUNCTION OF THE SKIN

1.1 Structure of the skin

Epidermis

Four layers

- Stratum corneum — keratinization
- Stratum granulosum
- Stratum spinosum
- Stratum basale

Cells

- Keratinocytes (95%)
- Merkel cells
- Melanocytes
- Langerhans' cells

Marked regional variation in thickness of epidermis

Dermoepidermal junction

- A barrier and a filter

Dermis

- 15–20% of body weight
- Variable thickness — 5 mm back, 1 mm eyelids
- Two protein fibres — collagen and elastin
- Supporting matrix/ground substance (proteoglycan (polysaccharide and protein))
- Rich blood supply

Cells

- Fibroblasts
- Mast cells
- Macrophages

Subcutaneous fat

Epidermal transit time: 52–75 days. Greatly decreased in hyperproliferative conditions, e.g. psoriasis

Palmoplantar skin: extra layer, stratum lucidum, present between stratum granulosum and stratum corneum

Two types of skin: glabrous skin on palms and soles and hair-bearing skin

1.2 Function of the skin

- **Barrier**: to the inward/outward passage of water and electrolytes
- **Mechanical**: depends on collagen and elastin fibres

- **Immunological**: cytokines, macrophages, lymphocytes and antigen presentation by Langerhans' cells
- **UV irradiation protection**: melanin is a barrier in the epidermis, protein barrier in the stratum corneum
- **Temperature regulation**: involves sweat glands and blood vessels in the dermis; heat loss by radiation, convection, conduction and evaporation
- **Sensory**: touch, pain, warmth, cold, itch
- **Respiration**: skin absorbs O_2 and excretes CO_2, accounting for 1–2% of respiration
- **Endocrine**: vitamin D_3 synthesized in stratum spinosum and stratum basale from previtamin D_3 due to UVB radiation

1.3 Skin biopsy

- For uncertain diagnosis, serious skin disorders, histological confirmation of diagnosis before treatment
- Usually a 3–4 mm punch biopsy under local anaesthetic. Stitch often not necessary
- Epidermolysis bullosa — needs special shave technique of unaffected rubbed skin

2. NEONATAL SKIN DISORDERS

2.1 Embryology

- **Nails**: form from 8 to 9 weeks onwards
- **Hair**: synthesis from 17 to 19 weeks
- **Keratinization**: of epidermis from 22 to 24 weeks
- **Epidermis**: all layers present from 24 weeks
- **Preterm**: (24–34 weeks) have poor epidermal barrier with thin stratum corneum directly correlating to degree of prematurity; increased skin losses and absorption; within 2 weeks skin is the same as that of term infant
- **Dermis**: is less thick in neonate compared to adult; collagen fibre bundles are smaller, elastin fibres are immature, vascular and neural elements are less well organized

2.2 Physiological lesions

- Cutis marmorata
- Physiological scaling
- Vernix caseosa
- Sebaceous gland hyperplasia
- Acrocyanosis (peripheral cyanosis)
- Harlequin colour change
- Sucking blisters
- Milia (large ones = pearls)
- Lanugo hairs in preterm baby

2.3 Differential diagnosis of vesiculopustular lesions

Transient rashes

- **Miliaria**: blockage of sweat ducts; vesicles (miliaria crystallina) or itchy red papules (miliaria rubra); first 2 weeks
- **Erythema toxicum neonatorum**: in first 48 hours; may recur beyond first month
- **Transient neonatal pustulosis melanosis**: superficial fragile pustules at birth, rupture easily leaving pigmented macule which lasts for up to 3 months
- **Infantile acropustulosis**: presents in first 3 months; recurrent crops of 1–4-mm vesicopustules usually on hands and feet; resolves by second to third year
- **Eosinophilic pustular folliculitis**: recurrent crops of papules on scalp, hands and feet; rare, usually in males
- **Neonatal acne**: relatively common, resolves by 3 months

Infections and infestations

Always take a swab to exclude *Staphylococcus aureus*/streptococcal infection and others in preterm infants or the immunocompromised. Scabies can occur in the first month of life.

Genetic and naevoid disorders

- **Epidermolysis bullosa**
- **Incontinentia pigmenti**: X-linked dominant, usually lethal in males; vesicular lesions in first 48 hours, verrucous lesions, streaky pigmentation and then atrophic pale lesions; associated with other abnormalities: **s**keletal, **e**ye, **C**NS and **d**entition (SEND)
- **Urticaria pigmentosa**: lesions in first year of life which urticate when rubbed; can be present at birth; systemic involvement is more common if presents > 5 years

2.4 Neonatal erythroderma

Causes of neonatal erythroderma

Skin disorders
- Seborrhoeic dermatitis
- Atopic eczema
- Psoriasis
- Ichthyosis
- Netherton's syndrome

Immunological disorders
- Omenn's syndrome
- Di George syndrome
- T-cell lymphoma
- Hypogammaglobulinaemia
- Graft-versus-host disease

Metabolic/nutritional deficiencies
- Zinc deficiency
- Cystic fibrosis
- Protein malnutrition
- Multiple carboxylase deficiencies
- Amino acid disorders

2.5   Developmental abnormalities

- Amniotic bands
- Aplasia cutis congenita: isolated defect commonly on posterior scalp; associations include epidermolysis bullosa, limb defects, spinal dysraphism, trisomy 13, Goltz syndrome and Adams Oliver syndrome

2.6   Neonatal lupus erythematosus

Presents in first few weeks of life. Erythematous scaly rash, typically around the eyes. May be associated with congenital heart block.

3.   BIRTHMARKS

3.1   Strawberry naevi (capillary haemangioma)

- Usually appear in first few weeks of life
- More common in preterm infants
- Precursor is an erythematous/telangiectatic patch +/– pale halo
- Three phases:
  - Proliferative (6–10 months)
  - Stabilization
  - Spontaneous resolution — pale centre initially
- Complications — ulceration, infection, bleeding, cardiac failure
- Treat if obstructs vital structures
- Often deep component: cavernous haemangioma

Multiple small diffuse haemangiomas in infants < 3 months of age may be associated with visceral involvement, particularly liver; high mortality if untreated

Kasabach–Merritt syndrome: thrombocytopenia, rapidly enlarging haemangioma, microangiopathic haemolytic anaemia, localized consumption coagulopathy

3.2   Salmon patch (stork bite)

Nape of neck, upper eyelids, glabella; 10–20% in occipital region persist whilst others resolve spontaneously

3.3   Port wine stain (naevus flammeus)

- Present at birth
- Capillary malformation

- Associations
  - Sturge–Weber syndrome
  - Klippel–Trenaunay–Weber syndrome
- Persists throughout life
- Can treat with pulse dye laser

3.4 Sebaceous naevi

Present at birth; scalp/face; flat/slightly raised and hairless; can undergo neoplastic change after puberty

3.5 Melanocytic naevi

Present in 1–2% at birth. Congenital usually > 5 mm, acquired < 5 mm. Giant melanocytic naevi (bathing trunk naevi) have increased melanoma risk (4–14%). May be associated with neurocutaneous melanosis (EEG abnormalities, raised intracranial pressure, hydrocephalus and space-occupying lesion).

4. DIFFERENTIAL DIAGNOSIS OF AN ITCHY, RED RASH

4.1 Atopic eczema

Affects 10–20% of children.

Multifactorial disease including

- Genetic factors: 70% of children have positive family history of atopy
- Immunological abnormalities: immunoglobulin E (IgE) dysregulation, skin immune abnormalities — altered cytokine secretion
- Altered pharmacological mechanisms

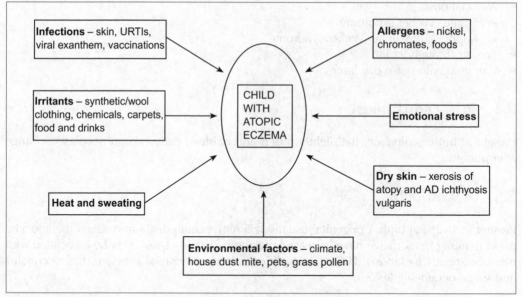

Exacerbating factors of atopic eczema (URTIs, upper respiratory tract infections; AD, autosomal dominant)

Features of atopic eczema

- **Age of onset**: usually in first 6 months, around 3 months most common
- **Site**: face/scalp initially, then flexures; extensor aspects may be involved
- **Erythematous macules/papules/plaques/oozing/crust formation**
- **Tendency to secondary infection**: *Staphylococcus aureus*, Group A beta haemolytic streptococcus, herpes simplex virus (HSV) (eczema herpeticum), warts, mollusca contagiosa
- **Skin colonization** with *S. aureus* in 90%
- **Lichenification**: chronic eczema
- **Resolves**: 50% by 6 years, 90% by 14 years

Associated conditions

- Ichthyosis vulgaris
- Keratosis pilaris
- Food intolerance and allergy
- Pityriasis alba
- Juvenile plantar dermatosis
- Asthma
- Cataract

Differential diagnoses

- **Lichen simplex chronicus**: asymmetrical lesion, chronic rubbing and scratching
- **Infantile seborrhoeic dermatitis**: usually in first 3 months, yellow greasy scales on scalp, forehead, napkin area and skin folds, lack of pruritus. Treat with emollients and 1% hydrocortisone if needed (see eczema treatments)
- **Contact dermatitis**
- **Hyper IgE syndrome (Job's syndrome)**: IgE > 2,000 IU/ml, recurrent cutaneous and sinopulmonary infections
- **Wiskott–Aldrich syndrome**: X-linked recessive, thrombocytopenia and recurrent pyogenic infections. Risk of malignancies, non-Hodgkin's lymphoma most common

Management of atopic eczema

General

- Avoid exacerbating factors
- Cut nails short, file edges
- Wear cotton clothes
- Use non-biological washing powders (and avoid fabric softeners)

Topical treatments

- **Emollients** — bath oil once or twice daily, soap substitute, moisturizer qds (e.g. aqueous cream, emulsifying ointment). Any of the moisturizers can be used as soap substitutes. Use antiseptic bath oils, e.g. Dermol 600, Oilatum Plus, and emollients, e.g. Dermol 500 lotion, if recurrent infection
- **Steroid creams/ointments** — weakest strength possible applied twice daily using fingertip unit (FTU) to control the eczema. In general; mild potency 1% hydrocortisone if < 2 years; moderate potency if needed, e.g. Eumovate, Betnovate 1 in 4, if > 2 years. Never use potent, e.g. Betnovate, or very potent, e.g. Dermovate, in children except in specialized centres. Some evidence that moderate potency three times weekly is as good as mild potency twice daily. Risk of side-effects increases with potency and includes skin thinning, irreversible striae and telangiectasia, acne, depigmentation and Cushing's syndrome
- **Bandages** — zinc impregnated, e.g. ichthopaste, worn with elasticated bandage such as Coban over the top. Change every 24–48 hours. Useful for chronic limb eczema
- **Wet wraps** — cotton tubular bandages of different sizes cut to make double body suit or ready-made vest and leggings (Tubifast/Comfifast). Make first layer wet with either water or cream. Wear at night. Either emollients used under wraps, e.g. aqueous cream, or dilute steroid cream, e.g. Betnovate, 1 in 10 in aqueous cream
- **Tacrolimus** (Protopic) 0.03% ointment and **Pimecrolimus** (Elidel) works on skin immune system, affecting cytokine release, new treatment for moderate or severe eczema not responding to conventional treatment. Use twice daily for 3 weeks then once daily. Not for continuous use of > 3–4 months because of concern of cancer risk
- **Antihistamines** — use with caution in children < 1 year
- **Antibiotics** — consider a 10-day course if eczema flares up. Flucloxacillin +/– penicillin

V or erythromycin. Beware of MRSA (methicillin-resistant *S. aureus*) and resistance to erythromycin in some hospital-acquired *S. aureus* infections

- **Aciclovir** — 1.5 g/m^2 per day intravenously for 5 days if eczema herpeticum (generalized HSV infection of atopic eczema). Oral aciclovir for HSV recurrences. Suspect eczema herpeticum if eczema deteriorates and vesicopustules or punched out lesions are present
- **Diet** — avoid obvious trigger foods. Give 3-month trial of cows' milk protein-free diet if severe eczema < 1 year. Involve paediatric dietitian
- **Systemic therapy** — severe eczema unresponsive to above therapies. Use prednisolone, starting around 2 mg/kg to control eczema, then weaning down to lowest alternate day dose which controls eczema. Short-course cyclosporin (up to 5 mg/kg per day) for 3–6 months also used, but monitor renal and liver function carefully
- **Alternative remedies** — many patients will use these, e.g. homeopathy, Chinese herbal medicine. Beware of potent steroid creams in Chinese herbal creams and monitor liver and renal function 3-monthly if taking herbs. Avoid in children < 2 years

4.2 Urticaria

Transient erythematous/oedematous itchy swellings of the dermis. Lasts from a few minutes to 24 hours. Clears leaving normal skin. 50% have angio-oedema (swelling of subcutaneous tissues). Histamine is the principal mediator released from mast cells.

Causes of urticaria

- **Infection**
  - Viral
  - *Streptococcus*
  - *Toxocara canis*

- **Drugs**
  - Penicillin/cephalosporins
  - Non-steroidal anti-inflammatory drugs (NSAIDs)

- **Food**
  - Cows' milk
  - Eggs
  - Nuts
  - Fish
  - Exotic fruits

- **Physical agents**
  - Cholinergic urticaria
  - Cold urticaria
  - Dermatographism

- **Idiopathic (50% cases)**

- **Associated with systemic disease**

4.3   Infections and infestations

Scabies

As a result of the mite *Sarcoptes scabiei humanis*. The mite can survive for 24–36 hours off the human host.

Variable intensely itchy skin eruption, about 1 month after infestation, is an immune response to the mite and includes:

- Burrows
- Excoriations
- Eczematization
- Papules
- Vesiculopustular lesions
- Bullae
- Secondary bacterial infection
- Nodules

Burrows common on palms, soles and sides of digits. Examine all family members if scabies is suspected. Treat all family at same time.

Management of scabies

- Use aqueous-based preparation (alcohol-based preparation will sting), e.g Malathion (Derbac M) and Permethrin 5%
- Treat all family members at the same time
- Two applications from the neck downwards at 7-day interval. Get under nails and in skin creases. Reapply after hand washing. Caution if < 1-year-old, applying for less time depending on age of child
- Apply to lesions on face if present (more common if < 1 year)
- Treat any secondary infection with systemic antibiotics
- Treat residual dry skin with emollients
- Wash all clothing, bedlinen and towels at the end of treatment

Pediculosis

- Usually *Pediculus humanus capitis* (head louse). May get lice on eyelashes and pubic hair
- Occurs in from < 10% to 40% of children
- Spread by head to head contact
- Pruritus, scratching and excoriation may lead to secondary bacterial infection and cervical lymph nodes
- Look for nits on hairs. Lice visible if recently had a blood meal
- Treat with two applications 7 days apart of malathion-based aqueous lotion or permethrin 5% cream (off licence use)
- Bug busting with wet combing – evidence varies of effectiveness

Viral infections

Tend to be maculopapular erythematous rashes which may be pruritic. Last from < 24 hours to a few weeks. Associated features include cough, runny nose, diarrhoea, vomiting and pyrexia.

Tinea

Erythematous, circular scaly lesions with clearly defined margin. *Microsporum canis* fluoresces with UV light, *Trichophyton tonsurans* (of human origin, common in inner cities) does not. Take skin scrapings.

Impetigo

Superficially spreading skin infection characterized by yellowish-brown crust. May be bullous. Peaks in late summer and is commonest in children < 5 years. Causative agent *S. aureus* or Group A beta haemolytic streptococcus. Treat with oral antibiotics.

Staphylococcal scalded skin syndrome

Caused by exotoxin-producing staphylococci. Localized infection becomes widespread after 24–48 hours. Characteristic signs are fever, skin tenderness, marked erythema, bullae and peeling of the skin. Treat with systemic antibiotics (flucloxacillin) and watch fluid balance.

Warts

Caused by human papillomavirus. Commonest on hands and feet (plantar warts/verrucas) but occur at any site. Most resolve spontaneously but can last for several years.

Treat with salicylic acid-based wart paint, e.g. Salactol, applying each night and rubbing wart down with an emery board until wart is flat. May need to treat for 3 months or longer. Freezing with liquid nitrogen is effective but often requires multiple treatments at monthly intervals. Poorly tolerated in children < 5 years.

Perianal warts

Usually innocently acquired but consider sexual abuse. Only treat if multiple and spreading. Use podophyllin 15%. May need surgery.

Mollusca contagiosa

'Water warts'. Caused by poxvirus. Dome-shaped papules with an umbilicated centre. Spread by autoinoculation. Resolve spontaneously but can last for several years. Treatments tend to be associated with scarring.

NB Both warts and mollusca contagiosa are more common in children who are immuno-suppressed and in those with underlying skin disorders such as atopic eczema.

4.4 Psoriasis

- **Onset**: < 2 years in 2% and at < 10 years in 10% of cases of psoriasis. In childhood onset tends to be between 5–9 years in girls and 15–19 years in boys
- **Increased epidermal turnover time**
- **Relapsing and remitting**: scaly rash, typically affects extensor surfaces and scalp (*Pityriasis amiantacea*)
- **Genetic predisposition**: risk of psoriasis is 10% if a first-degree relative is affected, risk is 50% if both parents are psoriatic; 73% monozygotic and 20% dizygotic twins have concordant disease; HLA Cw6 (B13 and B17) linked to 9–15 times risk, HLA B27 associated with psoriatic arthropathy
- **Nail involvement**: pits, onycholysis, subungual hyperkeratosis; may precede onset of skin lesions
- **Arthropathy**: may be severe; higher incidence in patients with nail changes

Recognized types of psoriasis

- **Common plaque**: chronic psoriasis, psoriasis vulgaris
- **Guttate psoriasis**: (raindrop psoriasis) multiple small lesions on trunk
- **Flexural sites**: intertriginous areas
- **Erythrodermic psoriasis**
- **Pustular psoriasis**: acute generalized form or chronic localized to hands and feet

Provoking factors

- **Trauma** (Koebner phenomenon)
- **Infection**: streptococcal disease especially in throat in guttate psoriasis; may also play a role in chronic plaque psoriasis
- **Endocrine**: peaks at puberty (and menopause); gets worse in postpartum period
- **Sunlight**: usually beneficial but makes a small number worse
- **Metabolic**: hypocalcaemia, dialysis
- **Drugs**: withdrawal of systemic steroids, β-blockers, antimalarials and lithium
- **Psychogenic factors**: stress
- **Human immunodeficiency virus**: psoriasis may appear for the first time or get dramatically worse

Differential diagnosis

- **Hyperkeratotic eczema**
- **Lichen planus**: flat-topped, purple polygonal papules with white reticulate surface (Wickham's striae); oral and nail changes may be present; rare in children; 90% resolve in 12 months
- **Pityriasis rosea**: larger herald patch, smaller lesions in Christmas tree distribution; clears in 6 weeks; linked to human herpes virus-7
- **Pityriasis lichenoides chronica**: excoriated papules on trunk and limbs in crops; lasts up to a few years

Management of psoriasis

- **Avoid triggering factors**
- **Treat streptococcal infection**
- **Topical treatment**
  - Emollients
  - Tar-based bath emollients, e.g. Polytar
  - Tar and salicylic acid ointments
  - Vitamin D-derivative creams — calcipotriol (Dovonex) for mild to moderate psoriasis (up to 40% of skin area affected)
  - Mild-potency topical steroid creams with tar, e.g. Alphosyl HC for delicate areas, e.g. face, flexures, ears, genitals
  - Carefully supervised dithranol preparations, e.g. dithrocream
  - Topical retinoids used but unlicensed
- **Phototherapy**: UVB phototherapy if child is old enough to comply. PUVA is contraindicated in young children
- **Systemic therapy**: severe psoriasis, acute pustular psoriasis, e.g. methotrexate, cyclosporin, acitretin

5. BLISTERING DISORDERS

Causes of blistering disorders

- **Inherited**
  - Epidermolysis bullosa
  - Incontinentia pigmenti
  - Bullous ichthyosiform erythroderma

- **Drugs**
  - Fixed drug eruptions
  - Photosensitivity reactions
  - Sulphonamides
  - Barbiturates

- **Autoimmune**
  - Chronic bullous disease of childhood
  - Pemphigoid
  - Epidermolysis bullosa acquisita
  - Dermatitis herpetiformis
  - Pemphigus

- **Mechanobullous**
  - Trauma/friction
  - Burns
  - Insect bites/papular urticaria

- **Contact dermatitis**

- **Infection**
  - Bullous impetigo
  - Herpes simplex virus
  - Varicella/zoster
  - Hand, foot and mouth disease
  - Scabies

- **Neonatal disorders**
  - Infantile acropustulosis
  - Miliaria

- **Others**
  - Erythema multiforme
  - Stevens–Johnson syndrome
  - Henoch–Schönlein purpura
  - Porphyria
  - Toxic epidermal necrolysis
  - Hartnup's disease
  - Pachyonychia congenita

- **Dermatoses**
  - Eczema
  - Lichen planus

5.1 Epidermolysis bullosa (EB)

Heterogeneous condition. Need skin biopsy for definitive diagnosis. First-trimester prenatal diagnosis is possible. Severe types at risk of nutritional deficiencies and anaemia.

There are three broad categories:

- **EB simplex**: mainly autosomal dominant (AD) — defect in basal layer of epidermis affecting keratins 5 and 14. Usually appears when child begins to crawl or walk, with blisters at friction sites, e.g. knees, hands and feet. Hair, teeth and nails not affected
- **Junctional EB**: autosomal recessive (AR) — lethal and non-lethal variants. Mucous membranes can be severely affected and teeth are often abnormal. Laminin-5 defect. Raw denuded areas show little tendency to heal. Hoarseness as a result of laryngeal involvement
- **Dystrophic EB**: AD and AR — subepidermal blister. Defect in collagen-VII production. Lesions heal with scarring. Hair and teeth are normal in dominant form, whilst involvement of mucous membranes, nails, hair and teeth may all be abnormal in recessive form. Web formation between digits leads to a useless fist. May develop squamous carcinoma

5.2 Drug eruptions

- **Fixed drug eruptions**: localized brown-purple plaques, may be bullous. Recur at fixed sites when drug is ingested. Hyperpigmentation may persist
- **Hypersensitivity syndrome reactions**: usually 7–28 days after first exposure to drug. Fever, maculopapular/pustular skin lesions, erythema, swelling. Can get nephritis, hepatitis and pneumonitis
- **Severe cutaneous adverse reaction**: erythema multiforme, Stevens–Johnson syndrome and toxic epidermal necrolysis
- **Toxic epidermal necrolysis**: bullae, extensive areas of skin necrosis, denuded areas, systemically toxic. May be 1–3-day prodome of high fever, sore throat, conjunctivitis and tender skin. Causative drugs similar to those for Stevens–Johnson syndrome. In toxic epidermal necrolysis there is full-thickness necrosis of epidermis whereas in staphylococcal scalded skin syndrome there is no necrosis and epidermal separation is just beneath the stratum corneum

5.3 Autoimmune blistering disorders

All rare. Listed in order of decreasing frequency.

Chronic bullous dermatosis of childhood

Usually > 3 years, mean age 5 years. Tense blisters like a string of pearls usually on abdomen and buttocks. May present as genital blisters/erosions. 40% have mucous membrane involvement. Clears after 3 years. Linear basement membrane IgA.

Bullous pemphigoid

Can be < 12 months. Palm and sole involvement common. 75% have mucous membrane changes. Lasts 2–4 years. Linear basement membrane IgG.

Dermatitis herpetiformis

Mean age 7 years. Affects buttocks, elbows, back of neck and scalp. Itchy. 15% resolve spontaneously. Skin changes can persist up to 18 months after gluten-free diet. IgA in papillary dermis.

Epidermolysis bullosa acquisita

Mechanobullous picture with blisters localized to areas of trauma. Remits in 2–4 years. Linear basement membrane IgG.

Pemphigus

Very rare. Flaccid blisters. Nikolsky's sign positive (i.e. a blister is induced by rubbing normal-appearing skin). Mucous membrane involvement in vulgaris type, with stomatitis the presenting sign in 50% of cases. Intercellular IgG.

6. ERYTHEMAS

6.1 Erythema multiforme

Acute self-limiting onset of symmetrical fixed red papules, some of which form target lesions. May blister. Can show Koebner phenomenon. May involve lips, buccal mucosa and tongue.

Cause of erythema multiforme

- **Infections**
  - Herpes simplex virus
  - Mycoplasma
  - Epstein–Barr virus
  - Chlamydiae
  - Orf
  - Deep fungal infections (histoplasmosis)

- **Drugs**
  - Sulphonamides
  - Penicillin

- **Collagen diseases**
  - Systemic lupus erythematosus
  - Polyarteritis nodosa

- **Underlying malignancy**

Stevens–Johnson syndrome

Causes as for erythema multiforme.

- Severe erosions of at least two mucosal surfaces
- Prodromal respiratory illness

- Extensive necrosis of lips and mouth
- Purulent conjunctivitis
- Variable skin involvement — red macules, bullae, skin necrosis and denudation

6.2 Erythema nodosum

Nodular, erythematous eruption on extensor aspects of legs, less commonly on thighs and forearms. Regresses to bruises. Lasts 3–6 weeks.

Causes of erythema nodosum

- **Infections**
  - *Streptococcus*
  - *Salmonella*
  - *Yersinia*
  - *Campylobacter*
  - Tuberculosis
  - Acnes
  - *Chlamydia*
  - Cat-scratch fever
  - Hepatitis B
  - Epstein–Barr virus
  - Mycoses

- **Gut disorders**
  - Ulcerative colitis
  - Crohn's disease

- **Malignancy**
  - Leukaemia
  - Lymphoma

- **Drugs**
  - Sulphonamides
  - Oral contraceptive pill

6.3 Erythema marginatum

Annular migratory erythema found in 10% of cases of rheumatic fever. Recurrent crops of lesions weekly. Active cardiac disease. Frequently precedes onset of migratory arthritis.

6.4 Erythema migrans

Lyme disease due to *Borrelia burgdorferi*. Red papule which develops with annular red ring around it.

7. PHOTOSENSITIVE DISORDERS

Causes of photosensitive disorders

- **Idiopathic**
  - Polymorphic light eruption
  - Actinic prurigo

- **Contact dermatitis** due to plants

- **Systemic lupus erythematosis**
  - Photosensitivity rash in 15–30%

- **Drugs**
  - Sulphonamides
  - Thiazides
  - Tetracycline

- **Genetic**

7.1 Genetic causes of photosensitivity

Phenylketonuria

AR. In addition to photosensitivity, skin changes include:

- Decreased pigmentation
- Eczema
- Fair hair
- Lightly pigmented eyes

Xeroderma pigmentosum

AR group of disorders caused by a DNA repair defect.

- Extreme photosensitivity
- Severe ophthalmological abnormalities
- Skin malignancies in childhood
- Neurological complications in 20%
- Freckling

Cockayne's syndrome

AD. Cells have increased sensitivity to UV light. Onset of symptoms is in the second year of life.

- Progressive neurological degeneration and growth failure
- Sensorineural hearing loss
- Skeletal abnormalities
- Dental caries
- Pigmentary retinopathy
- Cataracts

Trichothiodystrophy

AR. Hair has low sulphur content. Includes following defects — 'PIBIDS':

- **P**hotosensitivity
- **I**chthyosis
- **B**rittle hair
- **I**ntellectual impairment
- **D**ecreased fertility
- **S**hort stature

Rothmund–Thomson syndrome

AR. Characterized by poikiloderma (atrophic pigmented telangiectasia) by end of first year.

- Sparse hair
- Skeletal dysplasia
- Short stature
- Cataracts
- Hypogonadism
- Hypotrophic nails
- Increased risk of osteosarcoma and skin malignancy

Bloom's syndrome

AR.

- Growth retardation
- Immunodeficiency (IgA and IgM)
- Telangiectasia
- Pigmentary abnormalities
- Malignancies in third decade — leukaemia, lymphomas

Hartnup's disease

AR. Impaired amino acid transport in kidneys and small intestine. Most children asymptomatic.

- Photosensitivity with pellagra-like appearance is first sign
- Can form blisters
- Intermittent cerebellar ataxia
- Psychotic behaviour
- Mild mental retardation

Porphyrias

Group of diseases leading to accumulation of haem precursors. 5-aminolaevulinic acid (ALA) and porphobilinogen (PBG) have no cutaneous manifestations. Elevated porphyrins are associated with either acute photosensitivity or skin fragility with vesiculobullous and erosive lesions.

Erythropoietic protoporphyria (EPP)

Usually AD. Most common porphyria in children.

- Small pitted scars on nose and cheeks
- Burning/stinging sensation on exposed skin
- Photosensitivity less severe in adult life
- Gallstones in childhood
- Excess protoporphyrins in red cells and faeces (urine normal)

Congenital erythropoietic porphyria

AR. Presents at or shortly after birth. Acute episodes become less severe with time, leaving residual scarring, ulceration and marked deformity with sclerodactyly and loss of terminal phalanges.

- Severe photosensitivity
- Red staining of nappy
- Haemolytic anaemia
- Splenomegaly
- Hypertrichosis
- Teeth and bones may be red (fluoresce with UV light)

Porphyria cutanea tarda (PCT)

Familial or provoked by drugs, alcohol or infection.

- Skin fragility leading to vesicles/blisters and erosions
- Hypertrichosis
- Yellow/blue nails and onycholysis
- Systemic manifestations — anorexia, constipation, diarrhoea
- Urine dark brown

8. ICHTHYOSES

Disorders of keratinization, characterized by excessively dry and visibly scaly skin. Hereditary or associated with systemic disease.

8.1 Inherited ichthyoses

Ichthyosis vulgaris

AD. Variable range of expression; may affect in winter months only, affects 1 : 250. Fine, light scaling. Associated with keratosis pilaris and atopic eczema.

X-linked recessive ichthyosis (XRI, steroid sulphatase deficiency)

Occurs in 1 : 2,000 boys. Dark-brown scaling affecting limbs and trunk. Gene in Xp22.3 region.

- Cryptorchidism

- Corneal opacities
- Prolonged labour (placental sulphatase deficiency)

Lamellar ichthyoses

AD and AR. Large, dark, plate-like scales, reptilian appearance.

Bullous ichthyosiform erythroderma

AD. Erythroderma and severe blistering at birth. Mutations in keratin 1 or 10.

Non-bullous ichthyosiform erythroderma

AR. Generalized fine scaling and erythroderma.

Associated congenital ichthyoses

Sjögren–Larsson syndrome
AR. Fatty alcohol oxidation defect in fibroblasts. Spastic diplegia or tetraplegia, mental retardation. Onset of neurological signs at 4–13 months of age.

Refsum's disease
AR. Phytanic acid oxylase defect.

- Retinitis pigmentosa
- Peripheral neuropathy
- Anosmia
- Sensory deafness
- Variable ichthyosis — ichthyosis vulgaris-type appearance

Associated steroid sulphatase deficiency
X-linked recessive ichthyosis can be associated with:

- Kallmann's syndrome
- Pyloric stenosis
- Chondroplasia punctata
- Hypogonadism
- Mental retardation

Multiple sulphatase deficiency
AR. Lack of arylsulphatase A, B and steroid sulphatase.

- Neurodegenerative disease
- Coarse facies
- Hepatosplenomegaly
- Lumbar kyphosis

Trichothiodystrophy syndromes — Tay's syndrome and 'PIBIDS'
AR. Those with Tay's do not have photosensitivity. Hair has decreased sulphur content.

Netherton's syndrome

AR.

- Neonatal erythroderma
- Ichthyosis linearis circumflexa
- Atopy
- Faltering growth
- Recurrent infections
- Trichorrhosis invaginata — hair shaft abnormality

Happle's syndrome

X-linked dominant. Conradi–Hunermann syndrome is AD and is now thought not to have cutaneous manifestations.

- Chondroplasia punctata
- Cicatricial alopecia
- Cataracts
- Short stature
- Follicular atrophoderma

KID syndrome

Mode of inheritance uncertain — ? AD or AR.

- **K**eratitis
- **I**chthyosis
- **D**eafness

Neutral-lipid storage disease (Chanarin–Dorfman syndrome)

AR. Fatty changes of the liver, variable neurological and ocular involvement. Multiple lipid vacuoles in monocytes and granulocytes.

CHILD syndrome

Congenital **h**emidysplasia, **i**chthyosiform erythroderma and **l**imb **d**efects.

8.2   Collodion baby

Yellow, shiny, tight film covering skin at birth. 10% have normal skin. Film shed at 1–4 weeks of life. Can persist for 3 months. Biopsy after day 14 is helpful.

Disorders presenting as collodion baby include:

- Gaucher's disease
- Lamellar ichthyosis
- Trichothiodystrophy
- Sjögren–Larsson syndrome
- Non-bullous ichthyosiform erythroderma
- Neutral-lipid storage disease
- Chondroplasia punctata

- Ichthyosis vulgaris
- Netherton's syndrome

Neonatal problems of collodion baby and harlequin ichthyosis (see below)

- Hypothermia
- Dehydration
- Hypernatraemia
- Cutaneous infection
- Poor sucking

May need up to 250 ml/kg per day fluids. Nurse in high-humidity incubator with up to 1-hourly application of white soft paraffin and liquid paraffin 50 : 50.

8.3   Harlequin ichthyosis

AR. Problems are the same as for collodion babies. Most of the survivors have non-bullous ichthyosiform erythroderma. Need continued high-intensity skin care and high-calorie feeds, otherwise fail to thrive. Use of retinoids (acitretin) is thought to account for increasing survival of these children. Genetic mutation (*ABCA12*) recently identified. ABCA 12 is thought to play a critical role in formation of lamellar granules in the epidermis and the discharge of lipids into the intercellular spaces. This is defective in H1 and leads to the epidermal barrier defect.

> **Features of harlequin ichthyosis at birth**
>
> - Usually preterm
> - Erythroderma
> - Thick plate-like scales at birth — 'coat of armour'
> - Deep red fissures
> - Ectropion and eclabium (mouth pulled open with eversion of lips)
> - Hands and feet have tightly bound digits. Tips may be necrotic.
> - Nose and ears bound down
> - Respiratory distress depending upon prematurity and the degree of restriction of chest movement

9.   HAIR, NAILS AND TEETH

9.1   Hair

The hair has cyclical periods of growth throughout life. The three phases are:

- **Anagen**: growth phase
- **Catagen**: intermediate phase
- **Telogen**: resting usually 3 months before hair being shed

These phases occur randomly so that no one area is depleted of hair. Anagen lasts for variable lengths of time depending on site. Usually > 3 years on the scalp.

Genetic causes of hair loss (diffuse)

- Ectodermal dysplasias — AD/AR. Group of disorders with two or more abnormalities including teeth, nails, sweat glands and other ectodermal structures
- Acrodermatitis enteropathica
- Netherton's syndrome
- Cockayne's syndrome
- Hair-shaft abnormalities — monilethrix, pili torti, Menkes' kinky hair syndrome (X-linked recessive — copper transport defect)
- Hartnup's disease
- Homocystinuria

Causes of non-scarring alopecia (hair loss)

- **Telogen effluvium**
- **Trichotillomania**
- **Trauma** from rubbing or traction from pony tails
- **Endocrine causes**: hypothyroidism, hypopituitarism
- **Drugs**: oral contraceptive pill
- **Loose anagen syndrome**: young girls; hair increases in density and thickness as child gets older
- **Nutritional**: malnutrition, iron deficiency, zinc deficiency
- **Alopecia areata**
  - 2% prevalence. Usually > 5 years.
  - Family history in 5–25%
  - Associated with autoimmune disorders (thyroiditis, vitiligo) and Down's syndrome
  - Scalp is normal in appearance; exclamation-mark hairs are characteristic
  - Outcome unpredictable; most children have small patchy hair loss and outlook is good; the more extensive the disease the worse the prognosis

Causes of scarring alopecia

- Aplasia cutis congenita
- Systemic lupus erythematosus
- Fungal infection — tinea capitis, kerion
- Incontinenti pigmenti
- *Pachyonychia congenita*
- Epidermolysis bullosa
- Ichthyoses — CHILD syndrome, KID syndrome, syndromes with chondroplasia punctata

Causes of scalp scaling

- Seborrhoeic dermatitis
- Atopic eczema
- Fungal infection
- Psoriasis
- *Pityriasis amiantacea*
- Histiocytosis

Excessive hair growth

This is either androgen-independent 'hypertrichosis' or androgen-dependent 'hirsutism'.

Causes of hypertrichosis

- **Congenital**
  - Hypertrichosis lanuginosa
  - Cornelia de Lange syndrome
  - Rubinstein–Taybi syndrome
  - Hurler's syndrome
  - Porphyria — EPP, PCT

- **Endocrine**
  - Hyper/hypothyroidism

- **Acrodynia** (mercury poisoning)

- **Focal lesions — Becker's naevus**

- **Drugs**
  - Cyclosporin
  - Minoxidil
  - Phenytoin
  - Diazoxide
  - Streptomycin
  - Acetazolamide

- **Head trauma**

- **Dermatomyositis**

Causes of hirsutism

- **Adrenal**
  - Congenital adrenal hyperplasia
  - Cushing's syndrome
  - Virilizing adrenal tumours

- **Turner's syndrome**

- **Ovarian**
  - Polycystic ovary syndrome
  - Ovarian tumours
  - Gonadal dysgenesis

9.2   Nails

Development begins at the 9th week of gestation and is complete after the 22nd week. Toenail development lags behind that of fingernails.

Nail changes — normal variants

- **Koilonychia**: normal variant in early childhood due to thin nail-plate; commonly toenails; also associated with iron deficiency anaemia
- **Superficial longitudinal ridges**: normal variant
- **Beau's lines**: transverse depressions; can appear at 1–2 months of age and with any severe illness which affects nail growth
- **Longitudinal pigmented bands**: pigmented bands in dark-skinned children

Conditions affecting the nails

- **Acute paronychia**
- **Congenital malalignment of the big toe** (triangular shape to nail)
- **Atopic eczema**: pitting, Beau's lines, onycholysis
- **Parakeratosis pustulosa**: hyperkeratosis, onycholysis, pitting
- **Psoriasis**: nail pitting, onycholysis, salmon patches of nail-bed
- **Leukonychia**: liver disease, hypoalbuminaemia, hereditary and if punctate found following repetitive minor trauma
- **Twenty nail dystrophy**: many nails affected; spectrum of nail-plate surface abnormalities; may be associated with alopecia areata; regresses spontaneously
- **Lichen planus**: longitudinal ridging, pterygium
- **Nail–patella syndrome**: AD; nail hypoplasia, patella hypoplastic or absent, radial head abnormalities, iliac crest exostosis and nephropathy
- **Epidermolysis bullosa**: may be permanent nail loss
- **Pachyonychia congenita**: AD; severe nail-bed thickening as a result of hyperkeratosis; other features depend on type; include palmar plantar hyperkeratosis, cataracts, alopecia and bullae of palms and soles
- **Ectodermal dysplasias**: variable dystrophic nails depending on type
- **Alopecia areata**: nail pitting
- **Chronic mucocutaneous candidiasis**: nails are yellow–brown and are thickened; recurrence is common because of underlying immune defects
- **Fungal infection**
- **Dystrophy**: CHILD syndrome, congenital erythropoietic porphyria
- **Hypothyroidism**: decreased nail growth, ridging and brittleness
- **Rothmund–Thomson syndrome**: hypotrophic nails
- **Pityriasis rubra pilaris**: half-and-half nail; thickened curved and terminal hyperaemia
- **Incontinentia pigmenti**: nail dystrophy in 40%

9.3 Teeth

Always look at the teeth as part of a dermatological examination.

Conditions affecting the teeth

- **Ectodermal dysplasia**: hypodontia, small conical discoloured teeth and caries
- **Epidermolysis bullosa**: dental caries

- **Cockayne's syndrome**: dental caries, malocclusion, small mandible so teeth appear large
- **Dyskeratosis congenita**: poorly formed teeth, thin enamel. Degenerative disorder with reticulate skin pigmentation, atrophic nails, leukoplakia and bone marrow failure
- **Congenital syphilis**: Hutchinson's teeth (developmental abnormality of upper +/− lower incisors where teeth are notched/small); Mulberry molars (first molars have maldevelopment of cusps and look like a mulberry)
- **Congenital erythropoietic porphyria**: teeth may be pink/red and fluoresce with UV light
- **Incontinentia pigmenti**: 80% have dental abnormalities – hypodontia, delayed eruption, malformed crowns
- **Langerhans' cell histiocytosis**: premature eruption of teeth
- **Trichothiodystrophy**: enamel hypoplasia, caries

10. DISORDERS OF PIGMENTATION

Colour of the skin is the result of melanin produced by melanocytes in the basal layer of the epidermis.

10.1 Causes of hypopigmentation

Causes of hypopimentation

- **Nutritional deficiency**
  - Copper
  - Selenium
  - Kwashiorkor

- **Genetic**
  - Oculocutaneous albinism
  - Phenylketonuria
  - Homocystinuria
  - Apert's syndrome
  - Piebaldism
  - Waardenburg's syndrome
  - Tuberous sclerosis
  - Menke's kinky hair syndrome
  - Epidermolysis bullosa (at sites of bullae)
  - Hypomelanosis of Ito (incontinentia pigmenti achromians of Ito)

- **Autoimmune**
  - Vitiligo

- **Infection**
  - Pityriasis versicolor
  - Vaccination sites

- **Trauma sites**

- **Post-inflammatory**
  - Eczema
  - Psoriasis

Chediak–Higashi syndrome

AR. Incomplete oculocutaneous albinism, photophobia and severe recurrent infections.

Vitiligo

Total loss of pigment. Often symmetrical. Spontaneous repigmentation uncommon. Associated with autoimmune disorders.

10.2   Causes of hyperpigmentation

Causes of hyperpigmentation

- **Genetic**
  - Incontinentia pigmenti
  - Goltz syndrome (focal dermal hyperplasia)
  - Peutz–Jeghers syndrome
  - Albright's syndrome
  - Xeroderma pigmentosum

- **Metabolic**
  - Liver disease
  - Haemochromatosis
  - Wilson's disease
  - Porphyria
  - Congenital erythropoietic porphyria
  - Hepatic cutaneous porphyria

- **Infection**
  - Pityriasis versicolor

- **Drugs**
  - Minocycline
  - Tetracycline
  - AZT (Zidovudine)
  - Rifabutin
  - Clofazimine

- **Endocrine**
  - Addison's disease
  - Hyperthyroidism
  - Nelson's syndrome
  - Cushing's syndrome (ectopic ACTH production)

- **Nutritional**
  - Malabsorption
  - Pellagra (sun-exposed sites)
  - Kwashiorkor

- **Post-inflammatory**
  - Insect bites
  - Acne
  - Atopic eczema
  - Lichen simplex chronicus

Other pigmentary changes

Niemann–Pick type A

- Grey-brown/yellow–brown discoloration of sun-exposed areas

Metals

- Silver, bismuth and arsenic
- Slate-grey pigmentation

Mongolian blue spot

- Blue skin
- Typical site is lower back
- Common in Afro-Caribbean and Asian babies
- Increased numbers of melanocytes deep in dermis
- Tends to disappear by 4 years of age

10.3   Disorders associated with multiple café-au-lait macules

- Neurofibromatosis type I (NFI)
- NFII (minority of patients)
- Piebaldism
- Ataxia telangectasia
- Multiple endocrine neoplasia
- Russell–Silver syndrome
- McCune–Albright syndrome
- Tuberous sclerosis
- Noonan's syndrome
- Bloom's syndrome
- Tay's syndrome

10.4 Skin changes associated with tuberous sclerosis

- Earliest changes are forehead plaques, Shagreen patch and hypomelanotic macules. Shagreen patch occurs typically in lumbar region but can be at top of leg
- Facial angiofibromas (adenoma sebaceum): rare < 2 years. Present in 85% > 5 years
- Periungual fibromas: uncommon in first decade of life

11.   MISCELLANEOUS DISORDERS

11.1   Granuloma annulare

Ring of firm skin-coloured papules. Usually asymptomatic. May follow non-specific trauma in 25%. 50% clear in 2 years. 40% have recurrent eruptions. Link to diabetes mellitus controversial. Always test urine for glucose.

11.2   Dermatitis artefacta

Self-inflicted lesions on sites readily accessible to patient's hands. Take a variety of forms including blisters.

11.3 Nappy rash

Irritant contact dermatitis

- Common
- Due to urine and faeces
- Interogenous areas characteristically spared
- May be infected with *Candida albicans* (satellite lesions and skinfold involvement)

Other causes

- Seborrhoeic dermatitis
- Atopic eczema
- Psoriasis
- Scabies
- Acrodermatitis enteropathica
- Langerhans' cell histiocytosis
- Kawasaki's disease
- Child abuse
- Blistering disorders

11.4 Acne

Affects face and upper trunk. Lesions include comedones, papules, pustules, nodules and cysts. Usually 10–16 years. May get neonatal acne and infantile acne. Investigate for underlying cause if acne appears for the first time between 1 and 7 years.

Treatment

- Topical — benzoyl peroxide 2.5% to 10%, topical retinoids, topical antibiotics
- Oral antibiotics — erythromycin, oxytetracycline (not if < 12 years) taken bd
- Dianette (cyproterone acetate with ethinyloestradiol) for females
- Isotretinoin (Roaccutane) vitamin A derivative for severe acne. Causes dry mucous membranes and may cause depression. Council and assess for depression prior to therapy, which is started by a dermatologist only. Monitor lipids.

11.5 Spitz naevus

Pink/red, sometimes brown in colour. Benign lesion which can be difficult to distinguish from malignant melanoma. Excise if suspicious features, e.g. unusual pigmentation, rapid growth and size > 1 cm.

11.6   Keloids

Hypertrophic scar extending beyond boundary of original wound. More common in pigmented skin. Intralesional injections of steroid (triamcinolone) may help. Tend to recur if surgically excised.

11.7   Acanthosis nigricans

Hyperpigmentation is the earliest feature ('dirty skin'), preferentially in the flexures. May become hyperkeratotic and warty lesions occur elsewhere on the body. Occurs in families and is associated with obesity, syndromes of insulin resistance, hyperandrogenaemia and hypothyroidism.

11.8   Stings and snake bites

Bee/wasp stings

- **Local effects**: burning, pain, erythema, oedema. Subsides in a few hours
- **Systemic**: Usually due to multiple stings. Hypertension, generalized vasodilatation, severe headache, diarrhoea, vomiting, shock
- **Late onset reaction**: urticaria, serum-sickness-like reaction

Snake bites

- Depends on type of snake
- Local swelling/necrosis
- Haematological abnormalities including coagulation disturbance and complement depletion
- Treat with compression bandage and immobilization by splinting
- Important to identify venom (in urine, swab and kill snake) so that antivenom can be administered

12.   FURTHER READING

Ashcroft DM *et al.* 2005. Efficacy and tolerability of topical pimecrolimus and tacrolimus in the treatment of atopic dermatitis: meta-analysis of randomized controlled trials. *BMJ.* 330; 516–522.

Flohr C, Williams HC. 2004. Evidence based management of atopic eczema. *Arch Dis Child Educ Pract Ed* 89 ep35–9.

Burden AD. 1999. Management of psoriasis in childhood. *Clin Exp Dermatol* 24 341–5.

Pediatric Clinics of North America. 2000. *Pediatric Dermatology* Volume 47:4.

Higgins E, Du Vivier A. 1996. *Skin Disease in Childhood and Adolescence.* Blackwell Science.

Harper J, Oranje A, Prose N. 2005. *Textbook of Pediatric Dermatology* 2nd edition. Blackwell Scientific.

Chapter 6

Emergency Paediatrics

Serena Cottrell

CONTENTS

Emergency Paediatrics

1. INTRODUCTION

It is vital to have a structured approach when managing a critically ill child. A structured approach enables you to prioritize and stabilize most sick children even when the diagnosis is unknown. Preparation is useful, although not always possible, and good communication is essential both between members of the multidisciplinary team and with families. The structured approach concentrates on identifying and managing the immediate threats to life first: ABC, A for airway, B for breathing and C for circulation.

2. OUT-OF-HOSPITAL CARDIAC ARREST

Cardiac arrest should be suspected when a patient is found unconscious, is not breathing normally and when there are no signs of circulation or palpable pulses.

Traditionally the SAFE approach is taught.

- **S** shout for help
- **A** approach with care
- **F** free from danger
- **E** evaluate

Evaluation involves either verbal or physical stimulation, e.g. 'are you alright' to establish responsiveness.

- If there is any risk of cervical spine injury the neck should not be moved while establishing responsiveness.

Then the ABC approach with basic life support is established.

2.1 Airway opening procedures

An obstructed airway results in hypoxia and then cardiac arrest. The airway can be opened by either of two manoeuvres

- Head tilt with a chin lift (providing there is no risk of a cervical spine injury)
- Jaw thrust

2.2 Look, listen and feel

- **Look** for chest movement
- **Listen** for breath sounds
- **Feel** for the warmth of the breath

2.3 Rescue breaths

Up to five rescue breaths should be attempted to ensure two effective breaths. The chest should be seen to rise. This can be done with a bag and mask if available.

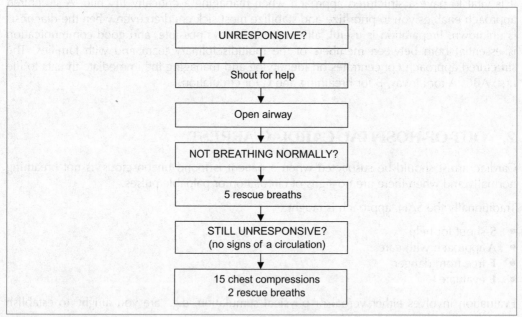

Algorithm for basic life support (Healthcare professionals with a duty to respond)

Call emergency services after 1 minute of CPR (cardiopulmonary resuscitation)

2.4 Checking the circulation

Take no more than 10 seconds to look for signs of circulation or to check the pulse.

These include:

- Any movement
- Coughing
- Normal breathing

Check the pulse only if you are trained and experienced. The brachial pulse is felt in an infant and the carotid pulse can be felt in a child.

If there are no signs of circulation, no pulse or a slow pulse, less than 60 beats per minute with poor perfusion, or you are unsure, start compressions.

2.5   Chest compressions

Compressions should be done at a rate of 100 per minute in all ages and should be sufficient to depress the sternum by approximately one-third of the depth of the chest.

The ratio is 15 compressions to two breaths in both the infant and the child when performed by health professionals. After puberty and in lay person performed resuscitation, the ratio becomes 30 compressions to two breaths.

Infant < 1 year

- Two fingers over the lower third of the sternum for the single rescuer
- Hands encircling the chest; two thumb technique for two rescuers

Child 1 year to puberty

- The heel of one or two hands may be used, depending on the size of the rescuer and the child

3.   IN-HOSPITAL CARDIAC ARREST

- Evaluate
- Initiate basic life support
- Shout for help

3.1   Airway adjuncts

- Oral and nasopharyngeal airways are often underused
- They are particularly useful to aid bagging while awaiting the arrival of a doctor with advanced airway skills or in the pre-arrest child
- **Oral airway**: to find the right size hold the flange of the airway at centre of incisors and the tip should reach to the angle of the mandible
- **Nasal airway**: can be sized by measuring the distance from the tip of the nose to the tragus of the ear

3.2 Oxygen

This should be:

- Administered immediately in all arrest scenarios
- Given by face mask or bag and mask with a flow of 15 litres per minute
- With a reservoir or non-rebreath bag attached

Make sure the arrest team and appropriate senior help are called.

3.3 Assessment of rhythm

Once effective ventilation is achieved with a patent airway and movement of the chest, assess the circulation, including use of monitoring and assessing the rhythm.

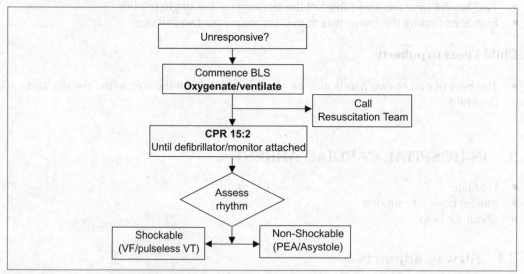

Algorithm for management of cardiac arrest in hospital

Asystole

This is the most common arrest rhythm in neonates and children and is usually secondary to hypoxia and acidosis from respiratory failure. It is often preceded by a bradycardia.

- Check the leads are attached correctly
- Increase the gain on the monitor
- Check the pulses if trained and experienced (no longer than 10 seconds)

Pulseless electrical activity

There are recognizable complexes on the ECG but no pulse.

200

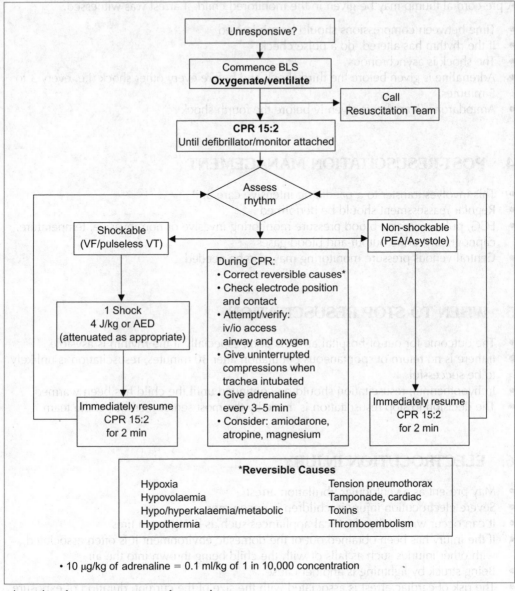

Algorithm for management of asystole

Ventricular fibrillation/pulseless ventricular tachycardia

This is an uncommon rhythm in children but can occur in:

- Hypothermia
- Electrocution injury
- Cardiac disease
- Poisoning with tricyclic antidepressants
- Hyperkalaemia

A pre-cordial thump may be given in the monitored child, if arrest was witnessed.

- Time between compressions should be minimized
- If the rhythm has altered, do a pulse check
- The shock is asynchronous
- Adrenaline is given before the third shock and before every other shock (i.e. every 3 to 5 minutes)
- Amiodarone (5 mg/kg) is given iv before the fourth shock

4. POST-RESUSCITATION MANAGEMENT

- This involves transfer to a paediatric intensive care unit
- Regular reassessment should be performed
- ECG, pulse oximetry, blood pressure monitoring invasive or non-invasive, temperature, capnography, urine output and blood gases
- Central venous pressure monitoring may also be needed

5. WHEN TO STOP RESUSCITATION

- The outcome for out-of-hospital arrest is poor, especially if the rhythm is asystole
- If there is no return of spontaneous circulation after 30 minutes, resuscitation is unlikely to be successful
- In hypothermia, resuscitation should be continued until the child has been warmed
- The decision to stop resuscitation is made by the most senior member of the team

6. ELECTROCUTION INJURY

- May present as a ventricular fibrillation arrest
- Severe electrocution injury in children is uncommon
- It can occur with faulty electrical appliances such as living room fires
- If the injury has been obtained out of the domestic environment it is often associated with other injuries such as falls or with the child being thrown into the air
- Being struck by lightning is another cause
- The risk of cardiac arrest is associated with the size of the current, duration of exposure and whether the current is AC (alternating current) or DC (direct current)
- Tetany can occur in the muscles which may make the child cling on to the electrical source e.g. the bar of an electric fire
- If tetanus occurs in the diaphragm and other respiratory muscles, it can lead to a respiratory arrest which continues until the child is disconnected
- Tetany occurs at currents < 100 mA. Defibrillators in resuscitation deliver about 10 A
- The child should be examined for entry and exit burns

- The path of the current can be estimated from the site of the entry and exit burns and by assuming the current will take the path of least resistance from the point of contact to the earth
- Fluid and blood have the least resistance whereas skin and bone have a high resistance
- The damage is caused by heat. Nerves, blood vessels, skin and muscle are damaged the most
- Swelling of tissues, especially muscles, can lead to compartment syndrome and myoglobinuria
- Myoglobinuria can lead to renal failure if unrecognized and untreated

6.1   Lightning injury

- Large direct current of short duration
- Can depolarize the myocardium and cause immediate asytole

6.2   Treatment of electrocution

- Disconnect from source of electrocution
- Immobilize cervical spine
- ABC: **A**irway, **B**reathing and **C**irculation
- Search for entry and exit points
- Consider other injuries
- Dysrhythmias may occur late
- Ventricular fibrillation is more common in this type of injury
- The external burn may look trivial but a greater fluid requirement is needed because of internal heat injury
- Myoglobinuria can occur as a result of massive internal thermic injuries with a relatively small external burn

6.3   Myoglobinuria

- Occurs after muscle injury such as a crush injury or electrocution
- Can be detected in the urine
- Treatment is maintaining a urine output of greater than 2 ml/kg per hour by fluid loading and diuretics, using mannitol if required
- Alkalinize the urine by using iv sodium bicarbonate to improve the excretion of myoglobin
- Alkalinization of the urine is used to keep a toxin in its ionized form, to reduce the amount of absorption in the renal tubule
- This is called forced alkaline diuresis and is also used for aspirin and phenobarbitone overdose

7. AIRWAY

The main aspects of airway that need to be addressed are:

- Obstruction
- Choking
- Failure to protect the airway from aspiration of gastric contents

7.1 Airway obstruction

- Obstruction of the airway can occur at all anatomical levels of the respiratory tract from the nose to the small airways. Obstruction of the upper airway is characterized by stridor, which is a high-pitched sound, heard on inspiration, whereas a lower airway obstruction produces an expiratory wheeze
- The upper and lower airways in children are smaller than in adults. Airway resistance is inversely proportional to the radius raised to the power of four. Therefore, halving the radius results in a 16-fold increase in resistance. This means that airway resistance is higher in small children
- Mucosal swelling and secretions are also more likely to obstruct the airway in infants, as the airways are small
- A bubbling or gurgling noise suggests pharyngeal secretions and is common in children with poor pharyngeal tone, as in cerebral palsy
- Poor pharyngeal tone also causes partial obstruction and snoring especially when the child is asleep or post-ictal
- Grunting is more likely to be heard in neonates and is the noise caused by expiration against a partially closed glottis. The lung volume at the end of expiration is almost equal to the closing volume in infants making atelectasis and areas of collapse common

Causes of airway obstruction

- Croup/laryngotracheobronchitis (stridor). There may be thick secretions, as in bronchitis, that may, rarely, obstruct the airway
- Epiglottitis (drooling, toxic, quiet stridor)
- Bacterial tracheitis
- Inhaled foreign body
- Asthma (wheeze or silent chest) or bronchiolitis
- Tracheobronchomalacia (prolonged expiratory phase)
- Extrinsic compression; vascular ring, mediastinal tumour
- Facial trauma and burns
- Anaphylaxis
- Angioneurotic oedema
- Retropharyngeal abscess, large tonsils and adenoids
- Diphtheria

Treatment of airway obstruction

If there is a concern about airway obstruction it is essential to get senior help with experience in airway skills. It may be necessary to move the child to theatre. Prior to the arrival of senior help the child should be kept calm, and be left in the position they find most comfortable, often on the parent's knee. They should be given high-flow oxygen and a saturation monitor should be attached. The saturations in air and high-flow oxygen should be recorded at regular intervals. It is important not to distress the child. An ENT surgeon may well be needed. Nebulized adrenaline (5 ml of 1 : 1000) with oxygen through a face mask, can be used while awaiting the arrival of experienced help. When experienced help arrives they will intubate using a gas induction anaesthetic of sevoflurane or halothane via an anaesthetic machine. This is usually done in theatre with the ENT surgeon present.

Once the child's airway is secured oral prednisolone, and antibiotics if a bacterial infection is suspected, can be commenced.

If the obstruction is the result of poor pharyngeal tone a soft nasal airway is useful for both opening the airway and for suctioning of secretions.

Airway obstruction can occur with an endotracheal tube in position and is either the result of obstruction distal to the tube or of secretions within the lumen of the tube. This presents as desaturation.

7.2   Choking

- A blind finger sweep should not be performed

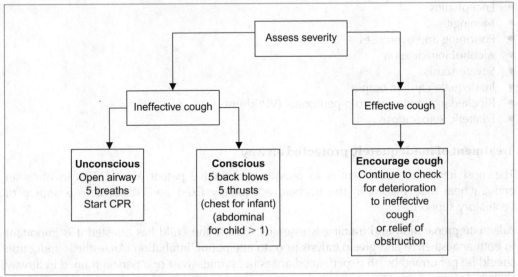

Infant choking protocol

- The baby is placed along one of the rescuer's arms in the head-down position with the rescuer's hand supporting the baby's jaw, keeping it open in the neutral position

- The rescuer then rests his or her arm along the thigh and delivers five back blows with the heel of the hand
- If the obstruction is not relieved, the baby is turned over and with head down is given five chest thrusts using the same landmarks as for cardiac compression
- The back blows and chest thrusts are at a rate of 1 per second
- If the infant is too large, place across the rescuer's lap and perform the same technique

Child choking protocol

- For the choking child, use abdominal thrusts instead of chest thrusts the rest of the protocol remains the same including the back blows
- The Heimlich manoeuvre can be performed in a child but never in an infant because of the risk of trauma to internal structures. The patient can be standing, sitting, kneeling or lying for the Heimlich manoeuvre

7.3 Inadequate airway protection

This is usually the result of decreased consciousness level and has several causes.

- Head injury associated with P on the AVPU scale, only responding to pain or a Glasgow Coma Scale score of 8 and below (A = Alert, V = responds to voice, P = responds to pain, U = unconscious)
- Fits
- Metabolic encephalopathy
- Hepatic encephalopathy
- Encephalitis
- Meningitis
- Poisoning and overdoses
- Alcohol intoxication
- Severe sepsis
- Inadequate cardiac output
- Blocked/infected ventriculo-peritoneal (VP) shunt
- Diabetic ketoacidosis

Treatment of inadequately protected airway

The most immediate treatment is to provide a definitive patent airway. This involves an endotracheal tube placed in the trachea, adequately fixed and attached to a source of ventilatory support.

Adequate preparation and training is essential. Unless the child has arrested it is important to both anaesthetize and give paralysis prior to attempting intubation. Anaesthetic induction should be performed by an experienced anaesthetist/intensivist or a person trained in airway skills.

If the child is not starved, a rapid sequence induction should be used with cricoid pressure to prevent aspiration of gastric contents.

If there is airway obstruction it is preferable to use a gas induction using sevoflurane or halothane.

It is important for the paediatrician to recognize airway compromise and to call for appropriate senior help. While awaiting help it is useful to draw up emergency drugs: adrenaline, atropine and suxamethonium, to get out appropriately sized endotracheal tubes and to know when and how to use basic airway adjuncts such as oral and nasopharyngeal airways.

An endotracheal tube in the right main bronchus, even for a short period of time, can cause right upper lobe collapse. It is therefore important to confirm the position of the endo-tracheal tube on a chest X-ray soon after placement. It is good practice to write in the notes the size of endotracheal tube used, the length at which it is taped or fixed at the nose or mouth as well as a comment on the view of the cords at intubation (a Grade 1 intubation is where the whole cords are viewed) and the degree of space round the tube at the cords.

8. RESPIRATORY FAILURE

Respiratory failure is defined as an inability of physiological compensatory mechanisms to ensure adequate oxygenation and carbon dioxide clearance resulting in either arterial hypoxia or hypercapnia, or both.

The most common causes of respiratory failure are an upper or lower respiratory tract illness; however, disorders of other systems can present with breathing difficulties and should be considered in the differential diagnosis.

Causes of respiratory failure

Neuromuscular disease	Muscle weakness	Respiratory failure
Gut disease e.g. peritonitis	Abdominal distension Pain	Respiratory failure
Cardiac failure	Pulmonary oedema	Tachypnoea
Head injury and fits	Central causes	Reduced respiratory drive
Diabetic ketoacidosis	Metabolic acidosis	Deep sighing respirations
Poisoning		↑ or ↓ respiratory drive

In children with respiratory infections the reduced lung compliance is reflected in recession, which is an indrawing of the ribs and is a useful clinical sign. Recession, however, reduces the efficiency of breathing and makes it harder to retain lung volume.

8.1 Apnoea

This is a common sign in neonates and small infants and has a wide differential diagnosis.

- Prematurity
- Bronchiolitis

- Pertussis
- Pneumonia
- Sepsis
- Severe gastro-oesophageal reflux
- Fits
- NAI (non-accidental injury)
- Vascular ring

8.2 Trauma and breathing difficulties

Chest injury following trauma can be difficult to differentiate from other causes of respiratory distress. Children's rib cages are much more compliant than adults and so rib fractures are far less common. If rib fractures are present it suggests severe chest injury and underlying lung contusion is almost inevitable. If they occur in the absence of a good story of trauma, non-accidental injury should always be considered although, it is important to exclude osteogenesis imperfecta or metabolic bone disease.

If there is a history of trauma, then inhalational injuries and, rarely, a fractured larynx should be considered as well as pneumothorax, tension pneumothorax, massive haemothorax and cardiac tamponade.

Abdominal pain and distension can present with breathing difficulties.

8.3 Management of acute severe asthma

The initial treatment of asthma is described in the respiratory chapter and is summarized as:

- Nebulized bronchodilators continuously (salbutamol)
- Add in nebulized atrovent
- Hydrocortisone iv
- Aminophylline iv
- Salbutamol iv up to a maximum of 5 µg/kg per minute
- Consider magnesium sulphate iv to keep magnesium levels at 1.5–2.5 mmol/l

In a child with asthma, ventilation should be avoided if possible but is necessary if the child is either hypoxic or exhausted.

If child is intubated

- Ketamine is the induction agent of choice as it is a bronchodilator
- Ketamine infusion can be added in
- Manual decompression of the chest on expiration gives an indicator of the severity
- Permissive hypercapnia is a ventilation strategy where the carbon dioxide levels are allowed to rise as long as the pH remains above 7.2
- Finding the ideal level of positive end-expiratory pressure (PEEP) is difficult in a ventilated asthmatic and is often done by trial and error. Measuring the auto-PEEP can help

- A slow respiratory rate is usually necessary, i.e. < 20
- It is important to remember that there is still mortality from asthma and so a respiratory paediatrician should be consulted in any child with asthma severe enough to need admission to the paediatric intensive care unit (PICU)

8.4 Ventilating children with bronchiolitis

There are three reasons to ventilate a child with bronchiolitis

- Apnoea
- Worsening blood gases, usually hypoxia despite maximum oxygen
- Exhaustion

Once a baby is ventilated they:

- Need enteral nutrition
- Usually need to remain ventilated for at least 4 days or until the basal crepitations have disappeared

Severe bronchiolitis can be confused with pertussis (history, raised lymphocyte count). Prophylactic immunization can be used in children at high risk of RIV bronchiolitis.

8.5 Children with pertussis needing admission to PICU

- Indications as for bronchiolitis
- Usually babies < 2 months of age
- Is associated with a high white-cell count
- May have a prolonged stay on PICU
- Occasionally needs extracorporeal membrane oxygenation (ECMO)

8.6 Cardiac causes of respiratory failure

The pulmonary vascular bed is also more muscular in infants and can lead to pulmonary hypertension or pulmonary vasoconstriction. This can lead to right-to-left shunting across a patent foramen ovale, can open up the ductus arteriosus or can cause shunting across any pre-existing cardiac defects such as an atrial or a ventricular septal defect. This results in cyanosis.

Children with cardiac disease with high pulmonary blood flow are more susceptible to pulmonary hypertension. Oxygen is a potent pulmonary vasodilator. It is also important to normalize the carbon dioxide levels and to avoid acidosis. Specific treatments such as inhaled nitric oxide or sildenafil can also be used. Pulmonary hypertension that does not respond to these treatments is called unreactive pulmonary hypertension and is a poor prognostic sign.

8.7 Treatment of respiratory failure

Some form of respiratory support is often needed. This includes

- Supplementary oxygen with or without an airway
- Non-invasive ventilation
- Conventional ventilation
- Oscillation
- ECMO

Airways

- The oropharyngeal or Guedel airway is poorly tolerated in the conscious patient and may cause vomiting
- The nasopharyngeal airway is better tolerated but may cause haemorrhage from the vascular nasal mucosa

Non-invasive ventilation

- Nasal prong or short-tube continuous positive airways pressure (CPAP) may be an intermediate intervention as is nasal or facial mask biphasic positive airway pressure (BIPAP)
- Non-invasive ventilation is particularly useful in children with neuromuscular disorders as an alternative to ventilation, or as part of the weaning process post extubation
- If there are areas of atelectasis or collapse, recruitment of the lung can be achieved with CPAP or BIPAP so avoiding the need for intubation

Oscillation

- Oscillation is used as a lung protective strategy to prevent damage to the lungs caused by high pressures and excessive shearing forces
- Oscillation uses a high mean airway pressure to recruit the lung and prevent alveolar collapse

ECMO

- ECMO or extracorporeal membrane oxygenation is a treatment used for reversible conditions where ventilation has become extremely difficult and the pressures required to adequately oxygenate are damaging to the lungs
- For respiratory disorders vein–vein ECMO is used, where both cannulas are inserted into veins
- It can also be used to support the heart either as a bridge to transplantation or if there is a reversible cardiac failure; this requires vein–artery ECMO where both a vein and an artery are cannulated
- ECMO is a very specialist therapy and is only performed in ECMO centres
- A cardiac surgeon inserts the cannulas for ECMO

9. CARDIOVASCULAR SYSTEM

9.1 The child with tachycardia

Tachycardia is one of the most useful clinical signs. There are multiple causes, so having a structured system is helpful. The following system is one of exclusion and is a useful bedside exercise.

There are seven main groups of causes for tachycardia

- Arrhythmia
- Inadequate cardiac output
  - Preload
  - Inotropic
  - Afterload
  - Tamponade
- Ventilation
  - Hypoxia
  - Hypercapnia
  - Anaemia
  - Blocked tube
  - Pneumothorax (usually tension)
- Central
  - Pain
  - Fits
  - Fever
  - Anxiety
- Pulmonary hypertension
- Drugs
- Poor ventricular function

The majority of these causes can be excluded on clinical signs or by simple measures such as giving some pain relief. It is then possible to decide whether it is necessary to get a cardiac opinion.

9.2 Supraventricular tachycardia

Supraventricular tachycardia (SVT) is the commonest tachyarrhythmia dealt with by paediatricians. It can often be difficult to differentiate from a sinus tachycardia. This is because the QRS complex is narrow and regular. The younger the child the more likely SVT will cause cardiovascular instability.

Symptoms include palpitations, heart failure and shock.

However with SVT:

- The onset is sudden as opposed to a gradual increase in rate
- There is no beat to beat variation
- The rate does not become slower with a bolus of fluid.

211

- Rate is usually greater than 220 beats per minute
- P waves, if visualized, are negative in leads II, III and AVF

Treatment of SVT

- ABC
- Vagal stimulation
  - Diving reflex; iced water on the face or immerse the face in iced water for 5 seconds
  - Carotid body massage on one side only
  - Valsalva manoeuvre in the older child

Drug management
Intravenous adenosine must be given quickly and into a large vein followed by a saline flush — the child must be ECG monitored.

- Start with a bolus of 100 µg/kg
- If unsuccessful after 2 minutes increase the dose to 200 µg/kg
- If unsuccessful after a further 2 minutes increase to 300 µg/kg
- The maximum total dose is
  - 300 µg/kg if child is < 1 month of age
  - 500 µg/kg if child is > 1 month — to a maximum of 12 mg single dose
- Side-effects are short lived though unpleasant (flushing, nausea, chest tightness, shortness of breath.) Some older children describe a feeling of impending doom
- It is important to involve a paediatric cardiologist
- They will consider cardioversion, especially if the child is shocked, or further drug treatment with flecanide, amiodarone, digoxin or β-blockers

Cardioversion

- This should be performed under anaesthesia using a synchronized DC shock
  - Initially use 1 J/kg
  - Follow with 2 J/kg if unsuccessful
  - Followed with 2 J/kg if still unsuccessful
- Hands-free defibrillation is a safe alternative to using the paddles
- A 12-lead ECG is essential to adequately diagnose any change in rhythm.

9.3 Causes of tachyarrhythmia

- Re-entrant tachycardia
- Cardiomyopathy
- Post cardiac surgery
- Drug-induced
- Long QT syndrome
- Metabolic disturbances
- Poisoning

9.4   Ventricular tachycardia

If the child is haemodynamically stable it is vital to consult a paediatric cardiologist.

- Treat electrolyte disturbances of potassium, calcium and magnesium
- Cardiologist may use amiodarone, often with a loading dose. However, this drug is negatively inotropic and can depress cardiac function
- Use anaesthesia for DC synchronized cardioversion
  - Use 1 J/kg, then 2 J/kg

If the child is pulseless follow ventricular fibrillation protocol.

9.5   Causes of bradyarrhythmia

The rate is slow and usually irregular. It is usually a pre-terminal sign.

If there has been a vagal stimulant to the bradycardia use atropine 20 µg/kg iv or via interosseous access.

- Pre-terminal event in hypoxia and shock
- Raised intracranial pressure
- Conduction damage post cardiac surgery
- Congenital heart block
- Myocarditis

9.6   Emergency management of severe heart failure

- Assess ABC
- Give high-flow oxygen
- Ventilation
- Diuresis
- Offload the heart
- Maximize oxygen-carrying capacity — exclude anaemia
- Inotropes

A child with a severe cardiomyopathy may need a dobutamine infusion. This can be given peripherally through an iv cannula. Non-invasive ventilation may also be useful.

The management of heart failure within the context of structural heart defects is discussed in Chapter 1 — Cardiology.

9.7   Recognizing low cardiac output state

- Tachycardia
- Low urine output or anuria
- Poor capillary refill
- Confusion

Late signs include:

- Hypotension
- Bradycardia
- Confusion can be a late sign
- ST depression on ECG

9.8 Inotropes

- An inotrope is used to improve the cardiac output
  - Cardiac Ouput = Heart Rate × Stroke Volume
- In the healthy adult the heart has the ability to change its stroke volume dramatically, this occurs during exercise and improves with training
- Neonates, however, have a more fixed stroke volume so need to increase their heart rate to improve the cardiac output
- Once a neonate or child becomes too tachycardic the heart no longer has time to fill and the cardiac output will reduce
- When a child is in sinus rhythm the atrial kick can provide between 10 and 25% of the cardiac output, if a child goes into atrioventricular block the blood pressure drops
- There is no perfect inotrope as all inotropes have unwanted effects such as increasing the metabolic demands of the heart

The best way to understand which inotrope to use when, is to understand which adrenoreceptor of the sympathetic nervous system each inotrope works on

- Stimulating β1-receptors increases both the heart rate and contractility of the heart
- Stimulating β2-receptors causes muscle relaxation in the smooth musculature of the airways, causing bronchodilatation, and also relaxes the peripheral vessels, causing a peripheral vasodilatation
- Stimulating α-receptors causes a peripheral vasoconstriction, increasing the peripheral vascular resistance

Most inotropes stimulate increased production of the enzyme adenyl cyclase to promote an increase in intracellular calcium, which results in increased contractility of the cardiac muscle.

Adrenaline

- Works on all the above receptors but its β1-receptor and α-receptor effects predominate
- Increases heart rate
- Increases cardiac contractility
- Increases blood pressure by increasing the peripheral vascular resistance

However,

- It makes the heart stiff, i.e. the ventricle is unable to fully relax in diastole
- It greatly increases the metabolic demands of the heart

These effects are also seen with other inotropes.

Dopamine

- Stimulates mainly β1-receptors at lower doses but at higher doses it has increasing α-receptor effects
- Increases heart rate
- Increases contractility
- There is probably a low-dose renal effect

However, dopamine is more arrhythmogenic than other inotropes.

Dobutamine

- Stimulates mainly β1- and β2-receptors at lower doses but at higher doses it has increasing α-receptor effects
- Increases heart rate
- Increases contractility of the heart
- Vasodilates at low doses and vasoconstricts at high doses
- Can bronchodilate
- Can be given peripherally

However, like dopamine, it is very arrhythmogenic.

Noradrenaline

- Stimulates mainly α-receptors, although in large doses it has some β-receptor effects
- Increases blood pressure by increasing the peripheral vascular resistance

Milrinone

- Is a phosphodiesterase inhibitor that works by preventing breakdown of adenyl cyclase. It is an inotrope that is used mainly with cardiac conditions
- It can be given peripherally
- It has a long half-life ($2\frac{1}{2}$ hours in adults)
- It causes peripheral vasodilatation
- It relaxes the ventricle in diastole (lusiotrophic action)
- It has an inotropic effect
- It is often termed an inodilator rather than an inotrope

When they are used for more than a few days in large amounts, inotropes become less effective as the receptors down-regulate. When this happens, either the inotrope is changed or steroids are given.

Decreasing the metabolic demands can have an inotrope-like effect. This is seen when a child is ventilated, pain is controlled and pyrexia is treated.

9.9 The child in shock

Shock is defined as inadequate perfusion and oxygenation of the tissues.

Causes of shock:

- Cardiogenic — e.g. cardiomyopathy, arrhythmias, myocarditis
- Hypovolaemic — e.g. haemorrhage, burns, gastroenteritis
- Distributive — e.g. anaphylaxis, sepsis
- Dissociative — e.g. severe anaemia, carbon monoxide poisoning
- Obstructive — e.g. tension pneumothorax, cardiac tamponade

Shock is further subdivided into

- Compensated
- Uncompensated
- Irreversible

The most common causes of shock in children are bleeding, septicaemia and gastro-enteritis.

Septic shock

- One of the most common causes of shock in children is meningococcal disease
- Systemic inflammatory response syndrome is seen, characterized by:
  - Vasodilatation
  - Pyrexia
  - Cascade of inflammatory markers
  - Coagulation disorder
  - Depressed myocardial function

Spinal shock

- Bradycardia
- Hypotension

Anaphylaxis

Allergy is an increasingly common problem and is immunologically mediated. It can present as respiratory distress with either stridor or wheeze, or as cardiovascular collapse.

Treatment

- Remove allergen
- Assess ABC
- Give high-flow oxygen
- Adrenaline im 10 µg/kg = 0.01 ml/kg of 1 in 1,000
- If complete obstruction,
  - Obtain a definitive airway

- If partial obstruction
  - Give nebulized adrenaline 5 ml of 1 in 1,000
  - Give hydrocortisone 4 mg/kg initial dose then 2–4 mg/kg 6-hourly
  - If wheeze present, give nebulized salbutamol,
  - Consider iv salbutamol 1–5 µg/kg per min
  - If shock present, give 20ml/kg fluid bolus, consider adrenaline infusion
  - Chlorpheniramine iv tds 250 µg/kg if < 1 year; > 1 year dose by age

10. MANAGING THE CHILD WITH SEVERE BURNS

The main issues to consider are

- Early first-aid measures are important, minimizing the duration of exposure to the heat; tepid water is used
- The airway can deteriorate rapidly and swelling of the airway can make intubation difficult, so early intervention and experienced airway help are necessary
- Shock in the first few hours is not the result of the burn injury and other causes of fluid loss, e.g. bleeding must be considered
- Fluid requirements are high and should be calculated from the time of injury and not from the time of arrival in the Emergency department
- Circumferential burns of the chest may restrict breathing so a burns surgeon should be consulted
- Burns are associated with other injuries, e.g. jumping out of windows in house fires or explosions, so consider that the cervical spine, for example, may be injured

10.1 Epidemiology

- Burn injuries are very common but the majority are minor
- 70% occur in children < 5 years
- Infants and children with learning difficulties are at increased risk
- House fires account for most fatal burn injuries and the cause of death is usually smoke inhalation
- In England and Wales 23 children died in 2001 from burns
- There is a strong link between burns and poverty
- Late infection is a significant cause of morbidity in children with burns injuries

10.2 Pathophysiology

- The severity of the burn depends on both the temperature and the time of contact with the burn
- Six hours contact at 44°C would be needed to cause cellular destruction, whereas at 54°C only 30 seconds contact is needed to cause injury. 30s at 54°C will cause cellular destruction

10.3   Assessment

- Signs of inadequate breathing include abnormal respiratory rate, abnormal chest movement and cyanosis, which is a late sign
- Reduced consciousness level may be the result of other injuries causing hypovolaemia, or of a head injury or it may be secondary to hypoxia
- Child protection issues should be considered

10.4   Indications of an inhalational injury

- History of exposure to smoke in a confined space
- Carbonaceous sputum (black sputum)
- Soot deposits around nose or mouth or on clothes

10.5   Assessment of the burn

- The severity of the burn is described by the percentage of the total body surface area affected and by the depth of burn
- The patient's palm and adducted fingers cover a surface area of approximately 1% of the total surface area
- The rule of nines for calculating the % burn is not applicable to children and a paediatric chart should be used
- Burns are classified as superficial, partial thickness and full thickness
  - Superficial burns cause injury only to the epidermis and are red and painful with no blisters
  - Partial thickness burns are also painful, blistered and the skin is pink or mottled
  - Full thickness burns are painless and both the dermis and epidermis are involved and sometimes deeper tissues. The skin is white or charred and feels leathery
- Special areas include the face, hands and feet, perineal burns and circumferential burns ie a burn that extends round the whole circumference of a limb or trunk which can act as a tourniquet round the limb or trunk as the burned skin contracts

10.6   Treatment

- High-flow oxygen
- Early airway assessment
- Ideally two intravenous cannulas should be placed in unburnt areas
- Early and adequate analgesia is important
- Burns of > 10% will need extra fluid in addition to their maintenance requirements. The estimated fluid = % burn × weight (kg) × 4 given over 24 hours. Half of this is given in the first 8 hours from the burn injury. Urinary catheters are essential in severe burns to assess adequate fluid resuscitation and urine output should be kept at 2 ml/kg per hour
- There is a high risk of rapid heat loss following a burn injury so after initial exposure the child should be re-covered and kept warm

- Circumferential burns may need surgical intervention (escharotomies)
  - Escharotomies are needed when the burn injury affects the whole of the dermis and the skin loses its ability to expand as oedema progresses. The burned wound is excised surgically down to the subcutaneous fat
- Carbon monoxide poisoning is discussed in Chapter 3 — Clinical Pharmacology and Toxicology.
- Inhalation of carbon monoxide may occur when a child has been in a house fire
- Inhalation of carbon monoxide induces the production of carboxyhaemaglobin which has a much higher affinity for oxygen than normal haemoglobin. Oxygen is therefore not given up to the cells and cellular hypoxia occurs
- The pulse oximeter may show a normal saturation
- The treatment is 100% oxygen or hyperbaric oxygen if very high levels are found

10.7   When to transfer to a burns centre

- 10% partial and/or full thickness burns
- 5% full thickness burns
- Burns to special areas; face, hands, feet or perineum
- Any circumferential burn
- Significant inhalational burn (excludes pure carbon monoxide poisoning)
- Chemical, radiation or high voltage burns

10.8   Chemical burns

- Alkali burns are more serious than acid burns because alkalis penetrate more deeply
- If dry powder is present, brush it off before irrigation
- Irrigate with water for 20 to 30 minutes

11.   INJURIES DUE TO SEVERE COLD

11.1   Frostbite

- Treatment for frostbite should be immediate to reduce the duration of injury unless there is a risk of re-freezing
- Provide warm blankets and a warm drink
- Place the injured part in circulating water at 40°C until pink in colour (periods of 20 minutes are recommended)
- Avoid dry heat
- Give analgesia because re-warming can be very painful
- Cardiac monitoring is required during re-warming

11.2 Systemic hypothermia

(see also Section 16.3 Core re-warming)

- Core body temperature is below 35°C
- Use special low-registering thermometer
- Decreased level of consciousness is a common sign
- Arrhythmias are common
- Clotting abnormalities occur
- Re-warming can lead to shock, especially if rapid, and should be carried out over the same time period as the initial cooling process
- Cardiac drugs and defibrillation are not usually effective if hypothermia is present, therefore only perform one cycle of defibrillation until the temperature is above 30°C
- Patients should not be pronounced dead until they have been re-warmed to 35°C

12. SEVERE HEAD INJURY

The aim of intensive care management in severe head injury is to prevent further brain injury. Therefore, it is important to:

- Maintain good oxygenation
- Avoid hypotension
- Avoid pyrexia
- Avoid hyper- or hypoglycaemia

The head is a closed box once the fontanelles have closed. If there is an expanding lesion within this closed box, such as a bleed or swelling of the brain, the pressure inside the box increases. This is called the Munro–Kelly doctrine.

The compartments in the closed box are

- Brain
- Cerebrospinal fluid (CSF)
- Arterial blood
- Venous blood

As the brain swells or a bleed increases in size, there is initial compensation. Venous blood and CSF are drained out of the head. Once this has occurred there is a decompensation where a small increase in volume causes a rapid increase in pressure.

The clinical signs of herniation include bradycardia, hypertension and enlarging pupils.

It is important to maintain the blood supply to the brain. This is measured by cerebral perfusion pressure (CPP)

$$CPP = MAP - ICP$$

where MAP = mean arterial blood pressure in mmHg and ICP = intracranial pressure in mmHg.

12.1 Maintaining an adequate cerebral perfusion pressure

This requires the blood pressure to be significantly higher than the intracranial pressure.

The CPP levels for different age groups are:

- 50 mmHg in infants
- 60 mmHg in a child
- 70 mmHg in a teenager

Often the child needs to be hypertensive to maintain adequate blood supply to the head

- A higher than normal blood pressure may be needed to maintain adequate blood supply to the head
- Inotropic support with noradrenaline

This means a child with a severe head injury will need ventilating, will need central and arterial access and a means of measuring the intracranial pressure.

- Intracranial bolt
- Ventricular drain
- A device to detect fits, e.g. a cerebral function analysis monitor

12.2 Reducing raised intracranial pressure

- Keep head central
- Keep head raised 20–30 degrees
- Maintain low to normal CO_2, aiming for 4–4.5 KPa
- Maintain high serum sodium levels > 140
- Maintain high serum osmolality, give mannitol or hypertonic saline
- Drain CSF from a ventricular drain
- Minimize stimulation to the brain by pain relief and sedation
- Give a paralysing drug
- Provide extra sedation for procedures such as suction
- Avoid seizures

The benefits of either cooling to 34°C and/or craniectomy are controversial.

The outcome following severe head injury is better in children than adults. The initial Glasgow Coma Scale at the scene is a useful guide. If it is 8 or less, it is essential to intubate. It is essential to evacuate any expanding bleed as soon as possible; however, speed should not exclude adequate resuscitation.

12.3 Complications in intensive care

- Neurogenic diabetes insipidus can occur and if the urine output is excessive, paired serum and urine osmolalities must be performed and vasopressin given
- Constipation
- Pneumonia

- Pressure sores
- Risk of infection in ventricular drains

12.4 Imaging

- Cervical spine injuries cannot be excluded by a normal X-ray or computerized tomograph (CT), but must be cleared clinically as well
- Regular CT scans of the head are used to monitor progress
- Thoracolumbar spinal X-rays exclude a fracture (if the spine is fractured in one place there is an increased risk of a second spinal fracture)
- Secondary survey must be documented in the notes. This is a top-to-toe examination for other injuries and is important as smaller non-threatening injuries can cause significant morbidity

13. THE CONVULSING CHILD AND PICU

- Generalized convulsive status epilepticus is defined as a generalized convulsion lasting 30 minutes or longer or when successive convulsions occur so frequently over a 30 minute period that the child does not recover consciousness in between them
- The protocol for the management of status epilepticus is described in Chapter 18, Neurology
- Mortality still occurs and is 4%. Death may be caused by airway obstruction, aspiration from vomiting, hypoxia, an overdose of medication, cardiac arrhythmias or the underlying disease process
- Complications of prolonged fitting include hyperthermia, arrhythmias, brain damage, hypertension, pulmonary oedema, diffuse intravascular coagulation and myoglobinuria

13.1 Pathophysiology

- Convulsions increase the cerebral metabolic rate
- Blood pressure and heart rate increase as a result of a surge in sympathetic activity
- Cerebral arterial regulation is impaired and as the blood pressure increases, there is increased cerebral blood flow, this is followed by a drop in blood pressure if fits are prolonged and therefore a reduction in cerebral blood flow
- There is an increase in lactate and subsequent cell death and oedema
- The intracranial pressure rises
- Calcium and sodium cellular metabolism is impaired

13.2 Treatment

- ABC and treat hypoglycaemia
- High-flow oxygen
- Follow flow chart in Chapter 18 – Neurology (p 731)

Rapid sequence induction

This is an anaesthetic procedure undertaken when there is a risk of aspiration of gastric contents. It involves the following sequence

- Pre-oxygenation with 100% oxygen
- Give induction agent thiopentone (4 mg/kg or less if the child is hypovolaemic) and muscle relaxant (suxamethonium 2 mg/kg)
- Cricoid pressure is applied by an assistant to occlude the oesophagus
- The child is not bagged during this process
- Intubation
- Assess chest movement to confirm tube position, and listen with a stethoscope in both axillae and over the stomach
- Release cricoid pressure

The child is then taken for a CT scan or to PICU with full monitoring including saturation monitoring, capnograph, ECG monitoring and blood-pressure monitoring

The majority of children with status epilepticus will stop fitting with these measures. A minority do not and then a thiopentone coma is considered.

Thiopentone coma

This usually involves a thiopentone infusion sufficient to achieve burst suppression on the EEG. The coma is continued for 1–3 days. Continuous cerebral function analysis monitoring is needed

- Intracranial pressure monitoring may be useful
- Standard neuroprotective measures may be needed if raised intracranial pressure is suspected

Complications include:

- Status epilepticus may persist or fits may restart
- Chest infection
- Hypotension secondary to thiopentone
- Renal impairment secondary to thiopentone infusion

Alternatives include high-dose midazolam or high-dose phenobarbitone

A paediatric neurologist must be consulted

Consider the differential diagnoses:

- Meningoencephalitis
- Pneumococcal meningitis
- Poisoning
- Metabolic disorder
- Electrolyte imbalance
- Trauma
- Pyrexia and infection
- Hypertension

- Non-accidental injury
- Pertussis in a neonate
- Apnoea in a neonate leading to hypoxia

Although a cause is often not found.

14. NON-TRAUMATIC COMA

PICU are often asked to see these children as there is either a concern that they will hypoventilate or that they will not adequately protect their airway.

In children coma is caused by a diffuse metabolic insult in 95% of cases and by structural lesions in the remaining 5%.

There are many investigations that need to be considered but this list gives the basic essential investigations when the cause of coma is unknown.

- History
- Examination including temperature and pupils
- Blood
  - Haematology
  - Full blood count and film
  - Erythrocyte sedimentation rate
  - Coagulation
- Biochemistry
  - Blood gas
  - Glucose
  - Urea and electrolytes and creatinine
  - Liver function tests (aspartate aminotransferase (AST), alkaline phosphatase (ALP), bilirubin, albumin)
  - Calcium, phosphate
  - C-reactive protein
  - Serum lactate
  - Ammonia
  - Amino acids (especially raised leucine in maple-syrup urine disease)
  - Creatine kinase
  - Drug levels, e.g. salicylate levels, anticonvulsant levels including thiopentone
- Septic screen
  - Culture and sensitivity; blood, urine, stool, bronchoalveolar lavage (BAL), NPA
  - Antibodies mycoplasma IgG
  - Viral titre Epstein–Barr virus, herpes virus and common respiratory viruses
  - Virus isolation from nasopharyngeal aspirate (NPA) and BAL, common respiratory viruses
  - Polymerase chain reaction for meningococcus, herpes simplex, pneumococcus

- Urine
  - Dipstick
  - Microscopy, culture and sensitivity (MC&S)
  - Toxicology
  - Myoglobin
  - Urine electrolytes
  - Organic acids
  - Ketones
- Chest X-ray
- ECG
- Cranial ultrasound
- EEG
- CT scan
- Poisoning is covered in Chapter 3 – Clinical Pharmacology and Toxicology

15. TRAUMA

15.1 Life-threatening extremity imjuries

- Crush injuries of the abdomen and pelvis
- Traumatic amputation of an extremity; partial amputation is often more life-threatening than complete amputation
- Massive open long-bone fractures

Crush injuries

- Splinting of the pelvis required
- Embolization of bleeding vessels may be useful
- Trauma to the internal organs is more likely in children than adults following crush injuries

Complete or partial amputation

- Compression over femoral or brachial artery may help but use of a tourniquet is now contraindicated
- Elevation of the limb
- Advice from a specialist centre

Long-bone fracture

- Splinting
- Consider vascular injury and compartment syndrome
- Consider tetanus immunization status

15.2 Gunshot wounds and stabbing

These are both rare in children but the following tips are useful aid memoires.

- Bullets usually follow the path of least resistance so do not assume the trajectory of the bullet is in a direct line from the entrance to the exit wound
- The entrance wound is often round or oval with a blackened area of burn
- The exit wound is often ragged because of tearing of tissues
- In both stabbing and gunshot wounds it is important to define which structures are likely to have been penetrated

16. DROWNING

- 450,000 people die per year world-wide as a result of drowning
- Drowning can occur in even small amounts of water, e.g. a few inches of rainwater in a bucket
- World-wide, for children < 15 years of age, drowning is the commonest cause of accidental death
- The majority of drownings are preventable
- Bradycardia and dsyrhythmias are common at this stage as a result of the severe hypoxia
- Hypoxia is usually the cause of death

16.1 Pathophysiology

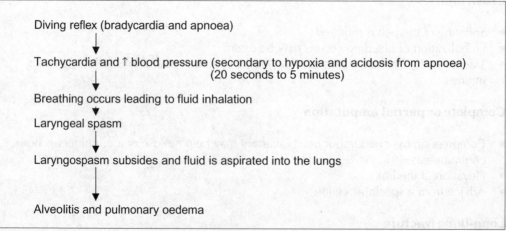

Pathophysiology of drowning

16.2   Treatment

- ABC

Consider:

- Hypothermia
- Hypovolaemia
- Spinal injury
- Electrolyte imbalance
- Other injuries
- Child protection issues
- Contaminated water can lead to infection with unusual organisms

Hypothermia can lead to disorders of coagulation and dysrhythmias and increased risk of infection.

- Remove from the water in a horizontal position to prevent venous pooling and distributive hypovolaemia
- Immobilize the spine
- Early and effective basic life support has been shown to improve outcome
- Secure an airway early and decompress the stomach with a nasogastric tube
- If core temperature is < 30°C prevent further cooling and re-warm
- Continue resuscitation until core temperature is > 35°C
- Below 30°C ventricular fibrillation may be refractory. Repeated shocks and inotropes should be delayed until the temperature is above this level, even in circulatory failure

16.3   Re-warming

(see also Section 11.2 Systemic hypothermia)

External re-warming

- Remove cold or wet clothes
- Supply warm blankets
- Use a heating blanket
- Use warm air
- Use an infrared radiant heat lamp

Core re-warming

- Only use warm fluids (warm to 39°C)
- Warm ventilator gases (42°C)
- Warm peritoneal dialysis fluids at 42°C
- Gastric or bladder lavage with normal saline
- Pleural or pericardial lavage
- Extracorporeal blood warming

External re-warming is appropriate for temperatures > 30°C.

During re-warming vasodilatation occurs, producing a relative hypovolaemia, often requiring fluid boluses.

Re-warming also increases the metabolic demands on the heart so myocardial dysfunction may become apparent on re-warming. Inotropes may be needed once the temperature is above 30°C.

16.4 Prognostic signs

Signs associated with a poor prognosis:

- Immersion for > 8 minutes
- If no respiratory effort has occurred after 40 minutes of full CPR the chances of survival are small — however, caveats to this are immersion in very cold water, a history of medication or alcohol intake
- It is unlikely for water in the UK to ever be cold enough to be neuroprotective
- Persisting coma
- pH of less than 7
- pO$_2$ < 8 despite treatment

Signs associated with a good prognosis

- If respiratory effort occurs within 3 minutes of starting CPR, the prognosis is good
- Provision of basic life support at the scene

Respiratory compromise may occur several hours after the drowning episode

17. FURTHER READING

APLS Manual 4th edition. 2005. BMJ Books.

Pearson G. *Handbook of Paediatric Intensive Care.* 2002. Saunders.

Shann F, Henning H. 2005. *Paediatric Intensive Care Guidelines*: 12th edition. Collective Pty Ltd.

Resuscitation Guidelines. 2005.Resuscitation Council (UK).

Chapter 7

Endocrinology

Heather Mitchell and Vasanta Nanduri

CONTENTS

Endocrinology

1. HORMONE PHYSIOLOGY

1.1 Introduction

Hormones are chemical messengers produced by a variety of specialized secretory cells. Their effects may be:

- Via transport to a distant site of action (endocrine)
- Direct, i.e. upon nearby cells (paracrine)

Plasma transport

- Most hormones are secreted into the systemic circulation, but those secreted from the hypothalamus are released into the pituitary portal system.
- Many hormones are bound to proteins when in the circulation. These binding proteins buffer against very rapid changes and act as a reservoir for the hormones — only free hormones can exert their biological action on tissues.

Examples of hormone–binding proteins

Hormone	Hormone binding proteins
Thyroxine	Thyroid-binding globulin, Albumin
Testosterone/oestrogen	Sex hormone-binding globulin
Insulin-like growth factor-1	Insulin-like growth factor-binding proteins
Cortisol	Cortisol-binding protein

1.2 Hormone–receptor interactions

Types of hormone

There are three main types of hormones:

- Amine — catecholamines, serotonin (5-hydroxytryptamine)
- Steroid — cortisol, aldosterone, androgens, oestrogen, progesterone
- Peptide — growth hormone (GH), insulin, thyroxine

Amine and peptide hormones have short half-lives (measured in minutes) and act on cell-surface receptors. Their secretion may be pulsatile and they often act via a second messenger (e.g. cyclic adenosine monophosphate (cAMP), calcium, etc.). Steroid hormones have longer half-lives (measured in hours) and act on intracellular receptors. They act on DNA to alter gene transcription and protein synthesis. Thyroxine is the exception to this rule as it acts as a steroid hormone and binds to intracellular receptors.

Intracellular messengers

- cAMP, e.g. glucagon, adrenocorticotrophic hormone (ACTH), luteinizing hormone (LH), follicle-stimulating hormone (FSH)
- Intracellular calcium, e.g. thyrotropin-releasing hormone (TRH), vasopressin, angiotensin II
- Tyrosine kinase, e.g. GH

G-protein receptors

Hormone receptors linked to cAMP do not generate cAMP directly, but act via a G-protein receptor on the cell surface. The G-proteins may be inhibitory — G_i (e.g. somatostatin) or stimulatory — G_s (e.g. all other hormones) to the formation of adenylate cyclase. Hormones that use intracellular calcium as an internal messenger activate the cytoplasmic enzyme phospholipase C (PLC), which then releases inositol triphosphate from membrane phospholipids, which in turn releases calcium from stores in the endoplasmic reticulum.

Second messengers

Insulin-like growth factor-1 (IGF-1) and IGF-2 are GH-dependent peptide factors. They are believed to modulate many of the anabolic and mitogenic actions of GH. IGF-1 is important as a post-natal growth factor, whereas IGF-2 is thought to be essential for fetal growth.

Disorders of hormone–receptor interactions

- Syndromes of G-protein abnormalities:
  - McCune–Albright syndrome
  - Pseudohypoparathyroidism

- Syndromes of receptor resistance:
  - Laron syndrome
  - Nephrogenic diabetes insipidus
  - Androgen insensitivity syndrome
  - Vitamin D-dependent rickets

1.3   Regulation

The effect and measured amount of a particular hormone in the circulation at any one time is the result of a complex series of interactions.

Control and feedback

Most hormones are controlled by some form of feedback. Insulin and glucose work on a feedback loop. Elevated glucose concentrations lead to insulin release, whereas insulin secretion is switched off when the glucose level decreases.

Receptor up- or down-regulation also occurs. Down-regulation leads to reduced sensitivity to a hormone and to a reduced number of receptors after prolonged exposure to high hormone concentrations. A good example of this is the administration of intermittent gonadotrophin-releasing hormone (GnRH), which induces priming and facilitates a large output of gonadotrophins, while continuous GnRH leads to a down-regulation of receptors and hence has a protective effect. However, this is not true of all pituitary hormones (e.g. ectopic ACTH secretion leads to receptor up-regulation, which is the reverse process).

Patterns of secretion

- Continuous — e.g. thyroxine
- Intermittent:
  - Pulsatile — FSH, LH, GH, prolactin
  - Circadian — e.g. cortisol
  - Stress-related — e.g. ACTH
  - Sleep-related — e.g. GH, prolactin

1.4   Investigation of hormonal problems

In view of the complexities of control on the concentration of a particular hormone and the various factors that influence its distribution and elimination, the use of a single random measurement of a hormone can be difficult to interpret. The plasma levels vary throughout the day because of pulsatile secretion, environmental stress, or circadian rhythms. They are also influenced by the values of the substrates they control. It is therefore often hard to define a normal range and dynamic testing may be required.

- Blood hormone concentration measurements:
  - Basal levels —those hormones in a steady state, e.g. thyroid function tests
  - Timed levels — those hormones whose levels need to be interpreted with a normal range for the time of day, e.g. cortisol measured at 0000 h and 0800 h
  - Stimulated — in suspected hormone deficiency, e.g. GH-stimulation tests
  - Suppression — in conditions of hormone excess as hormone-producing tumours usually fail to show normal negative feedback, e.g. dexamethasone suppression test for suspected Cushing's disease
- Urine concentrations:
  - Useful for identifying abnormalities in ratios of metabolites, e.g. diagnosis of the specific enzyme defect in congenital adrenal hyperplasia

2. HYPOTHALAMUS AND PITUITARY GLANDS

The hypothalamic–pituitary axis is of vital importance because it regulates many of the other endocrine glands in the body.

2.1 Anatomy

Hypothalamus

The hypothalamus extends from the pre-optic area (anteriorly) to the mamillary bodies (posteriorly) and includes the third ventricle. The hypothalamus has reciprocal connections with the frontal cortex and thalamus, and interacts with the limbic system and the brainstem nuclei involved in autonomic regulation, where it differentiates into discrete nuclei. The axonal processes extend down into the median eminence where regulatory hormones are secreted into the portal circulation.

Pituitary gland

Situated inferior to the hypothalamus within the pituitary fossa, above the sphenoid sinus, medial to the cavernous sinuses which contain the internal carotid arteries and cranial nerves III, IV and V. It is the combined product of an outgrowth of ectoderm from the buccal mucosa and the down-growth of neural tissue referred to as the 'infundibulum'.

The anatomical relationships of the anterior and posterior pituitary glands are important as tumours may arise from and/or compress surrounding structures.

- Above — optic chiasm, pituitary stalk, hypothalamus
- Below — sphenoid sinus, nasopharynx
- Lateral — cavernous sinus, internal carotid arteries, cranial nerves III, IV, V, VI
- Anterior lobe — derived from an invagination of oral mucosa (Rathke pouch)
- Posterior lobe — derived from neuronal tissue and contains neurones from the hypothalamus

Homeobox genes govern the embryonic development and gene expression. *PIT-1* is a homeobox gene that is necessary for the embryonic development of GH, prolactin and thyrotropin-producing cells.

2.2 Hormone physiology of the anterior pituitary

Gonadotrophins: LH and FSH

Structure

LH and FSH are glycoproteins composed of an α- and a β-subunit. The α-subunits are identical to other glycoproteins within the same species, whereas the β-subunits confer specificity.

Function

In the male, Leydig cells respond to LH, which stimulates the first step in testosterone production. In the female, LH binds to ovarian cells and stimulates steroidogenesis.

FSH binds to Sertoli cells in the male and increases the mass of the seminiferous tubules and supports the development of sperm. In the female, FSH binds to the glomerulosa cells and stimulates the conversion of testosterone to oestrogen.

Regulation

GnRH is released in a pulsatile fashion, which stimulates the synthesis and secretion of LH and FSH. Expression and excretion of FSH are also inhibited by inhibin, a gonadal glycoprotein. This has no effect on LH. In the neonate there are high levels of gonado-trophins and gonadal steroids. These decline progressively until a nocturnal increase occurs leading up to the onset of puberty (amplification of low-amplitude pulses).

Growth hormone (GH)

Structure

GH is a 191-amino acid peptide (22 kDa) secreted by somatotrophs. It circulates both in the unbound form and also bound to binding proteins, which are portions of the extracellular receptor domain.

Function

GH has direct effects on carbohydrate and lipid metabolism. The growth-promoting effects of GH are mediated by somatomedin C (otherwise known as IGF-1), which is produced in the liver cells following GH binding to cell-surface receptors which results in gene transcription. IGF-1 and IGF-2 are 70-amino acid peptides, structurally related to insulin. IGF-1 increases the synthesis of protein, RNA and DNA, increases the incorporation of protein into muscle, and promotes lipogenesis. The IGFs are bound to a family of binding proteins (IGFBP-1 to -6) of which IGFBP-3 predominates. These binding proteins not only act as transporters for the IGFs, but also increase their half-life and modulate their actions on peripheral tissues.

Regulation

GH secretion is pulsatile, consisting of peaks and troughs. Nocturnal release occurs during non-dreaming or slow-wave sleep, shortly after the onset of deep sleep. There is a gradual increase in GH production during childhood, a further increase (with increased amplitude of peaks) during puberty secondary to the effect of sex steroid, followed by a post-pubertal fall.

Three peptides are critical to the control of GH secretion:

- Growth hormone releasing hormone (GHRH)
- Growth hormone releasing peptide (GHRP) — ghrelin
- Somatostatin

These peptides mediate stimulation, inhibition and feedback suppression of GH secretion and form the final common pathway for a network of factors that influence the secretion of GH, which include sex steroids, environmental inputs and genetic determinants.

GHRH and somatostatin act via the activation of G-protein receptors on the somatotrophs, increasing or reducing cAMP and intracellular Ca^{2+}. GHRH stimulates GH release, whereas somatostatin inhibits both GH synthesis and its release. GH and IGF-1 exert a tight feedback control on somatostatin, and probably also on GHRH. GHRP — ghrelin — is an oligopeptide derivative of enkephalin and is a 28-peptide residue predominantly produced by the stomach. It requires fatty acylation of the N-terminal serine for biological activity and is released in response to acute and chronic changes in nutritional state. The concentrations of ghrelin fall post-prandially and in obesity and rise during fasting, after weight loss or gastrectomy and in anorexia nervosa. Both GHRP and GHRH act synergistically in the presence of a functioning hypothalamo-pituitary axis.

Prolactin

Structure
Prolactin has a similar amino acid sequence to GH, and acts via the lactogenic receptor, which is from the same superfamily of transmembrane receptors as the GH receptor.

Function
Prolactin is responsible for the induction of lactation and the cessation of menses during the puerperium. During the neonatal period, prolactin levels are high secondary to fetoplacental oestrogen; they then fall and remain consistent during childhood but there is a slight rise at puberty.

Regulation
Dopamine inhibition from the hypothalamus.

Thyroid-stimulating hormone (TSH)

Structure
TSH is a glycoprotein containing the same α-subunit as LH and FSH but a specific β-subunit.

Function
TSH is a trophic hormone and hence its removal reduces thyroid function to basal levels. It binds to surface receptors on the thyroid follicular cell and works via activation of adenylate cyclase to cause the production and release of thyroid hormone.

Regulation
TSH synthesis and release is modulated by TRH, which is produced in the hypothalamus and secreted into the hypophyseal portal veins, from where it is transported to the anterior pituitary gland. TRH secretion is influenced by environmental temperature, somatostatin and dopamine. Glucocorticoids inhibit TSH release at a hypothalamic level.

Adrenocorticotrophic hormone (ACTH)

Structure
ACTH is a 39-amino acid peptide cleaved from a large glycosylated precursor (pro-opiomelanocortin) which also gives rise to melanocyte-stimulating hormone and β-endorphin.

Function
ACTH is responsible for stimulation of the adrenal cortex and in particular the production of cortisol. Hypothalamic control of its function is evident in the late-gestation fetus. ACTH plays a role in fetal adrenal growth.

Regulation
Corticotropin-releasing hormone stimulates ACTH release via increasing cAMP levels. Arginine vasopressin (AVP) also stimulates ACTH release and potentiates the response to corticotropin-releasing hormone.

2.3 The neurohypophysis and water regulation

The body maintains its water balance by regulating fluid intake and output. There is a narrow range of normal serum osmolality between 280 and 295 mosmol/L.

Output
This is controlled by:

- Hypothalamic osmoreceptors and neighbouring neurones that secrete AVP
- Concentrating effect of the kidney

Input
This is controlled by:

- Hypothalamic thirst centre

Arginine vasopressin (AVP)

Structure
AVP is a nonapeptide containing a hexapeptide ring. It is produced as a pro-hormone in the supraoptic and paraventricular nuclei. Action potentials from the hypothalamus cause its release from the posterior pituitary gland into the circulation.

Regulation
This is largely by the osmolality of extracellular fluid and haemodynamic factors. The release of AVP is modulated by stimulatory and inhibitory neural input. Noradrenaline (norepinephrine) inhibits AVP release and cholinergic neurones facilitate it.

Physiology

The normal mature kidney is able to produce urine in a concentration range of 60–1100 mosmol/kg. The ability to vary urine concentration depends on the spatial arrangements and permeability characteristics of the segments of the renal tubules.

AVP regulates the permeability of the luminal membrane of the collecting ducts. Low permeability in the presence of a low AVP concentration leads to dilute urine.

2.4   Pituitary disorders

Anterior pituitary

Congenital

- Agenesis of the corpus callosum
- Structural abnormalities:
  - Septo-optic dysplasia
  - Pituitary hypoplasia
- Idiopathic hormonal abnormalities:
  - Isolated GH deficiency
  - Idiopathic precocious puberty

Acquired

- Excess, e.g. intracranial tumours:
  - Intracranial tumours
  - Cushing's disease — pituitary adenoma
- Deficiency, e.g. secondary to treatment with radiation or surgery:
  - Pituitary damage
  - Tumours
  - Surgery
  - Radiotherapy
  - Trauma

Septo-optic dysplasia (De Morsier syndrome)
A developmental anomaly of the midline structures of the brain. Classically characterized by:

- Absence of septum pellucidum and/or corpus callosum
- Optic nerve hypoplasia
- Pituitary hypoplasia with variable pituitary hormone deficiencies (most commonly this is GH deficiency which may either be isolated or progress to an evolving endocrinopathy)

Treatment is by hormone replacement and management of visual difficulties.

Craniopharyngioma
This is one of the most common supratentorial tumours in children. It commonly presents with headaches and visual field defects. On imaging, the tumour is frequently large and

cystic. Treatment is by resection plus radiotherapy if initial resection is incomplete or recurrence occurs.

Post-operative hormonal deficiencies are common, involving both anterior and posterior pituitary hormones. Treatment is by hormonal supplementation. There is also the risk of hypothalamic damage. Remember: the hypothalamus is responsible for other effects that are not so easily treated by replacement therapy, e.g. temperature, appetite and thirst control. The obesity associated with hypothalamic damage (secondary to hyperphagia) is very difficult to manage and has a poor prognosis. The maintenance of fluid homeostasis in children with the combination of diabetes insipidus and adipsia (loss of thirst sensation) can be a challenge.

Acquired endocrine problems secondary to tumours and/or their treatment

- Short stature
- Pubertal delay or arrest
- Precocious puberty
- Thyroid tumours
- Infertility
- Hypopituitarism — isolated or multiple
- Gynaecomastia

Posterior pituitary

Diabetes insipidus

Defined as insufficient AVP causing a syndrome of polyuria and polydipsia. With an intact thirst mechanism copious water drinking maintains normal osmolalities. However, problems with the thirst mechanism or insufficient water intake lead to hypernatraemic dehydration.

It is important to remember that cortisol is required for water excretion. Therefore, in children with combined anterior and posterior pituitary dysfunction, there is a risk of dilutional hyponatraemia if they are cortisol-deficient and receiving DDAVP (1-deamino-8-D-arginine vasopressin) treatment. Hence the emergency management of the unwell child is to increase their hydrocortisone treatment and to stop their DDAVP.

Causes of diabetes insipidus

- Central
  - Craniopharyngioma
  - Germinoma
  - Langerhans cell histiocytosis
  - Idiopathic
  - Trauma

- Nephrogenic
  - X-linked nephrogenic diabetes insipidus
  - Secondary to renal damage

Syndrome of inappropriate antidiuretic hormone (SIADH) secretion
Defined by the criteria of:

- Water retention with hypo-osmolality
- Normal or slightly raised blood volumes
- Less than maximally dilute urine
- Urinary sodium > sodium intake

Causes of SIADH

- Central nervous system disorders — meningitis, abscess; trauma; hypoxic–ischaemic insult
- Respiratory tract disease — pneumonia; cavitation
- Reduced left atrial filling — drugs
- Malignancies — lymphoma; bronchogenic carcinoma; idiopathic

Management of SIADH
Management focuses on treatment of the underlying cause and management of the fluid and electrolyte imbalance. Accurate input and output charts are required as are twice-daily weights in the initial period of assessment. Fluid restriction is the mainstay of management.

2.5 Investigation of hypothalamic and pituitary hormone disorders

Anterior pituitary stimulation tests

Many hormones (e.g. GH, LH and FSH) are secreted in a pulsatile fashion, and therefore a random measurement of the concentration of the circulating hormone is often inadequate for diagnosing a deficiency disorder.

Hormone measurement tests include:

- GH release/ACTH (via cortisol response) — insulin tolerance test/glucagon stimulation test
- TSH/prolactin response — TRH test
- FSH/LH response — LH releasing hormone (LHRH) test

GH tests
Provocation tests of GH are potentially hazardous. Insulin tolerance tests should only be performed in specialist centres because of the risk of severe hypoglycaemia. Other GH provocation tests include the use of glucagon, arginine and clonidine. Physiological tests of GH secretion include a 24-h GH profile and measurement of GH after exercise or during sleep.

Combined pituitary function test
The standard test involves the intravenous injection of either insulin or glucagon in combination with TRH and LHRH (in the pubertal child).

Blood samples are taken at 0 min (before stimulation) and at 20, 30, 60, 90 and 120 min after stimulation.

Following insulin administration, a profound hypoglycaemia results within 20 min which needs to be corrected by the use of an oral glucose solution or the judicious use of intravenous 10% dextrose. (**Remember**: the rapid correction of hypoglycaemia with a hypertonic glucose solution can result in cerebral oedema.)

GH concentrations rise at 30 min following insulin, or 60–90 min following glucagon injection. A rise to over 20 mU/L rules out GH deficiency.

A normal TSH response to TRH is a rise at 20 min post-dose and then a fall by 60 min. A continued rise of TSH at 60 min implies hypothalamic damage. Secondary hypothyroidism is demonstrated by a low baseline TSH level, whereas primary hypothyroidism is associated with a raised TSH.

A raised baseline prolactin level suggests a lack of hypothalamic inhibition of its release. Under normal circumstances following the administration of TRH, prolactin would be expected to rise at 20 min and then to be falling by 60 min.

In the absence of precocious puberty, the LHRH test will only demonstrate a rise in FSH and LH at 20 and 60 min during the first 6 months of life and in the peripubertal period. Raised baseline gonadotrophin levels reflect gonadal failure.

Posterior pituitary function tests

- Paired urine and serum osmolalities
- Water deprivation test

The child is weighed in the morning and is then deprived of water for a maximum of 7 h, during which time the child's weight, pulse rate and blood pressure and urine osmolality are measured hourly.

Plasma sodium levels and osmolality are measured every 2 h.

The test is terminated if the patient's weight falls by 5% from the starting weight, serum osmolality rises (> 295 mosmol/kg of water) in the face of an inappropriately dilute urine (< 300 mosmol/kg), or if the patient becomes significantly clinically dehydrated/clinically unwell.

A diagnosis of diabetes insipidus may be made in the presence of a plasma osmolality > 290 mosmol/kg of water with an inappropriately low urine osmolality.

The child is then given a dose of DDAVP and the urine and plasma osmolality are then measured. A rise in urine concentration confirms a diagnosis of central diabetes insipidus, whereas a child with nephrogenic diabetes insipidus will fail to concentrate urine after DDAVP.

2.6 Principles of management of hypothalamic–pituitary disorders

Treatment of anterior pituitary deficiencies

When specific hormones or their stimulating hormones are deficient the actual hormone may be replaced, e.g.:

- Lack of GH response — replace with GH

However, if the deficient hormone is a trophic or regulatory hormone then it is the target hormone that is replaced, e.g.:

- Lack of thyroid hormone — replace with thyroxine
- Low gonadotrophins — replace with testosterone in males, oestrogen in females
- ACTH — replace with hydrocortisone
- Vasopressin — replace with DDAVP

GH treatment

The following are the licensed indications for treatment with GH.

These recommendations have been endorsed by the National Institute for Clinical Excellence (NICE).

- Documented GH deficiency — congenital or acquired
- Turner syndrome
- Chronic renal failure
- Prader–Willi syndrome
- Small for gestational age

GH deficiency should be treated by a specialist who has experience of managing children with growth disorders. Most regimens involve daily injections with different doses of GH depending upon the indications. Close local/community liaison is required for this.

Panhypopituitarism

Panhypopituitarism is much less common than isolated hormone deficiency and may develop as an evolving endocrinopathy. Management includes replacement with GH, thyroxine, cortisol during childhood with induction and maintenance of puberty with the appropriate sex hormone (testosterone or estradiol). Parents of children who are cortisol- or ACTH-deficient should be given written instructions and training in the management of an acute illness and must have emergency supplies of intramuscular hydrocortisone available at all times.

Treatment of posterior pituitary deficiencies

Central diabetes insipidus
Treatment with DDAVP (desmopressin) either as a nasal spray or tablets.

3. GROWTH

3.1 Physiology of normal growth

Prenatal

Factors influencing intrauterine growth

- Nutrition
- Genetic
- Maternal factors (smoking, blood pressure)
- Placental function
- Intrauterine infections
- Endocrine factors — IGF-2

Postnatal growth

There are three principal phases of growth — infancy, childhood and puberty

Phases of postnatal growth	**Factors**
• Infancy	nutrition
• Childhood	GH (thyroxine)
• Puberty	sex hormones (GH)

Average growth during the pubertal phase is 30 cm (12 inches).

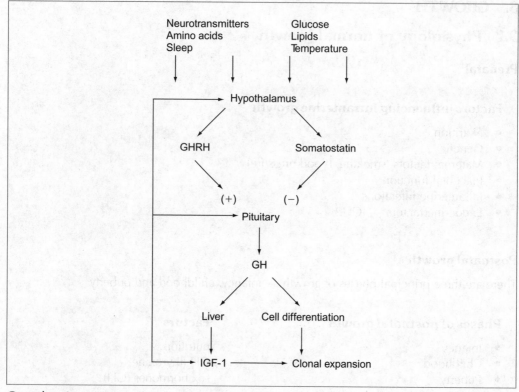

Growth axis

3.2 Assessment and investigation

The following parameters are important in the assessment of growth:

- Standing height
- Sitting height
- Head circumference
- Weight
- Skin-fold thicknesses
- Mid-arm circumference
- Pubertal status

Auxology

When measuring height, the optimal method is for the child to be measured by the same trained measurer, on the same equipment and at the same time of day on each occasion to minimize measurement error. A stadiometer should be used; supine height should be measured at < 2 years of age and standing height at > 2 years.

A child's height may be compared to the population using centile charts, and also considered in terms of his/her genetic potential by comparison with the mid-parental height.

Mid-parental height

- Add 12.6 cm to mother's height to plot on a boy's chart
- Subtract 12.6 cm if plotting a father's height on a girl's chart
- Mid-parental height is half-way between the plotted corrected parental heights

The measurement of skin-fold thicknesses (e.g. triceps, subscapular) gives important information about body fat distribution, which changes at different ages. For example, in puberty there is an increase in truncal fat but a reduction in limb fat. Mid arm circumference can be used to assess muscle bulk.

To estimate the rate at which a child is growing it is necessary to measure the height on two separate occasions (at least 4–6 months apart) and divide the change in height by the period of time elapsed. This is the height velocity and is expressed in cm/year. The height velocity can be plotted on standard reference charts.

3.3 Growth disorders

Short stature

Causes of short stature

- Familial

- Constitutional short stature, constitutional delay of growth and puberty

- Chronic illness:
  - Congenital heart disease
  - Respiratory disorders — e.g. cystic fibrosis
  - Renal failure
  - Gastrointestinal disorders — malabsorption, e.g. coeliac disease, Crohn's disease
  - Neurological — e.g. intracranial tumours

- Endocrine:
  - GH insufficiency
  - Hypothyroidism
  - Cushing syndrome

- Dysmorphic syndromes:
  - Turner syndrome
  - Down syndrome
  - Low birth weight, e.g. Russell–Silver syndrome
  - Prader–Willi syndrome

- Skeletal dysplasia:
  - Achondroplasia
  - Hypochondroplasia
  - Mucopolysaccharidoses
  - Spondyloepiphyseal dysplasia
- Psychosocial/emotional deprivation

As a general rule, if a child has a normal growth rate then the cause of the short stature is in the past history, whereas a child with a low growth rate requires thought as to what current process(es) are causing the growth failure.

Familial short stature

This remains one of the commonest causes of short stature, whereby the child takes after the parents' heights and grows along a centile that is appropriate for their genetic potential.

Constitutional short stature

This is a condition commonly seen in teenage boys who have a combination of delay in growth and in puberty. There is often a history of a similar pattern of growth in male members of the family. Bone-age assessment (see below) is often the only investigation initially required and usually shows a delay. Children do reach their genetic potential, but later than their peers. Management consists primarily of reassurance and, in certain circumstances, the use of a short (< 6-month) course of androgens to 'kick start' puberty.

NB: Constitutional delay of growth and puberty should not be diagnosed in girls without thorough investigation.

GH insufficiency

GH insufficiency (GHI) can be congenital or acquired.

- Congenital GHI can be inherited as an autosomal recessive trait which is very rare. More commonly it is the result of a structural abnormality of the hypothalamo–pituitary axis and may be isolated or associated with other midline developmental defects such as absent corpus callosum and septo-optic dysplasia. It may be an isolated phenomenon or associated with other anterior or posterior pituitary hormone deficiencies.
- Acquired GHI is associated with tumours or trauma in the hypothalamo–pituitary region. Surgery or radiotherapy to lesions in this region may also result in GHI.
- Deficiency can also occur as a genetic condition.
- Very rarely there may be high levels of GH associated with a clinical picture of severe GHI. This is the result of end-organ resistance (receptor abnormalities) resulting in low levels of IGF-1. This is know as Laron syndrome and is inherited as an autosomal recessive condition.

Common syndromes associated with short stature

Achondroplasia

- Inheritance:

- Autosomal dominant (but 50% new mutations)

Clinical features:
- Megalocephaly
- Short limbs
- Prominent forehead
- Thoracolumbar kyphosis
- Midfacial hypoplasia
- Disproportionate short stature

Radiology:
- Diminishing interpeduncular distances between L1 and L5
- Complications:
  - Short stature
  - Dental malocclusion
  - Hydrocephalus
  - Repeated otitis media

Hypochondroplasia

Definition:
- Rhizomelic short stature distinct from achondroplasia

Inheritance:
- Probable allelic autosomal dominant disorder

Clinical features:
- Affected persons appear stocky or muscular
- Usually recognized from 2 to 3 years of age
- Wide variability in severity

Radiology:
- No change in interpeduncular distances between L1 and L5

Complications:
- Short stature

Mucopolysaccharidoses (MPS)

Inheritance:
- Autosomal recessive, X-linked recessive

Clinical features — depend on type of MPS:
- Short spine and limbs
- Coarse facial features
- Reduced intelligence and abnormal behaviour in some forms
- Hurler syndrome — shortened lifespan
- Marked skeletal abnormalities and severe short stature in Morquio syndrome

Russell–Silver syndrome

Inheritance:
- Sporadic

Definition:
- Syndrome of short stature of prenatal onset

- Occurrence is sporadic and aetiology is unknown

Clinical features:

- Short stature of prenatal onset
- Limb asymmetry
- Short incurved fifth finger
- Small triangular face
- Café-au-lait spots
- Normal intelligence
- Bluish sclerae in early infancy

Turner's syndrome

Definition:

- A syndrome with a 45XO (or XO/XX or rarely XO/XY) karyotype associated with short stature, ovarian dysgenesis and dysmorphic features

Inheritance:

- Sporadic

Clinical features:

- Neonatal — lymphoedema of hands and feet
- Skeletal — short stature (mean adult height is 142 cm); widely spaced nipples, shield-shaped chest; wide carrying angle; short fourth metacarpal; hyperconvex nails
- Facial — prominent, backward-rotated ears; squint, ptosis; high arched palate; low posterior hairline, webbed neck
- Neurological — specific space–form perception defect
- Endocrine — autoimmune diseases (hypothyroidism); type 2 diabetes; infertility and pubertal failure
- Associations — horse-shoe kidneys; coarctation of the aorta; excessive pigmented naevi

Turner syndrome needs to be excluded in all girls whose height is below that expected for the mid-parental centile as not all girls with Turner syndrome show the classical phenotype.

Assessment of a child with short stature

Measure and plot the child's and parents' height and see if child is growing along predicted centile for genetic potential. Assess pubertal status according to Tanner stages (see below, Section 4.2). In teenage boys who are not yet in puberty, constitutional delay is the most likely.

History and clinical examination should identify an obvious chronic illness, which should then be specifically investigated. Features of recognized dysmorphic syndromes should be looked for. A child who is disproportionate should undergo skeletal survey to rule out a skeletal dysplasia.

Investigation of short stature

If above are ruled out, need:

- Full blood count
- Urea and electrolytes, C-reactive protein

- Coeliac antibodies screen
- Thyroid function tests
- Karyotyping
- IGF-1 levels
- Bone age
- GH provocation tests

Bone age
This is a measure of the maturation of the epiphyseal ossification centres in the skeleton. Bone age proceeds in an orderly fashion and therefore defines how much growth has taken place and the amount of growth left. A delayed bone age may be caused by constitutional delay of growth and puberty, GH deficiency or hypothyroidism. An advanced bone age is caused by precocious puberty, androgen excess (e.g. congenital adrenal hypoplasia) and GH excess.

Tall stature

Causes of tall stature in childhood

- Familial tall stature
- Constitutional obesity
- Precocious puberty
- Androgen excess:
  - Congenital adrenal hyperplasia
- GH excess
- Thyrotoxicosis
- Syndromes:
  - Cerebral gigantism
  - Marfan syndrome
  - Klinefelter syndrome

Familial tall stature
This is a child of tall parents whose height is following a centile line above, yet parallel, to the 97th centile, which is appropriate for the predicted mid-parental centile.

Constitutional obesity
Remember: if a child is tall and fat it is most probably the result of constitutional obesity. These children often have a slightly advanced bone age and go into puberty relatively early (not precocious) and thus end up appropriate (or slightly tall) for parents' heights.

Syndromes of tall stature

Marfan syndrome

Inheritance:
- Autosomal dominant
Clinical features:

- Skeletal — arachnodactyly; tall stature; scoliosis; high arched palate; pectus excavatum/carinatum; joint hypermobility
- Central nervous system — learning disabilities
- Ocular — lens dislocation
- Cardiovascular system — aortic dissection; mitral valve prolapse
- Respiratory — pneumothorax

Klinefelter syndrome

Definition:
- Karyotype 47XXY

Inheritance:
- Sporadic

Clinical features:
- Tall and slim
- Cryptorchidism
- Gynaecomastia
- Mental retardation
- Azoospermia and infertility
- Immature behaviour

Sotos syndrome (cerebral gigantism)

Inheritance:
- Sporadic

Clinical features:
- Birth weight and length > 90th centile
- Excessive linear growth during the first few years (which characteristically falls back)
- Head circumference is proportional to length
- Large hands and feet
- Large ears and nose
- Intellectual retardation
- Clumsiness

Assessment of a child with tall stature

Measure child's and parents' heights and compare with weight. Assess pubertal status. History and clinical examination should identify an obvious cause or syndrome that can then be investigated.

Investigation of tall stature

- Thyroid function
- Bone age
- Skeletal survey
- Karyotype

3.4 Genetics of growth

The genetics of growth is poorly understood but shows many characteristics of a polygenic model involving many genes. There are however, some single-gene growth defects, including defects of human GH and the human GH receptor.

4. PUBERTY AND INTERSEX DISORDERS

4.1 Physiology of normal puberty

The clinical manifestations of normal pubertal development occur secondary to sequential changes in endocrine activity.

Hormonal control of puberty

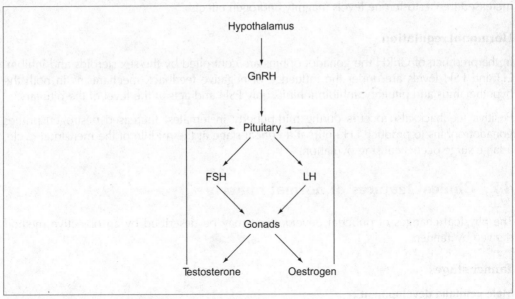

Hormonal control of puberty

The pulsatile release of GnRH from the hypothalamus leads to the secretion of LH and FSH from the gonadotrophin cells of the pituitary gland.

In the male, Leydig cells respond to LH, which stimulates the first step in testosterone production. In the female, LH binds to ovarian cells and stimulates steroidogenesis. FSH binds to Sertoli cells in the male where it increases the mass of the seminiferous tubules and supports the development of sperm. In the female, FSH binds to the glomerulosa cells and stimulates the conversion of testosterone to oestrogen.

Sex steroids

Testosterone is produced by the Leydig cells of the testes. It is present in the circulation bound to sex-hormone-binding globulin (SHBG). Free testosterone is the active moiety at the level of target cells. Testosterone is then either converted to dihydrotestosterone by 5α-reductase or to oestrogen by aromatase. Both dihydrotestosterone and testosterone attach to nuclear receptors, which then bind to steroid-responsive regions of genomic DNA to influence transcription and translation.

Oestrogen is produced by the follicle cells of the ovary. The main active form of oestrogen is oestradiol. This circulates bound to SHBG and causes growth of the breasts and uterus, the female distribution of adipose tissue and increases bone mineralization.

Inhibin

Inhibin is a glycoprotein produced by Sertoli cells in males and granulosa cells in females.

SHBG

Androgens reduce SHBG formation, and oestrogens stimulate its formation. Therefore increased free testosterone levels magnify androgen effects.

Hormonal regulation

In the presence of GnRH the gonadotrophins are controlled by the sex steroids and inhibin. LH and FSH levels are under the influence of negative feedback mechanisms in both the hypothalamus and pituitary. Inhibin inhibits only FSH and acts at the level of the pituitary.

Positive feedback also occurs during mid-puberty in females. Increased oestrogen primes gonadotrophins to produce LH until, at a critical stage at the middle of the menstrual cycle, a large surge occurs causing ovulation.

4.2   Clinical features of normal puberty

The physical changes of pubertal development may be described by an objective method derived by Tanner.

Tanner stages

Male genitalia development

Stage 1   Pre-adolescent
Stage 2   Enlargement of scrotum and testes and changes in scrotal skin
Stage 3   Further growth of testes and scrotum; enlargement of penis
Stage 4   Increase in breadth of penis and development of glans; further growth of scrotum and testes
Stage 5   Adult genitalia in shape and size

Female breast development

Stage 1   Pre-adolescent
Stage 2   Breast-bud formation

Stage 3   Further enlargement and elevation of breast and papilla with no separation of their contours

Stage 4   Projection of areola and papilla to form a secondary mound above the level of the breast

Stage 5   Mature stage with projection of papilla only

Pubic hair

Stage 1   Pre-adolescent

Stage 2   Sparse growth of long, slightly pigmented, downy hair

Stage 3   Hair spread over junction of the pubes, darker and coarser

Stage 4   Adult-type hair, but area covered is smaller

Stage 5   Adult in quantity and type

Axillary hair

Stage 1   No axillary hair

Stage 2   Scanty growth

Stage 3   Adult in quantity and type

Puberty starts on average at age 12 years in boys and 10 years in girls. As nutrition and health improve, the age of onset of puberty is becoming earlier with each generation.

In the male, acceleration in growth of the testes (from a prepubertal 2-ml volume) and scrotum are the first sign of puberty. This is followed by reddening and rugosity of scrotal skin, later by development of pubic hair, penile growth and axillary hair growth.

A 4-ml testicular volume signifies the start of pubertal change. Peak height velocity occurs with testicular volumes of 10–12 ml.

In the female, the appearance of the breast bud and breast development are the first signs of puberty and occur as the result of production of oestrogen from the ovaries. These are followed by the development of pubic and axillary hair, which is controlled by the adrenal gland. Peak height velocity coincides with breast stage 2–3. Menarche occurs late at breast stage 4, by which stage growth is slowing down. Most girls have attained menarche by age 13 years.

Body composition

Prepubertal boys and girls have equal lean body mass, skeletal mass and body fat. The earliest change in puberty is an increase in lean body mass.

Growth spurt

The pubertal growth spurt is the most rapid phase of growth after the neonatal period. This is an early event in girls and occurs approximately 2 years earlier than in boys, i.e. at a mean age of 12 years. The mean height difference between males and females of 12.5 cm is the result of the taller male stature at the time of the pubertal growth spurt and increased height gained during the pubertal growth spurt.

Adrenarche

Adrenal androgens, dehydroepiandrosterone sulphate (DHEAS) and androstenedione rise approximately 2 years before gonadotrophins and sex steroids rise. Adrenarche begins at 6–8 years of age and continues until late puberty. Control of this is unknown. Adrenarche does not influence onset of puberty.

Gynaecomastia

Gynaecomastia is physiological and occurs in 75% of boys to some degree (usually during the first stages of puberty), but most regress within 2 years. Management is by reassurance, support and weight loss if obesity is a factor.

Causes of gynaecomastia

- Normal puberty (common)
- Obesity (common)
- Klinefelter syndrome
- Partial androgen insensitivity

4.3 Abnormal puberty

- Early (precocious):
    - < 9 years in boys
    - < 8 years in girls
- Discordant (abnormal pattern)
- Delayed:
    - > 14 years in boys
    - > 13 years in girls

Precocious puberty

Definition

Central precocious puberty is consonant with puberty (i.e. occurs in the usual physiological pattern of development but at an earlier age). It is the result of premature activation of the GnRH pulse generator. In girls, often no underlying cause is found; however, it is almost always pathological in males.

Causes of true precocious puberty (gonadotrophin-dependent)

- Idiopathic
- Central nervous system tumour
- Neurofibromatosis
- Septo-optic dysplasia — in this rare condition precocious puberty may occur in the presence of deficiencies of other pituitary hormones (see Section 2.4).

Causes of gonadotrophin-independent precocious puberty

- McCune–Albright syndrome — usually because of ovarian hypersecretion
- Testicular/ovarian tumours
- Liver or adrenal tumours — may cause virilization

Useful tests for the investigation of precocious puberty

- Oestradiol/testosterone
- Adrenal androgens, including 17-hydroxyprogesterone
- LHRH stimulation test
- Bone age
- Pelvic ultrasound scan
- Brain magnetic resonance imaging (MRI)
- Abdominal computed tomography (CT) if adrenal/liver tumour suspected

Management of precocious puberty

Gonadotrophin-releasing hormone analogues (GnRHa) may be used to halt the progression of puberty. Children who enter puberty early are tall initially, but end up as short adults because of premature closure of the epiphyses. Although GH has been used in addition to GnRHa, there is no clear evidence that final height is improved.

Discordant puberty (abnormal pattern)

- Breast development only — gonadotrophin-independent precocious puberty, e.g. McCune–Albright syndrome
- Inadequate breast development, e.g. gonadal dysgenesis, Poland anomaly
- Androgen excess — pubic hair, acne, clitoral enlargement, e.g. congenital adrenal hyperplasia, Cushing's disease, polycystic ovarian syndrome, adrenal neoplasm
- Inadequate pubic hair, e.g. androgen insensitivity, adrenal failure
- No menarche, e.g. polycystic ovaries/absent ovaries or uterus
- No growth spurt, e.g. hypothalamic–pituitary disorders, skeletal dysplasias

Premature thelarche

- Usually in girls aged between 1 and 3 years
- Isolated breast development (never more than stage 3)
- No other signs of puberty
- Normal growth velocity for age
- Normal bone age
- Prepubertal gonadotrophin levels
- Progress to puberty at normal age

Delayed puberty

Definition

No signs of puberty at an age when pubertal change would have been expected.

Causes of delayed puberty

- Constitutional delay of growth and puberty
- Hypothalamic or pituitary disorders:
  - Hypogonadotrophic hypogonadism
  - Idiopathic
  - Pituitary tumours
  - Post-central irradiation
  - Post-intracranial surgery
  - Post-chemotherapy
- Anorexia nervosa
- Systemic disease
- Kallman syndrome — hypogonadotrophic hypogonadism with anosmia
- Gonadal dysgenesis:
  - Turner syndrome
- Hypothyroidism

Investigation of delayed puberty in boys

In otherwise well boys with short stature and delayed puberty the most likely cause is constitutional delay. Initially this requires no investigations apart from a bone age. If after a trial of treatment there is no progression of puberty, further investigations may be needed including:

- LH, FSH, testosterone
- LHRH test
- Karyotyping

Investigation of delayed puberty in girls

In girls, delayed puberty must always be investigated.

- Karyotyping
- LH, FSH, oestrogen
- LHRH test
- Pelvic ultrasound

Treatment

Constitutional delay

- Reassurance
- Androgens — oxandrolone orally daily or depot testosterone injection monthly
- Reassess at 4–6 months

Other causes of delayed puberty

- Treat underlying cause
- Induce and maintain puberty with testosterone in boys, ethinyloestradiol in girls

4.4 Intersex disorders (ambiguous genitalia)

Classification

- Virilized female
- Inadequately virilized male
- True hermaphrodite

Causes of a virilized female

- Androgens of fetal origin
- Congenital adrenal hyperplasia
- Androgens of maternal origin
- Drugs/maternal congenital adrenal hyperplasia
- Tumours of ovary or adrenal gland
- Idiopathic

Causes of an inadequately virilized male

- XY gonadal dysgenesis
- LH deficiency
- Leydig cell hypoplasia
- Inborn errors of testosterone synthesis
- 5α-reductase deficiency
- Androgen insensitivity

Useful investigations

- Karyotype
- Urine steroid profile
- Pelvic ultrasound
- 17-OH progesterone (day 3)
- LH/FSH testosterone/dihydrotestosterone
- Human chorionic gonadotrophin test

Management

This requires multidisciplinary assessment and management involving endocrinology, paediatric urology, gynaecology and psychology input.

4.5 Amenorrhoea

Amenorrhoea may be either primary or secondary. Patients with primary amenorrhoea have never menstruated, whereas those with secondary amenorrhoea have lost previously existing menstrual function.

Causes of amennorhoea

- Ovarian
  - Gonadal dysfunction
  - Secondary to irradiation/chemotherapy/surgery
  - Polycystic ovarian syndrome
- Genital tract
  - Müllerian dysgenesis
- Hypothalamopituitary
  - Hypogonadotophic hypogonadism
  - Secondary to tumours/irradiation/chemotherapy/surgery
- Functional
  - Weight loss
  - Exercise-induced
  - Chronic illness
  - Psychogenic

Management of amenorrhoea

Management of amenorrhoea depends on the underlying cause. Structural abnormalities may need surgical correction. Primary amenorrhoea may require pubertal induction with exogenous oestrogen. In secondary amenorrhoea the underlying cause needs to be identified and addressed.

5. THE ADRENAL GLAND

5.1 Anatomy

The adrenals are triangular in shape and located at the superior pole of the kidneys. Each adrenal gland comprises a cortex, arising from mesoderm at the cranial end of the mesonephros, and a medulla, which arises from neural crest cells.

The cortex consists of three zones:

- Zona glomerulosa — produces aldosterone
- Zona fasciculata — produces cortisol/androstenedione
- Zona reticularis — produces DHEAS

5.2 Physiology

Cortex

The adrenal cortex has three principal functions:

- Glucocorticoid production (cortisol)
- Mineralocorticoid production (aldosterone)
- Androgen production (testosterone, androstenedione)

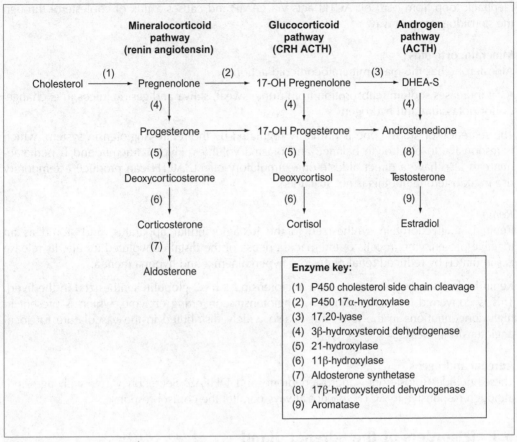

Pathways of adrenal hormone synthesis

Glucocorticoids

Cortisol is the principal glucocorticoid.

- It plays a vital role in the body's stress response
- It is an insulin counter-regulatory hormone increasing gluconeogenesis, hepatic glycogenolysis, ketogenesis
- It is necessary for the action of other hormones, e.g. noradrenaline (norepinephrine), adrenaline (epinephrine), glucagon
- It influences other organ physiology:
  - Normal blood vessel function
  - Cardiac and skeletal muscle
  - Nervous system
  - Inhibition of the inflammatory response of tissues to injury
  - Secretion of a water load

Cortisol secretion is under pituitary control from ACTH. ACTH has a circadian rhythm, being at its lowest at midnight and rising in the early morning. There is also a negative feedback loop from cortisol. ACTH acts via cAMP and causes a flux of cholesterol through the steroidogenic pathway.

Mineralocorticoids

Aldosterone has the main mineralocorticoid action:

- It increases sodium reabsorption from urine, sweat, saliva and gastric juices in exchange for potassium and hydrogen

The secretion of aldosterone is primarily regulated by the renin–angiotensin system, which is responsive to electrolyte balance and plasma volumes. Hyponatraemia and hyperkalaemia can also have a direct aldosterone stimulatory effect. ACTH can produce a temporary rise in aldosterone but this is not sustained.

Renin

Renin is a glycoprotein synthesized in the juxtaglomerular apparatus, and stored as an inactive pro-enzyme in cells of the macula densa of the distal convoluted tubule. Its release is stimulated by reduced renal perfusion, hyperkalaemia and hyponatraemia.

Renin hydrolyses angiotensin to form angiotensin I (an α2-globulin synthesized in the liver). This is converted to angiotensin II by angiotensin-converting enzyme, which is present in high concentrations in the lung, but is also widely distributed in the vasculature for local angiotensin II release.

Adrenal androgens

These include testosterone, androstenedione and DHEAS. Secretion varies with age and, although responsive to ACTH, do not always parallel the cortisol response.

5.3   Disorders of the adrenal gland

Medulla

Phaeochromocytoma

A catecholamine-secreting tumour. Malignancy is uncommon, but 10% are bilateral. Catecholamine excess leads to sustained hypertension. Phaeochromocytomas are associated with von Recklinghausen's disease, von Hippel–Landau disease and syndromes of multiple endocrine neoplasia.

Investigation is by

- MIBG (metaiodobenzylguanidine) isotope scans
- Plasma and urine catecholamine measurement

Management is by surgical excision. Pre-operative management requires both α- and β-adrenoceptor blockade to prevent an acute hypertensive crisis or cardiac dysrrhythmias.

Cortex

Adrenal insufficiency

Causes

Primary:
- Idiopathic
- Congenital adrenal hyperplasia
- Adrenal haemorrhage
- Addison's disease — tuberculosis; autoimmune disease
- Iatrogenic

Secondary:
- Pituitary hypoplasia
- Isolated ACTH deficiency
- Panhypopituitarism
- Tumour, e.g. craniopharyngioma

Addison's disease

Definition:
- Adrenal hypofunction

Aetiology:
- Autoimmune
- Secondary to tuberculosis
- Associated with adrenal leukodystrophy

Presentation:
- Often with non-specific symptoms of tiredness and abdominal pain
- May present with collapse related to a salt-losing crisis

Investigation of adrenal cortical insufficiency

- Synacthen test, which assesses the ability of the stimulated adrenal glands to mount a hormone response. A dose of synthetic ACTH is given and the cortisol level is measured after 30 and 60 min. A normal adrenal response would be a cortisol level > 450–550 nmol/L at 30 min.
- A 24-h blood cortisol profile assesses the natural secretion from the adrenal gland. This would be expected to show the normal diurnal rhythm of cortisol secretion, with an increase in the morning and a nadir at midnight.

Treatment

Glucocorticoid and mineralocorticoid replacement using hydrocortisone and fludrocortisone, respectively.

At times of illness, injury or acute stress, the body naturally increases the output of corticosteroids from the adrenal glands. A person on replacement hydrocortisone needs to mimic this process and to increase their hydrocortisone at these times. It is therefore important that a steroid-users card is carried at all times to alert medical professionals at the time of an emergency.

Adrenal steroid excess (Cushing syndrome)

Definition

- A syndrome of cortisol excess. Cushing's disease is the term used when this is secondary to a pituitary ACTH-producing tumour (adenoma)

Causes

- Primary — adrenal tumour
- Secondary — pituitary ACTH-secreting tumour; ectopic ACTH production
- Iatrogenic — exogenous administration of steroids

Clinical features

- Obesity — central distribution of fat — buffalo hump
- Purple striae
- Hypertension
- Osteoporosis
- Hypogonadism
- Growth failure
- Muscle wasting/hypotonia

Investigations

- 24-h urine cortisol
- 24-h profile (loss of circadian rhythm, no suppression of midnight cortisol level)
- Dexamethasone suppression test
- MRI brain/CT adrenals

Treatment

- Treat underlying cause

Congenital adrenal hyperplasia

Aetiology

- Deficiency of one of the enzymes in the biosynthetic pathway of the adrenal cortex. The classical type is deficiency of the enzyme 21-hydroxylase
- Other enzyme deficiencies result in non-classical CAH. These enzymes are listed in the figure on page 259 (Pathways of adrenal hormone synthesis)

Genetics

- Two genes encoding 21-hydroxylase expression have been localized to the short arm of chromosome 6, namely *CYP21B* and *CYP21A*. Deletion of *CYP21B* is associated with severe salt wasting and HLA B47, DR7 haplotype

Pathophysiology

- In classical CAH, there is a block in the production of cortisol and aldosterone with a build up of the 17-hydroxyprogesterone, the precursor before the block. The continuing

ACTH drive leads to the precursors being directed along the androgen biosynthetic pathway causing virilization

Presentation

- Ambiguous genitalia (in girls with 21-hydroxylase deficiency, and occasionally in boys with 3β-hydroxysteroid dehydrogenase deficiency)
- Salt-losing crisis and hypotension
- Hypertension may occur in 11β-hydroxylase deficiency
- Precocious puberty (in boys)
- Virilization

Investigation

- Karyotype
- 17-hydroxyprogesterone
- Urine steroid profile (metabolite pattern will help in diagnosing specific enzyme block)
- Adrenal androgen levels
- Bone age in older children

Treatment

Hydrocortisone and fludrocortisone replace the deficient steroids and also suppress the ACTH drive to the adrenal androgens. Growth is a good method of monitoring replacement therapy. Children who grow excessively fast with increased height velocity are either getting inadequate doses or may be non-compliant. Levels of 17-hydroxyprogesterone are also useful for monitoring treatment.

- It is important to teach parents to recognize signs of illness and to be able to administer emergency hydrocortisone
- Additional sodium chloride replacement is also required during the first year of life and electrolytes may need to be monitored over this period
- Surgery may be required in females with virilization

Side-effects of glucocorticoid treatment

When glucocorticoids are used in non-physiological doses, such as in asthma, chronic renal failure or rheumatological and immunological conditions, the following side-effects may be seen.

- Gastritis
- Osteoporosis
- Raised blood glucose/altered glucose tolerance
- Increased appetite and weight gain
- Increased susceptibility to infection
- Poor healing
- Menstrual irregularities
- Unpredictable mood changes
- Sleep disturbances
- Increased risk of glaucoma and cataracts

6. THE THYROID GLAND

6.1 Anatomy

The thyroid gland is formed from a midline outpouching of ectoderm of the primitive buccal cavity which then migrates caudally. It consists of follicles made of colloid surrounded by follicular cells and basement membrane. Thyroid hormone is synthesized at a cellular level and stored in thyroglobulin, a glycoprotein that is the main constituent of the colloid. Between the follicular cells are the parafollicular cells (C cells) which are of neurogenic origin and secrete calcitonin.

6.2 Physiology

The function of the thyroid gland is to concentrate iodine from the blood and return it to peripheral tissues in the form of thyroid hormones (thyroxine; tetra-iodothyronine, (T_4) and tri-iodothyronine (T_3)). In blood, the hormones are linked with carrier proteins, e.g. thyroxine-binding globulin and pre-albumin. T_4 is metabolized in the periphery into T_3 (more potent) and reverse T_3 (less potent).

Hormonogenesis

Steps include

- Iodide trapping by the thyroid gland
- Synthesis of thyroglobulin
- Organification of trapped iodine as iodotyrosines (mono-iodotyrosine (MIT) and di-iodotyrosine (DIT))
- Coupling of iodotyrosines to form iodothyronines and storage in the follicular colloid
- Endocytosis of colloid droplets and hydrolysis of thyroglobulin to release T_3, T_4, MIT and DIT
- Deiodination of MIT and DIT with intrathyroid recycling of the iodine

Thyroid hormone acts by penetrating the cell membrane and then binding to a specific nuclear receptor. It modulates gene transcription and mRNA synthesis. This leads to increased mitochondrial activity.

Functions of thyroid hormone

Thyroid hormone has multiple physiological actions. It is required for somatic and neuronal growth. Other actions include thermogenesis, stimulation of water and ion transport, acceleration of substrate turnover, amino acid and lipid metabolism. It also potentiates the actions of catecholamines.

Regulation

Thyroid hormone release is regulated by TSH and by iodine levels. TSH has both immediate and delayed actions on thyroid hormone secretion.

- Immediate actions:

- Stimulates binding of iodide to protein
- Stimulates thyroid hormone release
- Stimulates pathways of intermediate metabolism
- Delayed action (several hours):
  - Stimulates trapping of iodide
  - Stimulates synthesis of thyroglobulin

Physiological variations in iodide modulate trapping by the thyroid membrane.

Iodide inhibits the stimulation of cAMP by TSH and pharmacological doses block organification.

6.3   Disorders of thyroid function

Hypothyroidism

Causes of hypothyroidism

Primary

- Congenital:
  - Thyroid dysgenesis
  - Agenesis
  - Hypoplasia
  - Ectopic gland
  - Biosynthetic defects
- Acquired
  - Autoimmune
  - Post-surgery
  - Post-cervical irradiation
  - Systemic disorders
  - Iodine deficiency
  - Iodine overload

Secondary

- Congenital:
  - Congenital pituitary abnormalities
  - Receptor resistance
- Acquired:
  - Post-cranial irradiation
  - Post-tumour
  - Post-surgery

Screening for congenital hypothyroidism
TSH is measured as part of the newborn screening programme performed between the 5th and 7th days of life. A blood spot from a heel prick is put on a filter paper. Concentrations of TSH of over 10 mU/L are picked up by this test and abnormal results are immediately

notified by the test centre to the relevant local hospital/specialist unit or the general practitioner.

This screening programme detects > 90% of cases of congenital hypothyroidism. Those with secondary (pituitary) causes are picked up because TSH levels are low.

It is essential that treament with oral thyroxine is started as soon as the definitive measurements of TSH and free T_4 have been performed because delay may lead to a lower IQ and affect psychomotor development.

Hyperthyroidism

Causes of hyperthyroidism

- Autoimmune thyroiditis, e.g. Graves' disease
- Diffuse toxic goitre
- Nodular toxic goitre
- TSH-induced
- Factitious

Graves' disease

This is a multisystem, autoimmune disorder involving the eyes, hyperthyroidism and a dermopathy. There is an increased incidence in adolescence and it is six to eight times more common in girls than in boys. Thyroid-stimulating immunoglobulin may be demonstrated.

Neonatal thyrotoxicosis

This is a rare condition caused by the transplacental passage of thyroid-stimulating antibodies from mothers with either Graves' disease (active or inactive) or Hashimoto's thyroiditis. The neonate usually presents with a rapidly developing tachycardia, dysrhythmia, hypertension and weight loss. A goitre may be present. There may also be associated jaundice and thrombocytopenia. The condition is usually self-limiting in 4–12 weeks but severely affected neonates will require treatment with propranolol, carbamazepine and Lugol's iodine. A response is usually seen within 24–36 h.

Thyroid neoplasia

This usually presents as solitary nodules, of which 50% are benign adenomas or cystic lesions. The prevalence of malignancy in childhood is 30–40% and the risk increases following radiation to the neck during infancy or early childhood. Hyperfunctioning adenomas are rare and most (90%) are well-differentiated follicular carcinomas.

Medullary carcinoma may occur as part of multiple endocrine neoplasia type II (hyperparathyroidism and phaeochromocytoma) syndrome.

6.4 Investigation and management of thyroid disorders

Investigation

- Baseline blood tests:
  - Free T_4/T_3/TSH measurements
- Stimulation tests:
  - TRH test
- Thyroid ultrasound scan
- Radionuclide scans

In primary hypothyroidism, T_4 will be low and associated with a raised TSH. In hyperthyroidism, T_4 will be raised and TSH will be suppressed.

In secondary hypothyroidism, T_4 will be low in association with a low TSH. Further investigation is with a TRH test. This involves the injection of TRH followed by measurement of TSH at 30 and 60 min post-dose. In an individual with normal thyroid function, TSH would rise at 30 min but fall by 60 min. However, in patients with hypothalamic dysfunction, TSH would continue to rise at 60 min post-injection.

'Sick thyroid syndrome' refers to the scenario of a variety of abnormalities on thyroid function testing in an unwell patient but which spontaneously resolve as the illness improves. Usually there is a normal free T_4 level with raised TSH.

Management of thyroid disorders

Hypothyroidism

- Replacement of thyroxine in either congenital or acquired autoimmune thyroid hormone deficiency is with once-daily oral thyroxine tablets
- Babies with congenital hypothyroidism should be started on thyroxine replacement as early as possible to limit damage to the developing brain. Outcome is usually good. However, intrauterine damage cannot be completely corrected for and detailed psychometric testing may detect specific deficits
- Initial doses start at 25 μg per day with a gradual increase over the years
- The dose may be monitored by assessing the free T_4 and TSH levels at regular intervals

Transient neonatal hypothyroidism

Transient neonatal hypothyroidism may be seen in babies of mothers who have autoimmune thyroid disease. These babies do not usually require treatment.

Hyperthyroidism

Initial medical treatment:
- Suppression of thyroid hormone secretion using specific antithyroid treatments, e.g. carbimazole, propylthiouracil
- Blunting the peripheral effects of the thyroid hormones using α-blockade, e.g. propranolol

Definitive treatment:
- This is contemplated if there has been no remission in symptoms on medical

treatment, and may involve subtotal thyroidectomy or radioactive iodine, which is becoming an increasingly popular choice for teenagers

7. GLUCOSE HOMEOSTASIS

7.1 Physiology

The concentration of glucose in the blood is maintained by a balance between food intake or glucose mobilization from the liver and glucose utilization. Homeostatic mechanisms keep this within a narrow range.

In the fed state, insulin release is stimulated by a raised glucose and amino acid concentration. It is also stimulated by gut hormone release. In the fasting state, blood glucose concentrations fall and insulin production is turned off under the influence of somatostatin. A low glucose concentration is sensed by the hypothalamus, which regulates pancreatic secretion and stimulates the release of the counter-regulatory hormones glucagon, ACTH, GH, prolactin and catecholamines.

Actions of insulin

Liver:
- Conversion of glucose to glycogen
- Inhibits gluconeogenesis
- Inhibits glycogenolysis

Peripheral:
- Stimulates glucose and amino acid uptake by muscle
- Stimulates glucose uptake by fat cells to form triglycerides

Actions of the counter-regulatory hormones

- Inhibition of glucose uptake
- Stimulation of amino acid release by muscle
- Stimulation of lipolysis to release free fatty acids which can be oxidized to form ketones
- Stimulation of gluconeogenesis and glycogenolysis

7.2 Diabetes mellitus

Causes

Causes of diabetes mellitus
- Progressive loss of islet-cell function
- Insulin resistance
- Iatrogenic — e.g. post-pancreatic surgery

The most common cause of diabetes in childhood is type 1 autoimmune diabetes, although type 2 diabetes is increasingly being reported in association with obesity in teenagers. Type 2 diabetes is a combination of α-cell failure and insulin resistance.

Epidemiology

- UK — annual incidence is 20 per 100,000 children
- In many countries the incidence is rising, in some the incidence in children < 5 years of age is increasing
- Diabetes before 1 year of age is extremely rare. Incidence increases with age. Minor peak at age 4–6 years, major peak at 10–14 years
- No clear pattern of inheritance
- Increased risk if one family member is affected

Physiology of diabetes in β-cell failure

Low insulin levels ultimately lead to ketoacidosis through the following mechanisms:

- Liver glycogen mobilization to form glucose
- Muscle protein breakdown to form free amino acids
- Adipose tissue breakdown of triglycerides to form free fatty acids which are α-oxidized to form ketone bodies

Clinical effects

As the blood glucose level increases, the glucose in the glomerular filtrate exceeds the ability of the proximal tubules to reabsorb it. This leads to glycosuria. Polyuria then occurs, because the loop of Henlé is unable to concentrate the urine because the renal tubules are insufficiently hyperosmolar. Extracellular volume depletion leads to thirst and polydipsia.

Differential diagnosis of polyuria and polydipsia

- Diabetes mellitus
- Diabetes insipidus
  - Cranial — AVP deficiency
  - Nephrogenic — AVP insensitivity
- Habitual water drinking
- Drug-induced

Presentation of childhood diabetes

Children usually present acutely with polyuria (including nocturia and incontinence), thirst and poydipsia. About 40% have diabetic ketoacidosis. Other symptoms are weight loss, fatigue, infections (e.g. abscess, urinary tract infections), muscle cramps and abdominal pain.

Aetiology of diabetes in children

- Type 1 diabetes (95%) — autoimmune destruction of the pancreatic islet cells
- Type 2 Diabetes

- Cystic-fibrosis-related diabetes
- Maturity onset diabetes of the young
- Genetic syndromes (Down syndrome, Wolfram or DIDMOAD syndrome (diabetes insipidus, diabetes mellitus, optic atrophy and deafness))

Risk factors for Type 2 diabetes

- Family history of type 2 diabetes
- High-risk ethnic groups (African, Caribbean, Asian, Hispanic)
- Obesity
- Female sex
- Pubertal
- Clinical signs of insulin reistance (acanthosis nigricans, polycystic ovarian syndrome)
- Biochemical signs of insulin resistance (high insulin or c-peptide levels)
- No islet cell antibodies

Diagnosis

- Hyperglycaemia — random glucose > 11.1 mmol/L, fasting glucose > 7.6 mmol/L
- Glucose tolerance test is not routinely necessary for diagnosis.

Management of a child with newly diagnosed diabetes

There are a number of recent national publications regarding the management of children and young people with diabetes. In 2002 the National Service Framework for Diabetes was published and outlines the following standards.

In 2005 the National Institute for Clinical Excellence (NICE) published specific guidance on the management of type 1 diabetes in children and young people which included a protocol for the management of diabetic ketoacidosis.

A well child
A subcutaneous insulin regimen may be commenced as outlined below.

A child with diabetic ketoacidosis
In a child with diabetes, diabetic ketoacidosis is usually associated with hyperglycaemia (blood glucose > 11 mmol/L) and may be defined with the following parameters:

Definition

- pH < 7.2
- Bicarbonate < 15 mmol/L
- Raised blood/urinary ketones

Principles of management of diabetic ketoacidosis
National guidelines on the management of diabetic ketoacidosis in children and young people have been published by NICE in 2004. The principles are outlined below:

- Rehydration (slowly over 48 h) to prevent large fluid shifts and the risk of cerebral oedema. An initial fluid bolus can be used to resuscitate the child. Normal fluid requirements are calculated as maintenance + 10% deficit given evenly over 48 h

- Rule of thumb:
  - 6 ml/kg per hour for children weighing 3–9 kg
  - 5 ml/kg per h for children weighing 10–19 kg
  - 4 ml/kg per hour for children weighing > 20 kg
- This usually covers ongoing losses, but if excessive they need replacement
  - Initial fluid is 0.9% saline
  - When blood glucose is down to 15 mmol/L change to fluid containing glucose, e.g. 4% glucose + 0.45% saline
- Intravenous insulin 0.05–0.1 IU/kg per hour with the rate of infusion adjusted according to the blood glucose concentration
- Monitoring of glucose
- Replacement of potassium and monitoring of electrolytes

Long-term management of diabetes

The aims of management are to normalize blood glucose concentrations to prevent acute hypoglycaemia and to reduce the risk of developing long-term complications of diabetes. Monitoring is by capillary blood glucose measurements, glycated haemoglobin (HbA1c) and screening for complications. The NICE guidelines recommend a HbA1c value of < 7.5%.

Subcutaneous insulin regimens

Twice daily regimen of pre-mixed formulations of insulin are most common in paediatric practice. These are combinations of short/rapid-acting insulins and an intermediate-acting insulin. The insulin is usually delivered via a 'pen' device.

Intensive insulin regimens

Basal bolus regimen comprising of multiple insulin injections. This usually comprises a short/rapid-acting insulin as a meal-time bolus and a long/imtermediate-acting insulin once or twice daily as background.

Continuously via an insulin pump

The usual requirement is insulin 1 IU/kg per day and it is important to rotate insulin injection sites to prevent the formation of lipohypertrophied areas.

Diet

The aim is for a healthy diet containing adequate protein, small amounts of fat and complex carbohydrates that are digested slowly. The body cannot cope with sugary foods, the carbohydrate of which is rapidly absorbed, and these should be limited (including sugary drinks). The intensive insulin regimens allow for a more flexible eating pattern as the rapidly acting insulin can be adjusted according to the carbohydrate content of individual meals. However, the twice-daily insulin regimen requires a consistency of meal times with regular snacks and consistent carbohydate content of meals.

Exercise

Exercise is important not only to maintain cardiovascular fitness but also to reduce blood glucose levels.

Capillary blood glucose testing

Blood glucose testing multiple times daily is essential to monitor glycaemic control and enables insulin dose adjustment.

Hypoglycaemia in a child on insulin treatment

Hypoglycaemia in a person on glucose-lowering treament is defined as a blood glucose of < 4 mmol/L. The symptoms may be divided into neuroglycaemic and adrenergic and include weakness, trembling, dizziness, poor concentration, hunger, sweating, pallor, aggressiveness, irritability and confusion.

The initial management of hypoglycaemia is to have refined sugar, e.g. glucose tablets or a sugary drink, followed by a complex carbohydrate food, e.g. a biscuit or a sandwich. If the hypoglycaemic child is unconscious or unable to cooperate with glucose administration orally, then intramuscular glucagon may be administered.

Insulin administration during an intercurrent illness

A child with type 1 diabetes needs insulin to survive and will become insulin deficient if the insulin is stopped. This leads to increased ketone production and the risk of diabetic ketoacidosis. It is therefore important never to stop the insulin but to drink fluids and if there are concerns about hypoglycaemia an admission for the administration of intravenous fluids may be required.

Long-term complications of diabetes

Evidence shows that the more intensive treatment and monitoring regimens lead to improved control and a reduced risk of complications. These children are best managed by a multidisciplinary team including a paediatrician, dietitian, diabetic nurse and, ideally, a psychologist.

Long-term complications increase with time (> 10 years from onset of diabetes). They include nephropathy, retinopathy and neuropathy. All children with diabetes should have an annual review which includes 24-h urine collection for microalbuminuria and ophthalmology assessment.

7.3 Hypoglycaemia

Causes of hypoglycaemia

- Inadequate glucose production:
  - Counter-regulatory hormone deficiencies
  - Glycogen storage disease
  - Enzyme deficiency — e.g. galactosaemia

- Excessive glucose consumption — i.e. hyperinsulinism:
  - Transient
  - Infant of a diabetic mother
  - Beckwith–Wiedemann syndrome

- Persistent:
  - Persistent hyperinsulinaemic hypoglycaemia of infancy
  - Insulinoma
  - Exogenous insulin

Investigation of hypoglycaemia

Blood taken for a diagnostic screen is only useful if taken when the patient is hypoglycaemic (glucose < 2.6 mmol/L) and should include the following:

- Blood
  - Glucose
  - Insulin (C peptide)
  - Cortisol
  - GH
  - Lactate
  - Free fatty acids
  - Amino acids
  - Ketone bodies (β-hydroxybutyrate and acetoacetate)
- Urine
  - Organic acids

In hypoglycaemic states in the absence of ketones it is important to look at the free fatty acids (FFA). Normal FFA suggests hyperinsulinism and raised FFA suggests a fatty-acid oxidation defect. Hypoglycaemia in the presence of urinary ketones suggests either a counter-regulatory hormone deficiency or an enzyme defect in the glycogenolysis or gluconeogenesis pathways.

8. BONE METABOLISM

8.1 Physiology of calcium and phosphate homeostasis

- Principal regulators of calcium concentrations
  - Vitamin D (and its active metabolites)
  - Parathyroid hormone (PTH)
  - Calcitonin

- Regulators of phosphate concentrations
  - Main regulator is vitamin D
  - Less strictly controlled than calcium

Vitamin D

Vitamin D3 (cholecalciferol) is produced in the skin from a pro-vitamin as a result of exposure to ultraviolet light. Excess sunlight converts pro-vitamin D to an inactive compound thus preventing vitamin D intoxication. Vitamin D is also ingested and is a fat-soluble vitamin. Vitamin D is converted to its active form by hydroxylation — intially to its 25-hydroxyl form in the liver and the subsequent 1,25-hydroxylation occurs in the kidney.

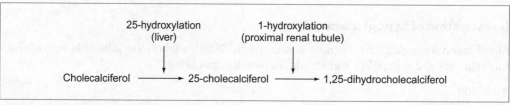

Vitamin D activation pathway

Vitamin D:

- Increases intestinal absorption of calcium
- Increases osteoclastic bone resorption
- Inhibits PTH secretion and hence increases 1α-hydroxylation

Parathyroid hormone

The *PTH* gene is located on chromosome 11. Active PTH is cleaved from a pro-hormone and then secreted by the parathyroid glands. Low calcium, cortisol, prolactin, phosphate and vitamin D all affect PTH secretion, but maximal PTH secretion occurs at a calcium concentration of < 2 mmol/L.

Immediate effects of PTH

- Reduction in renal calcium excretion. It promotes calcium reabsorption in the distal tubule by stimulating the 1α-hydroxylation of vitamin D
- Promotion of phosphaturia by inhibiting phosphate and bicarbonate reabsorption in the proximal tubule
- Mobilization of calcium from bone — together with vitamin A, the osteoblasts are stimulated to produce a factor that activates osteoclasts to mobilize calcium

Delayed effects of PTH

- Promotion of calcium and phosphate absorption from gut

Calcitonin

Produced by the C cells of the thyroid gland and synthesized as a large precursor molecule; its primary functions are:

- Inhibition of bone resorption
- Possible interaction with gastrointestinal hormones to prevent post-prandial hypercalcaemia

8.2   Disorders of calcium and phosphate metabolism

8.2.1   Hypocalcaemia

Causes of hypocalcaemia

- Transient neonatal hypocalcaemia
- Dietary
- Malabsorption
- Vitamin D deficiency
- Hypoparathyroidism
- Pseudohypoparathyroidism

8.2.2   Hypoparathyroidism

Causes

- Parathyroid absence or aplasia
- Di George syndrome (thymic abnormalities/cardiac defects/facial appearances)
- Autoimmune
- Associated with multiple endocrinopathy
- Iatrogenic — post-thyroid surgery

Treatment

In primary hypoparathyroidism, the management of neonatal tetany consists of intravenous calcium gluconate and oral 1,25-dihydroxycholecalciferol

Subsequent management is with vitamin D and an adequate intake of calcium

8.2.3   Pseudohypoparathyroidism

- Clinical features
  - Mental retardation
  - Short stature
  - Characteristic facies
  - Shortening of fourth and fifth metacarpal and metatarsal
  - Ectopic calcification
- Aetiology
  - Due to end-organ resistance
- Associations
  - TSH resistance and raised TSH levels

8.2.4   Pseudopseudohypoparathyroidism

Phenotypic features of pseudohypoparathyroidism are present but are not associated with the biochemical abnormalities.

8.2.5 Hypercalcaemia

Clinical features are non-specific, often with anorexia, constipation, polyuria, nausea and vomiting in a child with faltering growth.

Causes of hypercalcaemia

- Low PTH:
  - Vitamin D intoxication
  - Infantile hypercalcaemia
  - Transient
  - William syndrome
  - Associated with tumours
- High PTH:
  - Primary hyperparathyroidism
  - Familial hypocalciuric hypercalcaemia

Management of hypercalcaemia

This includes treatment of the underlying cause, hydration with intravenous saline, increasing urinary excretion of calcium using loop diurectics such as furosemide and the use of biophosphonates to inhibit osteoclast activity.

8.2.6 Rickets

Causes of rickets include:

- Hypocalcaemic
  - Calcium deficiency:
    - dietary
    - malabsorption
  - Vitamin D deficiency:
    - dietary
    - malabsorption
    - lack of sunlight
    - ~~liver disease~~
    - anticonvulsants
    - biosynthetic defect of vitamin D
    - 1α-hydroxylase deficiency
    - liver disease
    - renal disease
  - Defective vitamin D action
- Phosphopenic:
  - Renal tubular loss
    - isolated, e.g. X-linked hyphosphataemia
    - mixed tubular, e.g. Fanconi's syndrome
- Abnormal bones
- Renal osteodystrophy

8.3 Investigations of bone abnormalities

The basic investigations include

- Calcium, phosphate, alkaline phosphatase
- creatinine

In addition patients with hypocalcemia or rickets need

- 1,25-vitamin D, 25-vitamin D, concentrations

Where parathyroid abnormalities are suspected

- PTH
- urinary calcium, phosphate, creatinine and cAMP measurements

Other investigations depending on the underlying abnormality include

- X Rays
- Technitium bone scan
- bone mineral density scan (dual energy X-ray absorptiometry (DEXA) scanning)

9. MISCELLANEOUS ENDOCRINE DISORDERS

9.1 Obesity

Obesity is an excessive accumulation of fat. This may be because of an increase in size or in the number of adipocytes. There is no threshold value at which fatness becomes pathological.

Causes of obesity

- Nutritional:
    - Simple obesity/constitutional obesity
- Syndromes:
    - Down
    - Laurence–Moon–Biedl
    - Prader–Willi
- Endocrine:
    - Hypothalamic damage
    - Hypopituitarism, GH deficiency
    - Hypogonadism
    - Hypothyroidism
    - Cushing syndrome
    - Pseudohypoparathyroidism
    - Hyperinsulinism
    - Iatrogenic —glucocorticoids; oestrogens
- Inactivity
- Psychological disturbances

In general, simple constitutional obesity is associated with tall stature in childhood, whereas endocrine causes of obesity tend to be associated with short stature or a reduction in height velocity.

Consequences of obesity

- Childhood
  - Insulin resistance and abnormal glucose tolerance
  - Type 2 diabetes
  - Non-alcoholic steatohepatitis
  - Psychological problems
  - Orthopaedic problems
  - Obstructive sleep apnoea (pickwickian syndrome)
  - Increased cardiac diameter
- Adulthood — all the above plus:
  - Hyperlipidaemia
  - Hypertension
  - Diabetes
  - Increased risk of death from cardiovascular disease

Syndromes associated with obesity

Prader–Willi syndrome

- Genetics:
  - Deletion from paternally derived long arm of chromosome 15q
- Clinical features:
  - Neonatal hypotonia
  - Feeding difficulties in the newborn period
  - Obesity (food-seeking behaviour)
  - Hypogonadism
  - Tendency to diabetes mellitus
  - Strabismus
  - Facial features —narrow forehead; olive-shaped eyes; anti-mongoloid slant; carp mouth; abnormal ear lobes
  - Orthopaedic —small, tapering fingers; congenital dislocation of the hips; retarded bone age
  - IQ —reduced, usually 40–70
  - Behavioural difficulties —food-seeking
  - Endocrine — insulin resistance

Laurence–Moon–Biedl syndrome

- Clinical features:
  - Mental retardation
  - Obesity — marked by 4 years of age
  - Retinitis pigmentosa/strabismus
  - Polydactyly/clinodactyly
  - Moderate short stature

- Hypogonadism
- Associations:
  - Renal abnormalities
  - Diabetes insipidus

Beckwith–Wiedemann syndrome

- Clinical features:
  - Large birth weight
  - Transient hyperinsulinism
  - Macrosomia
  - Linear fissures on ear lobes
  - Umbilical hernia/exomphalos
  - Hemihypertrophy
- Associations:
  - Wilms' tumour

Assessment of the obese child

- Height, weight and pubertal assessment
- Body mass index (BMI): BMI = weight (kg)/height (m)^2; in children, the BMI should be compared to BMI centile charts for age because BMI varies during different phases of childhood. For adults the following ranges are used:
  - 20–25   healthy
  - 25–30   overweight
  - 30–40   clinically obese
  - >40   morbidly obese
- Identification of an underlying cause:
  - Thyroid function tests
  - 24 hr urinary cortisol and plasma cortisol measurements at midnight and 8 am as screening tests when Cushings syndrome is suspected
- Evidence of complications:
  - Respiratory function
  - Liver function
  - Orthopaedic problems
  - Blood pressure
  - Fasting lipids
  - Oral glucose tolerance test

Management of obesity

- Identification and treatment of underlying cause
- Dietary measures
- Reduction in sedentary behaviour
- Increased exercise
- Psychological support

9.2 Multiple endocrine neoplasia syndromes

Autosomal dominant syndromes:

- Type I (Wermer syndrome) — pancreatic (gastrinoma, insulinoma)/pituitary/parathyroid
- Type II (Sipple syndrome): — medullary thyroid cancer/parathyroid/phaeochromocytoma

Patients with multiple endocrine neoplasia type IIb have additional phenotypic features — marfanoid habitus, skeletal abnormalities, abnormal dental enamel, multiple mucosal neuromas

9.3 Autoimmune polyglandular syndromes

- Type 1 — Addison's disease, chronic mucocutaneous candidiasis, hypoparathyroidism
- Type 2 — Primary hypothyroidism, primary hypogonadism, type I diabetes, pernicious anaemia, Addison's disease, vitiligo

10. ENDOCRINE COMPLICATIONS OF OTHER DISORDERS

The endocrine glands may be affected by other chronic illnesses or their management regimens.

- Chronic pancreatitis
- Cystic-fibrosis-related diabetes
- Exogenous steroids (adrenal suppression/diabetes)
- Tumours — local erosion, radiotherapy, chemotherapy, surgical excision
- Thalassaemia (e.g. secondary iron overload as a result of multiple blood tranfusions)

11. FURTHER READING

Brook, CGD, Hindmarsh PC (eds). 2001. *Clinical Paediatric Endocrinology*, 4th edition. Oxford: Blackwell Science.

Creighton, S, Minto C. 2001. Managing intersex. *British Medical Journal* 323, 1264–6.

'Beneficial effects of intensive therapy of diabetes during adolescence: Outcomes after the conclusion of the Diabetes Control and Complications Trial (DCCT)' 2001. *Journal of Pediatrics*, 139(6), 804–812.

Hindmarsh, PC. 2002. Optimization of thyroxine dose in congenital hypothyroidism. *Archives of Disease in Childhood* 86, 73–5.

Hughes IA. 1989. *Handbook of Endocrine Investigations in Children*. Wright.

NICE Guideline. July 2004. *Type 1 Diabetes: Diagnosis and managment of Type 1 Diabetes in Children and Young People*. London: NICE.

Wright, CM, Booth, IW, Buckler, JMH. 2002. Growth reference charts for use in the United Kingdom. *Archives of Disease in Childhood* 86, 11–14.

Chapter 8

Ethics and Law

Vic Larcher and Robert Wheeler

CONTENTS

Ethics

Ethics

1. ETHICAL ISSUES, TECHNOLOGY AND LAW

This chapter provides an account of the ethical and legal principles that underpin good clinical practice. A sound knowledge of these principles will not remove or avoid ethical or legal dilemmas, but will assist their analysis and hopefully improve their resolution. Contemporary paediatric practice often demands high levels of technical expertise and may involve the application of advanced technology, the availability of which defines what **can** be done. Application of technology increasingly poses dilemmas about how, when and to whom it **should** be applied, that cannot be addressed or answered by appeal to scientific fact alone. Judgements as to what **should** be done need to be reasonable, transparent, accountable and based on sound ethical principles or theory. Such judgements must also conform to the Law. Although the Law is based on ethical principles, it has a different and more prescriptive function in decreeing what **must or must not** be done.

2. MORAL THEORIES AND PRINCIPLES

The following are some of the moral theories and principles that have been used in the analysis of ethical dilemmas and which can be used as the basis for justifying certain decisions and actions, with the strengths and weaknesses of each. Not all have considered the moral status of children but this does not preclude their use in the analysis of dilemmas arising in paediatrics.

2.1 Consequentialism/Utilitarian moral theory

In consequentialism the rightness or wrongness of an action, or its 'utility', is determined by its actual or foreseeable consequences. Utilitarianism is a type of consequentialism in which the best consequences are those in which human happiness is maximized and harms are minimized for all relevant persons involved. An action is morally correct if it maximizes welfare or individual preferences — 'the greatest good for the greatest number'. Some kind of formal calculation of risks/benefits is necessary and as such it justifies reflective, evidence-based, audited practice.

Strengths of utilitarianism

- Consequences of actions do matter
- Gives a clear answer to the question of what individuals should do

283

- Person neutral — no one counts as more than one, hence democratic
- Aspirational, promotes a happy society

Weaknesses of utilitarianism

- Difficult to predict consequences with precision
- No easily definable, universally agreed single measure of the components of the utilitarian calculus
- Some actions are wrong even if they lead to best consequences, e.g. use of torture to gain information to prevent harm
- Maximizing happiness of the majority may be unjust to the minority, especially the weak and vulnerable and those who lack capacity
- Which counts more — intensity or length of happiness?

Although the application of the principle of utility requires a potentially difficult calculation of the effects of uncertain consequences, this does not differ from any other exercise that involves balancing value judgements. Some form of calculation of harms/benefits is required in the distribution of health care to populations and in the allocation of scarce resources.

2.2   Deontology

Deontological theory is based on a doctrine of moral obligation or duty. To be moral is to do one's duty, or intend to do it, regardless of the consequences. To do one's duty involves obeying moral rules, which can be derived by rational consideration or discovery in the same way as natural laws, e.g. the laws of gravity or motion, can be deduced from physical events. Moral rules must be universal (apply to everyone), unconditional (no exceptions) and imperative (obligatory or absolutely necessary). Some obligations are deemed right regardless of consequences, e.g. truth telling, avoidance of harm to others.

Moral individuals should be capable of discerning rules (rational), able to formulate and carry out plans and govern their conduct by rules and values. A free choice must be available ('ought implies can'). Rational, autonomous beings have their own intrinsic value and are worthy of respect. They may not be used as means to further the ends of others, however laudable these may be. Thus if we wish to eliminate a disease in society by mass immunization programmes but do not obtain informed consent from subjects then we use them as means to achieving our ends without respecting their intrinsic worth.

Strengths of deontology

- General belief that some actions are wrong irrespective of consequences
- Upholds dignity and intrinsic value of individual
- Rational and supports equality
- 'Do as you would be done by'

Weaknesses of deontology

- Impossibility of truly free decisions — 'Autonomy is a philosopher's myth'
- Absolutist, austere, no place for duty of beneficence (obligation to benefit patients by acting in their best interests)
- Consequences do matter at times
- What if duties conflict? For example, the duties to avoid harms and to tell the truth

Societies may also regard other rights and obligations as important. Deciding between competing moral duties is difficult without taking some account of the consequences or likely consequences of actions.

2.3 Virtue ethics

Virtue ethics focuses on the characteristics that define the virtuous person — in this case the virtuous paediatrician. An action is right if it is what a virtuous person would do in the circumstances. A virtuous person is one who exhibits the human character traits (virtues) that are required for the best life overall (flourishing). It is associated with a deeper sense of happiness or well-being than that described by utilitarianism. Although ostensibly concerned with personal flourishing many of the virtues, e.g. kindness, generosity and tolerance, are not intrinsically selfish.

Strengths of virtue ethics

- It seems intuitively right to consider character in assessing right and wrong
- Explains why we might treat some people, e.g. family differently
- Provides a richer moral vocabulary than other theories
- Seemingly simple to operate
- Pluralistic — employing values that other theories ignore
- Enables physicians etc. to focus on developing moral characters that make them good doctors

Weaknesses of virtue ethics

- Unclear what should count as virtues and why it is good to have them
- How do we know what a virtuous person would do?
- Not independent of other moral theories, hard to analyse
- Egocentric
- May not provide a separate helpful analytical framework for addressing moral dilemmas
- May be too conservative, tied to cultural norms

2.4 Principles

An alternative approach to the day-to-day application of moral theories is the use of four prima facie moral principles that are compatible with a wide range of moral theories. There is widespread acceptance of the relevance and validity of using principles that transcend religious, cultural and philosophical differences.

When faced with an ethical dilemma it may be helpful to apply the following four moral principles that set out prima facie moral obligations. A prima facie moral obligation is one which in circumstances where duties conflict is the one which it is morally most important to follow.

The principles are:

- **Respect for autonomy** — this involves respecting the rights of patients to exercise as much self-determination as they are capable of exercising. It involves giving sufficient information to permit informed choice and a duty to respect decisions of autonomous patients even when they conflict with those of professionals
- **Beneficence** — an obligation to benefit patients by acting in their best interests, e.g. by providing treatments that are intended to produce net clinical benefits. In every day life we do not usually have an obligation to benefit others, apart from those with whom we have a special relationship e.g. family and close friends. In contrast doctors do have duties, which are often referred to as superrogatory to benefit their patients.
- **Non-maleficence** — an obligation not to cause net harm to patients even though some treatments may produce initial harms, e.g. chemotherapy. Applies to all, not just patients
- **Justice** — the obligation to act fairly and without discrimination, e.g. the distribution of healthcare resources

Strengths of principles approach

- Broad agreement that the four principles are valid and relevant
- Provides a moral checklist
- More flexible than moral theories
- More easily understood — easier to use

Weaknesses of principles approach

- Questionable moral origin of the principles — no overarching moral theory
- No hierarchy of principles to resolve conflicts between them
- Do not provide solutions but a means of analysis
- Different cultures may place different emphasis on different principles — non-uniform approach
- Regarded by some as formulaic — ethics by numbers
- Scope — to whom or to what are duties owed and how widely do they apply?

The application of four principles helps to clarify what ethical problems exist, but may not resolve dilemmas.

3. MORAL ANALYSIS OF CASES AND ISSUES

A moral philosopher's approach to dilemmas involves the application of classical moral theories or principles to deduce whether a proposed course of action is morally acceptable. Clinicians tend to approach problems in a different fashion, working from the facts of a given case to the general medical/nursing principles that might apply.

Ethical examination of cases can follow this approach by starting from the features of the particular case and seeking to recall similar cases, which might help in resolving it. For example, in dealing with a 15-year-old who is refusing further chemotherapy that his/her doctors recommend we might examine how similar cases were resolved and what ethical principles were relevant to them.

Whatever technique is used it is important that arguments used to justify positions adopted are fair-minded and are based on valid and sound reasoning. It is also important that there is a reflective equilibrium between intuitive or emotional responses to moral dilemmas and moral theory. Emotional responses to dilemmas — 'the yuk factor' — cannot be discounted altogether because emotional responses may be morally important, moral intuitions have a role in moral reasoning and emotional responses to others are an essential component of the doctor–patient relationship. Nevertheless, such emotional responses require rational analysis and justification

3.1 Moral duties of doctors

From the foregoing we can deduce that clinicians should:

- Save life, restore health and prevent disease
- Offer treatment that provides more net benefit than burden
- Offer evidence-based treatment derived from ethically conducted research
- Respect the autonomy of their patients by respecting their right to as much self-determination as they are capable of
- Respect the human dignity of all patients regardless of their abilities
- Obtain appropriately informed consent without coercion
- Carry out the above duties fairly and justly and with appropriate skill and care
- Act within the framework provided by national, and where relevant, international law

3.2 Best interests

These obligations can be further summarized by stating that all medical interventions should be in the best interests of the patient. The obligations to protect health and respect autonomy can and do conflict. In normal circumstances the respect that is accorded to the principle of autonomy means that great importance is placed upon respecting the wishes, beliefs and preferences of those who are capable of expressing and acting upon them. Most adults are capable of making informed choices to accept or refuse treatment but children may lack this capacity. An important moral issue that arises in paediatric practice is what constitutes the best interests of a child and who should determine what they are.

4. MORAL THEORY AND MORAL STATUS OF CHILDREN

Children are often regarded as lacking the characteristics that define autonomy and as such their moral status may not be sufficiently respected. Several approaches exist, which may be summarized:

- All children regardless of age have the same moral worth as adults
- All children are potential adults and should therefore be treated as such
- Society should grant children moral status because the consequences of doing so are better than treating them as though they have none
- Children's moral status depends on the extent to which they possess the qualities that we associate with personhood, e.g. consciousness, self-awareness, rationality, capacity for social interaction

The last approach accords with concepts of differing rates of growth and development with which paediatricians are familiar. It also seems an intuitive expression of respect for humanity to accord children more status than an animal with similar amounts of person-hood-satisfying characteristics.

4.1 Children's autonomy

- Children vary enormously — as do adults — in their possession of personhood-satisfying characteristics
- Autonomy may be affected by illness, its treatments or by moods
- Clinicians should enhance the development of as much autonomy as the child is capable of, e.g. by giving information and encouraging participation in decision-making
- Some children may not live long enough to develop autonomy, e.g. a child with glioblastoma
- Children may not achieve physical autonomy because of disability, e.g. muscular dystrophy
- Children may lack cognitive ability for self-determination, e.g. severe microcephaly, spastic quadriplegia
- Experience of illness may enhance autonomy, e.g. cystic fibrosis, Duchenne muscular dystrophy

5. PARENTAL RESPONSIBILITIES, RIGHTS, DUTIES AND POWERS

When children lack the capacity to express their views, others have ethical and legal authority to make decisions on their behalf until they are able to do so for themselves. In most cultures, religions and legal systems parents have this responsibility. In UK Law parental responsibility is 'all the rights, duties, power, responsibilities and authority which by law a parent of a child has in relation to the child and his property'.

Parents have moral obligations for their children's upbringing and for promotion and enhancement of their autonomy.

Application of both moral theory and law supports the autonomy of parents to rear their children in accordance with their own values provided they act in the child's best interests and do not harm them.

A family's concept of their child's best interests is likely to be determined by a number of factors that include:

- Their own ethical framework (see above)
- Social, cultural and spiritual influences
- Religious beliefs
- Political and cultural attitudes
- Peer pressure, e.g. religious groups, neighbours
- Life experiences and outside influences, e.g. media reports

These may conflict with:

- Values of professionals from different socio-economic backgrounds
- Children's need to make decisions that do not coincide with professional or parental choices

Conflicts may be exacerbated by:

- Power imbalances in professional–patient (child)–parent relationship
- Communication difficulties

6. CHILDREN'S RIGHTS

Rights are justifiable moral claims made on behalf of individuals that confer obligations on others. They provide status and protection for individuals, especially those who lack capacity or rationality. Rights are often regarded as being derived from fundamental moral principles or they may be part of a social contract. Possession of rights enables individuals to seek redress if their rights are infringed. Rights may be positive or negative and may be defined by special relationships, e.g. parent–child.

Positive rights	Negative rights
Welfare, institutional and legal rights	Natural or liberty rights
Require action by others	Entail an obligation not to infringe
Established by social contract	Natural, Constant
Change as our society changes	Take precedence over positive rights
Examples	*Examples*
Rights to information and	Freedom of movement
best available health care	speech, religious beliefs

The UN Convention of Rights of the Child sets out in a series of articles rights that apply to all aspects of a child's life. The World Medical Association (WMA) has codified those rights pertaining to health. Both endorse the development of a rights-based, child-centred healthcare system.

6.1 Key principles of UN Convention

- Any decision or action concerning children as individuals or a group must have their best interests as a primary consideration
- A child who is capable of forming his/her views has a right to express them freely
- A child's view should be given due weight in accordance with that child's age and maturity

Applied to medical practice this confers an obligation to consult children about treatment decisions and their implications, especially where cognitive ability is unimpaired, e.g. cystic fibrosis, cancer, renal failure and muscular dystrophy.

Other UN Convention articles confirm the right to

- Freedom of expression (A13)
- The highest attainable standards of health care and rehabilitation from illness (A24)
- Privacy (A16)
- Freedom from discrimination (A2) and the right to family life and to hold religious beliefs

In addition, there are obligations to provide families with the necessary support, advice and services in caring for their children.

The WMA document emphasizes children's rights to:

- Child-centred health care
- Encouragement to achieve their full potential
- Choose how much they should be involved in decision-making and how much information they wish to receive
- Help and support in decision-making
- Delegation of decision-making to others
- Confidentiality
- An explanation of reasons why their preferences cannot be met

The extent to which children are able to exercise their own rights is disputed. A child's capacity should not be underestimated but cannot be assumed as equal to an adult's. But parents, professionals or advocates make decisions from an adult perspective that may compromise a child's developing sense of personhood out of understandable desire to protect them. This may result in potential for personal choice being restricted, e.g. a teenage child with learning difficulties or muscular dystrophy who is prevented from mixing with the opposite sex. Some children may be unable to make a big choice, e.g. as to **whether** they will have a particular treatment but they can decide **where** they will have it.

Individual rights may conflict, e.g. the right to life as opposed to freedom from inhuman and degrading treatment, as may rights possessed by various parties, e.g. children, parents, clinicians. A child's right not to be harmed takes precedence over the rights to family life when the latter cannot be maintained without abuse or neglect. Resources may not allow rights to be exercised in full. It is not clear whose rights take precedence and mere appeal to rights may be insufficient to protect children's interests

7. WITHHOLDING OR WITHDRAWING LIFE-SUSTAINING TREATMENT

In most circumstances protecting and saving lives is in children's best interests because they can benefit from medical treatment; however, prolonging children's lives may impose more net burdens than benefits. Some children's lives may be regarded as having limited value to the extent to which certain qualities, e.g. the capacity for meaningful social interaction, may be lacking or lessened.

The moral and legal justification for considering withholding, withdrawing or limiting life-sustaining treatment (LST) must be that it is no longer in a child's best interests to continue to provide it.

There may be more uncertainty about the likely prognosis for a small child than there is for an adult with a comparable condition, compounded by uncertainties about their potential for growth and development. These factors may mean that children are given more chances to revive from or survive their illnesses than comparable adults, with the imposition of greater burdens.

There must be a frank discussion of the child's condition and prognosis and a decision to change the goals of treatment from cure to palliation. Both the process of initiating such discussions and their timing require skill and sensitivity and are intellectually and emotionally challenging but they are ethically justified provided that adequate and appropriate palliative care is available.

7.1 The legal framework for withholding or withdrawing LST

Deliberate killing is currently illegal however well justified ethically. Clinicians who deliberately act to shorten a child's life or take no action to save the life of patients whose death is foreseeable, may face prosecution for murder or manslaughter.

The following principles apply in UK Law and are derived from specific judgments in individual cases the effects of which have been to clarify the circumstances in which withholding or withdrawing LST may be considered not unlawful.

Courts have determined that the provision of LST is not in the best interests of patients in the following circumstances:

- If an infant has such a 'demonstrably awful life' that no reasonable person would want to live it
- Where death is imminent and irreversibly close, e.g. hydrocephalus and cerebral malformation
- Where the baby, although not close to death, had such severe disabilities that he would never be able to engage in any form of self-directed activity, e.g. severe spastic quadriplegia, with deafness, blindness and extremely limited capacity for interaction

- Clinicians cannot be forced to administer LST that they believe is not in the best interests of the child, even when the parents insist on it, e.g. severe brain damage as a consequence of microcephaly and cerebral palsy
- Permanent vegetative state, dependent on tube feeding for survival. The Court ruled that tube feeding was medical treatment and could be withdrawn because it was not in the best interests of the patient
- There is no legal distinction between withdrawing and withholding LST
- Non-provision of cardiopulmonary resuscitation was acceptable in circumstances of very severe brain damage
- Adults who are competent to do so may request that LST be withdrawn, especially if they face continuation of life that they regard as being worse than death
- Requests for assisted suicide or active euthanasia have been rejected by English Courts

The legality of withdrawal of fluids from children who are not close to death or in a permanent vegetative state remains unclear and many professionals have ethical concerns about it. Even considering UK Human Rights legislation, Courts appear to accept that there are circumstances in which the continued provision of LST no longer serves the broader concept of best interests, perhaps because of its intolerable burden.

7.2 Professional guidance

The Royal College of Paediatrics and Child Health (RCPCH) has published an ethical and legal framework within which decisions to withhold or withdraw LST might be made, and has provided advice on the process of decision-making and the resolution of conflicts. The RCPCH identified five situations in which withholding or withdrawing LST might be discussed. These were:

1 – Brain stem death
2 – Permanent vegetative state
3 – The 'no chance' situation when LST only marginally delayed death without alleviating suffering
4 – The 'no purpose' situation when survival is possible but only at the cost of physical or mental impairment, which it would be unreasonable to expect the child to bear. It was envisaged that such a child would never be capable of sufficient self-directed activity to make decisions for themselves (see legal criteria above)
5 – The intolerable situation where survival was again possible but, in the face of progressive and irreversible illness, the child and/or family believe that further treatment is more than the child and/or family can endure with any acceptable degree of human fulfilment. This situation clearly includes children with and without mental impairment

7.3 The process of decision-making

- All remediable causes for the child's condition must be excluded
- Absolute certainty over likely outcomes may not be possible and should be acknowledged
- There should be general acceptance that value judgments have to be made

- There should be openness and transparency in discussions within teams and with parents/children
- Consider second opinions to clarify position

7.4 Managing disputes/dissent

Disputes and dissent may arise within teams or with families as to what should be done. Where possible the reasons for this should be analysed so as to provide a means of resolution. Attention to or consideration of the following may be helpful:

- Communication
- Education/information sharing
- Negotiation/mediation/conciliation
- Trade offs — e.g. deferring to requests for benign treatment
- Consensus building
- Referral/second opinions
- Ethical review — e.g Clinical Ethics Committee
- Application to Courts

7.5 The extremely premature infant (< 24 weeks' gestation)

In some countries neonatal intensive care may not be routinely offered to extremely preterm infants. UK practice varies but withholding of LST should be justified by the ethical and legal principles outlined above and subject to parental agreement. If practicable, treatment options should be discussed with the family before the birth and decisions should be informed by the disclosure of both national and local survival figures and complication rates.

Decisions to withhold or withdraw LST are often viewed as psychologically and emotionally distinct; withholding treatment may deprive a child of treatment from which they may potentially benefit.

If there is doubt concerning parental wishes or lack of senior paediatric support the infant should be resuscitated and treated until a clearer picture of outcome emerges and parental views can be clarified.

Where disputes over the provision of LST cannot be settled by the above mechanisms a legal ruling on what is in the best interests of the child should be obtained before any action to withdraw LST.

Checklist for end of life decision-making

Individuals may find the following checklist helpful in formulating end of life care plans and obtaining consent for them.

The child's clinical condition

- Are sufficient and adequate medical facts available to make a diagnosis and give accurate prognosis?
- Has a potentially treatable condition been excluded?
- Is a second medical opinion necessary/desirable?
- Is there a need for a psychiatric or psychological assessment of the child?
- What are the problems in providing nursing care in the current situation?
- What are the views of nursing staff about changing goals for the child?
- What are the views of other therapists/professionals involved with the child?
- How has dissent in the team been handled?
- Is the child able to form a view about what he/she wants?
- Has he or she been consulted?

The family

- Is the family's understanding of their child's condition adequate?
- What are the family's relevant religious and cultural beliefs and values?
- Has there been a psycho-social assessment of the family?
- What the family's likely or actual views on changing goals of treatment?
- Do the family need the help of an advocate?

The decision-making process

- How has uncertainty about the outcome been addressed?
- Has there been an ethical review of the case?
- Has there been a strategy meeting or psychosocial meeting?
- Have human rights issues been properly considered?
- Is there a proportionate justification for any infringement of human rights?
- Is there a need for a legal opinion?
- Is there a properly formulated care plan?
- Has informed consent for this care plan been obtained?
- Do the notes adequately reflect the process?
- How is the process to be maintained/audited?

8. CONSENT (ETHICAL BASIS)

The need to obtain consent for medical treatment is morally justified because it respects the rights of patients to make informed choices as to what will be done to them, respects their autonomy and avoids treating them merely as a means. It is likely to have good consequences for those involved. To be ethically valid, consent should be sufficiently informed, given by a person who has the capacity to understand the issues involved and obtained freely.

Children may have the legal capacity to give consent but even if they do not they still have the right to information given in a form and at a pace that they can comprehend. If their views are to be overridden they should receive an explanation as to why this will happen. It is good practice to seek their assent, i.e. agreement, and where a treatment or intervention is not immediately necessary to delay it until they have had further opportunity to discuss it.

9. CONFIDENTIALITY

There is a general duty of confidentiality over the disclosure of personal information about patients (including children) to third parties.

In general such information should not be disclosed without the consent of the patient or those with parental responsibility in the case of children.

The ethical justifications for non-consensual disclosure are:

- Respect for children's autonomy and right for control over their own data
- Confidentiality is a professional duty — implied promise not to disclose
- The duty of the virtuous doctor is to keep patient details confidential
- Better consequences follow if patient's know they can trust their doctors not to reveal information

General principles of confidentiality:

- Wherever possible consent for disclosure should be sought
- Data should be made anonymous if unidentifiable data will serve the purpose
- Only information necessary for the purpose in question should be disclosed
- Information can be shared within healthcare teams unless patients specifically object because sharing of clinical and other information is implicit in and necessary for the effective delivery of health care.

Although there is no specific law of confidentiality the Law's approach to breaches of confidentiality is to consider whether there is a public interest in favour of breaching confidentiality or not breaching it.

Disclosure of information is a legal duty in certain circumstances:

- Notification of certain specified infectious diseases
- Notification of births and deaths
- If the Court makes a specific request for it

Disclosure of information is discretionary in circumstances where:

- There is risk of significant harm to a third party
- It is necessary to do so for detection or prevention of serious crime including child abuse

9.1 Confidentiality and children

Children are owed the same duty of confidentiality as are adults, irrespective of their legal status.

The disclosure of information usually depends on the consent of the child or a person with parental responsibility.

While children over 16 years are assumed competent to give consent, those under 16 may do so if they are able to understand what is involved and its consequences for their family. The principle that determines whether disclosure should take place is whether it is in the child's best interests to do so. Doctors may therefore ethically disclose information to parents of children of less than 18 years, even with the child's refusal, if they genuinely believe that it is in the young person's best interests to do so. This needs to be justified and the reasons for disclosure carefully explained.

9.2 Confidentiality and child protection

The paediatrician's primary duty is to the child not the carers. If a doctor has reasonable grounds to believe that a child is at risk of significant harm the facts should be reported to the appropriate statutory authority. Doctors have ethical and legal duties to assist statutory authorities in making relevant inquiries in such cases. Doctors must satisfy themselves that disclosure of information is in the child's best interests. Information about competent children can be disclosed without their consent if to do so is justified on the above grounds. Information about non-competent children can be disclosed without parental consent if it is necessary to protect the child. The child and or parents should normally be told about disclosure of information unless to do so would not be in the child's best interests or would expose them to risk of serious harm. All decisions about disclosure must be justifiable and reasonable.

10. CONTRACEPTION, CONSENT AND CONFIDENTIALITY IN TEENAGERS

Concern about teenage pregnancy rates stems from the ethical duty to protect children from harm. Ethical dilemmas arise when children under the age of 16 years seek contraceptive advice without the express consent or knowledge of their parents and are adamant that their parents should not be informed.

Ethical justifications for respecting the young person's wishes are:

- Respect for autonomy
- Duty to confer more benefits than harms
- Adverse consequences of failing to provide confidential advice, e.g. increased pregnancy rates, sexually transmitted diseases
- Respect for children's rights to health, information, identity

Although there may be ethical justification for the prescription of contraception in such circumstances, there has been dispute over its legality. It was held that 'Parental right...[to determine whether their child should undergo medical treatment]...terminates if...and when the child achieves sufficient understanding and intelligence to enable him or her to understand fully what is proposed'.

It is clear that children under the age of 16 may have the capacity to consent to medical treatment provided that they understand the nature and purpose of what is involved and its implications for themselves and their family.

The legal (Fraser's) criteria for the prescription of contraception (including emergency contraception) to adolescents are:

- Ability to understand implications for self and family
- There is a sustained and consistent refusal to discuss with parents
- The young person has made a decision to start or continue to have sexual intercourse, despite attempts at persuasion
- The adolescent's health will suffer or is likely to suffer if contraception is not given
- Prescribing contraception is in the young person's best interests

11. ABORTION

Children and young people may request abortion under the terms of the Abortion Act 1967 as amended in 1990. This provides that abortion may be carried out in pregnancies that do not exceed 24 weeks if:

- The continuation of the pregnancy would result in injury to the physical or mental health of the woman or any existing children in her family
- The termination is necessary to prevent that risk
- The continuation of the pregnancy would involve risk to the life of the mother, greater than if it were terminated
- There is a substantial risk that if the child were born it would suffer from such physical or mental abnormalities as to be seriously handicapped

Under the Act the young person needs to be assessed by two doctors who must be satisfied that the abortion is justified.

The ethical justifications for abortion in young women are essentially similar to those in adults but a more paternalistic approach with appeal to best interests is reasonable in those who cannot consent because they lack the capacity to do so.

12. ETHICS AND LAW

There may be tensions between ethical and legal obligations, e.g. in relation to end of life issues. It is important that, whatever ethical views are held, practice conforms to the law.

Child law

13. AN INTRODUCTION

It is not feasible, here, to state comprehensively the law pertaining to paediatric medicine, let alone the body of law applicable to children. This section simply touches on some of the legal topics that frequently vex doctors, and reviews child law in England and Wales. The stage is set by consideration of the very wide remit of the Children Act 1989. Subsequently, the status of the child and those with parental responsibility are considered, before discussing the most frequently exercised issue of medical law in childhood, namely the provision of valid consent.

14. CHILDREN ACT 1989

The underlying themes of this Act are that:

- The child's welfare is paramount
- The courts should impose orders on children only if
  - The imposition of an order would be better for the child than making no order at all
  - Any delays in decisions concerning the upbringing of a child are likely to prejudice the welfare of the child

The Act provides for state intervention in family matters, such as adjudication in issues of contact, residence, and in things that must and may not be done in relation to the child (i.e. Section 8 orders 'Contact, residence, Specific issue and Prohibited steps'). The Act ensures that local authorities provide services and support to families, and to 'children who are looked after by a local authority'. Finally, provision is made for the protection, care and supervision of children, establishing a 'threshold of harm' (Section 31(9): '"harm" means ill-treatment or the impairment of health or development including for example, impairment suffered from seeing or hearing the ill-treatment of another').

15. WHAT IS A CHILD?

15.1 'Full legal capacity'

Childhood ends on the 18th birthday. At this point, transition to 'Majority' occurs and the new adult assumes all decision-making powers (although applicants for adoption and holders of Public offices cannot generally be under 21 years), including the ability to make their own decisions concerning health care. The significance of the 21st birthday as a landmark occasion in our society derives in part from this being the age of majority, until legislation in 1969 (the Family Law Reform Act 1969). Under the same Act, 16- and 17-year-olds were given the legal right to agree to treatment independently of their parents, although the courts have not interpreted this statute as giving a right to refuse.

16. STATUS IN COURTS

Children traditionally have 'no voice' in courts (the word 'infant' derives from the Latin *infari*; no speech). This means that in civil litigation, the child's interests can only be represented through a litigation friend or a guardian ad litem; it is a parent's right and duty to perform these roles, and it can be seen how conflicts of interest may arise between adult and child in these circumstances.

This rule also applies in family proceedings, where 'children's guardians' now ensure that the feelings and wishes of the child are represented. However, it has been modified by the Children Act 1989, permitting a child with sufficient understanding to have an independent voice in matters such as residency and contact with family members.

17. WHO 'OWNS' THE CHILD?

17.1 Children Act 1989

Although it is clear that no-one owns a child, the title serves as a reminder that until 1989, the legal emphasis was on parental rights and influence. This legacy derived from times when the father had exclusive and total power over his child, while a mother was merely entitled 'only to reverence and respect'. Such power enabled unscrupulous fathers to earn money from the work of their children. Stealing children and effectively enslaving them reflected their economic value, and was legal until 1814. Progressive legislation addressed this appalling situation, but the central theme, of parental rights having overarching significance, was only finally reversed by the Act in 1989.

17.2 Parental responsibility

A key feature of the Act was to codify 'parental responsibility' as the central role of the adult who cares for the child. In most cases, it will obviously be the parents who have parental responsibility, but others may also share it, such as the local authority.

Defined as 'all the rights, duties, powers, responsibilities and authority, which by law a parent of a child has in relation to a child and his property', parental responsibility is automatically vested in the child's biological mother (although it should be noted that any of these basic rules would be invalidated by an adoption order). She, it is accepted in English law, is the person who gives birth to the child (as opposed to the genetic mother, in the case of some surrogates).

There is a legal presumption that the man who is married to the mother is the biological and thus legal father, whatever the truth of the situation. If married to the mother at the time of the birth, the father will have parental responsibility. An unmarried father whose name appears on the birth certificate on or after 1 December 2003 automatically has parental responsibility, and it can be acquired by other unmarried fathers by formal agreements with the mother, or the court.

Guardians, local authorities, adoption agencies and prospective adopters can share parental responsibility with the parents but the parents only surrender their parental responsibility when the child reaches majority, or is adopted away from them.

In terms of the residual 'rights' of parenthood, the naming of the child, the determination of education and religion, and the right to appoint a guardian remain. The other 'incidents' of parenthood (i.e. to provide a home, to protect and maintain, to provide for education, to discipline, etc.) would largely be viewed as duties or responsibilities, placed by the state on the parent.

17.3   Wardship

In ancient times, wardship described a right to have custody over an infant who was the heir to land. Combined with the sovereign's powers to act as the parent of any abandoned (or orphaned) child, it can be seen that this was a potent mechanism for a land-hungry monarch (*Parens patriae*: Latin: 'parent of the fatherland' or 'parent of the homeland'; in law, it refers to the power of the state to act as the parent of any child or the power to act on behalf of any individual who is in need of protection, such as an incapacitated individual or a child whose parents are unable or unwilling to take care of the child).

In the modern era, the High Court can use wardship as one means of exercising its *parens patriae* powers, to ensure that no important or major steps in the life of a ward of court can be taken without prior consent from the court. This certainly extends to medical treatments because for a ward of court, the court has parental responsibility. In general terms, one of the aims of the Children Act 1989 was to reduce the necessity for wardship proceedings, by incorporating its more worthwhile powers into the statute.

17.4   Guardians

Guardianship is confusing (see Bainham 2005), because there are several separate roles that adults play in relation to children which have acquired this label.

Natural or parental guardian

Over centuries, the legitimate father has been the **natural or parental guardian** of the child, not least because of the property rights this conferred. English literature is peppered with references to fathers exercising their rights of guardianship, rarely to the children's advantage. A father could exercise all parental rights, to the exclusion of the mother, until 1973, when mothers were given equal rights and authority. Fathers retained some residual rights of this **natural guardianship** even after 1973. This was reflected in their ability to prohibit the mother's unilateral wish for a change of a child's surname following divorce, even if they had lost custody of the child. This **natural or parental guardianship** has been abolished by the Children Act 1989, removing the final vestiges of parental legal inequality.

Guardians taking legal responsibility for a child after parental death

These **guardians** provide a vital, if under utilized, function. They can be appointed (commonly) by parents or (less commonly) by courts. When parents contemplate the sad reality that they may die together, in an accident, leaving children, they may well wish to have influence over who brings up their orphaned family. Appointing a guardian enables them to exercise this influence, because the guardian will assume parental responsibility on the death of the second parent. Guardians may be appointed with no more formality than a signed and dated letter, and this rather surprising theme of informality applies to several aspects of guardianship. Nevertheless, it permits parents to avoid the nightmare of having their children brought up by their least-favourite relative in the event of their untimely and simultaneous death.

The family court may have to intervene if the second parent has died without appointing guardians, particularly if there is a dispute within the family as to who should look after the children. Have you got appropriate arrangements in place?

Children's guardian

Children's guardians represent children in court during proceedings involving state intervention in the family; they are one of a number of individuals, collectively described as 'officers of the service', falling within the remit of the Children and Family Court Advisory and Support Service (CAFCASS). They are appointed on the basis of their expertise in social work and childcare law. Their role is to inform the court of the child's wishes and feelings, while providing all the information that may be relevant to the child's welfare. They are loosely equivalent to **guardians ad litem**, who represent children in civil litigation.

Special guardian

This is a new legal concept (introduced by the Adoption and Children Act 2002), providing legal security for permanent carers of children but falling short of adoption, for situations where adoption has been thought inappropriate for the child.

18. CONSENT

Those with parental responsibility have a duty to provide consent for the child's medical treatment.

Consent is required before any intervention, because society opposes the uninvited touch.

At its simplest, the outstretched hand, by implication, invites touching. However, the patient who consults their doctor does not assume that their very presence in the consulting room gives the doctor licence to touch them. The uninvited touch is, historically, an act of common assault. However, it is not the avoidance of this rather dramatic accusation that drives most contemporary doctors to obtain consent, although very occasionally the charge is still made.

What is far more relevant is the concept of negligence, where the doctor causes some harm by failing to deliver a reasonable standard of care to the patient, to whom there is undoubtedly a duty to provide such care.

One aspect of this standard of care is obtaining valid consent. This entails the provision of all necessary information for the patient to make an informed decision. Often, the only record of this provision is the annotated and signed consent form. This document thus acts both as a shield against a claim of assault, and objective evidence that some formal provision of information has occurred.

There are two excellent documents concerning consent which provide comprehensive guidelines (the DoH *Reference Guide* and the BMA report of the Consent working party). The main questions to be considered when obtaining consent may be summarized as follows.

When is consent required?
- Consent is required for any intervention

Who should obtain consent?
- The person who will perform the proposed treatment

In what form should consent be taken?
- There is no legal requirement for written consent, which can equally be verbal, or by acquiescence, provided the patient is correctly informed. However, a written document, which is signed by the patient, forms a piece of objective evidence that consent has been taken. Furthermore, if the document also records the details of the information given, it increases the certainty that relevant issues have been discussed. If the consent were verbal, it would be prudent to record the circumstances, topics discussed and outcome in the clinical notes

From whom should consent be obtained?
- Anyone with parental responsibility for a child may provide consent for his or her medical treatment. To consent to treatment, an individual must have the capacity (i.e. intelligence and understanding) fully to understand what treatment is being proposed (see below)
- It is assumed that a young person of 16 years has such capacity, and because the law provides that they can give valid consent, no additional consent from parents is required. In the period between 16 and 18 years, if the young person is incapacitated, their parents may consent on their behalf
- A child of less than 16 years may give consent if capacity can be established, but the test is relatively rigorous

In the absence of a parent, where a child is unable to consent because of lack of capacity, can the doctor treat in the emergency situation?
- If emergency treatment is necessary to save life or avoid a significant deterioration in health, the doctor may treat on the basis of this necessity. However, the views of the parents and the child (if known), the likelihood of improvement with treatment and the need to avoid restricting future treatment options where possible must all be considered in this situation

What information should be provided to obtain informed consent?

- The amount of information clearly depends upon the circumstances, and a balance must be found, to avoid either denying the patient relevant information or causing undue alarm. This should include the certainties of diagnosis; the options for treatment (including non-treatment); a balanced opinion of the likely outcome of these options; and the purpose, risks, benefits and side-effects of the intervention. The General Medical Council would also recommend ensuring that the name of the senior clinician is reiterated, together with a reminder that withdrawal from the treatment continues to be an option

19. CHILDREN'S CAPACITY

19.1   16-17 years

There is a legal presumption that these young people have the capacity to consent, so there is no requirement for clinicians to test capacity in this age group. However, if there is doubt that an individual is competent to provide consent, their competence should be assessed according to the criteria used for any adult (according to Re C (Adult: Refusal of Medical Treatment) [1994] 1 All ER 819). According to Grubb (2004) the patient must be able to:

- Comprehend and retain the relevant information
- Believe it
- Weigh it in the balance so as to arrive at a choice

Refusal of therapy, particularly if the treatment is for life-threatening disease, gives more difficulty, and legal advice should be sought. Despite wishing to uphold the autonomy of competent children, English courts effectively prohibit children from refusing treatment that will save them from death or serious permanent harm.

19.2   Preschool

It is self-evident that children in this age group are unable to provide valid consent but they still have autonomy and their interests should be considered. It is good practice to involve them where possible in the process of obtaining consent, particularly offering to answer their questions, and to remind them of the obvious consequences of a procedure (e.g. the scar).

19.3   The intervening years

The child who has yet to reach 16 years is presumed, by the law, to be incapable of providing consent. However, some children who quite clearly possess a degree of capacity may be able to demonstrate their competence. If they can, they may provide consent independently of their parents. However, it is both good manners and good practice to involve their parents; and it will be rare for such parental involvement to be inappropriate, unless confidentiality is an issue. In determining whether a child might have capacity for

303

consenting to a particular procedure, their age is probably the least consideration. The House of Lords have provided the means for the determination, in their ruling on the Gillick case (Gillick v West Norfolk & Wisbech AHA (1985) 3 All ER 402, HL). The child would need to:

- Understand that a choice exists
- Understand the purpose and nature of the proposed treatment
- Understand the risks, benefits and alternatives
- Understand the consequences of not undergoing the treatment

Furthermore, the child must:

- Be able to remember the information for long enough to make a considered decision
- Be free from undue pressure

It is clear that the ability of the child to pass this 'test' is entirely dependent on the proposed procedure, and the child's experience. It is not difficult to picture 14-year-olds with newly diagnosed leukaemia, bewildered and terrified, who would be entirely incapable of providing valid consent to a diagnostic lumbar puncture. On the other hand, a younger child who has spent months on the oncology ward, already had numerous similar procedures, and witnessed the consequences in many of his fellow patients, may well be competent.

It should be reiterated that the Gillick test, understandably, sets a high threshold for capacity that would probably be unattainable by many adults.

As with the 16- to 17-year-olds, the ability of Gillick-competent children to provide valid consent does not extend to a right to refuse.

19.4   Fraser Guidelines

Emerging from the House of Lords judgement, Lord Fraser also gave guidance on how the Gillick principle could be applied to the provision of contraceptives to young people. These guidelines emphasize the importance of parental support, acknowledging confidentiality and weighing the best interests of the child (see BMA 2004). They also take account of the risk that the patient may have unprotected sex if the contraception is denied, and the potential effects on their mental and physical health.

20.   FURTHER READING

Bainham A. 2005. *Children: The Modern Law*. London: Jordan Publishing.

BMA. 2001. *Report of the Consent Working Party March 2001*. London: Medical Ethics Department, BMA.

BMA. 2004. *Medical Ethics Today*. London: BMA Medical Ethics Department.

DoH 2001. Reference Guide to Consent for Examination or Treatment. www.doh.gov.uk/consent

Grubb A. 2004. *Principles of Medical Law*. Oxford: Oxford University Press.

Hope T, Savulescu J, Hendrick J. 2003. *Medical Ethics and Law: the Core Curriculum.* London: Churchill Livingstone.

Kennedy I, Grubb. A. 2000. *Medical Law Text and Materials,* 3rd edn. London: Butterworths.

Montgomery J. 2002. *Health Care Law,* 2nd edn. Oxford: Oxford University Press.

Raphael DD. 1994. *Moral Philosophy,* 2nd edn. Oxford: Oxford University Press.

RCPCH. 2004. *Withholding or Withdrawing Life Sustaining Treatment in Children; a framework for practice,* 2nd edn. Available on RCPCH web-site: www.rcpch. ac.uk

Sokol DK, Bergson G. 2000. *Medical Ethics and Law; Surviving the Wards and Passing Exams.* London: Trauma Publishing.

UK Clinical Ethics Network www.ethics-network.org.uk

Chapter 9

Gastroenterology and Nutrition

Mark Beattie

CONTENTS

Gastroenterology and Nutrition

1. BASIC ANATOMY AND PHYSIOLOGY

1.1 Anatomy

Oesophagus

Outer longitudinal and inner circular muscle layers with myenteric plexus in-between. Mucosa is lined by stratified squamous epithelium. Adult length 25 cm.

Stomach

Lined by columnar epithelium. Chief cells produce pepsin. Parietal cells produce gastric acid and intrinsic factor. Secretions in adults are 3 l/day. Gastric acid secretion is stimulated by vagal stimulation, gastrin and histamine via H_2 receptors on parietal cells. Secretion is inhibited by sympathetic stimulation, nausea, gastric acidity and small intestinal peptides. Blood supply from coeliac axis.

Small intestine

Main function is absorption, mostly in the duodenum and jejunum apart from bile salts and vitamin B_{12} which are absorbed in the terminal ileum. Blood supply from mid-duodenum onwards is the superior mesenteric artery. Adult length 2–3 metres.

Colon

Functions primarily for salt and water reabsorption. Blood supply from superior mesenteric artery until the distal transverse colon and then the inferior mesenteric artery after that. Approximately 1 m long in adults.

Pancreas

Retroperitoneal. Endocrine function (2% of tissue mass) and exocrine function (98%). Blood supply from coeliac axis.

1.2   Digestion

Carbohydrate digestion

- Carbohydrates are consumed as monosaccharides (glucose, fructose, galactose), disaccharides (lactose, sucrose, maltose, isomaltose) and the polysaccharides (starch, dextrins, glycogen)
- Salivary and pancreatic amylase break down starch into oligosaccharides and disaccharides. Pancreatic amylase aids carbohydrate digestion but carbohydrate digestion is not dependent upon it
- Disaccharidases (maltase, sucrase, lactase) in the microvilli hydrolyse oligo- and disaccharides into monosaccharides:
  - Maltose into glucose
  - Isomaltose into glucose
  - Sucrose into glucose and fructose
  - Lactose into glucose and galactose
- Monosaccharides are then absorbed, glucose and galactose by an active transport mechanism and fructose by facilitated diffusion

Protein digestion

- In the stomach, gastric acid denatures protein and facilitates the conversion of pepsinogen into pepsin
- Trypsin, chymotrypsin and elastase, secreted as the inactive precursors, are produced by the exocrine pancreas. Enterokinase (secreted in the proximal duodenum) activates trypsin and trypsin further activates trypsin, chymotrypsin and elastase
- These proteases convert proteins into oligopeptides and amino acids in the duodenum
- The small intestine absorbs free amino acids and peptides by active transport and these substances then enter the portal vein and are carried to the liver.

Fat digestion

- Entry of fats into the duodenum causes release of pancreozymin–cholecystokinin which stimulates the gallbladder to contract
- Hydrolysis of triglycerides by pancreatic lipase takes place
- Free fatty acids, glycerol and monoglycerides are emulsified by bile salts to form micelles which are then absorbed along the brush border of mucosal cells
- Short-chain fatty acids enter the portal circulation bound to albumin. Long-chain fats are re-esterified within the mucosal cells into triglycerides which combine with lesser amounts of protein, phospholipid and cholesterol to create chylomicrons
- Chylomicrons enter the lymphatic system and are transported via the thoracic duct into the bloodstream

Pancreatic function

The pancreas secretes more than a litre of pancreatic juice per day, which is bicarbonate-rich and contains enzymes for the absorption of carbohydrate, fat and protein. Faecal elastase is a commonly used screen for pancreatic function.

Gut hormones

The main gut hormones are:

- **Gastrin** — stimulated by vagal stimulation, distension of the stomach. Stimulates gastric acid, pepsin and intrinsic factor. Stimulates gastric emptying and pancreatic secretion
- **Secretin** — stimulated by intraluminal acid. Stimulates pancreatic bicarbonate secretion, inhibits gastric acid and pepsin secretion and delays gastric emptying
- **Cholecystokinin–pancreozymin** — stimulated by intraluminal food. Stimulates pancreatic bicarbonate and enzyme secretion. Stimulates gallbladder contraction, inhibits gastric emptying and gut motility

Other gut hormones include:

- **Gastric inhibitory peptide** — stimulated by glucose, fats and amino acids; inhibits gastric acid secretion, stimulates insulin secretion and reduces motility
- **Motilin** — stimulated by acid in the small bowel; increases motility
- **Pancreatic polypeptide** — stimulated by a protein-rich meal; inhibits gastric and pancreatic secretion
- **Vasoactive intestinal peptide** (VIP) — neural stimulation; inhibits gastric acid and pepsin secretion; stimulates insulin secretion; reduces motility

Enterohepatic circulation

Bile is produced by the liver and stored in the gallbladder. It is secreted into the duodenum following gallbladder contraction (stimulated by cholecystokinin–pancreozymin release). Bile acids aid fat digestion. They are formed from cholesterol. Primary bile acids are produced in the liver. Secondary bile acids are formed from primary bile acids through conjugation with amino acids by the action of intestinal bacteria. Primary and secondary bile acids are deconjugated in the intestine, reabsorbed in the terminal ileum and transported back to the liver bound to albumin for recirculation.

2. NUTRITION

2.1 Nutritional requirements

This is age dependent and there are standard tables available (Reference Nutrient Intake, RNI). The energy needs per kilogram of the infant are higher than the older child.

Daily requirements

Infant 0–3 months

- Fluid   150 ml/kg
- Calories   100 kCal/kg
- Protein   2.1 g/kg
- Sodium   1.5 mmol/kg
- Potassium   3 mmol/kg

12-year-old boy

- Fluid   55 ml/kg
- Calories   50 kCal/kg
- Protein   1 g/kg
- Sodium   2 mmol/kg
- Potassium   2 mmol/kg

Energy requirements list calories but nutrient and micronutrient requirements are also important to ensure that intake is balanced. It is essential for example to have an appropriate balance of fat, carbohydrate and protein. Calcium is essential for bone growth. Iron is required to prevent anaemia.

Energy requirements include Resting Energy Expenditure (Basal Metabolic Rate), which represents 60–70% of requirements and the component which arises as a consequence of physical activity (Physical Activity level).

Physical status (metabolic condition, bedridden, physical activity level) will impact on requirements

Requirements in disease are generally greater than requirements in health

2.2 Nutritional assessment

It is important to take a careful history, assess intake, consider requirements and weigh the patient.

- Body mass index is a useful marker of 'fatness' measured as (weight)/(height^2) in kg/m^2. The values need to be plotted against age on standard charts
- Other methods of assessing nutritional state include skin-fold thickness as an estimate of fat mass and mid-arm circumference as an estimate of lean body mass. Standard age-matched reference values are available
- Bio-impedance and indirect calorimetry as research tools are also used although less is known about the normal ranges
- Patients with chronic illness and those at risk for malnutrition should have detailed nutritional assessment

Important factors in the history

Consider the following

- Conditions that interfere with intake
- Conditions that interfere with absorption, e.g. intestinal resection
- Conditions associated with increased losses, e.g. diarrhoea, vomiting
- Condition associated with increased needs, e.g. fever, sepsis, tissue injury
- Conditions that restrict intake, e.g. cardiac disease, renal disease, food intolerance
- Gastrointestinal conditions, e.g. gastro-oesophageal reflux, constipation

Constipation, particularly if severe, can have a very major impact on nutritional intake. It is common in children with nutritional impairment from any cause.

Ensure that you understand relevant social and family factors that may impact on the child's nutrition.

2.3   Breast-feeding

Breast-feeding and infection

Ten per cent of the protein in mature breast milk is secretory immunoglobulin A (IgA). Lymphocytes, macrophages, proteins with non-specific antibacterial activity and complement are also present. There have been many studies in developing countries to show that infants fed formula milk have a higher mortality and morbidity particularly from gastrointestinal infection. In the UK, studies have shown:

- Breast-feeding for more than 13 weeks reduces the incidence of gastrointestinal and respiratory infections
- The response to immunization with the Hib vaccine is higher in breast-fed than formula-fed infants
- The risk of necrotizing enterocolitis in low-birth-weight babies is lower in those who are breast-fed

Breast-feeding and allergy

The incidence of atopic eczema in infants born to atopic mothers is reduced by breast-feeding. Overall, however, there is no definitive proven reduction in atopy apart from this specific circumstance.

Breast-feeding and neurological development

Although there are confounding variables which make study of this subject difficult, there is work that suggests that neurological development is enhanced in breast-fed infants.

Breast-feeding and diabetes

Infants who are breast-fed have a reduced risk of developing diabetes.

Breast-feeding and infantile colic

There is no good evidence to show that breast-feeding reduces the incidence of infantile colic.

Contraindications to breast-feeding

Maternal drugs and breast-feeding are discussed in Chapter 4 — Clinical Pharmacology and Toxicology, section 6.2 and in Chapter 16 — Neonatology.

- With regard to tuberculosis; infants can be immunized at birth with isoniazid-resistant BCG and treated with a course of isoniazid
- With regard to human immunodeficiency virus (HIV); the virus has been cultured from breast milk and is transmitted in it. In the Western world this makes breast-feeding contraindicated in HIV-positive mothers, as it will increase the perinatal transmission

rate. The problem is not so straightforward in the developing world where the risks of bottle feeding are high because of contaminated water supplies.

Term and pre-term formula

The principal differences are that pre-term formula contains more electrolytes, calories and minerals. All of the following are higher in pre-term than term formula; energy, protein, carbohydrate, fat, osmolality, sodium, potassium, calcium, magnesium, phosphate and iron.

Human (breast) milk and cows' milk

The energy content is the same. Human milk contains less protein than cows' milk — the cows' milk having a much higher casein content. The fat, although different qualitatively, is the same in amount. Human milk contains more carbohydrate. Cows' milk contains more of all the minerals except iron and copper.

2.4   Iron

- Dietary sources include cereals, red meat (particularly liver), fresh fruit, green vegetables
- Absorbed from the proximal small bowel. Vitamin C, gastric acid and protein improve absorption. 5–10% of dietary iron is absorbed
- Deficiency causes hypochromic microcytic anaemia. Associated with poor appetite and reduced intellectual function
- Common causes of deficiency include poor diet (particularly prolonged or excess milk feeding), chronic blood loss, malabsorption
- Low serum iron/high transferrin suggests deficiency; low iron/low transferrin suggests chronic disease. Ferritin is an indicator of total body stores but is also an acute-phase reactant
- Treatment is directed against the underlying cause. Dietary advice and iron supplements, of which numerous commercial preparations are available, are indicated in most patients. Side-effects of iron supplements include abdominal discomfort and constipation. Iron supplements can be fatal in overdose

2.5   Folate

- Dietary sources include liver, green vegetables, cereals, orange, milk, yeast and mushrooms. Excessive cooking destroys folate
- Absorbed from the proximal small bowel
- Deficiency causes megaloblastic anaemia, irritability, poor weight gain and chronic diarrhoea. Thrombocytopenia can occur
- The serum folate reflects recent changes in folate status and the red-cell folate is an indicator of the total body stores
- Treatment of deficiency is with oral folic acid
- Folate levels are not affected by the acute-phase response

Causes of folate deficiency

- Reduced intake
- Coeliac disease
- Tropical sprue
- Blind-loop syndrome
- Congenital folate malabsorption (autosomal recessive)
- Increased requirements (infancy, pregnancy, exfoliative skin disease)
- Increased loss (haemodialysis)
- Methotrexate
- Trimethoprim
- Anticonvulsants
- Oral contraceptive pill

2.6   Vitamin B$_{12}$

- Dietary sources include foods of animal origin, particularly meat
- Absorbed from the terminal ileum facilitated by gastric intrinsic factor
- Deficiency causes megaloblastic anaemia, low vitamin B$_{12}$, increased methyl-malonic acid in the urine
- Clinical features include anaemia, glossitis, peripheral neuropathy, subacute combined degeneration of the cord, optic atrophy
- Causes include pernicious anaemia (rare in childhood), gastric- and parietal-cell antibodies are usually positive
- Other causes of vitamin B$_{12}$ deficiency include poor intake (vegan diet) and malabsorption, e.g. blind-loop, post-resection
- Treatment is with vitamin B$_{12}$, usually given im once or twice a week initially then 3-monthly. Folic acid is also needed

2.7   Zinc

- Dietary sources include beef, liver, eggs and nuts
- Deficiency occurs secondary to poor absorption rather than poor intake
- Clinical features include anaemia, growth retardation, periorofacial dermatitis, immune deficiency, diarrhoea
- Responds well to oral zinc

Acrodermatitis enteropathica

- Autosomal recessive inheritance
- Basic defect is impaired absorption of zinc in the gut
- Presents with skin rash around the mouth and perianal area, chronic diarrhoea at the time of weaning and recurrent infections. The hair has a reddish tint, alopecia is characteristic. Superinfection with *Candida* sp. is common as are paronychia, dystrophic nails, poor wound healing and ocular changes (photophobia, blepharitis, corneal dystrophy)

- Diagnosis is by serum zinc levels and the constellation of clinical signs. This is difficult as the serum zinc is low as part of the acute-phase response. Measurement of white-cell zinc levels is more accurate. The plasma metallothionein level can also be measured. Metallothionein is a zinc-binding protein that is decreased in zinc deficiency but not in the acute-phase response
- Zinc deficiency in the newborn can produce a similar clinical picture
- The condition responds very well to treatment with oral zinc

2.8   Fat-soluble vitamins

Vitamin A

- Deficiency causes night blindness, poor growth, xerophthalmia, follicular hyperplasia and impaired resistance to infection
- Excess causes carotenaemia, hyperostosis with bone pain, hepatomegaly, alopecia and desquamation of the palms. Acute intoxication causes raised intracranial pressure
- Dietary sources are milk, fat, fruit and vegetables, eggs and liver
- Vitamin A has an important role in resistance to infection particularly at mucosal surfaces. In developing countries where vitamin A deficiency is endemic, vitamin A reduces the morbidity and mortality associated with severe measles.

Vitamin E

- Is an antioxidant
- Found in green vegetables and vegetable oils
- Deficiency causes ataxia, peripheral neuropathy and retinitis pigmentosa

Abetalipoproteinaemia

- Autosomal recessive inheritance
- Pathogenesis is failure of chylomicron formation with impaired absorption of long-chain fats with fat retention in the enterocyte
- Malabsorption occurs from birth
- Presents in early infancy with faltering growth, abdominal distension and foul smelling, bulky stools
- Symptoms of vitamin E deficiency (ataxia, peripheral neuropathy and retinitis pigmentosa) develop later
- Diagnosis is by low serum cholesterol, very low plasma triglyceride level, acanthocytes on examination of the peripheral blood film, absence of betalipoprotein in the plasma
- Treatment is by substituting medium-chain triglycerides for long-chain triglycerides in the diet. Medium-chain triglycerides are absorbed via the portal vein rather than the thoracic duct. In addition, high doses of the fat-soluble vitamins (A, D, E and K) are required. Most of the neurological abnormalities are reversible if high doses of vitamin E are given early

Vitamin K

- Is contained in cows' milk, green leafy vegetables and pork. There is very little in breast milk
- Deficiency in the newborn presents as haemorrhagic disease of the newborn. This usually presents on day 2 or 3 with bleeding from the umbilical stump, haematemesis and melaena, epistaxis or excessive bleeding from puncture sites. Intracranial bleeding can occur. Diagnosis is by prolongation of the prothrombin and partial thromboplastin times with the thrombin time and fibrinogen levels being normal. Treatment is with fresh-frozen plasma and vitamin K
- There is no proven association between intramuscular vitamin K and childhood cancer

2.9 Nutritional impairment

Energy balance

A positive energy balance implies that intake exceeds requirements and a negative energy balance implies that intake is less than requirements. It is important to remember that requirements during childhood include those needed for growth.

Pathogenesis of malnutrition

It is essential to think about the pathogenesis of malnutrition when assessing nutrition and looking at nutritional supplementation. Malnutrition can only result from:

- Inadequate intake or excessive losses
- Increased metabolic demand without increased intake
- Malabsorption

One or all of these may contribute to malnutrition in an individual.

A good example is cystic fibrosis in which:

- Pancreatic malabsorption causes increased losses
- Increased energy needs are caused by:
  - Chronic cough
  - Dyspnoea
  - Recurrent infection
  - Inflammation
- Reduced intake is caused by:
  - Anorexia
  - Vomiting
  - Psychological problems

Together, all of these factors result in an energy deficit. They all need to be taken into account when nutritional supplementation is considered.

2.10   Protein-energy malnutrition

Marasmus is characterized by muscle wasting and depletion of the body fat stores. **Kwashiorkor** is characterized by generalized oedema with flaky or peeling skin and skin rashes. Most children with malnutrition — rare in the Western world, exhibit a combination of the two. Micronutrient deficiencies are common in these children.

2.11   Faltering growth

Faltering growth (previously called 'failure to thrive') refers to the failure to gain weight at an adequate rate. It is common in infancy. It occurs because of one or a combination of the following:

- Failure of carer to offer adequate calories
- Failure of the child to take sufficient calories
- Failure of the child to retain adequate calories

Clearly this can be organic or non-organic. Insufficient calories may be offered as a consequence of parental neglect or because of a failure of the carer to appreciate the calorie requirements of the child. Insufficient calories may be taken as a consequence of feeding difficulties (for example, cerebral palsy) or increased needs (for example, cystic fibrosis) and calories may not be retained because of absorptive defects or loss through vomiting or diarrhoea.

The investigation of faltering growth is generally only fruitful when specific pointers to organic problems are elucidated in the history or on physical examination.

The management of non-organic faltering growth requires health visitor input and often dietary assessment. In difficult cases hospital admission is indicated for evaluation and to ensure an adequate weight gain can be obtained if sufficient calories are given.

2.12   Organic causes of faltering growth

This list provides examples only and is by no means exhaustive.

- Gastrointestinal — coeliac disease, cows'-milk-protein intolerance, gastro-oesophageal reflux
- Renal — urinary tract infection, renal tubular acidosis
- Cardiopulmonary — cardiac disease, cystic fibrosis, bronchopulmonary dysplasia
- Endocrine — hypothyroidism
- Neurological — cerebral palsy
- Infection/immunodeficiency — HIV, malignancy
- Metabolic — inborn errors of metabolism
- Congenital — chromosomal abnormalities
- ENT — adenotonsillar hypertrophy

3. NUTRITIONAL MANAGEMENT

3.1 Nutritional supplementation

Nutritional supplementation should be with the help of a dietitian. It is essential, however, to have some background information and to:

- Treat underlying pathology which may be a factor
- Assess the child's requirements
- Give additional calories either by increasing the calorie density of feed or giving feed by a different route, e.g. nasogastric tube, gastrostomy tube or parenterally

Enteral nutrition refers to that given either directly (by mouth) or indirectly (via nasogastric tube or gastrostomy) into the gastrointestinal tract. **Parenteral nutrition** is given either into the peripheral or central veins, usually the latter.

It may be helpful to consider specific scenarios.

A 6-month-old infant with congenital heart disease is failing to thrive — comment on his nutritional status. What nutritional supplementation would you recommend?

In this infant the poor nutritional state will be as a consequence of increased metabolic demands and poor intake secondary to breathlessness. Supplementation would be by increasing the calorie density of feeds and consideration of other methods of administration such as via a nasogastric tube. It is obviously also of importance to maximize medical therapy of the heart disease.

This 6-month-old infant has bronchopulmonary dysplasia and severe faltering growth. Comment on possible causes.

In this infant the above applies. In addition, other factors may be relevant such as chronic respiratory symptoms, gastro-oesophageal reflux and neurodevelopmental issues. Supplementation would be by increasing calorie density of feeds and considering using a nasogastric tube or gastrostomy to give the feed. In addition, investigation for problems like gastro-oesophageal reflux may be considered.

This 3-month-old infant, born at 29 weeks' gestation, had a massive resection for volvulus in the neonatal period and has poor feed tolerance, total parenteral nutrition (TPN) dependence and severe liver disease. What strategies are required in this child's subsequent management?

This child has intestinal failure with persistent TPN dependency and liver disease. The priority is to maximize enteral intake which will reduce the likelihood of progression of the liver disease. A hydrolysed feed given by continuous infusion will probably be tolerated best. TPN should only be weaned when the feed is tolerated and absorbed. Loperamide may reduce transit. Bacterial overgrowth is likely and should be managed with cyclical antibiotics. Macro- and micronutrients should be checked to ensure they are adequate. Attention should be given to promoting the child's oral feeding skills.

This 13-year-old boy has cerebral palsy. Comment on his nutritional status. What strategies could be used to improve his nutrition? Why do you think his nutritional status is so poor?

This child's principal problem is likely to be with intake, either because of reflux or secondary to bulbar problems or both. In addition to nutritional supplements, this child may benefit from help with feeding practices including the involvement of a dietitian, speech and language therapist, occupational therapist and neurodevelopmental paediatrician. Other medical problems may be relevant such as recurrent chest infections secondary to aspiration, intractable fits. Consideration needs to be given to feeding via nasogastric tube or gastrostomy tube if appropriate. In some instances a fundoplication will also be required.

This boy has cystic fibrosis. Comment on his nutritional status. What can be done to help?

The additional factor in this child is malabsorption for which pancreatic supplementation is required. Children with cystic fibrosis often dislike food and need either a nasogastric tube or gastrostomy to help with administration. The energy requirements are high and calorie supplementation with energy-dense supplements is required.

Nutritonal supplement

- Normal infant feeds or milk contain 0.7 kCal/ml
- Feeds can be concentrated
- Carbohydrate supplements can be used, usually as glucose polymer in powder form to add to feeds
- Combined carbohydrate and fat supplements can be used
- Feeds with a higher calorie density can be used, e.g. 1 kCal/ml, 1.5 kCal/ml
- Special feeds can be used, e.g. hydrolysed protein formula feeds, soya-based feeds, lactose-free feeds, medium-chain-triglyceride-based feeds
- Milk-based or juice-based supplements can be given
- There are many commercially available products available

3.2 Enteral nutrition

Enteral feeding strictly refers to enteral feed given directly into the gastrointestinal tract. For the purpose of this chapter, an enteral feed has been considered as a supplementary feed, i.e. not including foods normally taken by mouth, and therefore refers principally to feeds given either by nasogastric or gastrostomy tube or in rare cases via a jejunostomy.

Indications for enteral tube feeding

- Insufficient energy intake by mouth
- Wasting
- Stunting

Diseases for which enteral nutrition may be indicated

Gastrointestinal

- Short-bowel syndrome
- Inflammatory bowel disease
- Pseudo-obstruction
- Chronic liver disease
- Gastro-oesophageal reflux
- Glycogen storage disease types I and III
- Fatty-acid oxidation defects

Neuromuscular disease

- Coma and severe facial and head injury
- Severe mental retardation and cerebral palsy
- Dysphagia secondary to cranial nerve dysfunction, muscular dystrophy or myasthenia gravis

Malignant disease

- Obstructing disease
- Head and neck
- Oesophagus
- Stomach
- Abnormality of deglutition following surgical intervention
- Gastrointestinal side-effects from chemotherapy and/or radiotherapy
- Terminal supportive care

Pulmonary disease

- Bronchopulmonary dysplasia
- Cystic fibrosis
- Chronic lung disease

Congenital abnormalities

- Tracheo-oesophageal fistula
- Oesophageal atresia
- Cleft palate
- Pierre Robin syndrome

Other

- Anorexia nervosa
- Cardiac cachexia
- Chronic renal disease
- Severe burns
- Severe sepsis
- Severe trauma

Choice of feed type

A wide range of feeds is available and the decision about which to use is based on the child's needs. Factors that are of relevance include whether the enteral feed will be the sole source of feeding in which case the feed needs to be nutritionally complete or whether the feed is going to be given as a supplement. Feed tolerance and calorie requirements are relevant. A modified feed may be required, e.g. lactose-free in a child with carbohydrate intolerance. Factors such as fibre content and calorie density are also important particularly if supplementary feeding is going to be long term.

A hydrolysed protein is one that is broken down into oligopeptides and peptides. A hydrolysed protein milk formula is therefore one which does not contain whole protein (e.g. Pregestemil, Nutramigen, Prejomin, Pepti-junior). An elemental formula is a hydrolysed protein formula in which the protein is broken down into amino acids (e.g. Neocate and elemental EO28).

Hydrolysed protein formula feeds are used in children with cow's milk allergy, enteropathies, e.g. post gastroenteritis, post necrotizing enterocolitis, short-gut syndrome, severe eczema and Crohn's disease.

Choice of feed regimen

This will depend on a combination of requirements, tolerance and factors such as gastric emptying. Options include bolus feeding and continuous feeding or a combination of the two.

In the severely malnourished child, the volume and calorie density of a new feed regimen may need to be increased slowly, as tolerated, over a few days. This avoids metabolic upset (re-feeding syndrome) in the vulnerable child, e.g. severe postoperative weight loss, anorexia nervosa.

Dysmotility

The motility of the gut is a key factor in feed tolerance. Preterm infants, and children with cerebral palsy have delayed gastric emptying which impacts significantly on the ability to feed, particularly if nutrition is dependent upon nasogastric or gastrostomy feeding. Abdominal pain, bloating and constipation are common features of gut dysmotility.

Therapeutic strategies include the recognition of the problem, administration of a prokinetic agent such as Domperidone, laxatives and occasionally, if there is a need for distal gut deflation, suppositories. It may be necessary to give feeds by continuous infusion. Milk-free diets can be used and in difficult cases full gastrointestinal investigation including upper and lower gastrointestinal endoscopy, barium radiology, pH studies and scintigraphy may be indicated. A number of children, particularly those with cerebral palsy, respond to milk exclusion using a hydrolysed protein formula feed as an alternative.

Methods of feed delivery

Nasogastric tube feeding

This is the most commonly used route for short-term enteral feeding given either by bolus or continuously. There is a risk of reflux and aspiration pneumonia. Nasal irritation and inhibition of oral feeding sometimes occurs. Most infants will not tolerate nasogastric feeding long term.

Nasojejunal feeding

This is indicated when nasogastric feeding is not tolerated because of delayed gastric emptying or gross gastro-oesophageal reflux. Feed usually needs to be given continuously to avoid dumping. If nasojejunal feeding is required long term a jejunostomy can be fashioned.

Gastrostomy tube feeding

Gastrostomy is probably the best route for long-term feeding. Gastrostomy tubes are generally inserted endoscopically (percutaneous endoscopic gastrostomy) and the complications are few.

Indications for gastrostomy tube placement

- Chronic disease with nutritional impairment, e.g. cystic fibrosis, bronchopulmonary dysplasia
- For nutritional therapy, e.g. Crohn's disease
- Difficulties with feeding, e.g. cerebral palsy, particularly with an associated bulbar palsy. Some of these children may also have severe gastro-oesophageal reflux and require fundoplication
- Children long-term-dependent upon nasogastric feeding for any other reason

3.3   Total parenteral nutrition (TPN)

There are differences between children and adults particularly in terms of nutritional reserve.

- Adult can survive 90 days without food
- Preterm infant of 1 kg can survive 4 days
- Preterm infant of 2 kg can survive 12 days
- Term infant of 3.5 kg can survive 32 days
- One-year-old can survive 44 days

General principles of TPN

- It is important to use the gut where possible
- The complete exclusion of luminal nutrients is associated with atrophic changes in the gut, reduced pancreatic function, biliary stasis and bacterial overgrowth
- It is not usually necessary to use TPN for less than 5 days except in the extremely preterm

Benefits of minimal enteral nutrition in children who are TPN fed

- Stimulation of mucosal adaptation (trophic feeding)
- Protection against sepsis (normalize flora)
- Improved bile flow with decreased risk of cholestasis
- Reduced time to establish enteral feeds

Indications for TPN

Neonates
Absolute indications:

- Intestinal failure (short gut, functional immaturity, pseudo-obstruction)
- Necrotizing enterocolitis

Relative indications:

- Hyaline membrane disease
- Promotion of growth in preterm infants
- Possible prevention of necrotizing enterocolitis

Older infants and children
Intestinal failure:

- Short gut
- Protracted diarrhoea
- Chronic intestinal pseudo-obstruction
- Postoperative abdominal or cardiothoracic surgery
- Radiation/cytotoxic therapy

Exclusion of luminal nutrients:

- Crohn's disease

Organ failure:

- Acute renal failure or acute liver failure

Hypercatabolism:

- Extensive burns
- Severe trauma

Practical issues

TPN prescribing
There are standard regimens for TPN prescribing. This will include the starter regimen which then increases in nutrient density over the first few days. Protein is supplied as amino acid, carbohydrate as glucose and fat as a lipid emulsion. Electrolyte, calcium and phosphate content needs to be carefully controlled. Fat- and water-soluble vitamins and trace elements are added to the mix. Calorie density is increased through increase in carbohydrate and lipid as tolerated. It is important to use standard regimens adjusted according to fluid balance, electrolyte status and tolerance, e.g. of increases in glucose. It is important not to

push calorie density up too much without expert advice as this may result in poor tolerance and toxicity with a net reduction in metabolized energy intake. The use of a TPN pharmacist in conjunction with a nutrition team is essential in difficult cases.

Monitoring during TPN

The initial frequency will depend on the degree of electrolyte impairment and other factors, e.g. sepsis, liver disease. It is generally necessary in the acute situation to do at least routine biochemistry (including blood glucose and urine dipstix) daily until stable and then twice weekly. Urine biochemistry should be monitored twice weekly at least initially. Liver function, calcium and phosphate should be done weekly. Trace metals (copper, zinc, selenium, magnesium) should be checked monthly. In children on long-term TPN 6-monthly iron, vitamin B_{12}, red cell folate, fat-soluble vitamins, aluminium and chromium should be measured. Chest X-ray, liver ultrasound and echocardiography should be done 6- to 12-monthly.

Blood glucose should be monitored frequently during periods of increasing carbohydrate load.

Complications

Complications of TPN

- Phlebitis
- Infection
- Hypo- and hyperglycaemia
- Electrolyte disturbance
- Fluid overload
- Hypophosphataemia
- Anaemia
- Thrombocyte and neutrophil dysfunction
- Trace-element deficiencies
- Trace-element excess
- Vitamin deficiencies
- Hyperammonaemia
- Essential fatty-acid deficiency
- Cholestasis and hepatic dysfunction
- Metabolic acidosis
- Hypercholesterolaemia
- Hypertriglyceridaemia
- Granulomatous pulmonary arteritis

Complications of central venous catheter insertion

- Sepsis
- Air embolism
- Arterial puncture
- Arrhythmias
- Chylothorax
- Haemothorax
- Pneumothorax
- Haemo/hydropericardium
- Malposition of catheter
- Nerve injury
- Central venous thrombosis
- Thromboembolism
- Extravasation from fractured catheter
- Tricuspid valve damage
- Catheter tethering

Line infection

Infections are one of the potentially life-threatening hazards of TPN. Coagulase-negative staphylococcal infection is the most common. Children on TPN long term are at significant risk of life-threatening bacterial sepsis. A child on TPN should have cultures taken and antibiotics started promptly if there is a high fever. Children with short gut/enteropathy are at highest risk because of bacterial translocation; they should have regular gut decontamination particularly if infections are frequent. It is important that appropriate procedures are in place to ensure that lines are dealt with aseptically and only by trained personnel. Long-term feeding lines should not, for example, be used for blood letting.

TPN-induced liver disease

TPN-induced liver disease develops in 40–60% of infants who require long-term TPN for intestinal failure. The clinical spectrum includes cholestasis, cholelithiasis, hepatic fibrosis with progression to biliary cirrhosis, and the development of portal hypertension and liver failure. The pathogenesis is multifactorial and is related to prematurity, low birth weight, and duration of TPN. The degree and severity of the liver disease is related to recurrent sepsis, including catheter sepsis, bacterial translocation and cholangitis. Lack of enteral feeding leading to reduced gut hormone secretion, reduction of bile flow, and biliary stasis are important mechanisms in the development of cholestasis, biliary sludge and cholelithiasis. The management strategies for the prevention of TPN-induced liver disease include early enteral feeding, a multidisciplinary approach to the management of parenteral nutrition, and aseptic catheter techniques to reduce sepsis. The administration of ursodeoxycholic acid may improve bile flow and reduce gallbladder and intestinal stasis. Fat-soluble vitamin replacement is essential by the intravenous route when child is parenterally fed but may be given orally with regular monitoring during the transition to oral/enteral feeding.

Consequences of trace element abnormalities described during parenteral nutrition

Trace element	Deficiency	Excess
Zinc	Periorofacial dermatitis Immune deficiency Diarrhoea Growth failure	
Copper	Refractory hypochromic anaemia Neutropenia Osteoporosis Subperiosteal haematoma Soft tissue calcification	
Selenium	Cardiomyopathy Skeletal myopathy, pain and tenderness Pseudoalbinism	
Chromium	Glucose intolerance Peripheral neuropathy Weight loss	Renal and hepatic impairment
Manganese	Lipid abnormalities Anaemia	Liver toxicity Damage to basal ganglia
Molybdenum	Tachycardia Central scotomata Irritability Coma	
Aluminium		Anaemia Osteodystrophy Encephalopathy

3.4   Short-bowel syndrome

This is defined as intestinal failure secondary to massive resection.

Aetiologies:

- Neonatal — necrotizing enterocolitis, intestinal atresia, volvulus
- Older child — trauma, inflammatory bowl disease, vascular abnormalities

Factors that determine outcome

- Length of bowel resected and remaining bowel length — preterm bowel is likely to undergo further growth (bowel length increases by 100% in the third trimester)
- Less than 40 cm of residual small bowel is usually associated with a need for long-term nutritional support
- Quality of bowel remaining – ischaemic, distended, ileum greater potential to adapt than jejunum

- Presence of ileocaecal valve — loss of ileocaecal valve results in faster transit. Backflow (loss of the one-way valve) makes bacterial overgrowth more likely. There is a need for vitamin B_{12} replacement longer term
- Improved outcome if colon still present which facilitates salt and water resorption
- Coexistent disease, e.g. enteropathy is an adverse risk factor
- Presence of liver disease is an adverse risk factor

Management

There are three phases of intestinal adaptation – acute (TPN-dependent, postoperative ileus), adaptive (increasing enteral nutrition, can take months to years) and chronic. The priority is to maintain normal growth and development through adequate calorie, nutrient and micronutrient intake during these phases. The early introduction of enteral feeds promotes intestinal adaptation and will improve subsequent feed tolerance. Feeds are usually best given as a continuous infusion in the first instance and should only be increased if tolerated, i.e. no diarrhoea (or excess stoma output if present). Explosive stools imply feed intolerance which will increase the risk of metabolic upset and bacterial translocation leading to sepsis. TPN should not be weaned until feed is tolerated and absorbed. Weight needs careful monitoring during weaning of TPN. Artificial feeds (e.g. hydrolysed feeds) are often better tolerated although osmolality is higher. Liver disease is a serious complication of TPN and may lead to death from liver failure. It may be reduced by maximizing feeds, avoidance of sepsis, artificial bile salts (e.g. ursodeoxycholic acid) and vitamin supplementation. Bacterial overgrowth with the risks of malabsorption and bacterial translocation is common and requires treatment with oral antibiotics given in cycles, either metronidazole alone or in combination with gentamicin. Loperamide may help reduce gut transit and thus increase absorption. Monitoring of micronutrients and fat-soluble vitamins is essential during long-term TPN. Bowel lengthening surgery may reduce stasis and thus translocation. In severe cases, isolated liver transplant or intestinal transplantation may be considered. Multidisciplinary management is required, including attention to the child's oral skills, social and psychological development and the needs of the family.

4. FOOD INTOLERANCE

It is important to distinguish between allergy and intolerance. An allergy implies an immune-mediated reaction to food antigen (protein). Classically this is by IgE-mediated, type I hypersensitivity. The signs of this include anaphylaxis, urticaria and atopic dermatitis. Intolerance implies a reaction to food taken either in small quantity or in excess. It is a non-specific term. Examples range from symptoms as a result of a non-IgE-mediated immune reaction to food, such as coeliac disease, through to symptoms induced by simple over-indulgence. An intolerance does not necessarily need to be to a protein and includes, for example, lactose intolerance.

4.1 Cows' milk protein intolerance

There is a wide spectrum of clinical features induced by cows' milk protein and the condition is not always well defined, leading to concerns about both under- and over-diagnosis.

Clinical spectrum of cows' milk protein intolerance

- Acute type 1-mediated hypersensitivity
- Delayed-onset hypersensitivity
- Cows'-milk-sensitive enteropathy
- Cows' milk allergic colitis
- Non-specific symptoms possibly attributable to cows' milk

It is the latter group that presents the most difficulty and includes a wide variety of symptoms including colic, generalized irritability, chestiness, recurrent upper respiratory tract symptoms and constipation. Diagnosis is dependent on the clinical manifestations. A good history and, if possible, dietetic assessment is essential. To strictly diagnose allergy the Goldmann criteria should be met, which are that the attributable symptoms disappear on removal of the offending antigen and recur when it is reintroduced. Skin-prick testing and IgE radioallergosorbent testing (RAST) are sometimes useful. They test type I-mediated hypersensitivity. A negative result does not exclude allergy and a positive result can be seen in children who tolerate cows' milk protein without a problem. If either an enteropathy or colitis is suspected then it is useful to obtain histological confirmation.

Management

- Milk exclusion with a milk substitute. Soya preparations are commonly used and are palatable. There is, however, a cross-reactivity between cows' milk and soya protein of up to one-third and so hydrolysed protein formula feeds are preferred. Soya products should not be used in infants < 6 months
- The natural history of cows' milk intolerance is one of resolution with 80–90% back on a normal diet by their third birthday. It is sensible to challenge regularly. This will depend on the child's presentation. It is usual to organize challenges in hospital, particularly if the initial reaction was severe, because of the risk of anaphylaxis
- Children with a past history of anaphylaxis or severe respiratory symptoms following allergen ingestion require an adrenaline pen for use either in the home or school setting in the event of accidental exposure to the offending food antigen

It is common in children with milk allergy to see reactions to other foods, the most common of which are soya, egg, wheat and peanut.

Skin-prick testing and IgE RAST testing are most useful in children with peanut, nut and egg allergy.

4.2 Peanut allergy

Peanut and nut allergies are seen with increasing frequency. It is important to remember that peanuts are a vegetable rather than a true nut. However, between 60 and 80% of children with peanut allergy are also allergic to other nuts. Reactions vary from mild urticaria to life-threatening anaphylaxis. Skin-prick testing is useful with a high sensitivity and specificity. It is important to get the diagnosis right, many children have non-specific reactions during childhood and are labelled 'peanut-allergic'. Peanut avoidance is difficult and dietetic support is essential. Food contamination in food production, i.e. nuts are not an ingredient but there may be traces because of cross-contamination from other food production lines, is common. There is some controversy about whether all nuts should be avoided in peanut-allergic patients and about whether peanut oils should be given. The natural history suggests that children with early-onset allergy may grow out of it, although allergy in older children with symptomatic reactions is more likely to persist. Active management involves challenging peanut skin-prick-negative children. This is clearly not without risk and needs to be done in an inpatient setting with facilities for resuscitation.

Common other nuts that cause allergic reactions include brazil nut, cashew nut, hazelnut, walnut, almond and pistachio nut.

4.3 Food-induced anaphylaxis

Children who have had an anaphylactic reaction are at increased risk of a second reaction after second exposure, for which there is a significant mortality. These children benefit from an adrenaline pen. It is important that such children and their families are taught properly about the indications for use of the pen and subsequent action that should be taken. The school and all the main carers need to be involved. A medic-alert bracelet is useful. Children should also have antihistamines kept in their house. These are appropriate for minor reactions and some units advocate their use prior to potential accidental exposure.

It is essential to be aware of the guidelines for the management of an anaphylactic reaction.

4.4 Carbohydrate intolerance

Disorders of disaccharide absorption

Primary

- Congenital alactasia
- Congenital lactose intolerance
- Sucrose–isomaltase deficiency

Secondary (acquired)

- Post-enteritis (rotavirus), neonatal surgery, malnutrition
- Late-onset lactose intolerance

Disorders of monosaccharide absorption

Primary

- Glucose–galactose malabsorption

Secondary (acquired)

- Post-enteritis, neonatal surgery, malnutrition

Lactose intolerance

Carbohydrate intolerance is usually lactose intolerance and is usually acquired. The deficient enzyme is the brush-border enzyme lactase which hydrolyses lactose into glucose and galactose. The intolerance will present with characteristic loose explosive stools. The diagnosis is made by looking for reducing substances in the stool following carbohydrate ingestion. Clinitest tablets (which detect reducing substance in the stool) are used as the standard test, the detection of more than 0.5% is significant. Formal confirmation of the specific offending carbohydrate is through stool chromatography. Treatment is with a lactose-free formula in infancy and a reduced lactose intake in later childhood.

Following gastroenteritis, carbohydrate intolerance can be either to disaccharides or mono-saccharides. It is usually in children who have been infected with rotavirus. Both types of intolerance are usually transient and both respond to removal of the offending carbohydrate. Both mono- and disaccharide intolerance will result in tests for reducing substances in the stool being positive.

Glucose–galactose malabsorption

This is a rare autosomal recessively inherited condition, characterized by rapid-onset watery diarrhoea from birth. It responds to withholding glucose (stopping feeds) and relapses on reintroduction. The diagnosis is essentially a clinical one. Reducing substances in the stool will be positive and small-bowel biopsy and disaccharide estimation will be normal. Treatment is by using fructose as the main carbohydrate source. Fructose is absorbed by a different mechanism to glucose and galactose.

Sucrase–isomaltase deficiency

This is a defect in carbohydrate digestion, with the enzyme required for hydrolysis of sucrose and alpha-limit dextrins not present in the small intestine. Symptoms of watery diarrhoea and/or faltering growth develop after the introduction of sucrose or complex carbohydrate into the diet.

- Symptoms can be very mild
- Reducing substances in the stool are negative (non-reducing sugar)

Diagnosis is by stool chromatography. Management is by removal of sucrose and complex carbohydrate from the diet.

Hydrogen breath testing

The hydrogen breath test looks for carbohydrate malabsorption. Lactose is the usual substrate. The principle is that malabsorbed carbohydrate will pass to the colon where it is metabolized by bacteria and hydrogen gas is released. The gas is then absorbed and released in the breath. If there is a peak it suggests carbohydrate malabsorption. Other carbohydrates can be given as the substrate. Lactulose, which is a non-absorbable carbohydrate, can be used to assess transit time.

Other tests of gastrointestinal function

Xylose tolerance test

- Indirect method used to assess small-bowel absorption
- Xylose is a carbohydrate; a load (15 mg/m^2, maximum 25 g) is ingested and a blood level is taken after 1 hour, a level of less than 25 mg/dl is suggestive of carbohydrate malabsorption
- The test is neither sensitive nor specific
- False-positive results are obtained in pernicious anaemia and when there is gut oedema

Faecal α-1 antitrypsin

- Serum protein, not present in the diet
- Same molecular weight as albumin
- Faecal levels reflect enteric protein loss (e.g. protein-losing enteropathy)

Faecal calprotectin

- Neutrophil protein
- Stable in faeces
- Found in both adults and children to be a simple and non-invasive measure of bowel inflammation

Faecal elastase

- Pancreas-specific enzyme which is stable during intestinal transport
- Stable in faeces
- Reliable indirect marker of pancreatic function
- False-positives in short gut and bacterial overgrowth

5. GASTRO-OESOPHAGEAL REFLUX

Gastro-oesophageal reflux is common and implies passage of gastric contents into the lower oesophagus. It is a normal physiological phenomenon. It is common in infancy and is also seen in older children and adults, particularly after meals. It is secondary to transient relaxation of the lower oesophageal sphincter not associated with swallowing.

Differential diagnosis of gastro-oesophageal reflux

- Infection, e.g. urinary tract infection, gastroenteritis
- Intestinal obstruction, e.g. pyloric stenosis, intestinal atresia, malrotation
- Food allergy and intolerance, e.g. cows' milk allergy, soy allergy, coeliac disease
- Metabolic disorders, e.g. diabetes, inborn errors of metabolism
- Psychological problems, e.g. anxiety
- Drug-induced vomiting, e.g. cytotoxic agents
- Primary respiratory disease, e.g. asthma, cystic fibrosis

Symptoms and signs of gastro-oesophageal reflux disease

- **Typical**
  - Excessive regurgitation/vomiting
  - Nausea
  - Weight loss/faltering growth
  - Irritability with feeds, arching, colic/food refusal
  - Dysphagia
  - Chest/epigastric discomfort
  - Excessive hiccups
  - Anaemia — iron-deficient
  - Hamatemesis/Malaena
  - Aspiration pneumonia
  - Oesophageal obstruction due to stricture
- **Atypical**
  - Wheeze/intractable asthma
  - Cough/stridor
  - Apnoea/apparent life-threatening events/sudden infant death syndrome
  - Cyanotic episodes
  - Generalized irritability
  - Sleep disturbance
  - Neurobehavioural symptoms — breath holding, Sandifer syndrome, seizure-like events
  - Worsening of pre-existing respiratory disease
  - Secondary, e.g. post-surgery

Investigation of gastro-oesophageal reflux

The natural history of mild gastro-oesophageal reflux is resolution and many patients can be managed symptomatically with antacids and thickeners. More significant cases need further investigation, particularly if there are symptoms or signs of oesophagitis. There are various investigations available which need to be considered in conjunction with the clinical picture:

- Barium radiology — not particularly sensitive or specific but will pick up anatomical problems such as malrotation or stricture

- pH study — 'gold standard' for acid reflux, but unless dual pH recording is performed (i.e. simultaneous oesophageal and gastric pH monitoring) will miss alkaline reflux
- Nuclear medicine 'milk' scan which will assess acid or alkali reflux following a physiological meal, assess gastric emptying and it is possible to make a 24-hour film to look for evidence of aspiration (technetium-99m radioscintigraphy)
- Upper gastrointestinal endoscopy with biopsy

Scoring system for pH monitoring

- % of time pH < 4 (reflux index)
- Number of episodes > 5 minutes
- Duration of the longest episode
- Total number of reflux episodes

% of time pH < 4

- Mild reflux 5–10
- Moderate reflux 10–20
- Severe 20–30

Management of gastro-oesophageal reflux

General measures
Functional reflux does not require specific treatment

Simple measures

- Explanation and reassurance
- Review of feeding posture
- Review of feeding practice, e.g. too frequent feeds, large volume feeds
- Use of feed thickeners or an anti-reflux milk

Older children

- Life-style and diet
- Avoid excess fat, chocolate, tea, coffee, gaseous drinks
- Avoid tight-fitting clothes

Specific treatment

Antacids
Acid suppression

- H$_2$ blockers, e.g. ranitidine
- Proton-pump inhibitors, e.g. omeprazole, lansoprazole

Prokinetic drugs

- Metoclopramide
- Domperidone

- Erythromycin
- Cisapride

Cisapride is no longer licensed for use in children because of anxieties about potential cardiotoxicity. It can still be used on a named patient basis but seldom is.

Step-up approach to the treatment of gastro-oesophageal reflux

- Step 1 Life-style changes
- Step 2 Antacids /thickeners/H_2 blockers/?prokinetics
- Step 3 Proton-pump inhibitors
- Step 4 Add prokinetics if not already tried/consider change in diet
- Step 5 Surgery

Surgery is required for reflux resistant to medical treatment. High-risk groups include those with neurodisability or intractable respiratory symptoms exacerbated by reflux.

5.1 Differential diagnosis of reflux oesophagitis

- Cows' milk allergic oesophagitis
- Candidal oesophagitis
- Chemical oesophagitis from caustic ingestion
- Crohn's disease

5.2 Feeding problems in cerebral palsy

- Feeding difficulties may be secondary to bulbar weakness with oesophageal inco-ordination, primary or secondary aspiration or reflux oesophagitis
- Additional factors such as mobility of the patient, degree of spasticity, nutritional state and the presence of other conditions such as constipation are also relevant
- Children require careful multidisciplinary assessment by a feeding team including dietetics, speech and language therapy, occupational therapy and the neurodevelopmental paediatrician. A video barium assessment of the swallow is often indicated
- Gastro-oesophageal reflux disease is common and should be treated aggressively
- Attention to nutrition is of key importance and many children benefit from a feeding gastrostomy with or without an anti-reflux procedure

5.3 Barrett's oesophagus

- Presence of metaplastic columnar epithelium in the lower oesophagus
- Thought to be a consequence of long-standing gastro-oesophageal reflux
- Increase in the risk of adenocarcinoma of the oesophagus
- Rare in childhood

- Requires aggressive medical treatment, regular endoscopic assessment and because the risk of malignancy is felt to relate to the extent of persistent exposure of the distal oesophagus to acid, surgery is often considered

Notes

- Barium swallow assesses the oesophagus
- Barium meal assesses the stomach and proximal duodenum
- Barium meal and follow-through assess the stomach and small bowel to the terminal ileum
- Small-bowel meal (administered via an nasojejunal tube) assesses the small bowel only
- Barium enema assesses the colon
- A video barium can be used to assess the swallow and check for primary aspiration

6. PEPTIC ULCER DISEASE

6.1 *Helicobacter pylori* infection

Helicobacter pylori s a Gram-negative bacterium. Infection is usually acquired in childhood. Prevalence rates, however, are very variable. Persistent infection causes a chronic gastritis which may be asymptomatic. There is a strong relationship between Helicobacter infection and peptic ulceration in adults. *Helicobacter pylori* is also a carcinogen. There is no proven association between Helicobacter infection and recurrent abdominal pain. Transmission is faeco-oral and familial clustering is common.

Diagnosis is by the following:

- Serology — usually reverts to negative within 6–12 months of treatment
- Rapid urease tests — C13 breath test, CLO test
- Histology
- Culture (difficult)

Treatment is indicated for gastritis or peptic ulceration. There are various regimes. The most commonly used in children is omeprazole, amoxicillin and metronidazole for 2 weeks. Outcome following treatment is variable.

6.2 Other causes of antral gastritis and peptic ulceration

- Anti-inflammatory drugs
- Crohn's disease
- Zollinger–Ellison syndrome
- Autoimmune gastritis (adults)

6.3 Zollinger–Ellison syndrome

Gastrin-producing tumour of the endocrine pancreas, presenting with gastric acid hypersecretion resulting in fulminant and intractable peptic ulcer disease.

7. CHRONIC DIARRHOEA

Chronic diarrhoea refers to diarrhoea that has persisted for more than 2–3 weeks. Children with chronic diarrhoea and faltering growth need further assessment, as the underlying cause may be a malabsorption.

Common causes include:

- Coeliac disease
- Food intolerance
- Cystic fibrosis
- Infections/immunodeficiency
- Inflammatory bowel disease

In children with chronic diarrhoea who are thriving, alternative diagnoses such as constipation, carbohydrate intolerance and toddler's diarrhoea, should be considered. Chronic constipation is a common cause presenting as apparent diarrhoea which is in fact overflow soiling.

Protracted diarrhoea/intractable diarrhoea of infancy

This refers to persistent diarrhoea starting in infancy and is less common.

Examples include:

- **Congenital microvillous atrophy**
  - Intractable diarrhoea which is present from birth
  - Pathology is ultrastructural abnormality at the microvillous surface
  - Long-term nutritional support with total parenteral nutrition is required
- **Glucose–galactose malabsorption**
  - See Section 4.4
- **Congenital chloride diarrhoea**
  - Autosomal recessive
  - Severe watery diarrhoea starting at birth — often past history of polyhydramnios
  - Serum sodium and chloride are low with a high stool pH and stool chloride
  - Treatment is with sodium and potassium chloride supplements
  - Prognosis is good if diagnosis is made early
- **Autoimmune enteropathy**
  - Protracted diarrhoea presenting in infancy associated with the presence of circulating autoantibodies against intestinal epithelial cells
  - Severe villous atrophy with an inflammatory infiltrate
  - Associated with other autoimmune conditions
  - Treatment is with immunosuppression

Small-bowel biopsy

- Usually performed through a gastroscope — previously via a Crosby capsule
- Coeliac disease results in total villous atrophy with characteristic features (see Section 7.1); partial villous atrophy, which is less commonly seen, has a wide differential diagnosis

---

Differential diagnosis of partial villous atrophy

- Coeliac disease
- Transient gluten intolerance
- Cows' milk sensitive enteropathy
- Soy protein sensitive enteropathy
- Gastroenteritis and post-gastroenteritis syndromes
- Giardiasis
- Autoimmune enteropathy
- Acquired hypogammaglobulinaemia
- Tropical sprue
- Protein energy malnutrition
- Severe combined immunodeficiency
- Antineoplastic therapy

7.1 Coeliac disease

The prevalence is between 1 : 300 and 1 : 1000 (precise prevalence data are much debated) in the UK, higher in Northern Europe. There are associations with HLA DQ2 and DQ8. There is an increased incidence in first-degree relatives (approximately 1 : 10). Intolerance is to gliadin in gluten, which is present in wheat, rye, barley and oats (oat is probably not a primary cause but is cross-contaminated with the other grains during production).

Coeliac disease presents after 6 months of age (i.e. after gluten has been introduced into the diet). Chronic diarrhoea and poor weight gain (short stature in older children) generally occur. Other features include anorexia, lethargy, generalized irritability, abdominal distension and pallor. Atypical presentations with less specific symptoms including recurrent abdominal pain are increasingly common and picked up early with the advent of antibody screening. With family screening, silent coeliac disease (i.e. disease in the absence of overt symptoms) is increasingly recognized.

Diagnosis is by small-bowel biopsy (endoscopic duodenal or jejunal). The characteristic features on biopsy are of subtotal villous atrophy, crypt hypertrophy, intraepithelial lymphocytosis and a lamina propria plasma-cell infiltrate. It is of crucial importance that the child's gluten intake is adequate at the time of the biopsy otherwise a false-negative result may be obtained.

Treatment is with a gluten-free diet for life. There is a long-term risk of small-bowel lymphoma and other gastrointestinal malignancies if the diet is not adhered to. The gluten-free diet itself has no long-term complications, although in the young child its use should be supervised by a paediatric trained dietitian.

The standards for the diagnosis of coeliac disease are set out by the European Society of Paediatric Gastroenterology. Diagnosis is confirmed by characteristic histology and a clinical remission on a gluten-free diet. There are indications for a subsequent gluten challenge and these include initial diagnostic uncertainty and when the diagnosis is made under the age of 2 years. The latter being because at that age there are other causes of a flat jejunal biopsy (see above). A gluten challenge involves an initial control biopsy on a gluten-free diet followed by a period on gluten with a repeat biopsy after 3–6 months and then again after 2 years, sooner if symptoms develop. The response to a challenge can be monitored by antibody screening. There are reports of late relapse following gluten challenge.

Antibody testing in the screening of children with faltering growth or other gastrointestinal symptoms in whom coeliac disease is a possibility and in the ongoing management of children with coeliac disease is helpful. The biopsy, however, currently remains the 'gold standard' for diagnosis.

Antibody tests available

- IgG anti-gliadin
- IgA anti-gliadin
- IgA anti-reticulin
- IgA anti-endomysial
- IgA anti-tissue transglutaminase

The IgA anti-tissue transglutaminase antibody is the most sensitive and specific. The sensitivity and specficity of the IgA anti-endomysial antibody test is similar although the assay is more difficult to perform. However, false-negatives occur in children who are IgA-deficient. This means that IgA levels should be measured routinely alongside the antibody test. IgG tissue transglutaminase levels are now done in same centres.

Children who are IgA deficient with features suggestive of coeliac disease require consideration of small-bowel biopsy.

The IgA anti-tissue transglutaminase/endomysial antibody will turn negative in a child with coeliac disease on a gluten-free diet. This can be used as a marker of compliance.

Conditions with an increased prevalence of coeliac disease

- Type 1 diabetes
- Autoimmune thyroiditis
- Down syndrome
- Turner syndrome
- William syndrome
- Selective IgA deficiency
- First-degree relatives

Associations of coeliac disease

- Dermatitis herpetiformis
- Dental enamel hypoplasia of permanent teeth
- Osteoporosis
- Short stature
- Delayed puberty
- Iron-deficiency anaemia not responsive to iron supplements
- Infertility
- Increased incidence of small-bowel malignancy, especially lymphoma

There is weaker evidence for an association with hepatitis, arthritis and epilepsy with occipital calcification.

There is an increased recognition that at-risk groups should be screened. Silent coeliac describes children with abnormal small-bowel mucosa with no symptoms. Latent coeliac disease refers to positive serology in the absence of an enteropathy. A number of such cases will probably develop coeliac disease. Screened high-risk asymptomatic patients have been found to be negative on initial serological screening but positive subsequently.

7.2 Cows' milk protein sensitive enteropathy

Implies enteropathy secondary to cows' milk protein and improves following withdrawal of cows' milk protein with a longer term history of resolution in most cases (see Section 4.1).

7.3 Giardiasis

- *Giardia* is a protozoal parasite which is infective in the cyst form. It also exists in the trophozoite form and is found in contaminated food and water
- Clinical manifestations vary; can be asymptomatic, acute diarrhoeal disease, chronic diarrhoea. Partial villous atrophy is occasionally seen
- Diagnosis is by stool examination for cysts or examination of the duodenal aspirate at small-bowel biopsy
- Treatment is with metronidazole and is often given blind in suspicious cases

7.4 Cystic fibrosis

This subject is well covered in Chapter 21, Respiratory. It is important to remember the gastrointestinal manifestations.

Gastrointestinal manifestations of cystic fibrosis

- **Pancreatic**
  - Insufficiency occurs in up to 90%
  - Pancreatitis
  - Abnormal glucose tolerance in up to 10% by the second decade
  - Diabetes mellitus
- **Intestinal**
  - Meconium ileus
  - Atresias
  - Rectal prolapse
  - Distal obstruction syndrome
  - Strictures, perhaps secondary to high-dose pancreatic supplementation
- **Hepatobiliary**
  - Cholestasis in infancy
  - Fatty liver
  - Focal biliary fibrosis
  - Multilobular cirrhosis
- **Abnormalities of the gallbladder**
  - Cholelithiasis
  - Obstruction of the common bile duct

7.5 Schwachman–Diamond syndrome

- Autosomal recessive
- Incidence 1 : 20 to 1 : 200,000
- Main features — pancreatic insufficiency, neutropenia and short stature
- Other features include metaphyseal dysostosis, mild hepatic dysfunction, increased frequency of infections, further haematological abnormalities (including thrombocytopenia, increased risk of malignancy)

7.6 Bacterial overgrowth (small bowel)

- Repeated courses of antibiotics are a risk factor
- Stasis causes bacterial proliferation with the emergence of resistant strains
- Malabsorption results with steatorrhoea and fat-soluble vitamin malabsorption
- Diagnosis is by a high index of suspicion — particularly in patients with risk factors, e.g. previous gastrointestinal surgery, short-bowel syndrome. Hydrogen breath testing may be useful. Radioisotope-labelled breath testing may also have a role. Barium radiology should be performed if obstruction is suspected. Culture of the duodenal juice can be taken at endoscopy if performed
- Treatment involves appropriate management of the underlying cause. Metronidazole, which is effective orally and intravenously, is the antibiotic of first choice. Probiotics have been used.

7.7   Intestinal lymphangiectasia

- Functional obstruction of flow of lymph through the thoracic duct and into the inferior vena cava
- Leads to fat malabsorption and a protein-losing enteropathy
- Treatment is with medium-chain triglycerides — absorbed directly into the portal vein
- Can be primary or secondary to other causes of lymphatic obstruction

8.   RECURRENT ABDOMINAL PAIN

Recurrent abdominal pain is very common in childhood, affecting up to 10% of the school-age population. In the majority of cases the aetiology is non-organic. The condition is more common in girls than boys and a family history is common. The pain is usually periumbilical and rarely associated with other gastrointestinal symptoms such as diarrhoea, blood per rectum or weight loss.

Abdominal pain accompanied by other symptoms is suggestive of organic pathology. Night pain is suggestive of oesophagitis or peptic ulceration. Diarrhoea with blood per rectum suggests a colitis and diarrhoea associated with weight loss suggests a malabsorption syndrome.

Children with chronic abdominal pain lasting for longer than 3 months should have a basic blood screen, including inflammatory markers and coeliac disease serology.

There are three syndromes:

- Isolated paroxysmal abdominal pain
- Abdominal pain associated with symptoms of dyspepsia (functional dyspepsia)
- Abdominal pain associated with altered bowel habit (irritable bowel syndrome)

Factors that suggest an organic cause

- Age < 5 years
- Constitutional symptoms — fever, weight loss, poor growth, joint symptoms, skin rashes
- Vomiting — particularly if bile stained
- Pain that awakens the child from sleep
- Pain away from the umbilicus +/− referred to back/shoulders
- Urinary symptoms
- Family history of inflammatory bowel disease, peptic ulcer disease
- Perianal disease
- Occult or gross blood in the stool
- Abnormal screening blood tests

8.1   Functional abdominal pain

This implies non-organic pain. It is more common in girls than boys. Children are usually older than 5 years. Peak age 8–9 years. Pain is usually gradual in onset, of variable severity with symptom-free periods, periumbilical, lasts 1–3 hours, type of pain (e.g. burning, stabbing) unclear, rarely causes a child to wake from sleep, not usually related to meals, activity or bowel movement. Loose diagnostic criterion is three or more episodes in 3 months. Pain interferes with normal activity, e.g. results in time off school. Extraintestinal symptoms common (e.g. headache). Family history common. Child often offered positive reinforcement for symptoms.

Normal examination. Normal investigations.

Associations

- Timid, nervous anxious characters
- Perfectionists — over achievers
- Increased number of stresses and more likely to internalize problems than other children, but no increase in the risk of depression or other psychiatric problems when compared with children with organic pain
- School absence common — may be a degree of school refusal — may be issues at school

Remember children with organic pathology can suffer from non-organic pain and children with non-organic pain can also have organic pathology.

Management of functional abdominal pain

1. Positive diagnosis

2. Education

3. Realistic expectation of treatment

- Pain is real not psychogenic or imaginary
- Goal of management cannot be total freedom from pain
- Support the child
- Avoid environmental reinforcement
- Review associated symptoms (e.g. headache)
- Dietary triggers (fibre, lactose, chocolate)
- Life-style issues (e.g. exercise, school attendance)
- Diary of symptoms occasionally useful in severe cases

A number of children in this group benefit from the diagnostic label 'irritable bowel syndrome'. A number of children with recurrent abdominal pain in childhood go on to develop either migraine or recurrent tension headache as adults.

9. INFLAMMATORY BOWEL DISEASE

The recent British Paediatric Surveillance Unit survey suggests that the incidence of inflammatory bowel disease in children under 16 years is 5 : 100,000, with Crohn's disease being twice as common as ulcerative colitis.

9.1 Crohn's disease

Crohn's disease is a chronic inflammatory disorder of the bowel involving any region from mouth to anus. The inflammation is transmural with skip lesions. There has been an increase in incidence over the past 10 years. 25% of cases present in childhood, usually in the second decade. The commonest presenting symptoms are abdominal pain, diarrhoea and weight loss. Growth failure with delayed bone maturation and delayed sexual development is common. The diagnosis is made on the basis of clinical symptoms, raised inflammatory indices and diagnostic tests including barium radiology, gastroscopy and ileocolonoscopy with biopsy. White-cell scanning is not useful as a diagnostic test as it is not sufficiently sensitive, particularly in small-bowel disease. Treatment is difficult as the disease often runs a chronic relapsing course. The aim of management is to induce a disease remission and facilitate normal growth and development.

The most widely used treatment in children is enteral nutrition, used as an exclusion diet for up to 8 weeks, followed by a period of controlled food reintroduction. The type of enteral nutrition used varies and can be either elemental (protein broken down into peptide chains or amino acids) or polymeric (whole protein). This induces remission in up to 85% of patients. Maintenance is with 5 ASA derivatives and continued nutritional support. Unfortunately disease relapse is common and either repeated courses of enteral nutrition or corticosteroids are usually required. Corticosteroid dependence or resistance can occur and additional immunosuppression or surgery is indicated. The most commonly used additional immunosuppressive agent is azathioprine which will reduce steroid requirements in 60–80% of patients, and in many of those will induce a long-term remission. Important toxicity includes the risk of myelosuppression and so regular blood counts are required. Other medications tried include thalidomide, methotrexate and monoclonal antibodies to tumour necrosis factor-α. Surgical resection is indicated for disease resistant to medical therapy particularly if there is growth failure, although there is a high risk of recurrence following surgery.

Extraintestinal manifestations of Crohn's disease

*   Joint disease in 10% — ankylosing spondylitis rarely
*   Skin rashes — erythema nodosum, erythema multiforme, pyoderma gangrenosum
*   Liver disease (rare in childhood) — sclerosing cholangitis, chronic active hepatitis, cirrhosis
*   Uveitis
*   Osteoporosis

9.2 Ulcerative colitis

*   Ulcerative colitis is an inflammatory disease limited to the colonic and rectal mucosa. It is the more distal bowel that is the most involved. Inflammation is neither pan-enteric or transmural as is seen in Crohn's disease. A backwash ileitis into the terminal ileum is often seen. The characteristic histology in the colon is of mucosal and submucosal inflammation with goblet-cell depletion, cryptitis and crypt abscesses but no granulomas. The inflammatory change is usually diffuse rather than patchy

- Aetiology is unknown. Disease is more common in females than males
- The gut disease can be mild, moderate or severe. The symptoms of colitis are diarrhoea, blood per rectum and abdominal pain. Systemic disturbance can accompany more severe disease; tachycardia, fever, weight loss, anaemia, hypoalbuminaemia and leukocytosis
- Although unusual, the disease can present with predominantly extraintestinal manifestations, including growth failure, arthropathy, erythema nodosum
- The presentation can be more indolent with occult blood loss, non-specific abdominal pain, cholangitis and raised inflammatory indices
- Complications of ulcerative colitis include toxic megacolon, growth failure, cholangitis, carcinoma, non-malignant stricture. The cancer risk reflects the disease severity and duration of disease. Regular screening is carried out in adult life
- Diagnosis is by endoscopy and biopsy with the classical histological features being shown. A small number of children have an indeterminate or unclassified colitis. The differential diagnosis of colitis is wide and a list of the causes of a non-infective and an infective colitis are listed in section 9.3. It is, for example, crucial to exclude infection in a child presenting with acute colitis which is more likely, particularly if the disease is of short duration. Management is with 5 ASA derivatives, local or systemic steroids, azathioprine to reduce steroid toxicity in steroid-dependent patients. Surgical resection is indicated in resistant cases. Surgery is a colectomy with ileostomy. Reversal is possible in early adult life by ileoanal anastomosis and pouch formation.
- Management of toxic colitis involves intravenous fluids, antibiotics and corticosteroids.

Differences between Crohn's disease and ulcerative colitis

Crohn's	Ulcerative colitis
Panenteric	Colon only
Skip lesions	Diffuse
Transmural	Mucosal
Granulomas	Crypt abscesses
Perianal disease	

Colitis can be indeterminate, i.e. the histological features are consistent with inflammatory bowel disease but not diagnostic of either Crohn's disease or ulcerative colitis.

9.3   Differential diagnosis of colitis

Causes of infective colitis
Salmonella spp.
Shigella spp.
Campylobacter pylori
Escherichia coli 0157 (and other *E. coli*)
Clostridium difficile (pseudomembranous colitis)
Yersinia spp.
Tuberculosis
Cytomegalovirus
Entamoeba histolytica

Causes of non-infective colitis
Ulcerative colitis
Crohn's disease
Necrotizing enterocolitis
Microscopic colitis
Behçet disease
Food allergic colitis
Enterobius vermicularis

9.4   Pseudomembranous colitis

- Occurs secondary to infection with *Clostridium difficile* — a Gram-positive anaerobe
- Risk factor is disruption of the normal intestinal flora by antibiotics
- Clinical features vary from asymptomatic carriage to life-threatening
- Pathogenesis is through toxin production
- Treatment is with vancomycin (oral) or metronidazole (intravenous or oral); probiotics may have a role
- Relapse rate is 15–20%

9.5   Behçet syndrome

- Orogenital ulceration with/without non-erosive arthritis, thrombophlebitis, vascular thromboses or central nervous system abnormalities including meningoencephalitis
- Treatment of orogenital ulceration is often unsatisfactory; however, local and/or systemic steroids may be used acutely
- Other drugs that have been used in prophylaxis include azathioprine and thalidomide

10. GASTROINTESTINAL BLEEDING

This can present as haematemesis (usually upper gastrointestinal source), melaena (partially digested blood) or frank blood per rectum.

10.1 Causes of gastrointestinal bleeding

- Anal fissure
- Volvulus
- Intussusception
- Peptic ulcer
- Polyp
- Meckel's diverticulum
- Inflammatory bowel disease
- Haemolytic–uraemic syndrome
- Infective colitis
- Henoch–Schönlein purpura
- Vascular malformation
- Oesophagitis/varices
- Epistaxis/swallowed blood — including swallowed maternal blood in the neonatal period
- Necrotizing enterocolitis
- Haemorrhagic disease of the newborn
- Trauma/sexual abuse

10.2 Intussusception

- Peak incidence aged 6–9 months. Male to female ratio 4 : 1
- Usually presents with spasmodic pain, pallor and irritability. Vomiting is an early feature and rapidly progresses to being bile stained. Passage of blood-stained stools often occurs and a mass is frequently palpable. The presentation, however, is often atypical
- The intussusception is usually ileocaecal, the origin being either the ileocaecal valve or the terminal ileum
- An identifiable cause is commoner in those who present later — Meckel's diverticulum, polyp, reduplication, lymphosarcoma and Henoch–Schönlein purpura being examples.
- Diagnosis is usually on clinical grounds. Confirmation is by plain abdominal X-ray, ultrasound or air-enema examination.
- Treatment is either with air-enema reduction if the history is short or surgically at laparotomy. Resuscitation with saline is often required. Contraindications to air enema include peritonitis and signs of perforation.

10.3   Meckel's diverticulum

- Remnant of the vitellointestinal duct
- Present in 2% of individuals
- 50% contain ectopic gastric, pancreatic or colonic tissue
- Distal ileum on the anti-mesenteric border within 100 cm of the ileocaecal valve and is around 5–6 cm long
- Presents with intermittent, painless blood per rectum; bleeding can be quite severe and may require a blood transfusion; other presentations include intussusception (commoner in older males), perforation and peritonitis
- The technetium scan is used to look for ectopic gastric mucosa

10.4   Polyposis

Juvenile polyps

These make up 85% of the polyps seen in childhood. Present at age 2–6 years with painless blood per rectum. Most polyps are solitary and located within 30 cm of the anus. Not premalignant. Juvenile polyposis refers to multiple juvenile polyps and can be premalignant.

Peutz–Jeghers syndrome

Autosomal dominant inheritance. Diffuse gastrointestinal hamartomatous polyps associated with hyperpigmentation of the buccal mucosa and lips. Premalignant.

Gardener syndrome and familial adenomatous polyposis coli

Best considered together. Both conditions are inherited as an autosomal dominant. Gardener syndrome is familial adenomatous polyposis plus bony lesions, subcutaneous tumours and cysts. Both conditions carry a very high risk of colonic carcinoma and prophylactic colectomy at the end of the second decade is advised.

11.   GASTROENTERITIS

Gastroenteritis is a common problem. The majority of cases can be managed at home. Oral rehydration therapy is the mainstay of treatment, with rapid rehydration over 4–6 hours with reassessment and the early reintroduction of normal feeds after that. Breast-feeding should not be stopped. Antimicrobials are only of use in very specific circumstances. Antidiarrhoeal agents are of no use. Complications such as carbohydrate intolerance and chronic diarrhoea and faltering growth are relatively rare.

Composition of oral rehydration solution (ORS)

Oral rehydration therapy, which has probably saved more children's lives world-wide than any other medical intervention, remains the mainstay of treatment. The World Health Organization ORS contains 90 mmol/l of sodium and is specifically designed for cholera treatment. European ORS contain between 35 and 60 mmol/l sodium with varying concentrations of glucose and potassium. There remains controversy over the best combination but it would appear that all of the available formulations are effective and safe. Home-made solutions, usually with an excess of salt, put children at risk of hypernatraemic dehydration.

Causes of gastroenteritis

- **Unknown** — in both the developed and developing world, no pathogens are identified in up to 50% of cases, even when the condition is fully investigated
- **Viral** — rotaviruses (commonest), adenovirus, small-round viruses and astroviruses
- **Bacterial** — *Campylobacter* spp. (commonest), *Shigella* spp., *Salmonella* spp., enteropathogenic *E. coli*, enterotoxigenic *E. coli* 0157:H7 (rare but associated with haemolytic–uraemic syndrome), *Vibrio cholerae*, *Yersinia enterocolitica*
- **Protozoa** — *Cryptosporidium* sp. (particularly in the immunocompromised host), *Giardia* sp., which has a varied presentation ranging from the asymptomatic carrier state to chronic diarrhoea with growth failure, *Entamoeba histolytica* (amoebic dysentery)

Differential diagnosis

This is potentially wide and includes many other potential conditions including:

- Other infections, e.g. otitis media, tonsillitis, pneumonia, septicaemia, urinary tract infection, meningitis
- Gastro-oesophageal reflux
- Food intolerance
- Haemolytic–uraemic syndrome
- Intussusception
- Pyloric stenosis
- Acute appendicitis
- Drugs, e.g. laxatives, antibiotics

Assessment of dehydration

% Dehydration	Severity	Clinical features
3		Undetectable
3–5	Mild	Slightly dry mucous membranes
5	Moderate	Decreased skin turgor, slightly sunken eyes, depressed fontanelle, circulation preserved
10	Severe	All the above plus more marked, drowsiness, rapid weak pulse, cool extremities, capillary refill time greater than 2 seconds
12–14		Moribund

Children with 10% dehydration usually require intravenous fluid resuscitation

Remember

- Less than 3% of dehydration is clinically not apparent
- A normal capillary refill time (< 2 seconds) makes severe dehydration very unlikely (measured by pressing the skin and measuring the time taken for the skin to re-perfuse)
- Useful signs include reduced skin turgor, dry oral mucosa, sunken eyes and altered consciousness level

Hospital admission should be considered when:

- Diagnosis is unclear/complications have arisen, e.g. carbohydrate intolerance (see Section 4.4)
- Home management fails/unable to tolerate fluids/persistent vomiting
- Severe dehydration
- Significant other medical condition, e.g. diabetes, immunocompromised
- Poor social circumstances
- Hydration difficult to assess, e.g. obesity
- Inability to reassess

11.1 Post-gastroenteritis syndromes

Acute gastroenteritis usually resolves in 7–10 days. Chronic diarrhoea is defined as diarrhoea lasting > 3 weeks, particularly if associated with poor weight gain/weight loss (should be referred for investigation). The continuing diarrhoea may be secondary to a second infection or reflect the 'unmasking' of another pathology, for example coeliac disease, cows' milk protein intolerance or cystic fibrosis.

12. CONSTIPATION

Childhood constipation is common. Most children do not have an underlying cause and their constipation is functional.

Many factors can trigger constipation including:

- Intercurrent illness with poor fluid and food intake
- Perianal pathology such as anal fissure or streptococcal infection resulting in stool withholding
- Difficult early toilet training resulting in stool withholding

If associated with a mega rectum then soiling is common. A plain abdominal X-ray may be helpful in the assessment of such patients with the potential to assess severity and extent. This can be helpful particularly in the obese patient when clinical assessment is often difficult. The soiling occurs because the normal sensory process of stool being in the rectum, resulting in distension and the urge to defecate, is lost when the rectum is permanently distended. This should be distinguished from encopresis in which stool is passed in to the pants at inappropriate times and in inappropriate places with no underlying constipation — the latter being a primarily psychological problem.

Underlying physical causes need to be considered for the purpose of the examination, including Hirschsprung disease, endocrine causes such as thyroid disease and meconium ileus equivalent or distal intestinal obstruction syndrome seen in children with cystic fibrosis.

Hirschsprung disease is very rare in children who have at some stage of their life had a normal bowel habit and usually presents in the neonatal period.

Most constipation is short term and is readily treated with bulk and/or stimulant laxatives.

The management of chronic functional constipation is more difficult and often requires a multidisciplinary approach. Many factors are often involved in the perpetuation of the problem including local pathology such as anal fissure, lower abdominal pain, poor diet, poor fluid intake, lack of exercise, previous difficult toileting experiences, and psychosocial problems. High doses of stimulant and bulk laxatives are required, usually for a prolonged period. Enema therapy, which can reinforce difficult toileting experiences, should be reserved for the more difficult cases. An essential part of management is explanation and reassurance and practical advice and support in the institution of a toileting regimen. Children need to sit on the toilet regularly, this is best 15–30 minutes after meals.

Commonly used laxatives include lactulose, sodium docussate, Senokot, sodium picosulphate. Enemas are occasionally required but can exacerbate the stool withholding cycle.

Constipation is common in children with nocturnal and diurnal enuresis and treatment of the constipation frequently results in a significant improvement in the wetting.

12.1 Perianal streptococcal infection

- Common cause of perianal redness
- Can present as constipation or perianal pain
- Secondary to group A streptococcal infection
- Treatment is with penicillin, there may be a need for continuing laxatives

Other causes of perianal soreness

- Poor perineal hygiene
- Soiling/encopresis
- Threadworm infestation
- Lactose intolerance (acidic stool)
- Anal fissure
- Sexual abuse (rare)

12.2 Hirschsprung disease

- Absence of ganglion cells in the myenteric plexus of the most distal bowel
- Males more than females. 1 in 5,000. Gene on chromosome 10
- Long-segment Hirschsprung disease is familial with equal sex incidence
- Associated with Down syndrome; high frequency of other congenital abnormalities

- Usually presents in infancy, failure to pass meconium with presentation in the older child being rare — the diagnosis in this group usually being chronic functional constipation; most children with Hirschsprung will have never had a normal bowel habit
- Enterocolitis commonly can occur before or after surgery
- Definitive test is by rectal biopsy to confirm the absence of ganglion cells in the submucosal plexus; histochemistry will demonstrate excessive acetylcholinesterase activity and the absence of ganglion cells
- Surgery is excision, usually with temporary colostomy followed by pull-through at a later stage
- Ultrashort-segment Hirschsprung disease is very rare and can present significant diagnostic difficulty

13. FURTHER READING

Ball PA, Booth IW, Holden CE, Puntis JW (Eds). 1998. *Paediatric Parenteral Nutrition*, 3rd edn. Pharmacia and Upjohn Nutrition.

Bremner AR, Beattie RM. 2002. Therapy of Crohn's disease in childhood. *Expert Opinion in Pharmacotherapy* 3:7, 809–25.

Goulet O, Ruemmele F, Lacaille F, Colomb V. 2004. Irreversible intestinal failure. *Journal of Paediatric Gastroenterology and Nutrition* 38, 250–69.

Preedy V, Grimble G, Watson R (Eds). 2001. *Nutrition in the Infant: Problems and Practical Procedures*. Greenwich Medical Media Ltd.

Plunkett A, Beattie RM. 2005. Recurrent abdominal pain in childhood. *Journal of the Royal Society of Medicine* 98, 101–6.

Shulman R, Phillips S. 2003. Parenteral nutrition in infants and children. *Journal of Paediatric Gastroenterology and Nutrition* 36, 587–607.

Walker WA, Goulet OJ, Kleinman RE, Sherman PM, Schneider BL, Sanderson IR (Eds). 2004. *Paediatric Gastrointestinal Disease. Pathophysiology, Diagnosis and Management*, 4th edn. BC Decker Inc.

Walker-Smith JA, Murch SH. 1999. *Diseases of the Small Intestine in Childhood*, 4th edn. Isis Medical Media.

Wyllie R, Hyams JS (Eds). 2006. *Paediatric Gastrointestinal and Liver Disease*, 3rd edn. Elsevier.

Chapter 10

Genetics

Louise Wilson

CONTENTS

353

Genetics

1. CHROMOSOMES

Background

Within the nucleus of somatic cells there are 22 pairs of autosomes and one pair of sex chromosomes. Normal male and female karyotypes are 46,XY and 46,XX respectively. The normal chromosome complement of 46 chromosomes is known as **diploid**. Genomes with a single copy of each chromosome or three copies of each are known respectively as **haploid** and **triploid**. A karyotype with too many or too few chromosomes, where the total is not a multiple of 23, is called **aneuploid**.

Chromosomes are divided by the centromere into a short '**p**' arm ('petit') and a long '**q**' arm. **Acrocentric** chromosomes (13, 14, 15, 21, 22) have the centromere at one end.

Lyonization is the process whereby in a cell containing more than one X chromosome, only one is active. Selection of the active X chromosome is usually random and each inactivated X chromosome can be seen as a Barr body on microscopy.

Mitosis occurs in somatic cells and results in two **diploid** daughter cells with nuclear chromosomes which are genetically identical both to each other and the original parent cell.

Chromosomes replicate forming 2 chromatids joined at the centromere, and condense

Homologous chromosomes align independently on the spindle

Chromatids move to opposite poles and cell divides

2 diploid daughter cells, genetically identical to each other and the parent cell

Mitosis

355

Meiosis occurs in the germ cells of the gonads and is also known as '**reduction division**' because it results in four **haploid** daughter cells, each containing just one member (homologue) of each chromosome pair and all genetically different. Meiosis involves two divisions (**meiosis I and II**). The reduction in chromosome number occurs during meiosis I and is preceded by exchange of chromosome segments between homologous chromosomes called **crossing over**. In males the onset of meiosis and spermatogenesis is at puberty. In females, replication of the chromosomes and crossing over begins during fetal life but the oocytes remain suspended prior to the first cell division until just before ovulation.

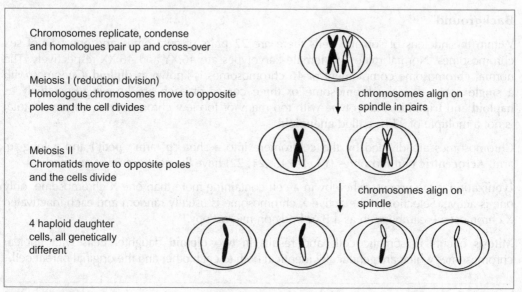

Chromosomes replicate, condense and homologues pair up and cross-over

Meiosis I (reduction division)
Homologous chromosomes move to opposite poles and the cell divides

chromosomes align on spindle in pairs

Meiosis II
Chromatids move to opposite poles and the cells divide

chromosomes align on spindle

4 haploid daughter cells, all genetically different

Meiosis

Translocations

- **Reciprocal** — exchange of genetic material between non-homologous chromosomes
- **Robertsonian** — fusion of two acrocentric chromosomes at their centromeres, e.g. (14;21)
- **Unbalanced** — if chromosomal material has been lost or gained overall
- **Balanced** — if no chromosomal material has been lost or gained overall

Carriers of balanced translocations are usually phenotypically normal but are at increased risk for having offspring with chromosomal imbalance.

Carriers of a Robertsonian translocation involving chromosome 21 are at increased risk of having offspring with translocation Down syndrome. For female and male (14;21) translocation carriers the observed offspring risks for Down syndrome are ~15% and 5%, respectively. Remember, they can also have offspring with normal chromosomes or offspring who are balanced translocation carriers like themselves.

1.1 Common sex chromosome aneuploidies

Turner syndrome (karyotype 45,X)

This affects 1 in 2,500 liveborn females but it is a frequent finding amongst early miscarriages. Patients are usually of normal intelligence. They have streak ovaries which result in failure of menstruation, low oestrogen with high gonadotrophins, and infertility. Normal secondary sexual characteristics may develop spontaneously or can be induced with oestrogens. Short stature throughout childhood with failure of the pubertal growth spurt is typical. Final height can be increased by early treatment with growth hormone. Other features may include:

- Webbed or short neck
- Low hairline
- Shield chest with widely spaced nipples
- Cubitus valgus (wide carrying angle)
- Cardiovascular abnormalities (particularly aortic coarctation in 10–15%)
- Renal anomalies (e.g. horseshoe kidney, duplicated ureters, renal aplasia) in one-third
- Non-pitting lymphoedema in one-third

Triple X syndrome (karyotype 47,XXX)

These patients show little phenotypic abnormality but tend to be of tall stature. Whilst intelligence is typically reduced compared to siblings it usually falls within normal or low–normal limits; however, mild developmental and behavioural difficulties are more common. Fertility is normal but the incidence of early menopause is increased.

Klinefelter syndrome (karyotype 47,XXY)

This affects 1 in 600 newborn males. Phenotypic abnormalities are rare prepubertally other than a tendency to tall stature. At puberty, spontaneous expression of secondary sexual characteristics is variable but poor growth of facial and body hair is common. The testes are small and associated with azoospermia, testosterone production is around 50% of normal and gonadotrophins are raised. Gynaecomastia occurs in 30% and there is an increased risk of male breast cancer. Female distribution of fat and hair and a high pitched voice may occur but are not typical. Intelligence is generally reduced compared to siblings but usually falls within normal or low–normal limits. Mild developmental and behavioural problems are more common.

47,XYY males

These males are phenotypically normal but tend to be tall. Intelligence is usually within normal limits but there is an increased incidence of behavioural abnormalities.

1.2   Common autosomal chromosome aneuploidies

Down syndrome (trisomy 21)

Down syndrome affects 1 in 700 livebirths overall and is usually secondary to meiotic non-disjunction during oogenesis, which is commoner with increasing maternal age. Around 5% of patients have an underlying Robertsonian translocation, most commonly between chromosomes 14 and 21. Around 3% have detectable **mosaicism** (a mixture of trisomy 21 and karyotypically normal cells) usually resulting in a milder phenotype.

Phenotypic features include:

* Brachycephaly
* Upslanting palpebral fissures, epicanthic folds, Brushfield spots on the iris
* Protruding tongue
* Single palmar crease, fifth finger clinodactyly, wide sandal gaps between first and second toes
* Hypotonia and moderate mental retardation

The following are more common in patients with Down syndrome:

* Cardiovascular malformations in 40%, particularly atrioventricular septal defects
* Gastrointestinal abnormalities in 6%, particularly duodenal atresia and Hirschsprung disease
* Haematological abnormalities, particularly acute lymphoblastic, acute myeloid and transient leukaemias
* Hypothyroidism
* Cataracts in 3%
* Alzheimer disease in the majority by 40 years of age

Edward syndrome (trisomy 18)

This typically causes intrauterine growth retardation, a characteristic facies, prominent occiput, overlapping fingers (second and fifth overlap third and fourth), rockerbottom feet (vertical talus) and short dorsiflexed great toes. Malformations, particularly congenital heart disease, diaphragmatic hernias, renal abnormalities and dislocated hips, are more common. Survival beyond early infancy is rare but associated with profound mental handicap.

Patau syndrome (trisomy 13)

Affected infants usually have multiple malformations including holoprosencephaly and other central nervous system abnormalities, scalp defects, microphthalmia, cleft lip and palate, post-axial polydactyly, rockerbottom feet, renal abnormalities and congenital heart disease. Survival beyond early infancy is rare and associated with profound mental handicap.

1.3 FISH testing

FISH (**F**luorescent **I**n **S**itu **H**ybridization) is a technique used to assess the copy number of specific DNA sequences in the genome. Fluorescently labelled probes are designed which are complementary to the DNA sequences being assessed, and they are allowed to hybridize to the chromosome spread. The number of copies can then be visualized as fluorescent spots using confocal microscopes. FISH can be performed much more rapidly than formal karyotyping. The main clinical uses are:

- Rapid trisomy screening (for chromosomes 21, 13, 18)
- Rapid sexing
- Detection of specific microdeletion syndromes

1.4 Microdeletion syndromes

These are caused by chromosomal deletions which are too small to see on standard microscopy but which involve two or more adjacent (contiguous) genes. They can be detected using specific **FISH testing**.

Examples of microdeletion syndromes:

- **DiGeorge syndrome** (parathyroid gland hypoplasia with hypocalcaemia, thymus hypoplasia with T-lymphocyte deficiency, congenital cardiac malformations particularly interrupted aortic arch and truncus arteriosus, cleft palate, learning disability) due to microdeletions at 22q11. There appears to be an increased incidence of psychiatric disorders, particularly within the schizophrenic spectrum
- **Williams syndrome** (supravalvular aortic stenosis, hypercalcaemia, stellate irides, mental retardation) due to microdeletions involving the elastin gene on chromosome 7
- **WAGR syndrome** (association of **W**ilms tumour, **a**niridia, **g**enitourinary abnormalities and mental **r**etardation) due to deletions of chromosome 11p13

1.5 Genetic counselling in chromosomal disorders

As a general rule:

For parents of a child with trisomy 21

Recurrence risks will be around 1% above the maternal age-related risks for which there are tables. At age 36 years the background risk for Down syndrome is 0.5%.

For parents of a child with any other trisomy

Recurrence risks in future pregnancies for that specific trisomy will be < 1%. However, couples are generally counselled that there is a 1% risk for any chromosome abnormality in future offspring which takes into account the small risks that one parent may be mosaic or may have an increased risk of chromosome mis-segregation at meiosis.

For parents of a child with a microdeletion

Parental chromosomes should be checked. If they are normal, recurrence risks will be < 1%. If one parent carries the microdeletion then recurrence risks will be 50%.

For parents of a child with any other chromosome abnormality

Parental chromosomes should be checked. If they are normal then recurrence risks are usually small (< 1%). If one parent carries a predisposing translocation then recurrence risks will be higher, depending on the nature of the translocation.

Prenatal karyotyping is available for any couple who have had a previous child with a chromosome abnormality.

2. MENDELIAN INHERITANCE

2.1 Autosomal dominant (AD) conditions

These result from mutation of one copy of a gene carried on an autosome. All offspring of an affected person have a 50% chance of inheriting the mutation. Within a family the severity may vary (**variable expression**) and known mutation carriers may appear clinically normal (**reduced penetrance**). Some conditions, such as achondroplasia and neurofibromatosis type 1, frequently begin de novo through new mutations arising in the egg or (more commonly) sperm.

> **Example of autosomal dominant conditions:**
> | | |
> |---|---|
> | Achondroplasia | Marfan syndrome |
> | Alagille syndrome | Myotonic dystrophy |
> | Ehlers–Danlos syndrome (most) | Neurofibromatosis types 1 and 2 |
> | Facioscapulohumeral dystrophy | Noonan syndrome |
> | Familial adenomatous polyposis coli | Porphyrias (except congenital |
> | Familial hypercholesterolaemia | erythropoietic which is AR) |
> | Gilbert syndrome | Tuberous sclerosis |
> | Huntington chorea | von Willebrand disease |
>
> Conditions pre-fixed 'hereditary' or 'familial' are usually autosomal dominant.

2.2 Autosomal recessive [AR] conditions

These result from mutations in both copies of an autosomal gene. Where both parents are carriers, each of their offspring has a 1 in 4 (25%) risk of being affected, and a 2 in 4 (50%) chance of being a carrier.

Examples of autosomal recessive conditions:

Alkaptonuria	Glycogen storage diseases
Ataxia telangiectasia	Homocystinuria
β-Thalassaemia	Haemochromatosis
Congenital adrenal hyperplasias	Mucopolysaccharidoses (all except Hunter)
Crigler–Najar (severe form)	Oculocutaneous albinism
Cystic fibrosis	Phenylketonuria
Dubin–Johnson	Rotor (usually)
Fanconi anaemia	Sickle-cell anaemia
Galactosaemia	Spinal muscular atrophies
Glucose-6-phosphatase	Wilson disease
deficiency (von Gierkes)*	Xeroderma pigmentosa

*Do not confuse with glucose-6-phosphate dehydrogenase deficiency (favism) which is X-linked recessive. Most metabolic disorders are autosomal recessive – remember the exceptions.

Risk calculations for autosomal recessive disorders

Remember:

- People who have no family history of an autosomal recessive disorder have the background population carrier risk
- The parents of a child with an autosomal recessive disorder are assumed to be carriers
- Where both parents are known to be carriers for an autosomal recessive disorder, any of their children who are known to be unaffected are left with a two-thirds carrier risk (because if the possibility they are affected is discounted, only three possibilities remain).

Autosomal recessive inheritance and consanguinity

It is believed that everybody carries some deleterious autosomal recessive genes. First cousins share on average one-eighth of their genes because they share one set of grand-parents. As a result, they are more likely to be carrying the same autosomal recessive disorders. For consanguineous couples in a family with a known autosomal recessive disorder, specific risks should be calculated and appropriate testing should be arranged. For first-cousin parents who have no known family history of any autosomal recessive disorder, their offspring have around a 3% increased risk above the general background risk of any genetic abnormality of 2% (i.e. a 5% overall risk). Screening should be offered for any autosomal recessive disorder which is available and known to be common in their ancestral ethnic group, e.g.:

- Caucasians — cystic fibrosis
- African/Afro-Caribbean — sickle-cell anaemia
- Mediterranean/Asian — thalassaemia
- Jewish — Tay–Sachs disease

2.3 X-linked recessive (XLR) conditions

These result from a mutation in a gene carried on the X chromosome and affect males because they have just one gene copy. Females are usually unaffected but may have mild manifestations as a result of lyonization. New mutations are common in many XLR disorders which means that the mother of an affected boy, with no preceding family history, is not necessarily a carrier. XLR inheritance is characterized by the following:

- No male-to-male transmission — an affected father passes his Y chromosome to all his sons
- All daughters of an affected male are carriers — an affected father passes his X chromosome to all his daughters
- Sons of a female carrier have a 50% chance of being affected and daughters have a 50% chance of being carriers

Examples of X-linked recessive conditions:

Alport syndrome (usually XLR; some AR forms)   Hunter syndrome (MPS II)
Becker muscular dystrophy   Lesch–Nyhan disease
Duchenne muscular dystrophy   Ocular albinism
Fabry disease   Red–green colour blindness
Fragile X syndrome   Testicular feminization syndrome
Glucose-6-phosphate dehydrogenase deficiency   Wiskott–Aldrich syndrome
(favism)
Haemophilias A and B (Christmas disease)

2.4 X-linked dominant (XLD) conditions

These are caused by a mutation in one copy of a gene on the X-chromosome but both male and female mutation carriers are affected. Because of lyonization, females are usually more mildly affected and these disorders are frequently lethal in males. New mutations are common. For the reasons outlined above:

- There is no male-to-male transmission
- All daughters of an affected male would be affected
- All offspring of an affected female have a 50% chance of being affected

Examples of X-linked dominant conditions include:

Goltz syndrome   Rett syndrome
Incontinentia pigmenti   Vitamin D-resistant rickets

2.5 Constructing a pedigree diagram (family tree)

The basic symbols in common usage are shown in the figure below. Occasionally symbols may be half shaded or quarter shaded. This generally means that the individual manifests a specified phenotypic feature denoted in an accompanying explanatory key, e.g. lens dislocation in a family with Marfan syndrome.

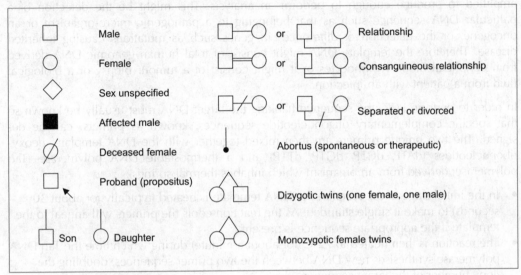

Basic symbols used in pedigree diagrams

3. MOLECULAR GENETICS

3.1 DNA (Deoxyribonucleic acid)

DNA is a **double-stranded** molecule composed of purine (adenine + guanine) and pyrimidine (cytosine and thymine) bases linked by a backbone of covalently bonded **deoxyribose sugar** phosphate residues. The two anti-parallel strands are held together by hydrogen bonds which can be disrupted by heating and reform on cooling:

- **Adenine (A) pairs with thymine (T)** by two hydrogen bonds
- **Guanine (G) pairs with cytosine (C)** by three hydrogen bonds

3.2 RNA (Ribonucleic acid)

DNA is **transcribed** in the nucleus into messenger RNA (mRNA) which is **translated** by ribosomes in the cytoplasm into a polypeptide chain. RNA differs from DNA in that it is:

- **Single-stranded**
- Thymine is replaced by **uracil**
- The sugar backbone is **ribose**

3.3 Polymerase chain reaction (PCR)

This is a widely used method for generating large amounts of the DNA of interest from very small samples. PCR can be adapted for use with RNA providing the RNA is first converted to DNA.

PCR is a method by which a small amount of target DNA (the template) is selectively amplified to produce enough to perform an analysis. This might be the detection of a particular DNA sequence such as that belonging to a pathogenic micro-organism or an oncogene, or the detection of differences in genes such as mutations causing inherited disease. Therefore the template DNA might consist of total human genomic DNA derived from peripheral blood lymphocytes or it might consist of a tumour biopsy or a biological fluid from a patient with an infection.

In order to perform PCR, the sequence flanking the target DNA must usually be known so that specific complementary oligonucleotide sequences, known as primers, can be designed. The two unique primers are then mixed together with the DNA template, deoxyribonucleotides (dATP, dCTP, dGTP, dTTP) and a thermostable DNA polymerase (Taq polymerase, derived from an organism which inhabits thermal springs).

- In the initial stage of the reaction the DNA template is heated (typically for about 30 seconds) to make it single stranded. As the reaction cools the primers will anneal to the template if the appropriate sequence is present.
- The reaction is then heated to 72°C (for about a minute) during which time the Taq DNA polymerase synthesises new DNA between the two primer sequences, doubling the copy number of the target sequence.
- The reaction is heated again and the cycle is repeated. After 30 or so cycles (each typically lasting a few minutes) the target sequence will have been amplified exponentially.

The crucial feature of PCR is that to detect a given sequence of DNA it only needs to be present in one copy (ie. one molecule of DNA): this makes it extremely powerful.

Clinical Applications of PCR

- Mutation detection
- Single cell PCR of in vitro fertilised embryo to diagnose genetic disease before implantation
- Detection of viral and bacterial sequences in tissue (Herpes Simplex Virus in CSF, Hepatitis C, HIV in peripheral blood, meningococcal strains).

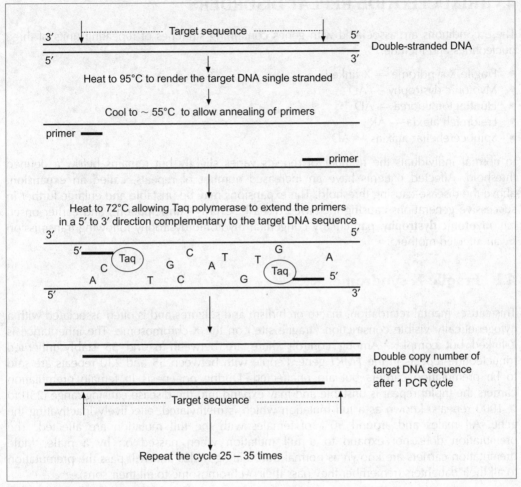

Polymerase chain reaction

3.4 Reverse Transcription PCT (rt PCR)

This is a modification of conventional PCR used to amplify messenger RNA (mRNA) sequence in order to look at the expression of particular genes within a tissue. mRNA is single-stranded, unstable, and is not a substrate for Taq DNA polymerase. For that reason it must be converted to complementary DNA (cDNA) using reverse transcriptase, a retroviral enzyme, which results in a double stranded DNA copy of the original RNA sequence. PCR can then be performed in the normal way.

4. TRINUCLEOTIDE REPEAT DISORDERS

These conditions are associated with genes containing stretches of repeating units of three nucleotides and include:

- Fragile X syndrome — X-linked
- Myotonic dystrophy — AD
- Huntington chorea — AD
- Freidreich ataxia — AR
- Spinocerebellar ataxias — AD

In normal individuals the number of repeats varies slightly but remains below a defined threshold. Affected patients have an increased number of repeats, called an **expansion**, above the disease-causing threshold. The expansions may be unstable and enlarge further in successive generations causing increased disease severity ('**anticipation**') and earlier onset, e.g. **myotonic dystrophy**, particularly congenital myotonic dystrophy following transmission by an affected mother.

4.1 Fragile X syndrome

This causes mental retardation, macro-orchidism and seizures and is often associated with a cytogenetically visible constriction ('fragile site') on the X-chromosome. The inheritance is X-linked but complex. Among controls there are between 6 and 55 stably inherited trinucleotide repeats in the *FMR1* gene. People with between 55 and 230 repeats are said to be premutation carriers but are unaffected. During oogenesis in female premutation carriers the triplet repeat is unstable and may expand into the disease-causing range (230 to > 1000 repeats) known as a full mutation which is methylated, effectively inactivating the gene. All males and around 50% of females with the full mutation are affected. The premutation does not expand to a full mutation when passed on by a male. Male premutation carriers are known as normal transmitting males and will pass the premutation to all their daughters (remember they pass their Y-chromosome to all their sons).

5. MITOCHONDRIAL DISORDERS

Mitochondria are **exclusively maternally inherited**, deriving from those present in the cytoplasm of the ovum. They contain copies of their own **circular 16.5-kilobase chromosome** carrying genes for several respiratory chain enzyme subunits and transfer RNAs. Mitochondrial genes differ from nuclear genes in having no introns and using some different amino acid codons. Within a tissue or even a cell there may be a mixed population of normal and abnormal mitochondria known as **heteroplasmy**. Different proportions of abnormal mitochondria may be required to cause disease in different tissues, known as a **threshold effect**. Disorders caused by mitochondrial gene mutations include:

- **MELAS** (**m**itochondrial **e**ncephalopathy, **l**actic **a**cidosis, **s**troke-like episodes)
- **MERRF** (**m**yoclonic **e**pilepsy, **r**agged **r**ed **f**ibres)
- Mitochondrially inherited diabetes mellitus and deafness

- Leber hereditary optic neuropathy (NB Other factors also contribute)

6. GENOMIC IMPRINTING

For most genes both copies are expressed but for some genes, either the maternally or paternally derived copy is preferentially used, a phenomenon known as genomic imprinting. The best examples are the Prader–Willi and Angelman syndromes both caused by either cytogenetic deletions of the same region of chromosome 15q or by **uniparental disomy** of chromosome 15 (where both copies of chromosome 15 are derived from one parent with no copy of chromosome 15 from the other parent).

Prader-Willi	Angelman
Clinical	
Neonatal hypotonia and poor feeding	'Happy puppet', unprovoked laughter/clapping
Moderate mental handicap	Microcephaly, severe mental handicap
Hyperphagia + obesity in later childhood	Ataxia, broad-based gait
Small genitalia	Seizures, characteristic EEG
Genetics	
70% deletion on **p**aternal chromosome 15	80% deletion on maternal chromosome 15
30% maternal uniparental disomy 15 (i.e. no paternal contribution)	2–3% paternal uniparental disomy 15 (i.e. no maternal contribution) remainder due to subtle mutations

Other imprinting disorders

Russell–Silver syndrome
Prenatal onset growth retardation, relative macrocephaly, triangular facies, asymmetry, fifth finger clinodactyly and normal IQ associated with maternal uniparental disomy for chromosome 7 in a proportion. The cause in the remainder is not yet known.

Beckwith–Wiedemann syndrome
Prenatal onset macrosomia, facial naevus flammeus, macroglossia, ear lobe creases, pits on the ear helix, hemihypertrophy, nephromegaly, exomphalos (omphalocele) and neonatal hypoglycaemia. There is an increased risk of Wilms tumour, adrenocortical and hepatic tumours in childhood. The condition appears to result from abnormalities of chromosome 11p15 which contains several imprinted genes including the *IGF-2* (insulin-like growth factor 2) gene.

7. GENETIC TESTING

Genetic tests can be thought of as diagnostic, predictive or for carrier status. Informed verbal, and increasingly written, consent (or assent) should be obtained prior to genetic testing.

Diagnostic tests

Those where the diagnosis is already suspected on clinical grounds but genetic testing is useful for confirmation, or for counselling or predictive testing in the wider family.

Predictive tests

When an individual is clinically normal but is at risk for developing a familial disorder. Predictive testing is not usually offered without a formal process of genetic counselling over more than one consultation with time built in for reflection. Where there are intervening relatives whose genetic status may be indirectly revealed there are additional issues which must be taken into consideration. Written consent for predictive testing is required by most laboratories. Nationally agreed guidance is that predictive testing in children for disorders which have no implications in childhood should not be undertaken until the child is old enough to make an informed choice.

Carrier tests

These are usually undertaken in autosomal recessive or X-linked recessive disorders where the result has no direct implications for the health of the individual, but is helpful in determining the risks to their offspring. Carrier status may be generated as a by-product of diagnostic or prenatal testing. National guidance is that specific testing for carrier status should be avoided in children until they are old enough to make an informed choice.

8. IMPORTANT GENETIC TOPICS

This section includes short notes on conditions which form popular examination topics.

8.1 Ambiguous genitalia

Normal development of the reproductive tract and external genitalia

A simplified outline is shown below.

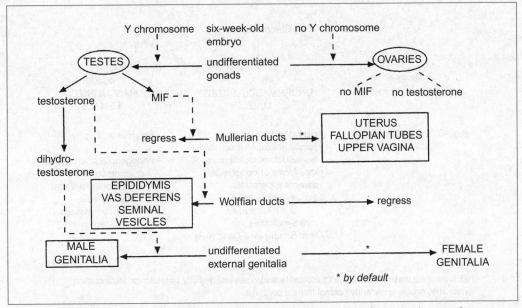

Outline of the normal development of the reproductive tract and external genitalia

The 6-week embryo has undifferentiated gonads, Müllerian ducts (capable of developing into the uterus, Fallopian tubes and upper vagina), Wolffian ducts (capable of forming the epididymis, vas deferens and seminal vesicles) and undifferentiated external genitalia.

In the presence of a Y chromosome the gonads become testes which produce testosterone and Müllerian inhibiting factor (MIF). Testosterone causes the Wolffian ducts to persist and differentiate and, after conversion to dihydrotestosterone (by 5α-reductase), masculinization of the external genitalia. MIF causes the Müllerian ducts to regress.

In the absence of a Y chromosome the gonads become ovaries which secrete neither testosterone nor MIF and in the absence of testosterone the Wolffian ducts regress and the external genitalia feminize. In the absence of MIF, the Müllerian ducts persist and differentiate.

The causes of **ambiguous genitalia** divide broadly into those resulting in undermasculinization of a male fetus, those causing masculinization of a female fetus, and those resulting from mosaicism for a cell line containing a Y chromosome and another which does not. They are summarized in the diagram below.

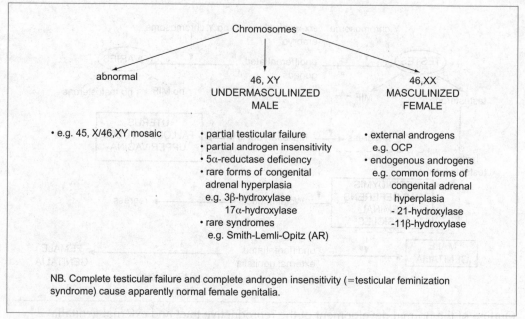

Ambiguous genitalia — outline of causes

8.2 Cystic fibrosis

This results from mutations in the *CFTR* (cystic fibrosis transmembrane regulator) gene. The $\Delta F508$ mutation (deletion of three nucleotides coding for a phenylalanine residue at amino-acid position 508) accounts for 75% of mutations in Caucasians. Most laboratories now screen for 31 common mutations including $\Delta F508$. Such testing identifies 90% of Caucasian cystic fibrosis mutations, but a much smaller proportion in many other ethnic groups. Therefore, negative molecular testing cannot exclude a diagnosis of cystic fibrosis.

8.3 Duchenne and Becker muscular dystrophy

These result from different mutations within the dystrophin gene on chromosome Xp21.

Important distinguishing features of Duchenne and Becker muscular dystrophy

	Duchenne	Becker
Immunofluorescent dystrophin on muscle biopsy	undetectable	reduced/abnormal
Wheelchair dependence	95% at < 12 years	5% at < 12 years
Mental handicap	20%	rare

In around one-third of boys with Duchenne muscular dystrophy, the condition has arisen as a new mutation.

8.4 Neurofibromatosis (NF)

There are two forms of NF which are clinically and genetically distinct:

	NF1	NF2
Major features	≥ 6 Café-au-lait patches	Bilateral acoustic neuromas
	Axillary/inguinal freckling	(vestibular schwannomas)
	Lisch nodules on the iris	Other cranial and spinal tumours
	Peripheral neurofibromas	
Minor features	Macrocephaly	Café-au-lait patches (usually < 6)
	Short stature	Peripheral schwannomas
		Peripheral neurofibromas
Complications	Plexiform neuromas	Deafness/tinnitus/vertigo
	Optic glioma (2%)	Lens opacities/cataracts
	Other cranial and spinal tumours	Spinal cord and nerve compressions
	Pseudarthrosis (especially tibial)	Malignant change/sarcomas
	Renal artery stenosis	
	Phaeochromocytoma	
	Learning difficulties	
	Scoliosis	
	Spinal cord and nerve compressions	
	Malignant change/sarcomas	
Gene	Chromosome 17	Chromosome 22
Protein	Neurofibromin	Schwannomin

8.5 Tuberous sclerosis (TS)

There are at least two separate genes which cause TS, on chromosomes 9 (*TSC1*; hamartin) and 16 (*TSC2*; tuberin).

Clinical features of tuberous sclerosis
Skin/nails

- Ash-leaf macules
- Shagreen patches (especially over the lumbosacral area)
- Adenoma sebaceum (facial area)
- Subungual/periungual fibromas

Eyes

- Retinal hamartomas

Heart

- Cardiac rhabdomyomas, detectable antenatally, usually regressing during childhood

Kidneys

- Renal cysts

Neurological

- Seizures
- Mental handicap

Neuroimaging

- Intracranial calcification (periventricular)
- Subependymal nodules
- Neuronal migration defects

8.6   Marfan syndrome

This results from mutations in the fibrillin 1 (*FBN1*) gene on chromosome 15. Intelligence is usually normal.

> **Clinical features of Marfan syndrome**
> **Musculoskeletal**
>
> - Tall stature with disproportionately long limbs (dolichostenomelia)
> - Arachnodactyly
> - Pectus carinatum or excavatum
> - Scoliosis
> - High, narrow arched palate
> - Joint laxity
> - Pes planus
>
> **Heart**
>
> - Aortic root dilatation and dissection
> - Mitral valve prolapse
>
> **Eyes**
>
> - Lens dislocation (typically up)
> - Myopia
>
> **Skin**
>
> - Striae

8.7   Homocystinuria

(see also Chapter 15 – Metabolic Medicine)

This is most commonly the result of cystathione-β-synthase deficiency and causes a Marfan-like body habitus, lens dislocation (usually down), mental handicap, thrombotic tendency and osteoporosis. Treatment includes a low methionine diet +/– pyridoxine.

8.8   Noonan syndrome

This is an autosomal dominant condition. Around 40% of individuals with Noonan syndrome have mutations in the *PTPN11* (protein-tyrosine phosphatase, non-receptor-type 11) gene on chromosome 12. In the remaining 60% the causative gene(s) is not yet known. The karyotype is usually normal.

Clinical features of Noonan syndrome
Cardiac

- Pulmonary valve stenosis
- Hypertrophic cardiomyopathy
- Septal defects (atrial and ventricular septal defects)
- Branch pulmonary artery stenosis

Musculoskeletal

- Webbed or short neck
- Pectus excavatum or carinatum
- Wide-spaced nipples
- Wide carrying angle (cubitus valgus)
- Short stature in 80%

Other features

- Ptosis
- Low-set and/or posteriorly rotated ears
- Small genitalia and undescended testes in boys
- Coagulation defects in 30% (partial factor XI:C, XIIC, and VIIIC deficiencies, von Willebrand disease, thrombocytopenia)
- Mild mental retardation in 30%

8.9 Achondroplasia

A short-limb skeletal dysplasia resulting from specific autosomal dominant mutations in the *FGFR3* (fibroblast growth factor receptor 3) gene on chromosome 4. There is a high new mutation rate. Important complications are hydrocephalus, brain-stem or cervical cord compression resulting from a small foramen magnum, spinal canal stenosis, kyphosis and sleep apnoea.

8.10 Alagille syndrome

A variable autosomal dominant disorder resulting from deletions of or mutations in the *JAG1* (jagged) gene on chromosome 20. Major features of the syndrome include:

- Cardiac — peripheral pulmonary artery stenosis +/– complex malformations
- Eye — posterior embryotoxon, abnormalities of the anterior chamber
- Vertebral — butterfly vertebrae, hemivertebrae, rib anomalies
- Hepatic — cholestatic jaundice, paucity of intrahepatic bile ducts

8.11 CHARGE syndrome

A malformation syndrome including:

Colobomas

Heart malformations

Atresia of the choanae

Retardation of growth and development (mental handicap)

Genital hypoplasia (in males)

Ear abnormalities (abnormalities of the ear pinna, deafness)

Cleft lip/palate and renal abnormalities are also common.

In the majority of patients with CHARGE syndrome it results from mutations or deletions of the *CHD7* (chromodomain helicase DNA-binding protein 7) gene on chromosome 8. Most affected individuals have new autosomal dominant mutations.

8.12 VATER (VACTERL) Association

A sporadic malformation syndrome including:

Vertebral abnormalities

Anal atresia +/− fistula

Cardiac malformations

Tracheo-oesophageal fistula

Renal anomalies, **r**adial ray defects

Limb anomalies, especially radial ray defects
The cause is not yet known.

8.13 Goldenhar syndrome

Also known as oculo-auriculo-vertebral spectrum, or first and second and branchial arch syndrome. It is mainly sporadic and the cause is unknown. Major features include:

*   Craniofacial — asymmetry, hemifacial microsomia, micrognathia
*   Ears – malformed pinnae, deafness, pre-auricular tags
*   Eyes – epibulbar (scleral) dermoid cysts, microphthalmia
*   Oral – macrostomia, cleft lip/palate
*   Vertebral – hemivertebrae
*   Cardiac – cardiac malformations
*   Renal – renal malformations

8.14   Pierre Robin sequence

An association of micrognathia and cleft palate which may occur alone, but a proportion will have 22q11 deletions or Stickler syndrome.

8.15   Potter sequence

Oligohydramnios as a result of renal abnormalities, urinary tract obstruction or amniotic fluid leakage may lead to secondary fetal compression with joint contractures (arthrogryposis), pulmonary hypoplasia and squashed facies known as the Potter sequence.

9.   FETAL TERATOGENS

9.1   Maternal illness

Maternal diabetes

Maternal diabetes is associated with fetal macrosomia, neonatal hypoglycaemia and increased risk of a wide variety of malformations, particularly cardiac (transposition of the great arteries, aortic coarctation, septal defects, cardiomyopathy), vertebral (sacral abnormalities, hemivertebrae), renal (agenesis, duplex collecting systems), intestinal (imperforate anus, other atresias), limb abnormality (short femurs, radial ray abnormalities).

Maternal myasthenia gravis

This is associated with fetal arthrogryposis.

Maternal phenylketonuria (PKU)

Although the fetus is unlikely to be affected by PKU (which is autosomal recessive), if an affected mother has relaxed her low phenylalanine diet, the fetus is at risk of microcephaly and learning disability secondary to exposure to the raised maternal phenylalanine levels.

Maternal systemic lupus erythematosus (SLE)

Maternal SLE with anti-Ro and anti-La antibodies is associated with an increased risk of fetal bradycardia and congenital heart-block for which pacing may be required. A self-limiting neonatal cutaneous lupus may also occur.

9.2   Infectious agents

The following agents are associated with increased fetal loss in the first trimester; hepatosplenomegaly, jaundice and thrombocytopenia in the neonate; and abnormalities particularly those affecting the central nervous system, vision and hearing.

Fetal cytomegalovirus

Infection may be associated with microcephaly, intracranial calcification, chorioretinopathy, deafness and mental handicap.

Fetal toxoplasmosis

Infection with *Toxoplasma*, a protozoan, may be associated with microcephaly, hydrocephalus, intracranial calcification, chorioretinopathy, and mental handicap.

Fetal rubella

Infection with rubella virus is most often associated with deafness particularly in the first and early second trimesters, but cardiac abnormalities (persistent ductus arteriosus, peripheral pulmonary stenosis, septal defects), microcephaly, chorioretinopathy, cataract, and learning disability are also associated.

Congenital syphilis, herpes and varicella

See Chapter 14 — Infectious Diseases, Section 11.1

9.3   Other teratogens

Fetal alcohol syndrome

Pre- and postnatal growth retardation, neonatal irritability, microcephaly, learning disability, hyperactivity in childhood, cardiac defects (particularly ventricular and atrial septal defects), small nails on fifth fingers and toes, facial anomalies (short palpebral fissures, ptosis, smooth philtrum, thin upper lip) and a variety of less common, often mid-line, malformations. It is likely that the effects on any one fetus are determined by the degree, timing and duration of exposure as well as the susceptibility of the fetus which is probably genetically determined.

Fetal retinoic acid

Exposure to retinoic acid (which is used in the treatment of acne) is associated with structural brain abnormalities, neuronal migration defects, microtia, and complex cardiac malformations.

Fetal valproate syndrome

Fetuses exposed to valproate have an increased risk of cleft lip and palate, neural tube defects, cardiac defects, radial ray defects, learning disability and facial anomalies (frontal narrowing including metopic craniosynostosis, thin eyebrows, infraorbital skin grooves, long philtrum, thin upper lip).

Fetal warfarin syndrome

Fetuses exposed to warfarin typically have nasal hypoplasia, stippled epiphyses, and are at risk of learning disability and brain, eye, cardiac and skeletal malformations.

10. PRENATAL TESTING

- **Chorionic villus sampling or biopsy** (CVS or CVB) — a small piece of placenta is taken either transabdominally or transvaginally. CVS testing can be safely performed from 10–11 weeks' gestation.
- **Amniocentesis** — amniotic fluid is taken, containing cells derived from the surfaces of the fetus and amniotic membranes. Amniocentesis is usually performed from 15–16 weeks' gestation.
- **Cordocentesis** — a method of obtaining fetal blood which can be performed from 18 weeks' gestation.

Chromosome and DNA testing can be performed on any of the above types of sample. Each method carries a small risk of miscarriage.

11. PREIMPLANTATION GENETIC DIAGNOSIS (PIGD)

This technique is being pioneered for couples whose offspring are at risk of a specific genetic disorder, where the family mutation(s) or chromosome rearrangement is known, and where prenatal testing with termination of affected fetuses is not acceptable to them. Embryos are generated by in vitro fertilization (IVF). At the 8–16 cell stage a single cell is removed for testing. Only embryos predicted to be unaffected are re-implanted into the mother. PIGD is technically difficult. It is not routine and the rate of achieving viable pregnancies is lower than for routine IVF. Availability in the UK is restricted to a small number of conditions.

12. FURTHER READING

Kingston, HM. 2002. *ABC of Clinical Genetics*. BMJ Publishing.

Harper, PS. 1998. *Practical Genetic Counselling 5th Edition*. Butterworth Heinemann.

Jones, KL. 1997. *Smith's Recognizable Patterns of Human Malformation 5th Edition*. WB Saunders.

Chapter 11

Haematology and Oncology

Michael Capra

CONTENTS

Haematology and Oncology

1. HAEMOGLOBIN (HB)

1.1 Haemoglobin synthesis

Erythropoietic activity is regulated by erythropoietin, a hormone secreted by the peritubular complex of the kidney (90%), the liver and elsewhere (10%). The stimulus to erythropoietin production is the oxygen tension within the kidney. Mitochondria of the developing erythroblast are the main sites for the synthesis of haem.

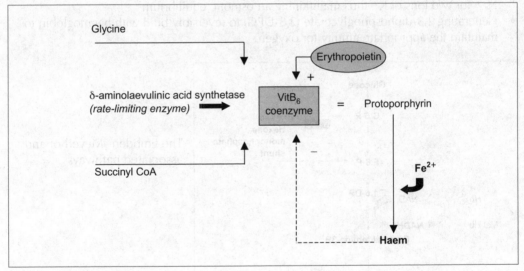

Haem synthesis

- The cofactor vitamin B_6 is stimulated by erythropoietin and inhibited by haem
- The Fe^{2+} is supplied by circulating transferrin
- Globin chains, comprising a sequence of polypeptides, are synthesized on ribosomes
- A tetramer of four globin chains, each with its own haem group attached, is formed to make a molecule of haemoglobin

1.2   Red cell physiology

The 8-μm diameter red cell has three challenges:

- To pass through the microcirculation of capillaries (diameters of 3.5 μm)
- To maintain haemoglobin in the reduced state
- To maintain an osmotic equilibrium despite a high concentration of protein (five times that of plasma)

It achieves this by:

- The protein, spectrin, which enables it to have a flexible biconcave-disc shape
- Generating reducing power in the form of nicotinamide adenine dinucleotide (NADH) from the Embden–Meyerhof pathway and NADPH (reduced NADP) from the hexose monophosphate shunt; this reducing power is vital in preventing oxidation injury to the red cell and for reducing functionally dead methaemoglobin (oxidized haemoglobin) to functionally active, reduced haemoglobin (see figure below)
- Generating energy in the form of ATP from the Embden–Meyerhof pathway; this energy is used to drive the cell membrane Na^+/K^+ pump to exchange three ions of intracellular Na^+ for two ions of K^+ thus maintaining an osmotic equilibrium
- Generating 2,3-diphosphoglycerate (2,3-DPG) to reversibly bind with haemoglobin to maintain the appropriate affinity for oxygen.

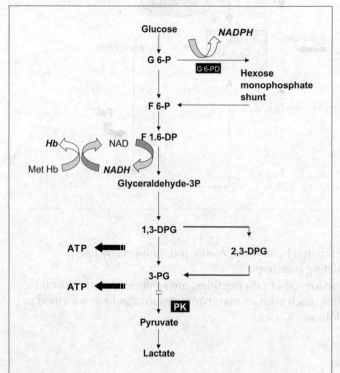

The Embden–Meyerhof and associated pathways

2,3-DPG, 2,3-diphosphoglycerate;
F 6-P, fructose 6-phosphate;
F 1,6-DP, fructose 1,6-diphosphate;
G 6-P, glucose 6-phosphate;
G 6-PD, glucose 6-phosphate dehydrogenase;
Met Hb, methaemoglobin;
PK, protein kinase

1.3 Oxygen-dissociation curve

When oxygen is unloaded from a molecule of oxygenated haemoglobin, the β-chains open up, allowing 2,3-DPG to enter. This results in the deoxygenated haemoglobin having a low affinity for oxygen, preventing haemoglobin from stealing the oxygen back from the tissues. This 2,3-DPG-related affinity for oxygen gives the oxygen-dissociation curve its nearly sinusoidal appearance rather than that of a straight line.

Factors that cause this dissociation curve to shift are summarized in the figure below.

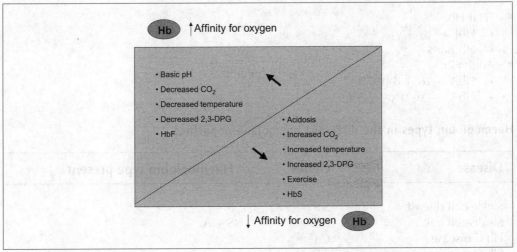

Factors shifting the oxygen-dissociation curve: HbF, fetal haemoglobin; HbS, sickle-cell haemoglobin

Shift of the curve by changes in the blood CO_2 is important to enhance oxygenation of the blood in the lungs and also to enhance the release of oxygen from the blood to the tissues. This is the **Bohr effect**.

As CO_2 diffuses from the capillaries into the alveoli within the lungs, $p(CO_2)$ is reduced and the pH increases. Both of these effects cause the curve to shift left and upwards. Therefore the quantity of oxygen that binds with the haemoglobin becomes considerably increased, so allowing greater oxygen transport to the tissues. When the blood reaches the capillaries the exact opposite occurs. The CO_2 from the tissues diffuses into the blood, decreasing the pH and causing the curve to shift to the right and downwards; that is, the curve shifts to the right in the tissues and to the left in the lungs.

2. HAEMOGLOBIN ABNORMALITIES

These result from the synthesis of an abnormal haemoglobin (haemoglobinopathy) or from a decreased rate of synthesis of normal α- or β-globin chains (thalassaemia). The chain structure is determined by a pair of autosomal genes. The genes for β-, σ- and γ-chains are carried on chromosome 11, while chromosome 16 carries the α-chain. Haemoglobinopathy and thalassaemia genes are allelomorphic (different genes can occupy the same locus on a chromosome) — which is the reason why mixed haemoglobinopathies can occur in one patient. For example, HbS and thalassaemia may occur in one patient.

2.1 Thalassaemia

Thalassaemia results from a genetically determined imbalanced production of one of the globin chains. α-, β-, σ- and γ-globin chains make up normal fetal and adult haemoglobin in the following combinations:

- Fetal Hb:
  - HbF — $\alpha_2 + \gamma_2$
  - Hb Barts — γ_4
- Adult Hb:
  - HbA — $\alpha_2 + \beta_2$ (97%)
  - HbA$_2$ — $\alpha_2 + \sigma_2$ (2.5%)

Haemoglobin types in the different haemoglobinopathies

Disease	Genes	Haemoglobin type present
Sickle-cell disease	S/S	S + F
Sickle-cell trait	S/A	S + A
Hb C disease	C/C	C
Hb C trait	C/A	C + A
Hb D disease	D/A	D
Hb E disease	E/A	E + F
Sickle-cell — Hb C disease	S/C	S + C + F
Sickle-cell — thalassaemia	S/β^+	S + F (also A if β^+, if β^0 then no A)
Hb C — thalassaemia	C/β^+	C + F (also A if β^+, if β^0 then no A)
Hb E — thalassaemia	E/β^+	E + F (also A if β^+, if β^0 then no A)

Clinical management of thalassaemia

Safe blood transfusion programmes with effective iron-chelation therapy have transformed the outlook for children with thalassaemia.

Red cell transfusions

The aim here is to eliminate the complications of anaemia and ineffective erythropoiesis, which will allow the child to grow and develop normally. The decision to commence on a transfusion programme can be difficult but generally the recommendation is to start when the haemoglobin concentration is ≤ 6.0 g/dl over 3 consecutive months. The desired maintenance haemoglobin level is around 9.5 g/dl, with care being taken not to increase the iron burden too much.

Chelation treatment

The challenge here is to balance the complications of iron overload (cardiac failure is the leading cause of death) with the inherent challenges of desferrioxamine, currently the chelating agent of choice although not an ideal drug. It is not absorbed orally, it has an extremely short half-life, it is expensive and it has significant complications. It is estimated that approximately two-thirds of the world's 72,000 patients with thalassaemia do not have access to desferrioxamine. As a result, the search for a less toxic, more affordable and more effective chelator continues. Although promising, the benefit of the new oral chelator Deferiprone (L1) remains controversial despite it being licensed for use in the European Union but not in North America.

When to initiate chelation therapy remains unclear but it is recommended that a liver biopsy is performed after 1 year of a transfusion programme to establish the iron burden. Serum ferritin, although helpful, is not entirely accurate especially at the high levels seen in such patients.

Curative treatment

Bone marrow transplant remains the only curative option but this treatment option must be carefully balanced against the morbidity (and significant mortality) associated with allo-geneic transplantation. Lawson (see further reading) report on 55 children with β-thalassae-mia who received allogeneic bone marrow transplants in two major UK centres over the 10-year period between 1991 and 2001 who had 8-year overall survival and thalassaemia-free survival rates of 95% and 82% respectively. The thalassaemias are likely to benefit from specific gene therapies in the future although to date no such treatment option is available.

2.2 Sickle-cell disease (SCD)

- It primarily affects people of African, Afro-Caribbean, Middle Eastern, Indian and Mediterranean descent
- In parts of Africa, 30% of the population have sickle-cell trait
- It is caused by a single-base mutation of adenine to thiamine, resulting in a substitution of valine for glutamic acid (at the sixth codon) on the β-globin chain
- HbS is insoluble and forms crystals when exposed to low oxygen tension
- The symptoms of anaemia are mild relative to the severity of the anaemia, as HbS shifts the oxygen–haemoglobin curve to the right (see figure on p. 383)
- It presents after the age of 6 months — the time at which the production of haemoglobin should have switched from HbF to HbA
- The clinical picture is variable, although usually it is one of a chronic severe haemolytic anaemia punctuated by crises
- Crises may be visceral, aplastic, haemolytic and painful (see below) and are precipitated by infection, acidosis, dehydration and deoxygenation from whatever cause
- Patients are susceptible to infections with *Pneumococcus*, *Haemophilus* and *Salmonella* spp.

Sickle-cell disease — clinical entities and appropriate management

Acute painful episodes (vaso-occlusive crises)

- Most frequent complication of SCD
- Common sites include bone and abdomen
- Pathophysiology — ischaemic tissue injury from the obstruction of blood flow by sickled erythrocytes
- Precipitating factors — infection, fever, acidosis, hypoxia, dehydration, sleep apnoea and exposure to extremes of heat and cold
- Diagnosis is based strictly on the history and clinical findings only

Treatment includes the following:

- Pain relief
- Antibiotic treatment if fever is present and perform blood culture
- Ensure patient is adequately hydrated — intravenous fluid is recommended
- Check haematological parameters and crossmatch blood

Acute chest syndrome

This is responsible for up to 25% of all deaths in children with SCD. Aetiology is variable and may include both infectious and non-infectious causes (pulmonary infarction, hypoventilation secondary to rib/sternal infarction, fat embolism, pulmonary oedema secondary to fluid overload).

Treatment includes:

- Pain relief
- Oxygen
- Hydration

Intravenous antibiotic (third-generation cephalosporin initially, adding erythromycin if the child is ≥ 5 years old because *Mycoplasma* spp. may be present). Consider blood transfusion if the haemoglobin level is ≥ 1.5 g/dl less than baseline. If severe and condition is deteriorating, an exchange transfusion is indicated.

Aplastic crisis

Occurs when red cell production is temporarily reduced while the ongoing haemolytic process continues — resulting in severe anaemia. Parvovirus is usually the aetiological agent. The haemoglobin can fall to 3 g/dl and is the cause of presentation — malaise, lethargy, syncope and congestive heart failure. Urgent transfusion is necessary but must be performed slowly because the patient may develop cardiac failure acutely.

Acute splenic sequestration crisis

This is characterized by pooling of large quantities of red blood cells in the spleen with sudden enlargement of the spleen and a precipitous decline in haemoglobin. It occurs most commonly in infants and young children between 6 months and 5 years. Treatment is in the form of a blood transfusion and treatment of any underlying causes.

Stroke

Stroke occurs in 5–10% of people with SCD, with the highest risk being between the ages of 1 and 9 years. Treatment should follow the general principles for SCD — infection control, oxygen, hydration and blood parameters. In addition, an exchange transfusion is indicated as soon as possible.

2.3 Other haemoglobinopathies

Sickle-cell trait

Individuals are usually asymptomatic as long as they are maintained with good oxygenation — an important point during anaesthesia.

Hb C disease

- Is the result of a substitution of lysine for glutamic acid in the β-globin chain at the same point as the substitution in HbS
- Milder clinical course than HbS
- Prevalent in West Africa

Hb D and Hb E disease

- Hb D is prevalent on the north-west coast of India, while Hb E is in south-east Asia — both demonstrate mild anaemia only

Sickle-cell–Hb C disease

- Typically has a similar clinical picture to that of HbS, although fewer infections and fewer crises are described
- Associated with avascular necrosis of the femoral head and vascular retinal changes

Asplenia

- Definition — loss of splenic function can be partial (splenic hypofunction) or complete (asplenia)
- Causes — surgical resection of the spleen, autosplenectomy (due to infarction secondary to haemoglobinopathy), congenital (e.g. Ivemark syndrome (asplenia syndrome))
- Management — there are four important management areas:
  - Penicillin is the antibiotic of choice — given twice a day. When to discontinue prophylactic antibiotics remains controversial. Some centres discontinue at 5 years of age while others continue for life
  - Appropriate immunization — routine immunization should be followed. In addition, pneumococcal and meningococcal vaccination is recommended. For pneumococcal vaccination in children < 2 years use conjugated heptavalent; in children ≥ 2 years use 23 valent conjugated vaccination. For meningococcal vaccination use polysaccharide quadrivalent vaccination (NB this does not offer protection against *Neisseria meningitidis* serogroup B)
  - Aggressive management of suspected infection — patients with suspected infection

must be evaluated promptly, appropriate specimens for bacterial culture must be obtained and empirical intravenous broad-spectrum antibiotics should be commenced

- Parent education — parents must be educated to seek medical assistance immediately on suspicion of an infection and must be informed of the potential life-threatening complications of such infections

3. BLOOD GROUP ANTIBODIES

Approximately 400 red blood cell group antigens have been described, of which the ABO and rhesus (Rh) groups are of major clinical significance. Kell, Duffy, Kidd and Lutheran groups occasionally cause reactions, while the remaining groups rarely do.

3.1 ABO system

This consists of three allelic genes — A, B and O. Each gene codes for a specific enzyme that will result in the production of a carbohydrate residue. This residue will attach itself to one of the three respective lipid and sugar chains — H-antigen, A-antigen and B-antigen chains on the red cell membrane. The O gene is an amorph and therefore does not transform the H antigen.

The A gene encodes for a carbohydrate residue that will attach itself to the end of the A-antigen chain, thereby blocking the distal glycoprotein antigenic portion. Similarly, the B gene encodes for a carbohydrate residue that will block the antigenic portion of the chain (see figure overleaf).

ABO blood groups

A, B, AB and O blood groups

Group	O	A	B	AB
Genotype	OO	AA or AO	BB or BO	AB
Antigens	O	A	B	AB
Naturally occurring antibodies	anti-A and anti-B	anti-B	anti-A	none
Frequency in the UK	46%	42%	9%	3%

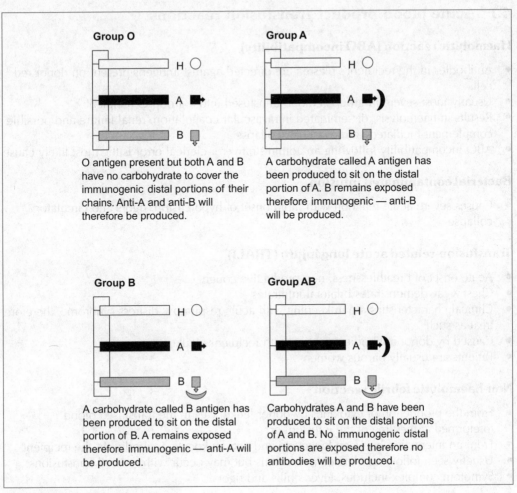

Group O

H ◯

A ◼➡

B ⬇

O antigen present but both A and B have no carbohydrate to cover the immunogenic distal portions of their chains. Anti-A and anti-B will therefore be produced.

Group A

H ◯

A ◼➡)

B ⬇

A carbohydrate called A antigen has been produced to sit on the distal portion of A. B remains exposed therefore immunogenic — anti-B will be produced.

Group B

H ◯

A ◼➡

B ⬇︶

A carbohydrate called B antigen has been produced to sit on the distal portion of B. A remains exposed therefore immunogenic — anti-A will be produced.

Group AB

H ◯

A ◼➡)

B ⬇︶

Carbohydrates A and B have been produced to sit on the distal portions of A and B. No immunogenic distal portions are exposed therefore no antibodies will be produced.

A, B, AB and O blood groups

4. BLOOD PRODUCT TRANSFUSION

Paediatricians prescribing, and administering, blood product transfusions, must be familiar with the principles of blood product replacement therapy and with how to manage adverse transfusion reactions.

Serious or life-threatening acute reactions are rare; however new symptoms or signs that occur during a transfusion must be taken seriously as they may be the first warning of a serious reaction.

4.1 Acute blood product transfusion reactions

Haemolytic reaction (ABO incompatibility)

- Antibodies in the recipient's plasma are directed against antigens present on donor red cells
- Usually most severe in group A blood transfused into a group O recipient
- Results in haemolysis, disseminated intravascular coagulation, renal failure and possible complement-mediated cardiovascular collapse
- ABO incompatibility following an administrative or clerical error is the most likely cause

Bacterial contaminated infusion

- Causes severe acute reaction with rapid onset of hypotension, rigors and circulatory collapse

Transfusion-related acute lung injury (TRALI)

- Acute onset of breathlessness, non-productive cough
- Chest X-ray demonstrates bilateral infiltrates
- Clinical characteristics are in keeping with acute respiratory distress syndrome, therefore treat as such
- Caused by donor antibodies reacting with recipient's leukocyte
- Patients are usually parous women

Non-haemolytic febrile reaction

- From the production of cytokines by donor leukocytes in the transfused blood (preformed at the time of the infusion) or
- From an interaction between leukocyte and anti-leukocyte antibodies in the recipient
- Usually seen following platelet transfusions but may occur with red cell transfusions
- Symptom complex includes: fever, chills and rigors

Anaphylactic reaction

- A rare but life-threatening complication
- Increased risk with transfusion containing large volumes of plasma, e.g. fresh-frozen plasma or platelets
- Clinical presentation — hypotension, bronchospasm, periorbital and laryngeal oedema, vomiting, erythema, urticaria, conjunctivitis, dyspnoea, chest/abdominal pain
- Occurs in patients pre-sensitized to allergen-producing immunoglobulin E (IgE) antibodies, less commonly with IgG or IgA antibodies

4.2 Massive transfusion reactions

A massive transfusion, defined as replacement of more than half of the patient's blood volume at one time or the replacement of the entire blood volume within a 24-hour period, may be complicated by:

- Coagulopathy (secondary to a relative thrombocytopenia and platelet dysfunction)
- Volume overload
- Hypothermia
- Hypokalaemia (the potassium-depleted donor's red cells have the ability to absorb serum potassium)
- Hypocalcaemia (secondary to citrate toxicity — citrate is used as an anticoagulant to prevent coagulation of stored blood).

Details of blood products for transfusion

Blood product	Indication	Content description	Dose	Predicted increment	Special precautions
Packed RBC	Correct inadequate tissue O_2 delivery	RBC concentrate	10–15 ml/kg	2–3 g/dl	Cross-match Must be ABO compatible
Fresh frozen plasma	Coagulopathy DIC Warfarin reversal Viatmin K deficiency	All coagulation factors and complement	10 ml/kg		Should be ABO compatible
Cryoprecipitate	vWD hypo-fibrinogemia F XIII deficiency	10 ml contains > 80 U F VIII and > 150 mg fibrinogen	10–50 ml/kg		Should be ABO compatible
Platelet concentrate	Thrombocyto-penia	6.5×10^{10} platelets/U	1 U/5 kg max. 6 U	5×10^9 to 10×10^9/l	Should be ABO compatible Monitor recipient's response

RBC, red blood cells; U, unit; DIC, disseminated intravascular coagulopathy; vWD, von Willebrand disease; F VIII, factor VIII; F XIII, factor XIII.

5. ANAEMIA

Anaemia can be classified by decreased substrate, abnormal production and destruction of red cells, as below.

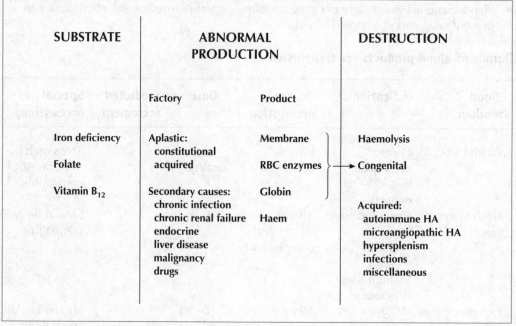

SUBSTRATE	ABNORMAL PRODUCTION		DESTRUCTION
	Factory	Product	
Iron deficiency	Aplastic: constitutional	Membrane	Haemolysis
Folate	acquired	RBC enzymes	Congenital
Vitamin B$_{12}$	Secondary causes: chronic infection	Globin	
	chronic renal failure	Haem	Acquired: autoimmune HA
	endocrine		microangiopathic HA
	liver disease		hypersplenism
	malignancy		infections
	drugs		miscellaneous

Working classification of anaemia

5.1 Iron deficiency anaemia

The major part of body iron is in the form of haem — essential for the delivery of oxygen to the tissues. Iron can exist in both the reduced (electron-gain) or oxidized (electron-loss) state, the vital property for electron-transfer reactions. A useful mnemonic is LEO = loss of an electron is oxidation. As iron is a major constituent of many important respiratory chain enzymes it is therefore directly involved in the production of cellular energy in the form of ATP. Deficiency of iron results in widespread non-haematological effects: for example, reduced central nervous system (CNS) higher functions, diminished T-cell function and cell-mediated immunity as well as diminished muscle performance.

- Iron deficiency anaemia (Hb < 11 g/dl) occurs in 10 to 30% of preschool children living in inner cities in the UK

Causes of iron deficiency

- Dietary insufficiency, e.g. unfortified milk
- Increased physiological requirement — infancy/adolescence
- Blood loss — gastrointestinal
- Malabsorption — coeliac disease

The most common reason in infancy is the early weaning to cows' milk. Giving an infant iron-supplemented formula milk instead of cows' milk not only prevents anaemia but reduces the decline in developmental performance observed in those given only cows' milk.

Causes of a microcytic anaemia

Definition: mean corpuscular volume (MCV) < 72 fl in children < 2 years or < 78 fl in older children (where fl = femtolitres).

- Iron deficiency
- Anaemia of chronic disorders — infection, malignancy
- Disorders of globin synthesis — thalassaemia trait, homozygous haemoglobinopathies
- Lead poisoning
- Sideroblastic anaemia

5.2 Aplastic anaemia

Classification of aplastic anaemia

- Constitutional (30%)
  - Fanconi anaemia
  - Familial marrow aplasia in association with hand anomalies, deafness, ataxia, immune deficiencies
  - Dyskeratosis congenita — ectodermal dysplasia, X-linked
  - Shwachman–Diamond syndrome — pancreatic insufficiency
  - Amegakaryocytic thrombocytopenia
  - Reticular dysgenesis
- Acquired
  - Idiopathic — majority of cases
  - Drugs, e.g. acetazolamide, chloramphenicol
  - Infections, e.g. Epstein–Barr virus (EBV), viral hepatitis, parvovirus
  - Toxins, e.g. glues, dichlorodiphenyltrichloroethane (DDT)
  - Paroxysmal nocturnal haemoglobinuria

Steroids and/or anti-thymocyte globulin have some beneficial effects in a few cases. The prognosis is invariably poor in severe cases, with bone marrow transplantation the only viable treatment option available.

5.3 Hereditary haemolytic anaemias

For an understanding of hereditary haemolytic anaemias, one has to consider the membrane, red cell enzyme and haemoglobin defects involved.

Membrane defects

Hereditary spherocytosis

- Commonest hereditary haemolytic anaemia in north Europeans
- Autosomal dominant
- Complex defect but involves the spectrin structural protein
- Diagnosis made on appearances of blood film — the presence of spherocytes identified by demonstrating that the cells are osmotically active using the osmotic fragility test
- The serum bilirubin and lactate dehydrogenase (LDH) may be elevated
- Treatment, by splenectomy, is reserved for severe cases

Hereditary elliptocytosis

- Usually autosomal dominant
- Most cases are asymptomatic

Red cell enzyme defects

Although a deficiency of any enzyme involved in the Embden–Meyerhof pathway may cause haemolysis, the two most commonly occurring deficiencies are:

Glucose 6-phosphate dehydrogenase (G6PD) deficiency

- G6PD helps to maintain glutathione in a reduced state, thus protecting the red cell from oxidative injury
- It is X-linked
- Different mutations of the gene are all found in different racial groups — Black Africans: 10% incidence, Mediterranean races: up to 35% incidence
- Neonatal jaundice may be the first sign
- Precipitating causes include infections, acidosis, favism, drugs
- Diagnose by assaying G6PD enzyme

Drugs to avoid in G6PD deficiency are:

- Analgesics/antipyretics: aspirin, probenecid
- Antimalarials: chloroquine
- Sulphonamides: dapsone
- Antibiotics: co-trimoxazole, nitrofurantoin, nalidixic acid, chloramphenicol
- Cardiovascular drugs: procainamide

- Miscellaneous: ascorbic acid, methyldopa, urate oxidase

Pyruvate kinase (PK) deficiency

- Deficiency of PK blocks the Embden–Meyerhof pathway — see figure on p. 382)
- PK deficiency causes a rise in 2,3-DPG, which causes a shift to the right on the oxygen-dissociation curve and consequent improvement in oxygen availability (figure on p. 383). Patients can therefore tolerate very low Hb levels
- It is autosomal recessive
- Infections, especially parvovirus, can produce dramatic haemolysis
- Splenectomy may be beneficial

5.4   Haemoglobin defects

See also Section 2 — Haemoglobin abnormalities.

Autoimmune haemolytic anaemia (AIHA)

- Coombs test (anti-human globulin) positive (see page 396)
- Uncommon in childhood, but if present is usually the result of an intercurrent infection — predominantly viral but occasionally mycoplasmal in origin
- In the older child, AIHA may be a manifestation of a multisystem disease, e.g. systemic lupus erythematusus (SLE)
- Causes include drugs (high-dose penicillin), infections (non-specific viral, measles, varicella, EBV), multisystem disease (SLE, rheumatoid arthritis) and lymphoproliferative disease (Hodgkin lymphoma)
- Can be divided into warm and cold types depending on the temperature at which the causative cell-bound antibody is best detected
  - Warm (usually IgG) — multisystem disease
  - Cold (usually IgM) — infective causes

Microangiopathic haemolytic anaemia

- A rapidly developing haemolytic anaemia with fragmented red cells and thrombocytopenia
- Occurs in haemolytic–uraemic syndrome and thrombotic thrombocytopenic purpura

Hypersplenism

- The red cell lifespan is decreased by sequestration in an enlarged spleen for whatever cause

Infections

- Malaria
- Septicaemia

Miscellaneous

- Burns
- Poisoning
- Hyperphosphataemia
- A-betalipoproteinaemia

The Coombs (anti-globulin) test

Anti-human globulin (AHG) is produced in many animal species following the injection of human globulin. When AHG is added to human red cells that have been coated (sensitized) by immunoglobulin or complement components, agglutination of the red cells will occur, indicating a positive test.

There are two anti-globulin tests:

Direct antiglobulin test

This is used to detect antibody or complement on the red cell surface where sensitization has occurred **in vivo**.

A positive test occurs in:

- Haemolytic disease of the newborn
- Autoimmune haemolytic anaemia
- Drug-induced immune haemolytic anaemia
- Haemolytic transfusion reactions

Indirect antiglobulin test

This is used to detect antibodies that have coated the red cells **in vitro**. It is a two-stage procedure. The first stage involves incubation of test red cells with serum. The second stage involves washing these red cells with saline to remove free globulins. AHG is then added to the washed red cells. Agglutination implies that the original serum contained antibody, which has coated the red cells in vitro.

This indirect anti-globulin test is used in the following circumstances:

- Routine cross-matching procedures — to detect antibodies in the patient's serum that will be directed towards the donor red cells
- Detecting atypical blood group antibodies in serum during screening procedures
- Detecting blood group antibodies in a pregnant woman
- Detecting antibodies in serum in autoimmune haemolytic anaemia

6. THE WHITE CELLS: PHAGOCYTIC CELLS

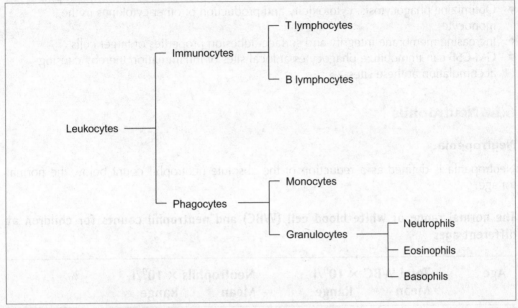

White cells or leukocytes can broadly be classified into groups.

The primary function of the white cells, in conjunction with immunoglobulins and complement, is to protect the body against infection.

Granulocytes and **monocytes** comprise the phagocytic (myeloid) group of white cells. They originate from a common precursor cell. It takes between 6 and 10 days for the precursor cell to undergo mitosis and maturation within the bone marrow. The immature **neutrophil** remains in the bone marrow as a reserve pool until required in peripheral blood. Bone marrow normally contains more myeloid than erythroid precursors — in a ratio of up to 12 : 1 and between 10 and 15 times more the number of granulocytes than in peripheral blood. Granulocytes spend only a matter of hours within the bloodstream before going into tissues. There are two pools of cells within the bloodstream — the circulating pool (what is included in the blood count) and the marginating pool (not included in the blood count as these cells adhere to the endothelium).

Formation, proliferation, differentiation and function

Growth factors are produced in stromal cells (endothelial cells, fibroblasts and macrophages) and from T lymphocytes. Under the influence of specific growth factors — stem-cell factor, interleukin-1 (IL-1), IL-3 and IL-6 — a haematopoietic stem cell is produced. Granulocyte–monocyte colony-stimulating factor (GM-CSF) increases the commitment of this stem cell to differentiate into a **phagocyte**. Further differentiating and proliferating stimulus is required from G-CSF for **neutrophil** production, from IL-5 for **eosinophil** production and from M-CSF for **monocyte** production.

In addition, growth factors affect the function of the mature myeloid cells:

- Optimizing phagocytosis, superoxide generation and cytotoxicity in the neutrophil
- Optimizing phagocytosis, cytotoxicity and production of other cytokines in the monocyte
- Increasing membrane integrity and surface-adhesion properties of target cells
- GM-CSF can immobilize phagocytes at local sites of inflammation thereby causing accumulation at these sites

6.1 Neutrophils

Neutropenia

Neutropenia is defined as a reduction of the absolute neutrophil count below the normal for age.

The normal range of white blood cell (WBC) and neutrophil counts for children at different ages

Age	Total WBC × 10^9/l		Neutrophils × 10^9/l		%
	Mean	Range	Mean	Range	
Birth	18	9.0–30	11	6.0–26	61
1 week	12	5.0–21	5.5	1.5–10	45
1 month	10.8	5.0–19.5	3.8	1.0–9	35
6 months	11.9	6.0–17.5	3.8	1.0–8.5	32
1 year	11.4	6.0–17.5	3.5	1.5–8.5	31
6 years	8.5	5.0–14	4.3	1.5–8	51
16 years	7.8	4.5–13	4.4	1.8–8	57

Neutropenia can be divided according to the severity, indicating the likely clinical consequences:

- Mild — 1.0–1.5 (10^9/l) — Usually no problem
- Moderate — 0.5–1.0 (10^9/l) — Clinical problems more common
- Severe — < 0.5 (10^9/l) — Potentially severe and life-threatening, especially if prolonged beyond a few days

Bacterial infections such as cellulitis, superficial and deep abscess formation, pneumonia and septicaemia are the commonest problems associated with isolated neutropenia, while fungal, viral and parasitic infections are relatively uncommon.

The typical inflammatory response may be greatly modified with poor localization of infection, resulting in a greater tendency for infection to disseminate.

Although challenging in some cases, it is important to identify the cause of the neutropenia, see following box, especially for the two following reasons:

- The clinical significance of the neutropenia will depend upon whether or not there is underlying marrow reserve
- Identifying the cause can help in predicting the duration of the neutropenia and therefore effect subsequent management

Marrow suppression (decreased production) will usually cause a severe neutropenia. The majority of children treated with chemotherapy will be in this group. Increased consumption or sequestration will cause mild to moderate neutropenia.

Causes of Neutropenia

Decreased marrow production

Congenital
Kostmann syndrome
Reticular dysgenesis

Acquired
Aplastic anaemia
Fanconi anaemia
    Drug suppression
    Cyclical neutropenia
    Vitamin B_{12}, folate, copper deficiency
    Chronic benign neutropenia
    Myelofibrosis
    Osteopetrosis

Export
Metabolic conditions:
    Propionic, isovaleric and
    Methylmalonic acidaemia
    Hyperglycinaemia

Consumption
Autoimmune antibodies
Neonatal isoimmune haemolytic disease
Infection/endotoxaemia

Sequestration
Immune complexes
Viral
SLE
Felty syndrome
Sjögren syndrome
Hypersplenism

Associated with immune deficiency
X-linked hypogammaglobulinaemia
Selective immunoglobulin deficiency states

Associated with phenotypically abnormal syndromes
Shwachman syndrome
Chediak–Higashi syndrome
Cartilage hair hypoplasia
Dyskeratosis congenita

The risk of infection is directly proportional to the duration of neutropenia. If the duration of neutropenia is predicted to be prolonged, preventive measures against possible future infective episodes may be considered, for example:

- Good mouth care and dental hygiene
- Prophylaxis against *Pneumocystis* spp. (co-trimoxazole)
- Prophylaxis against fungal infections (fluconazole)
- Prophylaxis against recurrent herpes simplex virus infection (aciclovir)
- Regular throat and rectal swabs looking for Gram-negative colonization
- Dietary avoidance of unpasteurized milk and salads
- Avoidance of inhaling building/construction dust because of the risk of acquiring *Aspergillus* infection

Neutrophilia

The neutrophil count can be increased in one of the following three ways:

- Increased production of neutrophils as a result of increased progenitor cell proliferation or an increased frequency of cell division of committed neutrophil precursors
- Prolonged neutrophil survival within the plasma as a result of impaired transit into tissues
- Increased mobilization of neutrophils from the marginating pools or bone marrow

Acute neutrophilia

Neutrophils can be mobilized very quickly, within 20 minutes of being triggered, from the marginating pool. A stress response (acute bacterial infection, stress, exercise, seizures and some toxic agents) releases adrenaline (epinephrine) from endothelial cells which decreases neutrophil adhesion. This results in the neutrophils adhering to the endothelial lining of the vasculature (the marginating pool) being dragged into the circulation.

The bone marrow storage pool responds somewhat slower (a few hours) in delivering neutrophils in response to endotoxins, released from micro-organisms, or complement.

Corticosteroids may inhibit the passage of neutrophils into tissues, thereby increasing the circulating number.

Chronic neutrophilia

The mechanism in chronic neutrophilia is usually an increased marrow myeloid progenitor-cell proliferation. The majority of reactions last a few days or weeks. Infections and chronic inflammatory conditions (e.g. juvenile chronic arthritis, Kawasaki disease) are the predominant stimulators of this reaction. Less common causes include malignancy, haemolysis or chronic blood loss, burns, uraemia and post-operative states.

Splenectomy or hyposplenism may result in a reduced removal of increased neutrophils from the circulation.

6.2   Eosinophils

Eosinophils enter inflammatory exudates and have a special role in allergic responses, in defence against parasites and in removal of fibrin formed during inflammation. Eosinophils are proportionately reduced in number during the neonatal period. The causes of eosinophilia are extensive but some of the major causes are:

- Allergic diseases, e.g. asthma, hay fever, urticaria
- Parasitic diseases, e.g. worm infestation
- Recovery from infection
- Certain skin diseases, e.g. psoriasis, dermatitis herpetiformis
- Pulmonary eosinophilia
- Drug sensitivity
- Polyarteritis nodosa
- Hodgkin disease

6.3   Basophils

Basophils, the least common of the granulocytes, are seldom seen in normal peripheral blood. In tissues they become mast cells. They have attachment sites on their cell membrane for IgE — which, when attaching, will cause degranulation to occur resulting in the release of histamine.

6.4   Monocytes

Monocytes, the largest of the leukocytes, spend a short time in the bone marrow and an even shorter time in the circulation (20–40 hours) before entering tissues where the final maturation to a phagocyte takes place. A mature phagocyte has a lifespan of months to years.

7.   THE WHITE CELLS: LYMPHOCYTES

Lymphocytes, divided into **T lymphocytes** and **B lymphocytes**, are the immunologically active cells which help the phagocytes to defend the body from an infective or other foreign invasion by aiding specificity.

Formation

The bone marrow and thymus are the two primary sites in which lymphocytes are produced, not by specific antigens but by non-specific cytokines. Thereafter they undergo specific transformation in secondary or reactive lymphoid tissue — the lymph nodes, spleen, the circulating lymphocytes and the specialized lymphoid tissue found in the respiratory and gastrointestinal tracts.

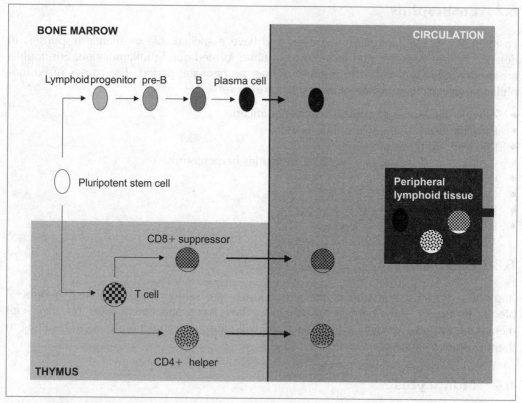

Diagrammatic illustration of immunocyte production

T cells are produced in the bone marrow and undergo transformation in the thymus, whereas the exact location where the B lymphocytes are transformed remains unknown.

In peripheral blood 80% of the lymphocytes are T cells, while only 20% are B cells. T cells are responsible for cell-mediated immunity (against intracellular organisms and transplanted organs). B cells and plasma cells (differentiated B cells) are responsible for humoral immunity by producing immunoglobulins.

8. PLATELETS

Megakaryocytes, produced in the bone marrow, develop into platelets by a unique process of cytoplasm shedding. As the megakaryocyte matures the cytoplasm becomes more granular, these granules develop into platelets and are released into the circulation as the cytoplasm is shed.

Platelet production is under the control of growth factors, particularly thrombopoietin and IL-6, while GM-CSF and IL-3 have megakarocyte colony-stimulating factor (MG-CSF) properties.

The main function of platelets is the formation of mechanical plugs during the normal haemostatic response to vascular injury.

8.1 Thrombocytopenia

A useful classification of thrombocytopenia is listed below.

Thrombocytopenia — causes

Impaired production
- Congenital
- Thrombocytopenia and absent radius (TAR) syndrome
- Fanconi anaemia
- Wiskott–Aldrich syndrome
- Acquired
  - Aplastic anaemia
  - Bone marrow replacement, for example infiltration by malignant disease

Decreased platelet survival
- Immune-mediated
  - Immune (idiopathic) thrombocytopenic purpura (ITP)
  - Neonatal isoimmune thrombocytopenia
  - Alloimmune neonatal thrombocytopenia
  - Neonatal ITP
  - Infections
  - Drug-induced
  - Autoimmune disorders (e.g. SLE)
  - Malignancy
- Non-immune-mediated
  - Disseminated intravascular coagulation
  - Haemolytic–uraemic syndrome
  - Thrombotic thrombocytopenic purpura (TTP)
  - Kasabach–Merritt syndrome
  - Cyanotic congenital heart disease
  - Liver disease
  - Drug-induced
  - Miscellaneous

8.2 Immune thrombocytopenic purpura

Immune thrombocytopenic purpura (ITP) is a generic term used to describe an immune-mediated thrombocytopenia that is not associated with drugs or other evidence of disease. It is not a specific condition in that the cause and pathology are poorly understood. It may follow a viral infection or immunization and is caused by an inappropriate response of the immune system.

ITP does not have a predictable course, although it usually follows a benign self-limiting course. Approximately 20% of cases, in older girls predominantly, fail to remit over 6 months (chronic ITP).

Investigations

- A bone marrow biopsy is not indicated in a typical case, but when the diagnosis is uncertain it is a necessity
- Autoantibodies against platelet surface glycoprotein can be commonly detected, although they are neither a useful diagnostic test nor a useful prognostic indicator

Management

- No clear benefit of inpatient management
- Written information about ITP, sensible advice (avoidance of contact sports, what to do in the event of an accident, etc.) and a contact person to call are usually sufficient
- Treatment to raise the platelet count is not always required as the few remaining platelets, even if profoundly low in number ($< 10 \times 10^9$/l), function more efficiently. The risk of serious bleeding from ITP, as compared to that from thrombocytopenia related to marrow failure syndromes, is low
- Less than 1% of cases suffer an intracranial haemorrhage. In a recent national audit in the UK (performed over a 14-month period in 1995) no intracranial bleeds were reported in 427 patients

Treatment includes the following modalities:

Intravenous immunoglobulin (IVIG)

IVIG is the treatment of choice in severe haemorrhage as it raises the platelet count the fastest — usually within 48 hours. The most practical and effective administration of IVIG is a single dose of 0.8 g/kg, although side-effects are common at this dose. Traditionally, 0.4 g/kg/day has been given over 5 days.

Side-effects with IVIG are common and, as IVIG is a pooled blood product, a risk of viral transmission does exist.

Steroids

Given at a dose of 1–2 mg/kg daily for up to 2 weeks. There is evidence that a higher dose of 4 mg/kg for 4 days may raise the platelet count as quickly as IVIG.

Anti-D

This has been shown to be effective in children who are Rh-positive. It is a rapid single injection, although it may cause significant haemolysis.

Splenectomy

Rarely required and is only indicated in a patient with chronic ITP who has significant bleeding unresponsive to medical treatment. The failure rate after splenectomy is at least 25%.

Transfusions

Platelet transfusions are generally not indicated in ITP as it is a consumptive disorder.

Other agents

Vincristine, cyclophosphamide and cyclosporin have all been used with varying degrees of success. The combination of cyclophosphamide and rituximab (an anti-CD2O antibody) is currently demonstrating promising results.

Neonatal isoimmune thrombocytopenia

Babies may be born thrombocytopenic as a result of the transplacental passage of maternal antiplatelet antibodies. This can occur in two ways.

Alloimmune neonatal thrombocytopenia (ANT)

- Maternal antibodies are produced as a result of direct sensitization to fetal platelets (analogous to haemolytic disease of the newborn)
- Nineteen human platelet alloantigen (HPA) systems have been documented, the most important one (causing 85% of ANT cases) is HPA-1a. Only 3% of the population does not express HPA-1a, therefore if a mother does not express HPA-1a the chances of her partner expressing HPA-1a is high — resulting in an HPA-1a-positive fetus. Only 6% of such mothers will become sensitized, and then not all sensitized mothers will produce a thrombocytopenic baby
- Antibodies against HPA-1a are IgG and therefore can cross the placenta, bind to fetal platelets and decrease their survival time
- Not only is it possible but it is common that ANT occurs in the first born
- The diagnosis of ANT is suspected when a low platelet count is demonstrated in an otherwise healthy term neonate with a normal clotting screen
- Treatment is in the form of an urgent platelet transfusion if severe (platelet count $< 20 \times 10^9$/l) because the risk of an intracerebral bleed is high in the first few days of life.
- Treatment of the fetus with periumbilical transfusions of immunologically compatible platelets (maternal platelets can be used) or maternal infusions of IgG and/or corticosteroids are possible — but are not without significant risks
- Genetic counselling, identification of the paternal genotype (heterozygous for HPA-1 results in a 50% chance of a positive genotype fetus) and close liaison between the haematologist, obstetrician and neonatologist is essential

8.3 Neonatal isoimmune thrombocytopenia

- Occurs in babies born to mothers with active or previous ITP
- Clinically identical presentation to ANT but treatment is different, in that maternal platelets cannot be used because they would be consumed
- Maternal steroid therapy prior to delivery may improve the fetal platelet count

Drug-induced thrombocytopenia

An immune thrombocytopenia may occur with the following commonly prescribed drugs:

- Sodium valproate
- Phenytoin
- Carbamazepine
- Co-trimoxazole
- Rifampicin
- Heparin (non-immune mechanisms also possible)

8.4   Functional abnormalities of platelets

Before classifying these abnormalities it is important to understand the normal function of platelets. To achieve haemostasis, platelets undergo the following reactions of adhesion, secretion or release reaction, aggregation and procoagulation.

Adhesion

Adhesion of platelets to the subendothelial lining requires interactions between platelet membrane glycoproteins, elements of the vessel wall (e.g. collagen) and adhesive proteins such as von Willebrand factor (vWF) and fibronectin.

Release reaction

Collagen exposure results in the release or secretion of the contents of platelet granules: fibrinogen, serotonin, ADP, lysosomal enzymes, heparin-neutralizing factor. The cell membrane releases an arachidonate derivative which transforms into thromboxane A_2 — a stimulus for aggregation as well as being a powerful vasoconstrictor.

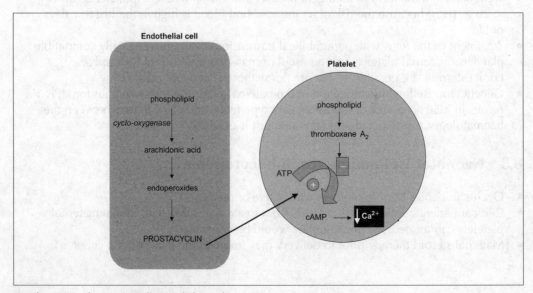

Production of prostacyclin and thromboxane

Aggregation

The contents of the platelet granules, specifically ADP and thromboxane A_2, cause additional platelets to aggregate at the site of the injury.

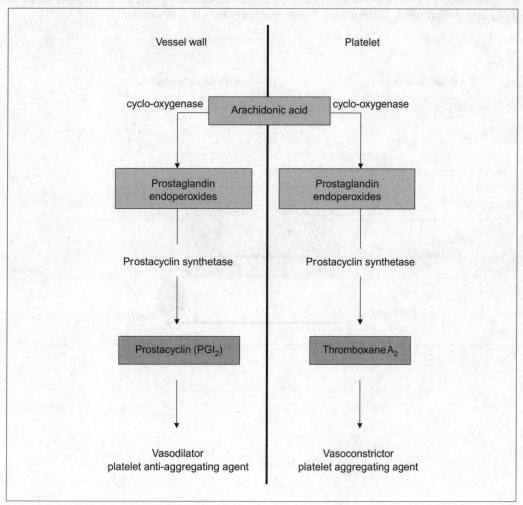

Function of prostacyclin and thromboxane

Platelet procoagulation activity

After secretion and aggregation have taken place a phospholipid (platelet factor 3) becomes exposed on the platelet membrane, thereby making itself available for its surface to be used as a template for two important coagulation protein reactions — the conversion of factor X to X_a and prothrombin to thrombin. These reactions are Ca^{2+}-dependent.

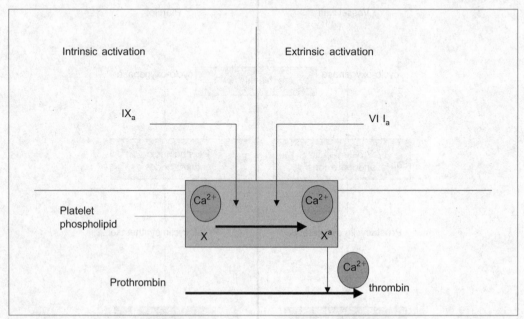

Procoagulant activity

Functional platelet abnormalities — classification

Congenital
Defects of platelet membrane

- Glanzmann thrombasthenia
  - rare, autosomal recessive, failure to aggregate, normal platelet count and morphology
- Bernard–Soulier syndrome
  - rare, autosomal recessive, failure of adhesion, no receptor to bind to vWF, giant platelets, moderate platelet count reduction

Deficiency of storage granules

- Wiskott–Aldrich syndrome
- Chediak–Higashi syndrome

Defects of thromboxane deficiency

- e.g. thromboxane synthetase deficiency
  — cyclo-oxygenase deficiency

Acquired
- Renal failure
- Liver failure
- Myeloproliferative disorders
- Acute leukaemia, especially myeloid
- Chronic hypoglycaemia
- Drugs
- Aspirin, non-steroidal anti-inflammatory drugs (NSAIDs), penicillin, cephalosporin, sodium valproate

Investigations

- A prolonged bleeding time and normal or moderately reduced platelet count are the characteristic hallmarks of a congenital/hereditary platelet disorder (or von Willebrand disease)
- Platelet size followed by tests of aggregation and secretion in response to ADP, collagen, arachidonate and ristocetin will be necessary

9. BLOOD FILM

9.1 Approach to a blood film at MRCPCH level

Is the pathology in the red or white blood cell?

This is the first and most vital question you need to ask yourself when presented with a blood film to interpret. Apart from the accompanying history being important in helping you to answer this question, the other clue will be the number of white cells seen. If there is an abundance of white cells the likelihood that the pathology will be in the white cells is very high, and I will go as far as to say that acute lymphoblastic leukaemia will be top of your differential diagnosis. If only an occasional white cell is seen then red cell pathology is likely. Platelet pathology will be unlikely at MRCPCH level — the only real possibility is one of giant platelets (same size as a red cell, or bigger) in Bernard–Soulier syndrome.

Red cell pathology?

Once you have decided on red cell pathology then look at the following parameters.

Shape

- Sickle-shaped cells, as in sickle-cell disease
- Fragments of red cells (e.g. helmet cells, etc.) indicative of microangiopathic haemolysis such as in the haemolytic–uraemic syndrome
- All different shapes, i.e. poikilocytosis as in thalassaemia, sickle-cell, iron deficiency anaemia

Size

- Small cells or microcytosis in iron deficiency anaemia
- Large cells or macrocytosis in vitamin B_{12} and/or folate-deficient anaemia
- Different sizes: anisocytosis (haemoglobinopathies, anaemias)

Amount of central pallor in red cell

- No central pallor: spherocytosis (hereditary spherocytosis, haemolytic conditions, burns for example)
- Large central pallor: hypochromic anaemia
- 'Halo' central pallor: target cells (haemoglobinopathies, hyposplenism)

Red cell inclusions

- Malaria: most commonly *Plasmodium falciparum*, seen as a 'signet-ring' inclusion
- Howell–Jolly bodies: remnants of nuclear fragments, seen in hyposplenism
- Heinz bodies: denatured haemoglobin, resulting from oxidant stress (e.g. G6PD) or haemolysis; can only be seen with a special stain, so if normal staining was used then it is most likely a Howell–Jolly body
- Basophilic stippling: multiple small inclusions in a red cell — e.g. lead poisoning

White cell pathology?

The abundance of white cells is most likely to be leukaemia at the MRCPCH level. A lymphoblast cell is recognized by its size (large), with a large nucleus taking up nearly the entire cell with only a rim of cytoplasm remaining (in contrast, a mature neutrophil has a multilobed small nucleus). The morphological differentiation between acute lymphoblastic leukaemia (ALL) and acute myeloid leukaemia (AML) is not realistic at this level, but remember the relative incidence of each, 4 : 1, respectively.

10.   COAGULATION

A representation of the coagulation cascades is shown below. It consists of an extrinsic pathway (tissue thromboplastin is the initiator) and the intrinsic pathway (what happens in the blood when it clots away from the body). These two pathways share a common final pathway resulting in the production of a fibrin clot.

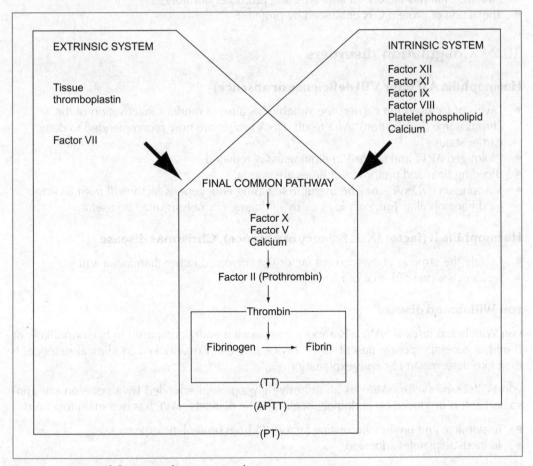

Representation of the coagulation cascades

The system can be divided into boxes, each box representing one of the following three basic screening tests of coagulation:

- **Prothrombin time** (PT) measures the extrinsic system and common pathway
- **Activated partial thromboplastin time** (APTT) measures the intrinsic system and common pathway
- **Thrombin time** (TT) measures the final part of the common pathway, it is prolonged by the lack of fibrinogen and by inhibitors of this conversion, e.g. heparin and fibrin degradation products

10.1 Natural anticoagulants

It is important that thrombin is limited to the site of injury. This is achieved by circulating inhibitors of coagulation:

- Antithrombin III — the most potent inhibitor, heparin potentiates its effect markedly
- Protein C inhibits factors Va and VIIIa and promotes fibrinolysis
- The action of protein C is enhanced by protein S

10.2 Coagulation disorders

Haemophilia A (factor VIII deficiency or absence)

- Levels of factor VIII in carriers are variable because of random inactivation of the X chromosome (lyonization). As a result, DNA probes are now recommended to detect carrier status
- Prolonged APTT and factor VIII clotting assay reduced
- Bleeding time and prothrombin times are normal
- Vasopressin (DDAVP) may be useful in releasing endogenous factor VIII from its stores in mild haemophilia. Tranexamic acid, by inhibiting fibrinolysis, may be useful

Haemophilia B (factor IX deficiency or absence), Christmas disease

- Exactly the same as above, except factor IX is involved rather than factor VIII
- Incidence is one-fifth that of haemophilia A

von Willebrand disease

von Willebrand disease (vWD) is a more complicated entity compared to haemophilia A or B and is generally poorly described — hence it is often overlooked in clinical practice. It therefore deserves an in-depth explanation.

von Willebrand factor (vWF), is an adhesive glycoprotein encoded by a gene on chromosome 12. It is produced by endothelial cells and by platelets. vWF has two main functions:

- To stabilize and protect circulating factor VIII from proteolytic enzymes
- To mediate platelet adhesion

vWD will therefore result when the synthesis of vWF is reduced or when abnormal vWF is produced.

The clinical presentation of vWD will include the following:

- Mucous membrane bleeding
- Excess bleeding following surgical/dental procedures
- Easy bruising

Three types (at least) have been described

Type 1 vWD

- Most common, accounts for at least 70% of vWD
- Due to a partial deficiency of vWF
- Autosomal dominant

Type 2 vWD

- Due to abnormal function of vWF

Type 3 vWD

- Due to the complete absence of vWF

Can often be mistaken for haemophilia A because factor VIII levels will be low as there is no vWF to protect factor VIII from proteolysis. Laboratory results are important in distinguishing the types of vWD and in the differentiation from haemophilia. In vWD type 1 the following results will be expected:

- Platelet count   N
- Bleeding time   N/↑
- Factor VIII   ↓
- vWF   ↓
- Ristocetin cofactor activity   ↓

Ristocetin, an antibiotic, is now confined to laboratory-only use after it was documented to cause significant thrombocytopenia. Ristocetin, when added to a patient's plasma, will bind vWF and platelets together causing platelet aggregation (hence, the clinical thrombocytopenia). In the absence of vWF, no platelet aggregation will be seen (vWF type 3). In the presence of decreased vWF, diminished aggregation will ensue (vWD type 1). Hence, when faced with the clinical picture of haemophilia A (bruising, normal platelet count, slightly increased bleeding time and a decreased factor VIII), the ristocetin cofactor test will be able to differentiate between vWD (decreased) and haemophilia A (normal).

Haemorrhagic disease of the newborn

- Vitamin K-dependent factors are low at birth and fall further in breast-fed infants in the first few days of life

- Other factors associated with this deficiency include:
  - Liver-cell immaturity
  - Lack of gut bacterial synthesis of the vitamin K
  - Low quantities in breast milk
- Haemorrhage is usually between day 2 and day 4 of life
- PT and APTT are both abnormal, while the platelet count and fibrinogen levels are normal. Fibrin degradation products will not be detected
- Treatment is with vitamin K, either administered intramuscularly at birth or orally on day 1, followed by interval dosing thereafter
- Prophylactic vitamin K remains controversial — see further reading

11. MALIGNANT PATHOLOGY

- There are 1,200 new cases of malignancy diagnosed each year in the UK in children under 15 years of age (an incidence of 1 in 600 children < 15 years)
- The relative incidence rates for the different tumour types is illustrated below
- Leukaemia, together with lymphoma, accounts for nearly 50% of all cases
- Brain and spinal cord tumours are the most commonly occurring solid tumours
- Overall, childhood cancer is about one-third more common in boys than girls

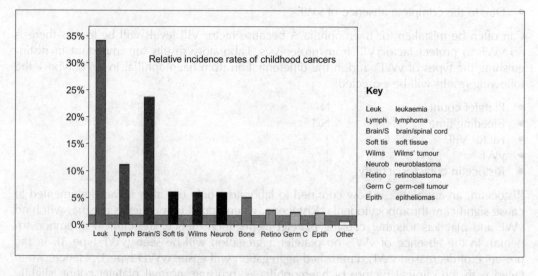

Relative incidence rates of childhood cancers

Key

Leuk	leukaemia
Lymph	lymphoma
Brain/S	brain/spinal cord
Soft tis	soft tissue
Wilms	Wilms' tumour
Neurob	neuroblastoma
Retino	retinoblastoma
Germ C	germ-cell tumour
Epith	epitheliomas

Environmental factors predisposing to cancer

- Ultraviolet radiation — skin cancer, particularly malignant melanoma
- Ionizing radiation
  - Preconceptual paternal exposure — remains controversial
  - In vitro exposure — increased incidence of leukaemia
  - Postnatal exposure — leukaemia
- Electromagnetic fields — remains controversial

Syndromes/conditions predisposing to cancer

Syndrome	Cancer
Down	Acute leukaemia 20 times more susceptible than population
Neurofibromatosis type 1	Brain tumours, including optic glioma Juvenile myelomonocytic leukaemia Phaeochromocytoma
Li–Fraumeni	Soft tissue sarcomas in children born to families who have the Li–Fraumeni syndrome (mutation of p53)
Klinefelter	Germ-cell tumours, including dysgerminoma
Tuberous sclerosis	Benign tumours in organs
von Hippel–Lindau disease	Cerebellar haemangioblastomas — multiple Retinal angiomas Renal-cell carcinoma Phaeochromocytoma
Familial adenomatous polyposis (FAP)	Hepatoblastoma — children born to a parent with FAP have an increased risk of developing hepatoblastoma
WAGR (Wilms' tumour, aniridia genitourinary abnormalities, mental retardation)	Wilms' tumour
Beckwith–Wiedemann (macroglossia, organomegaly, omphalos, hemihyertrophy)	Wilms' tumour
Denys–Drash (pseudohermaphroditism, Wilms' tumour, nephrotic syndrome)	Wilms' tumour
Perlman (phenotypically similar to Beckwith–Wiedemann)	Wilms' tumour
Xeroderma pigmentosum	Basal- and squamous-cell skin carcinoma
Ataxia telangiectasia	Leukaemia and B-cell lymphoma

11.1 Leukaemia

The leukaemias can be divided into acute and chronic leukaemia. Chronic leukaemia accounts for less than 5% of all leukaemias in childhood — all of these cases would be chronic myeloid leukaemia (CML) as chronic lymphoblastic leukaemia does not exist in childhood.

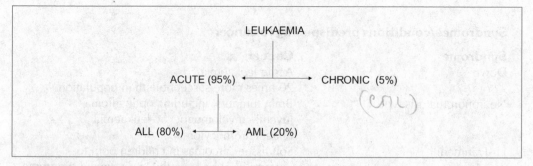

- In acute leukaemia, a differentiating white cell undergoes a structural and/or numerical change in its genetic make-up, causing a failure of further differentiation and dysregulated proliferation and clonal expansion
- Aetiology remains unknown, although associations or risk factors have been identified
  - Chromosomal breakage or defective DNA repair mechanisms (e.g. Fanconi anaemia, ataxia telangiectasia)
  - Chemotherapy — second tumour effect
  - Immunodeficiency syndrome, for example Wiskott–Aldrich
  - Trisomy 21
  - Identical twin, especially if twin contracted leukaemia in infancy
  - Ionizing radiation
- Clinical presentation is related to bone marrow failure and possibly to extramedullary involvement

Acute lymphoblastic leukaemia

Acute lymphoblastic leukaemia (ALL) is divided into B-cell or T-cell ALL depending on which cell line (determined by immunophenotyping) is affected. The majority of cases (>80%) originate from the B-cell line with early pre-B, or common ALL (cALL), being the commonest. About 15% are T-cell ALL with 2% demonstrating mixed lineage. cALL has the most favourable prognosis out of all the immunophenotypes.

Poor prognostic signs in ALL include:

- Presenting white cell count (WCC) greater than $50 \times 10^9/l$
- Outside the age range 2–9 years
- Males do less well than females
- Chromosomal abnormalities/translocations: rearrangement of the Mixed Lineage Leukaemia (*MLL*) gene (11q23), e.g. t(4:11) purports a poor prognosis, while t(9:22) involving the Philadelphia chromosome carries a dismal prognosis
- Normal diploid number of chromosomes in blast cell (hyperdiploidy carries a more favourable prognosis)
- Afro-Caribbean ethnicity
- CNS disease

The poor risk or prognostic factors above are now used to tailor treatment, i.e. a child with a high WCC will receive more intensive treatment than if the WCC had been normal. Treatment is in the form of intensification blocks with ongoing maintenance therapy in between. Cytotoxic/chemotherapy agents used in the treatment of leukaemia include the following: corticosteroids (prednisone and/or dexamethasone, vincristine, asparaginase, daunorubicin/doxorubicin, cytarabine, cyclophosphamide, methotrexate, mercaptopurine, CNS-directed treatment is a vital component of treatment because lymphoblasts can be protected from standard chemotherapy by being on the 'other-side' of the blood–brain barrier. In standard-risk children this will comprise intrathecal chemotherapy at regular intervals; but for higher risk children, high-dose intravenous methotrexate (at a sufficient dose to cross the blood–brain barrier) or craniospinal radiotherapy may be required. The latter is the most effective in sterilizing the CNS of lymphoblasts, but it has a high price to pay in that the neurocognitive side-effects can be profound. Treatment is over 2.5–3 years. Bone marrow transplantation is generally reserved for specific patients with relapsing ALL or with extremely poor prognosis ALL. The 5-year survival rate for standard-risk ALL is now approximately 80%.

Acute myeloid leukaemia (AML)

- Is divided into seven subtypes depending on morphology (FAB — French, American, British classification) and immunophenotyping characteristics — M1 to M7
- Chromosomal abnormalities occur in at least 80% of cases, with translocations the most common
- Treatment is with a more intensive, but shorter (6 months) chemotherapy regimen than that used for ALL
- Bone marrow transplantation plays a much more prominent role in the treatment of AML although its use remains controversial in some subsets of patients because the increased complete remission rates with this modality need to be weighed up against the increased mortality of the transplantation procedure
- Five-year survival figures are now in excess of 50%

11.2 Lymphoma

Two types of lymphoma are recognized: non-Hodgkin lymphoma (NHL) and Hodgkin lymphoma (HL). In NHL the originating cell is either a B or T lymphocyte or an immature form thereof, while in HL the originating cell is a B-lineage lymphoid cell. Histologically, the presence of the Reed–Sternberg cell remains pathognomonic of HL.

Non-Hodgkin lymphoma

- NHL is the term adopted to describe a heterogeneous group of malignant proliferations of lymphoid tissue
- The classification of NHL is complicated, and controversial. A practical way of classifying NHL is to divide the entities into immature forms (T- or B-cell acute lymphoblastic lymphoma), mature form (e.g. Burkitt lymphoma – a mature B-cell NHL) and large cell lymphomas (e.g. anaplastic large cell lymphoma, diffuse B-cell large cell lymphoma, peripheral T-cell lymphoma)
- The acute lymphoblastic lymphoma form of NHL is derived from the same T- and B-lineage lymphoid cells as ALL, but an important difference exists between these two

entities. In ALL, 80% of cases are pre-B-cell-derived; while 20% are T-cell-derived. In NHL this is reversed, with T-cell tumours predominating

The following sites are commonly affected, in descending order of frequency:

- Abdomen — usually with B-cell disease
- Mediastinum — typically T cell in origin
- Head and neck — no specific cell

Chemotherapy is the mainstay of treatment because NHL is a systemic disease, despite the apparent local sites of disease

Hodgkin lymphoma (HL)

- Painless cervical lymphadenopathy is the most frequent presenting symptom
- The EBV-related causal hypothesis remains unproven
- An excision biopsy of the entire lymph node, not just a biopsy of a portion of the node, is necessary to examine lymph node architecture and stromal cellular elements
- Combined modality treatment with chemotherapy and radiotherapy remains the treatment of choice with attempts now being made to decrease treatment intensity (specifically radiotherapy) in an attempt to minimize treatment-related side-effects. Patients with HL have the highest incidence of such complications compared to children with any other type of malignancy.

11.3 Tumour-lysis syndrome

- High-count ALL (especially T-cell) and B-cell NHL (specifically Burkitt lymphoma) have the potential for bulky disease — a high cell mass, which will undergo lysis with treatment, resulting in the intracellular contents of potassium, phosphate and nuclear debris being released into the circulation
- Lymphoblast cells have four times the amount of phosphate compared to normal white cells
- Uric acid crystals and phosphate (precipitating out with calcium) crystals may cause acute renal failure and the following:
  - Fluid overload ↑
  - Phosphate ↑
  - Potassium ↑
  - Urea and creatinine ↑
  - Calcium ↓

Treatment involves:

- Hyperhydration
- Uric acid-lowering agents — allopurinol or uricozyme (urate oxidase)
- Treatment of hyperkalaemia
- Consideration of fluid filtration or dialysis

11.4   Tumours of the CNS

- The anatomical grouping together of brain tumours masks their diverse biological differences
- Brain tumours in children tend to be located in the posterior fossa, in the midline, have greater differentiation and have slightly better survival figures than their counterparts in adults
- Brain tumours as a general rule do not metastasize out of the CNS
- They are notoriously difficult to diagnose because of their varied and often non-specific presentations. The mean time from onset of symptoms to diagnosis is 5 months.

Presenting symptoms of brain tumours

Presenting symptoms	% of children
Vomiting	65
Headache	64
Changes in personality and mood	47
Squint	24
Out-of-character behaviour	22
Deterioration of school performance	21
Growth failure	20
Weight loss	16
Seizures	16
Developmental delay	16
Disturbance of speech	11

Astrocytoma

- Most commonly occurring brain tumour
- Range from low-grade (benign) tumours, usually in the cerebellum, to high-grade (malignant) tumours, usually supratentorial and brainstem
- The glioblastoma multiforme tumour has a near-fatal prognosis

Medulloblastoma (primitive neuroectodermal tumour (PNET) occurring in the cerebellum)

- 20% of brain tumours
- The most commonly occurring high-grade tumour
- Commonly metastasizes within the CNS, and it is the one tumour that can metastasize out of the CNS
- Prognosis is in the region of a 50% 5-year survival

Brainstem glioma

- 20% of brain tumours
- Can either be diffuse (e.g. diffuse pontine glioma) or local
- Less than 10% survival

Craniopharyngioma

- 8% of all brain tumours
- Situated in the suprasellar region predominantly
- Presenting features may be in the form of raised intracranial pressure, visual disturbances, pituitary dysfunction and psychological abnormalities

Treatment remains controversial but usually involves surgery and/or radiotherapy

11.5 Retinoblastoma

Retinoblastoma can be hereditary or sporadic.

Hereditary

- 40% of retinoblastomas
- Deletion of a tumour-suppressor gene at chromosome 13q14
- Behaves in an autosomal dominant fashion (with a high degree of penetrance) but requires inactivation of remaining allele at the cellular level
- Usually multifocal disease
- Early onset (mean 10 months)
- Increased risk of developing a second primary tumour

Sporadic

- 60% of retinoblastomas
- Unifocal
- Late onset (mean 18 months)

11.6 Neuroblastoma

- Aggressive tumour originating from neural crest-derived sympathetic nerve cells (e.g. sympathetic chain, adrenal medulla)
- Presenting symptoms often non-specific and can mimic commonly occurring conditions; symptoms are the result of the numerous possible tumour sites, metastases and the associated metabolic disturbances (caused by catecholamine secretion: sweating, pallor, diarrhoea, hypertension)
- Urinary and plasma catecholamine metabolites (vanillyl mandelic acid (VMA)) and homovanillic acid (HVA)) may be raised

Prognostic factors are:

- Tumour stage: inversely proportional to outcome, with the exception of Stage 4S — a local primary tumour with dissemination to liver, skin or bone marrow occurring in infancy in which spontaneous regression occurs in approximately 85% of patients

- Age: inversely proportional to outcome — patients younger than 12–18 months have superior survival rates compared to children older than 18 months.
- Histopathological characteristics, specifically the characteristics of the stroma
- Molecular biology: presence of the following confers a poor prognosis:
  - N-*myc* amplification
  - 1p deletion
  - DNA ploidy – diploid worse than hypo/hyperdiploid
  - Unbalanced chromosome rearrangement resulting in partial gain of chromosome 17

11.7   Wilms' tumour (nephroblastoma)

- Presents in a well child with a painless (or minimal discomfort) abdominal mass, haematuria and hypertension (independently or collectively)
- Patients with Beckwith–Wiedemann syndrome have an increased propensity for developing Wilms' tumours.
- Intensity of treatment is relative to the staging and the histology of the tumour
- Very good overall prognosis — in excess of 90% 5-year survival

11.8   Bone tumours

Osteosarcoma

- Twice as common as Ewing sarcoma
- Predominantly in the metaphyses of long bones, 50% occurring in the femur
- Presentation peaks in teenage years, suggesting a relationship between rapid bone growth and tumour formation
- 80% of all patients develop lung metastases

Ewing sarcoma

- Occurs more commonly in flat bones (e.g. pelvis, ribs, vertebra) than osteosarcoma, although long bones can be affected
- Can be extraosseous in rare cases

11.9   Soft-tissue sarcomas

These are a group of tumours derived from contractile, connective, adipose and vascular tissue. **Rhabdomyosarcoma** is the most common of these, arising from cells destined to be striated muscle cells. Rhabdomyosarcomas can occur anywhere in the body, with the common sites being genitourinary, parameningeal and orbit.

11.10   Malignant germ-cell tumours

Tumours derived from germ cells (cells giving rise to gonadal tissue) can be gonadal (30%) or extragonadal (70%).

- Extragonadal sites are the sacrococcygeal region, retroperitoneum, mediastinum, neck and the pineal area of the brain
- As gonadal tissue can give rise to any cell type, tumours derived from such cells may express any cell line in any stage of differentiation. This gives rise to a range of tumours, from an undifferentiated embryonal carcinoma to a benign and fully differentiated mature teratoma
- Serum markers α-fetoprotein and β-human chorionic gonadotrophin are useful in diagnosing and monitoring disease state

11.11   Hepatoblastoma

- Hepatoblastoma, an embryonal tumour of the liver, occurs in an otherwise normal liver (compared to hepatocellular carcinoma) and generally presents in children under the age of 2 years
- Patients with Beckwith–Wiedemann syndrome or familial adenomatous polyposis have an increased incidence of hepatoblastoma
- There is evidence to suggest that low-birth-weight babies are predisposed to hepatoblastoma
- Treatment involves chemotherapy and surgery (partial liver resection or in some cases liver transplantation)
- Overall survival figures of 70–80% have been reported

11.12   Langerhans-cell histiocytosis

- Langerhans cell histiocytosis is a clonal accumulation and proliferation of abnormal bone-marrow-derived Langerhan cells. These cells, functioning as potent antigen-presenting cells, together with lymphocytes, eosinophils and normal histiocytes form infiltrates, in various organs, causing inflammatory tissue damage responsible for the morbidity, and in some cases mortality, associated with this disease
- Any age group may be affected
- Patients can have localized disease (to skin, bone, or lymph node) or multi-system disease (with spleen, lung, liver and bone marrow involvement carrying a worse prognosis)
- The disease course is unpredictable — varying from spontaneous regression to rapid progression and death or repeated recurrences
- Treatment is with a combination of corticosteroids, vinblastine, methotrexate, 6-mercaptopurine

11.13 Haemophagocytic lymphohistiocytosis

- Haemophagocytic lymphohistiocytosis (HLH) is a rare disease resulting from abnormal proliferation of histiocytes (macrophages) in tissues and organs, and carries a high fatality rate
- Classified into familial or secondary HLH
- **Familial HLH** is an autosomal recessive condition and involves a mutation in the peforin gene (other gene defects are suspected but are not yet proven) resulting in a defect in the natural killer cell and T-cell cytotoxic function. It is thought that this causes strong immunological activation of phagocytes and mediators of inflammation, resulting in multi-system pathology that may, if untreated, be fatal. Active treatment with corticosteroids and chemotherapy is required in the acute phase followed by definitive treatment with a bone marrow transplant
- **Secondary HLH**, or its other commonly used term, macrophage activating syndrome, is not inherited but has a similar pathophysiological process usually precipitated by infection or rheumatological disorders
- Typical findings of HLH are fever, hepatosplenomegaly, cytopenia, hypertriglyceridaemia, coagulopathy, hypofibrinogenaemia, liver dysfunction, elevated ferritin and serum transaminases, and neurological symptoms.

11.14 Role of bone marrow transplantation

The three broad areas in which bone marrow transplantation is a possibility are:

- To replace a missing enzyme, e.g. mucopolysaccharidosis, adrenoleukodystrophy
- To restore bone marrow function following high-dose or bone marrow ablative chemotherapy, e.g. chemotherapy for neuroblastoma
- To treat and/or immunomodulate a disease process, e.g. AML, juvenile CML (now myelomonocytic — JMML), high-risk ALL (e.g. Philadelphia chromosome +ve)

Bone marrow transplant can be:

- Autologous— the patient receives his/her own bone marrow
- Allogeneic — patient receives donated marrow from either a sibling (matched related donor) or an unrelated donor (matched unrelated donor)

The technique of harvesting peripheral-blood stem cells from a patient prior to ablative chemotherapy and returning them post-chemotherapy now provides an alternative to bone marrow harvesting. Currently, the use of cord-blood stem cells is becoming an option for bone marrow transplant.

11.15 Principles of managing malignancy

The ultimate goal of oncological treatment is to cure the patient, i.e. to ensure the patient is in life-long remission, while at the same time keeping treatment-related side-effects to the minimum.

The first step in achieving this goal in patients with haematological malignancies, such as leukaemia, is to get the patient into remission. This is achieved with induction chemotherapy, usually over a 4-week period. To ensure that this remission is durable, further treatment in the form of consolidation, intensification and maintenance chemotherapy is required.

Patients with solid-tumour malignancies, on the other hand, generally require sequential multimodal treatment. The tumour, depending on multiple factors including histological type, stage, size, anatomical location, age of patient and degree of resectability, is either surgically resected at the start of treatment, with adjuvant treatment in the form of chemotherapy and/or radiotherapy required thereafter to ensure complete eradication of remaining tumour cells. If the localized primary tumour is too large to be safely resected or in cases of metastatic disease, chemotherapy and/or radiotherapy are commenced to shrink the tumour, thereby enabling resection at a later stage of treatment.

11.16 Late effects of cancer treatment

Chemotherapy

Second malignancies
Leukaemia and lymphoma are the two most likely secondary malignancies to occur — particularly AML with topoisomerase II inhibitors (e.g. etoposide) while alkylators (e.g. nitrogen mustard, cyclophosphamide) may cause either.

Cardiac
Cardiomyopathy is the most likely complication, particularly with anthracycline-containing chemotherapy, which is commonly used in treating solid tumours and, to a lesser extent, leukaemia. This toxicity is exacerbated by thoracic radiotherapy.

Reduced fertility or infertility
Diminished fertility potential with increasing cumulative doses of alkylating chemotherapy (particularly with procarbazine, which at high doses will render all males infertile), for example in Hodgkin disease.

Pulmonary
Pulmonary fibrosis may result from bleomycin chemotherapy used, for example, in Hodgkin disease and germ-cell tumours.

Neurocognitive
There are insufficient data at present to claim a definite association between chemotherapy and neurocognitive difficulties, although this may very well exist. Methotrexate is the one exception where an association has been made.

Auditory
Ototoxicity may result from platinum-containing agents, for example, cisplatinum and carboplatinum, used commonly in the treatment of CNS and other solid tumours.

Renal

Decreased renal function as measured by the glomerular filtration rate (GFR) may be caused by the same platinum-containing agents as above. In addition, a Fanconi syndrome with electrolyte abnormalities may result from numerous chemotherapeutic agents.

Radiotherapy

The developing child is extremely susceptible to the damaging effects of radiotherapy, particularly in the following areas:

- Neurocognitive — especially in the younger child
- Endocrine abnormalities — particularly growth and hypothyroidism
- Second malignancies — particularly sarcomas and lymphoma
- Musculoskeletal atrophy
- Organ damage — for example, cardiac, lung, gastrointestinal

12. FURTHER READING

Bolton-Maggs PHB. 2000. Idiopathic thrombocytopenic purpura. *Archives for Diseases in Childhood* 83, 220–2.

Cunningham MJ, Nathan DG. 2005. New developments in iron chelators. Review. *Current Opinions in Hematology* 12, 129–34.

Lawson SE, Roberts IA, Amrolia P, Dokal I, Szydlo R, Darbyshire PJ. 2003. Bone marrow transplantation for beta-thalassaemia major: the UK experience in two paediatric centres. Review. *British Journal of Haematology* 120:2, 289–95.

Lilleyman J, Hann I, Blanchette V (Eds). 2000. *Paediatric Haematology*: London, Churchill Livingstone.

Ouwehand WH, Smith G, Ranasinghe E. 2000. Management of severe alloimmune thrombocytopenia in the newborn. *Archives for Diseases in Childhood Fetal Edition* 82, F173–5.

Pinkerton CR, Plowman PN (Eds). 1997. *Paediatric Oncology*. Chapman and Hall Medical.

Stiller CA, Eatock EM. 1999. Patterns of care and survival for children with acute lymphoblastic leukaemia diagnosed between 1980 and 1994. *Archives for Diseases in Childhood* 81, 202–8.

Tripp JH, McNinch AW. 1998. The vitamin K debacle – cut the Gordian knot but first do no harm (Annotations). *Archives for Diseases in Childhood* 79, 295–7.

Williams J, Wolff A, Daly A, MacDonald A, Aukett A, Booth I. 1999. Iron supplemented formula milk related to reduction in psychomotor decline in infants from inner city areas. *BMJ* 318, 693–8.

Chapter 12

Hepatology

Nancy Tan and Anil Dhawan

CONTENTS

Hepatology

1. JAUNDICE IN INFANCY

See also Chapter 16 — Neonatology, Section 10.

1.1 Bilirubin metabolism

- Unconjugated bilirubin is a product of haem metabolism and is transported by albumin to the hepatocytes
- Hepatocyte uptake is via membrane receptor carriers or by simple passive diffusion
- Conjugation with glucuronic acid by esterification to make it water soluble (enzyme – bilirubin uridine diphosphate glucuronosyltransferase UGT1A1)
- Secretion of conjugates against a concentration gradient through the canalicular membrane into the bile

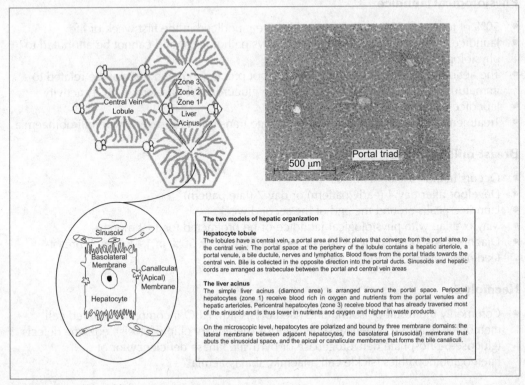

The two models of hepatic organization

Hepatocyte lobule
The lobules have a central vein, a portal area and liver plates that converge from the portal area to the central vein. The portal space at the periphery of the lobule contains a hepatic arteriole, a portal venule, a bile ductule, nerves and lymphatics. Blood flows from the portal triads towards the central vein. Bile is collected in the opposite direction into the portal ducts. Sinusoids and hepatic cords are arranged as trabeculae between the portal and central vein areas

The liver acinus
The simple liver acinus (diamond area) is arranged around the portal space. Periportal hepatocytes (zone 1) receive blood rich in oxygen and nutrients from the portal venules and hepatic arterioles. Pericentral hepatocytes (zone 3) receive blood that has already traversed most of the sinusoid and is thus lower in nutrients and oxygen and higher in waste products.

On the microscopic level, hepatocytes are polarized and bound by three membrane domains: the lateral membrane between adjacent hepatocytes, the basolateral (sinusoidal) membrane that abuts the sinusoidal space, and the apical or canalicular membrane that forms the bile canaliculi.

The two models of hepatic organization

1.2   Approach to a jaundiced infant

- 30–50% of normal term neonates experience jaundice
- Physiological and breast-milk jaundice (unconjugated hyperbilirubinaemia) account for the majority of cases in the first weeks of life
- Approximately 1 in every 2500 infants is affected with cholestatic jaundice (conjugated hyperbilirubinaemia)
- Up to 15% of neonates can be jaundiced at 2 weeks of age and need to be investigated

1.3   Unconjugated hyperbilirubinaemia

- The commonest causes include:
  - Physiological jaundice
  - Breast-milk jaundice
  - Haemolysis
  - Congenital hyperbilirubinaemia
- Unconjugated bilirubin is normally tightly bound to albumin
- Kernicterus may result from high levels of unconjugated bilirubin
- Management strategy is with phototherapy (if serum bilirubin > 250 µmol/l in term babies), adequate hydration, and identification and treatment of the underlying causes

Physiological jaundice

- 50% of term and 80% of preterm babies are jaundiced in the first week of life
- Jaundice within the first 24 h of life is always pathological and cannot be attributed to physiological jaundice
- The aetiology of physiological jaundice is not precisely known but may be related to immaturity of bilirubin uridine diphosphate glucuronosyl transferase (UGT) activity
- Jaundice peaks on day 3 of life
- Treatment is by phototherapy or by exchange transfusion for severe hyperbilirubinaemia

Breast-milk jaundice

- Occurs in 0.5–2% of neonates
- Develops after day 4 (early pattern) or day 7 (late pattern)
- Jaundice peaks around the end of the second week
- May overlap with physiological jaundice or be protracted for 1–2 months
- Diagnosis is supported by a drop in serum bilirubin (≥ 50% in 1–3 days) if breast-feeding is interrupted for 48 hours

Haemolysis

- Commonly the result of isoimmune haemolysis (Rh, ABO incompatibility), red cell membrane defects (congenital spherocytosis, hereditary elliptocytosis), enzyme defects (glucose-6-phosphate dehydrogenase or pyruvate kinase deficiency) or of haemoglobinopathies (sickle cell anaemia, thalassaemia)

- Findings of jaundice in the presence of anaemia and a raised reticulocyte count would necessitate further investigation for the cause of haemolysis

Inherited disorders of unconjugated hyperbilirubinaemia

This spectrum of disease depends on the degree of bilirubin UGT deficiency. Liver function tests and histology are normal.

Gilbert syndrome

- Mild deficiency ($\geqslant$ 50% decrease of UGT activity) occurring in 7% of population
- Polymorphism with TA repeats in the promoter region (TATA box) in Whites compared to exon mutations in Asians on chromosome 2q37
- Correlation between hepatic enzyme activity and serum bilirubin levels is unpredictable because up to 40% of patients with Gilbert syndrome have a reduced red blood cell life-span
- Higher incidence of neonatal jaundice and breast-milk jaundice
- Usually presents after puberty with an incidental finding of elevated bilirubin on blood tests or jaundice after a period of fasting or intercurrent illness
- More common in males
- No treatment required, compatible with normal life span

Crigler–Najjar type II

- Moderate deficiency
- May require phototherapy and phenobarbitone

Crigler–Najjar type I

- Severe deficiency of UGT
- High risk of kernicterus
- Requires life-long phototherapy or even liver transplantation

Autosomal recessive inheritance. Both Gilbert syndrome and Crigler–Najjar type II can also have autosomal dominant transmission.

Causes of neonatal unconjugated hyperbilirubinaemia

Increased production of unconjugated bilirubin from haem
Haemolytic disease (hereditary or acquired)

- Isoimmune haemolysis (neonatal; acute or delayed transfusion reaction; autoimmune)
  - Rh incompatibility
  - ABO incompatibility
  - Other blood group incompatibilities
- Congenital spherocytosis
- Hereditary elliptocytosis
- Infantile pyknocytosis

- Erythrocyte enzyme defects
  - Glucose-6-phosphate dehydrogenase deficiency
  - Pyruvate kinase deficiency
- Haemoglobinopathy
  - Sickle cell anaemia
  - Thalassaemia
  - Others
- Sepsis
- Microangiopathy
  - Haemolytic–uraemic syndrome
  - Haemangioma

Ineffective erythropoiesis
Drugs
Infection
Enclosed haematoma
Polycythaemia

- Diabetic mother
- Fetal transfusion (recipient)
- Delayed cord clamping

Decreased delivery of unconjugated bilirubin (in plasma) to hepatocyte
Right-sided congestive heart failure
Portocaval shunt

Decreased bilirubin uptake across hepatocyte membrane
Presumed enzyme transporter deficiency
Competitive inhibition

- Breast-milk jaundice
- Lucy–Driscoll syndrome
- Drug inhibition (radiocontrast material)

Miscellaneous

- Hypothyroidism
- Hypoxia
- Acidosis

Decreased storage of unconjugated bilirubin in cytosol (decreased Y and Z proteins)
Competitive inhibition
Fever

Decreased biotransformation (conjugation)
Physiological jaundice
Inhibition (drugs)
Hereditary (Crigler–Najjar)

- Type I (complete enzyme deficiency)
- Type II (partial deficiency)

Gilbert disease
Hepatocellular dysfunction

Enterohepatic recirculation
Intestinal obstruction

- Ileal atresia
- Hirschsprung disease
- Cystic fibrosis
- Pyloric stenosis

Antibiotic administration

Breast-milk jaundice

1.4   Conjugated hyperbilirubinaemia

- Jaundice, dark urine, pale stools and hepatomegaly or hepatosplenomegaly
- Baby may be acutely ill with hypoglycaemia, acid–base imbalance, electrolyte imbalance, coagulopathy and liver failure
- Biochemical definition is direct bilirubin > 20% of total
- Top causes are:
  - 'Idiopathic' neonatal hepatitis (40%)
  - Extrahepatic biliary atresia (25–30%)
  - Intrahepatic cholestasis syndromes (20%), e.g. Alagille syndrome, progressive familial intrahepatic cholestasis (PFIC)
  - α_1-antitrypsin deficiency (7–10%)

Work-up of conjugated hyperbilirubinaemia

Investigations	Pathology
General investigations Liver function tests	Type and level of jaundice Degree of liver failure Normal GGT levels (PFIC1, PFIC2 and defects of bile acid synthesis)

Investigations	Pathology
General investigations (continued)	
Full blood count and peripheral blood film	Marrow suppression (familial haemophagocytic lymphohistiocytosis, lysosomal storage diseases) Anaemia/acanthocytosis/thrombocytosis (HFI) Vacuolated lymphocytes (Wolman disease)
PT/PTT, INR	Coagulopathy (liver failure) Vitamin K deficiency
Blood glucose	Hypoglycaemia (liver failure, metabolic disorders)
Renal function test	Impaired renal function (liver failure, Zellweger syndrome)
Lipid profile	Hypercholesterolaemia and hypertriglyceridaemia (Wolman syndrome, Alagille syndrome, PFIC)
Blood gas	Metabolic acidosis (metabolic disorders)
Infections	
Urine cultures	Urinary tract infection
Herpes, toxoplasma, CMV, rubella, syphilis, parvovirus B19 serology	Intrauterine infection
Hepatitis B and A serology HIV	Hepatitis B and rarely hepatitis A
Enterovirus serology, CSF for PCR or cultures	Neonatal systemic infection
Blood cultures, CSF cultures	Systemic bacterial infection
Endocrine	
Thyroid function test	High TSH, low T4, free T4 and T3 (hypothyroidism, hypopituitarism)
Cortisol	Low cortisol (hypopituitarism, septo-optic dysplasia)

Investigations	Pathology
Metabolic	
Serum α_1-antitrypsin levels and PI type	Low level and PI ZZ (α_1-antitrypsin deficiency)
Galactose-1-phosphate uridyl transferase (Gal-1-PUT)	Deficiency (galactosaemia)
Lactate	Elevated (HFI, mitochondrial disorders)
Urine-reducing substances	Positive (galactosaemia, HFI)
Ferritin	Grossly elevated (neonatal haemochromatosis)
α-fetoprotein	Grossly elevated (tyrosinaemia)
Plasma amino acid, urine amino acid	$3\times \uparrow$ plasma tyrosine, phenylalanine, methionine, $\uparrow$ urinary succinylacetone (tyrosinaemia)
Urinary organic acid	Organic aciduria (tyrosinaemia, peroxisomal enzyme deficiency, mitochondrial hepatopathies)
Urinary bile acid intermediates	Elevated (primary disorders of bile acid synthesis, Zellweger syndrome)
Very long chain fatty acids (VLCFA)	Elevated (peroxisomal enzyme deficiency)
Plasma transferrin isoforms	Characteristic patterns in congenital disorders of glycosylation
Sweat chloride	Abnormal chloride levels (cystic fibrosis, PFIC)
Genetic testing	
Karyotyping	Trisomy (trisomies 21 and 18) Duplication of chromosome 22 (cat eye syndrome)
Specific mutations	
Immune	
Autoantibodies	Anti-Ro and anti-La antibodies (neonatal lupus erythematosus)

Investigations	Pathology
Biopsy	
Liver	Biliary atresia
	Giant cell hepatitis
	Immunostaining for PFIC
	Bile duct paucity (syndromic and non-syndromic causes)
	Gaucher cells (Gaucher syndrome)
	Foamy histiocytes (Niemann–Pick, Wolman)
Lip	Extrahepatic siderosis (neonatal haematochromatosis)
Skin biopsy and fibroblast culture studies	Sea blue histiocytes (Wolman disease)
	Accumulation of intracytoplasmic unesterified cholesterol (Niemann–Pick C)
	Glucocerebrosidase deficiency (Gaucher)
	Sphingomyelinase deficiency (Niemann–Pick A, B)
	Acid lipase deficiency (Wolman)
	α1,4-glycan-6-glycosyltransferase deficiency (GSD IV)
Muscle biopsy	Steatosis and ragged red fibres, respiratory chain enzyme analysis (mitochondrial)
Bone marrow aspirate	Gaucher cells (Gaucher)
	'Foam' cells (Niemann–Pick, Wolman)
	Erythrophagocytosis (familial phagocytic lymphohistiocytosis)
Imaging	
Hepatobiliary ultrasound	Adrenal calcification (Wolman)
	Triangular cord sign and absent or small irregular gall bladder (biliary atresia)
	Structural abnormalities (e.g. choledochal cyst)
HIDA scan	Normal excretion excludes biliary atresia. Delayed or no excretion usually seen in neonatal hepatitis

Investigations	Pathology
Eye examination	Cherry red spot (Niemann–Pick)
	'Oil-drop' cataracts, intraocular haemorrhage and retinal detachment (galactosaemia)
	Corneal clouding, cataracts, pigmentary retinopathy (Zellweger syndrome)
	Coloboma (cat-eye syndrome)
	Posterior embryotoxon, optic disc drusen (Alagille syndrome)

GGT, γ-glutamyl transferase; PT/PTT, prothrombin time/partial thromboplastin time; INR, international normalized ratio; CMV, cytomegalovirus; HIV, human immunodeficiency virus; CSF, cerebrospinal fluid; PCR, polymerase chain reaction; TSH, thyroid-stimulating hormone; T3, tri iodothyronine; HFI, hereditary fructose intolerance; T4, thyroxine; PI, protease inhibitor.

Idiopathic neonatal hepatitis

- Diagnosis of exclusion
- Associated with low birth weight or prematurity
- Histology
  - Hepatocellular swelling (ballooning), focal hepatic necrosis and multinucleated giant cells
  - Bile duct proliferation and bile duct plugging are usually absent
- Factors predicting poor prognosis
  - Severe jaundice beyond 6 months
  - Acholic stools
  - Familial occurrence
  - Persistent hepatosplenomegaly
- 90% do well with no long-term liver disease

Biliary atresia (BA)

- Incidence: 1 per 16,000 live births
- Slight female preponderance
- Exact pathogenesis is unknown
- 25% associated with other congenital malformations
- Anatomical variants
  - Type I — obliteration of the common bile duct
  - Type II — obliteration is extended to the common hepatic duct
  - Type III — obliteration of the entire extrahepatic biliary tree (commonest form)

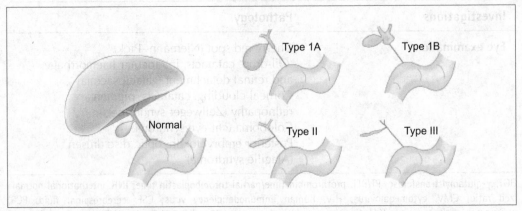

The three variants of biliary atresia

- Diagnosis is suggested by
  - Hepatobiliary ultrasound (*fasting*) — will show absent gallbladder or irregular outline and triangular cord sign
  - Radionuclide imaging (*phenobarbitone priming*) — no excretion indicates possible biliary atresia; excretion indicates that it is not biliary atresia
  - Liver biopsy — expanded portal tracts with bile duct proliferation, bile plugs and fibrosis
  - Gold standard for diagnosis is exploratory and operative cholangiography
- Portoenterostomy (Kasai operation) should be offered to all children unless there is decompensated liver disease
- Between 70 and 80% achieve partial bile flow with 50% becoming jaundice free after surgery
- Ascending bacterial cholangitis follows the first year of surgery in 45–50%
- It is a progressive disease even with a successful Kasai although prognosis may be better if procedure is performed within 8 weeks of birth
- Majority (80%) require liver transplantation by 20 years of age
- Fat-soluble vitamin supplementation is essential
- Role of choleretic agents like phenobarbitone and ursodeoxycholic acid and steroids is unproven

Alagille syndrome (arteriohepatic dysplasia)

- Autosomal dominant
- Incidence is 1 per 100,000 live births
- Defect of the *JAG1* gene on chromosome 20p12
- Intrahepatic biliary hypoplasia
- Characteristic facies (may not be prominent at birth)
  - Broad forehead
  - Deep-set eyes
  - Mild hypertelorism
  - Small chin

- Skeletal abnormalities
  - Thoracic hemivertebrae/'butterfly' vertebrae
- Eye findings
  - Posterior embryotoxon
  - Retinal changes
- Cardiac disease
  - Peripheral pulmonary artery stenosis
  - Other congenital cardiac malformations
- Intrauterine growth retardation and faltering growth with severe malnutrition occur in 50%
- Others
  - Renal disease
  - Delayed puberty or hypogonadism
  - Mental retardation, learning difficulties or psychosocial dysfunction
  - Vascular abnormalities
  - Hypothyroidism and pancreatic insufficiency
  - Recurrent otitis media, chest infection
  - Hypercholesterolaemia
- Variable phenotype, severe liver disease may require liver transplantation

Progressive familial intrahepatic cholestasis (PFIC)

Group of inherited diseases which present as neonatal hepatitis, faltering growth, pruritis and progressive liver disease, requiring liver transplantation in the first few years of life.

Type 1

- Byler disease
- Mutation of the *FIC1* gene on chromosome 18q21-22
- Pancreatitis, persistent diarrhoea, short stature and sensorineural hearing loss
- Normal GGT, serum cholesterol
- Elevated serum bile salts, sweat chloride
- Low chenodeoxycholic acid in bile

Type 2

- Mutations on chromosome 2q24, bile salt export pump (*BSEP*) gene
- Normal GGT

Type 3

- Mutations in the P-glycoprotein MDR-3 gene (*ABCB4*)
- Elevated GGT
- Bile phospholipids 15% of normal

α1-Antitrypsin deficiency

- Commonest inherited cause of conjugated jaundice
- Autosomal recessive

- Incidence is 1 in 1600–2000 live births
- Mutation at the protease inhibitor (PI) locus on chromosome 14
- More than 75 variants are known but not all mutations result in disease
- The most common disease phenotype is PI ZZ, homozygous for a point mutation in which glutamic acid is replaced by glycine at position 342. This causes abnormal folding of the α1-antitrypsin molecule so that it becomes trapped in the endoplasmic reticulum, causing liver damage
- Associated with intrauterine growth retardation
- Hepatomegaly at presentation is common
- Cholestasis may be severe enough to produce totally acholic stools
- Approximately 2% of infants will present with vitamin K-responsive coagulopathy
- Diagnosis is from
  - low α1-antitrypsin levels
  - phenotype (PI) by isoelectric focusing
- Replacement with recombinant α1-antitrypsin is not helpful because abnormal protein continues to accumulate in the endoplasmic reticulum
- Prognosis — 50% of children presenting with neonatal hepatitis develop chronic liver disease with half of them requiring a liver transplant in the first 10 years of life.

Causes of conjugated jaundice

Infections
Bacterial

- Urinary tract infection
- Septicaemia*
- Syphilis
- Listeriosis
- Tuberculosis

Parasitic

- Toxoplasmosis
- Malaria

Viral

- Cytomegalovirus
- Herpes simplex virus*
- Human herpes virus type 6*
- Herpes zoster virus
- Adenovirus
- Parvovirus*
- Enterovirus
- Reovirus type 3
- Human immunodeficiency virus
- Hepatitis B virus*
- ? Hepatitis A
- ? Rotavirus

Metabolic disorders
Carbohydrate metabolism

- Galactosaemia*
- Fructosaemia*
- Glycogen storage type 4
- Congenital disorders of glycosylation*

Protein metabolism (amino acid)

- Tyrosinaemia*
- Hypermethioninaemia
- Urea cycle defects (arginase deficiency)

Lipid metabolism

- Niemann–Pick disease (type C)
- Wolman disease*
- Cholesterol ester storage disease

Bile acid disorders*
Fatty acid oxidation defects*
Disorders of oxidative phosphorylation*
Zellweger's syndrome
Other mitochondrial disorders*

Endocrine disorders
Hypothyroidism
Hypopituitarism (with or without septo-optic dysplasia)

Chromosomal disorders
Down syndrome
Trisomy E
Patau syndrome
Leprechaunism

Other genetic–metabolic defects
α1-Antitrypsin deficiency
Cystic fibrosis
Familial cholestasis syndromes

- Alagille syndrome
- Byler syndrome (PFIC 1)
- Bile salt export protein defect (BSEP defect, PFIC 2)
- Multidrug resistant 3 deficiency (MDR 3, PFIC 3)
- Hereditary cholestasis with lymphoedema (Aagenaes syndrome)

Metals and toxins
Neonatal haemochromatosis*
Copper-related cholestasis*
Parenteral nutrition
Drugs

Haematological disorders
Haemophagocytic lymphohistiocytosis*
Langerhans' cell histiocytosis
Inspissated bile syndrome

Biliary tree disorders
Biliary atresia
Mucus plug
Bile duct stenosis/stricture
Spontaneous perforation of common bile duct
Neonatal sclerosing cholangitis
Caroli disease
Compression of bile duct by a mass
Inflammatory pseudotumour at porta hepatis

Immunological disorders
Neonatal lupus erythematosis
Giant cell hepatitis with Coomb's positive haemolytic anaemia*
Graft-versus-host disease
Adenosine deaminase deficiency

Vascular anomalies
Haemangoendothelioma
Congenital portocaval anomalies

Idiopathic
Familial
Non-familial (good prognosis)

Miscellaneous
Hypoperfusion of liver*
Dubin–Johnson syndrome

*Conditions that can also present as acute liver failure

2. ACUTE HEPATITIS

Acute hepatitis is characterised by liver inflammation and necrosis. The underlying trigger varies, including infective, autoimmune, toxic (e.g. drugs) and metabolic causes.

2.1 Acute infective hepatitis

Acute infection of the liver may result from many pathogens. Complete recovery from an infection is dependent on the host's ability to eliminate the infective agent, resolution of liver inflammation and prevention of infection by effective antibody production.

Symptoms in hepatitis may include:

- Prodrome of malaise
- Anorexia
- Nausea
- Vomiting
- Fever
- Tender hepatomegaly
- Splenomegaly
- Lymphadenopathy
- Rash
- Jaundice

Viruses are the commonest cause of acute infective hepatitis.

Causes of acute infective hepatitis

Viruses	Bacteria
Hepatotropic viruses	*Bartonella hensele/Quintana*
Hepatitis A	*Brucella melitensis*
Hepatitis B	*Legionella pneumophilia*
Hepatitis C	*Leptospira ictohaemorrhagica*
Hepatitis D	*Listeria monocytogenes*
Hepatitis E	*Mycobacterium tuberculosis*
Non-hepatotropic viruses	*Salmonella typhi*
Paramyxovirus (measles)	
Togavirus (rubella)	**Protozoa**
Enterovirus	*Toxoplasma gondii*
Echovirus	
Cosackievirus	
Flavivirus	**Helminths**
Marbug virus	Cestodes (tapeworms)
Ebola virus	*Echinococcus multilocularis*
Arenavirus (Lassa fever)	*Echinococcus granulosus*
Parvovirus B19	Nematodes (roundworms)
Adenovirus	*Ascaris lumbricoides*
Herpesvirus	*Toxocara canis*
Herpes simplex type 1	*Toxocara catis*
Herpes simplex type 2	Trematodes (flukes)
Varicella zoster virus	*Schistosoma mansoni*
Cytomegalovirus	*Schistosoma japonicum*
Epstein–Barr virus	*Fasciola hepatica*
Human herpes virus 6	

Hepatitis A infection

- Commonest form of acute viral hepatitis, accounting for 20–25% of all clinically apparent hepatitis world-wide
- Picornavirus family, RNA virus
- Orofaecal route of spread
- Incubation period 2–6 weeks
- Infectivity from faecal shedding begins during the prodromal phase, peaks at the onset of symptoms and then rapidly declines. Shedding may persist for up to 3 months
- Usually asymptomatic, less than 5% of infected people have an identifiable illness
- Symptomatic infection increases with age of acquisition
- Mortality is 0.2–0.4% of symptomatic cases and is increased in individuals > 50 or < 5 years
- Morbidity and mortality are associated with:
  - Fulminant hepatic failure
  - Prolonged cholestasis
  - Recurrent hepatitis
  - Extrahepatic complications
  - Neurological involvement — Guillain–Barré syndrome, transverse myelitis, postviral encephalitis, mononeuritis multiplex
  - Renal disease — Acute interstitial nephritis, mesangioproliferative glomerulonephritis, nephrotic syndrome, acute renal failure
  - Acute pancreatitis
  - Haematological disorders — autoimmune haemolytic anaemia, red cell aplasia, thrombocytopaenic purpura
- Non-specific elevation of conjugated bilirubin and aminotransferase enzymes. Degree of elevation does not correlate with severity of illness or likelihood of complications
- Confirmation of diagnosis relies on detection of:
  - Anti-HAV IgM — indicator of recent infection; peak levels occur during acute illness or early convalescent phase; persists for 4–6 months after infection
  - Anti-HAV IgG — appears early; peaks during convalescent phase; persists lifelong, conferring protection
- Supportive symptomatic treatment and adequate hydration. Complete recovery is usual within 3–6 months
- Active immunization with a formaldehyde-inactivated vaccine is available
- Passive immunization with human normal immunoglobulin offers up to 6 months of protection and is effective if given within 2–3 weeks of exposure

2.2 Drug induced liver disease

Most drugs are lipophilic and are detoxified and excreted in bile. This is achieved by oxidation or demethylation by the cytochrome P450 enzyme system or conjugated by glucuronidation or sulphation by specific transferases. Intermediate metabolites can be potentially harmful and may be detoxified by the binding of gluthathione, catalysed by gluthathione-S-transferase.

Mechanism of drug-induced liver disease
  - Direct hepatotoxicity — usually dose dependent

- Adverse drug reaction — unpredictable and idiosyncratic

Spectrum of drug-induced liver disease
- Enzyme induction without disease
- Acute hepatitis/hepatocellular necrosis (commonest) — acetaminophen, methyldopa, isoniazid, halothane, phenytoin
- Cholestasis — erythromycin, cotrimoxazole
- Granulomatous hepatitis — carbemazepine
- Drug-induced chronic hepatitis — methyldopa, nitrofurantion
- Fatty liver — microvesicular (aspirin, valproate, tetracycline) or macrovesicular (amiodarone)
- Fibrosis — methotrexate, vitamin A, actinomycin D
- Vascular disorders — sinusoidal dilatation (oestrogen) or veno-occlusive disease (6-mercaptopurine)
- Hepatic tumours — oral contraceptives

Diagnosis of drug-induced liver disease is usually based on circumstantial evidence and exclusion of other causes
Withdrawal of the causative drug is the most effective treatment
Specific therapy is available for paracetamol (*N*-acetylcysteine)

3. ACUTE LIVER FAILURE

Acute liver failure or fulminant hepatitis is rare in childhood. Mortality is 70% without appropriate management or liver transplantation. It is the indication for liver transplant in about 10–20% of paediatric recipients in major transplant centres. One-year survival rate is in the range of 60–70%.

It is a multisystemic disorder, defined as:

- Severe impairment of liver function (INR > 2 and unresponsive to vitamin K)
- ± encephalopathy (not essential to make diagnosis)
- Associated hepatocellular necrosis
- No previous underlying recognizable liver disease

The commonest causes of acute liver failure are:

In the neonate:
- Neonatal haemochromatosis
- Disseminated herpes simplex infection
- Haemophagocytic lymphohistiocytosis
- Metabolic causes

In the older child:
- Viral hepatitis
- Metabolic causes
- Acetaminophen toxicity
- Autoimmune hepatitis
- Wilson disease
- Idiopathic

Causes of acute liver failure

Infective

Viral

    Viral hepatitis — A, B, B + D, E

    Non-A–E hepatitis (seronegative hepatitis)

    Adenovirus, Epstein–Barr virus, cytomegalovirus

    Echovirus

    Varicella, measles viruses

    Yellow fever

    Rarely Lassa, Ebola, Marburg viruses, dengue virus, Toga virus

Bacterial

    Salmonellosis

    Tuberculosis

    Septicaemia

Others

    Malaria

    Bartonella

    Leptospirosis

Drugs

Acetaminophen

Halothane

Idiosyncratic reaction

Isoniazid

Non-steroidal anti-inflammatory drugs

Phenytoin

Sodium valproate

Carbamazepine

Ecstasy

Troglitazone

Antibiotics (penicillin, erythromycin, tetracyclines, sulphonamides, quinolones)

Allopurinol

Propylthiouracil

Amiodarone

Ketoconazole

Antiretroviral drugs

Synergistic drug interactions

Isoniazid + rifampicin

Trimethoprim + sulfamethoxazole

Barbiturates + acetaminophen

Amoxycillin + clavulinic acid

Toxins
Amanita phalloides (mushroom poisoning)
Herbal medicines
Carbon tetrachloride
Yellow phosphorus
Industrial solvents
Chlorobenzenes

Metabolic
Galactosaemia
Tyrosinaemia
Hereditary fructose intolerance
Neonatal haemochromatosis
Niemann–Pick disease type C
Wilson disease
Mitochondrial cytopathies
Congenital disorders of glycosylation
Acute fatty liver of pregnancy

Autoimmune
Type 1 autoimmune hepatitis
Type 2 autoimmune hepatitis
Giant cell hepatitis with Coombs-positive haemolytic anaemia

Vascular/Ischaemic
Budd–Chiari syndrome
Acute circulatory failure
Heat stroke
Acute cardiac failure
Cardiomyopathies

Infiltrative
Leukaemia
Lymphoma
Haemophagocytic lymphohistiocytosis

> **Causes of neonatal acute liver failure**
> Perinatal herpes simplex virus infection
> Neonatal haemochromatosis
> Galactosaemia
> Tyrosinaemia
> Haemophagocytic lymphohistiocytosis
> Septicaemia
> Mitochondrial cytopathies
> Congenital disorders of glycosylation
> Severe birth asphyxia

Biochemistry of acute liver failure

- ↑ prothrombin time (does not improve with parenteral vitamin K)
- ↑ direct and indirect bilirubin
- ↑ aminotransferase activities (AST), then ↓ as patient deteriorates
- ↑ serum ammonia

Complications of acute liver failure

- Encephalopathy
  - May be absent or difficult to recognize in children
  - Stage 1 — mild confusion/anxiety, disturbed or reversal of sleep rhythm, shortened attention span, slowing of ability to perform mental tasks (simple addition or subtraction). In young children, irritability, altered sleep pattern, unexplained bursts of excessive crying
  - Stage 2 — drowsiness, confusion, mood swings with personality changes, inappropriate behaviour, intermittent disorientation of time and place, gross deficit in ability to perform mental tasks. In young children, excessive sleepiness, inability to interact with or recognize parents, lack of interest in favourite toys or activities
  - Stage 3 — pronounced confusion, delirious but arousable, persistent disorientation of time and place, hyperreflexia with a positive Babinski sign
  - Stage 4 — comatose with or without decerebrate or decorticate posturing, response to pain present (stage 4a) or no response to pain (stage 4b)
- Renal insufficiency/failure
  - 10–15% have renal failure, 75% have renal insufficiency as a result of hepatorenal syndrome, direct kidney toxicity or acute tubular necrosis
  - 50% require haemodialysis or haemofiltration support
- Cardiovascular
  - Early hyperdynamic circulation with decreased peripheral vascular resistance
  - Late haemodynamic circulatory failure as a result of falling cardiac output, depression of brainstem function or cardiac arrythmias
- Pulmonary

- Aspiration, intrapulmonary shunting, atelectasis, infection, intrapulmonary haemorrhage, respiratory depression or pulmonary oedema
- Metabolic
  - Hypoglycaemia
  - Acid–base imbalance
    - Respiratory alkalosis, metabolic alkalosis and metabolic acidosis
  - Electrolyte imbalance
- Coagulopathy
  - ↓ synthesis of clotting factors
  - ↑ fibrinloysis and ↓ clearance of activated factors and fibrin degradation products
  - Thrombocytopenia (correlates with risk of haemorrhage)
- Infections
  - Poor host defences, poor respiratory effort, multiple invasive lines and tubes
- Others
  - Adrenal hyporesponsiveness, pancreatitis, aplastic anaemia

Management of acute liver failure involves management of complications, and elucidation and treatment of the cause.

- Discuss/refer to a liver centre
- No sedation unless patient is on assisted ventilation
- Ventilate for respiratory failure, agitation with grade I or II encephalopathy or severe encephalopathy (grade III or IV)
- No coagulation support unless bleeding or for invasive procedures
- Monitoring should involve
  - Continuous oxygen saturation monitoring
  - At least 6-hourly — neurological observations/vital signs (may need invasive monitoring)/urine output/blood glucose (maintain > 4 mmol/l)
  - At least 12-hourly — acid–base/electrolytes/PT/PTT, INR
  - Gastric pH (>5)
  - Daily or more often — haemoglobin and platelet count
- Fluid balance
  - 75% maintenance with 0.45% (or less) saline with dextrose
  - Maintain circulating volume with colloid, crystalloids or blood products as appropriate
  - Haemofiltration if there is renal failure
- Coagulation
  - Fresh frozen plasma when bleeding
  - Keep platelet count > 50 × 10^9/dL
- Drugs
  - H_2 blockers or proton pump inhibitors (prevent gastrointestinal bleed)
  - Lactulose to achieve two or three stools per day
  - N-acetylcysteine as experimental for non-paracetamol-induced acute liver failure
  - Intravenous broad-spectrum antibiotics and anti-fungals as prophylaxis

- Nutrition
  - Enteral feeding (1–2 g protein/kg per day)
  - Parenteral nutrition is rarely indicated
- Specific therapy
  - Acetaminophen toxicity — *N*-acetylcysteine (100 mg/kg per day)
  - Hereditary tyrosinaemia — NTBC
  - Neonatal haemochromatosis — iron chelation and antioxidant cocktail/*N*-acetylcysteine (100 mg/kg per day intravenous infusion)/selenium (3 µg/kg per day intravenous)/desferrioxamine (30 mg/kg per day intravenous)/prostaglandin E1 (0.4–0.6 µg/kg per hour intravenous)/vitamin E (25 U/kg per day intravenous/oral)
  - Mushroom poisoning — benzylpenicillin (1,000,000 U/kg per day) or thiotic acid (300 mg/kg per day)
  - Hepatic support with liver assist devices such as molecular adsorbent recirculating system (MARS) are still under investigation
  - Emergency liver transplantation

3.1 Paracetamol (acetaminophen) poisoning

- Mainly one large dose in a suicidal attempt, occasionally accidental over-ingestion over several days.
- Direct dose dependent hepatotoxic effect
- Metabolism

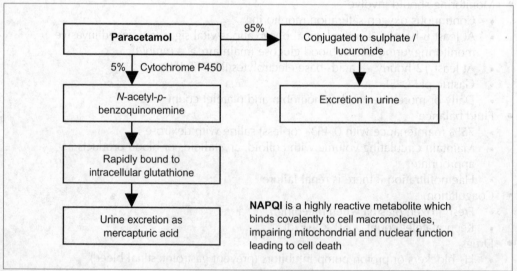

Metabolism of paracetamol

- With overdosage, gluthathione is depleted and NAPQI is not detoxified
- Acute ingestion of 150 mg/kg is likely to cause significant hepatotoxicity
- Triphasic clinical course
  - Stage 1 (0–24 h) — nausea, vomiting, anorexia
  - Stage 2 (24–48 h) — liver enlarged and tender from hepatic necrosis
  - Stage 3 (48–96 h) — acute liver failure
  - If patient survives stage 3, resolution of liver dysfunction within 4 days to 2 weeks
- Prognosis is bad if:
  - Arterial pH < 7.3
  - PTT > 100 s or INR > 6.6, creatinine > 300 mmol/l, grade III–IV encephalopathy (all three)
- Management
  - Discuss with a liver centre
  - N-acetylcysteine infusion 100 mg/kg per day until INR < 1.5

3.2   Wilson disease

An autosomal recessive disease with incidence of 1 in 50, 000; caused by a mutation of the *ATP7B* gene at 13q14.3 (commonest H1069Q).

Clinical presentation is as follows:

- Asymptomatic
  - Family screening
- Hepatic (5–12 years)
  - Insidious onset with vague symptoms followed by jaundice
  - Abnormal liver function tests
  - Acute hepatic failure
  - Acute hepatitis
  - Chronic liver disease
  - Cirrhosis and portal hypertension
- Neurological (second decade)
  - Deteriorating school/work performance
  - Mood/behaviour changes
  - Incoordination (e.g. deterioration of handwriting)
  - Resting and intention tremors
  - Dysarthria, excessive salivation
  - Dysphagia
  - Mask-like facies
- Others
  - Sunflower cataracts
  - Acute haemolytic anaemia
  - Renal, cardiac, skeletal abnormalities

Diagnosis is suggested by:
- ↓ plasma caeruloplasmin (< 200 mg/l)
- ↓ urinary copper
- > 5 µmol/24 h (baseline)
- > 25 µmol/24 h (after penicillamine challenge)
- ↑ liver copper concentration (> 250 µg/g dry weight of liver)
- Mutation analysis
- Kayser–Fleischer rings

Treatment
- Penicillamine 20 mg/kg per day (gradually increased from 5 mg/kg per day)
- Pyridoxine 10 mg/week
- Other drugs include: triethylene tetramine dihydrochloride (trientine), zinc sulphate/ acetate, tetrathiomolybelate
- Liver transplantation
  - fulminant hepatic failure
  - chronic, progression of hepatic dysfunction despite treatment

4. CHRONIC LIVER DISEASE AND END-STAGE LIVER FAILURE

Chronic liver diseases of childhood lead to cirrhosis and/or cholestasis. The resulting fibrosis and regenerative nodular formation distorts the liver architecture and compresses hepatic vascular and biliary structures, resulting in portal hypertension and a vicious cycle of events that worsen the hepatic injury.

Diagnostic considerations

Confirming the presence and type of liver disease
- Compensated — may be asymptomatic
- Decompensated — presence of liver synthetic failure and occurrence of complications
- End-stage — a persistent rise in bilirubin, prolongation of the INR > 1.3, persistent fall in serum albumin to < 35 g/l, faltering growth despite intensive nutritional support, severe hepatic complications such as chronic hepatic encephalopathy, refractory ascites, intractable pruritus, or recurrent variceal bleeding despite appropriate medical management

Determining aetiology
Assessing complications

Complications and management

Malnutrition and growth failure
- Specialized formula (↓Na ↑MCT (medium chain triglycerides))
- Supplement vitamins A, D, K, and E
- ↑ Caloric density of enteral feeds
- Continuous nocturnal nasogastric or nasojejunal feeds

- Parenteral nutritional support

Portal hypertension
- Major cause of morbidity and mortality (30–50%)
- Portal vein pressure > 5 mmHg or portal vein to hepatic vein gradient > 10 mmHg
    - splenomegaly → hypersplenism
    - oesophageal, gastric and rectal varices
    - ascites
    - encephalopathy
- Prevention and management of oesophageal variceal bleeding
    - sclerotherapy
    - variceal ligation
    - surgical porto-systemic shunts
    - transjugular intrahepatic porto-systemic shunt (TIPS)
    - oesophageal transection and devascularization
    - pharmacotherapy, e.g. propanolol
- Factors that predict bleeding
    - portal vein–hepatic vein gradient > 12 mmHg
    - large, tense varices
    - red wale marks, red spots on varices
    - severity of underlying liver disease

Ascites
- 50% of patients will die within 2 years of developing ascites
- Treatment
    - Step 1 — sodium restriction (1–2 mmol/kg per day)
    - Step 2 — spironolactone
    - Step 3 — ± chlorthiazide/frusemide and fluid restriction
- Spontaneous bacterial peritonitis can occur insidiously and causes high mortality

Coagulopathy
- Vitamin K malabsorption/deficiency
- Vitamin K-dependent coagulation protein deficiencies (factors II, VII, IX and X)
- Hypofibrinogenaemia and dysfibrinogenaemia
- Thrombocytopenia
- Consumption coagulopathy
- Parenteral vitamin K and transfusion of fresh frozen plasma (prothrombin time > 40 s) or platelets (< 40×10^9/l)

Hepatopulmonary syndrome
- Triad of:
    - Liver dysfunction
    - Intrapulmonary arteriovenous shunts
    - Arterial hypoxaemia — arterial oxygen pressure of < 70 mmHg in room air and an alveolar/arterial gradient of > 20 mmHg
- Type 1 — functional shunt
- Type 2 — anatomical
- Should be suspected if there is increasing history of breathlessness, cyanosis, clubbing and platypnoea
- Site and extent of shunt is assessed by:

- arterial blood gas analysis
- technetium 99m-labelled macroaggregated albumin (^{99m}Tc MAA) study
- contrast echocardiogram
- Definitive treatment is with liver transplantation

Portopulmonary hypertension

- Mean pulmonary artery pressure > 25 mmHg, pulmonary capillary wedge pressure of < 15 mmHg in the absence of any secondary causes of pulmonary hypertension

---

Comparison of hepatopulmonary syndrome and portopulmonary hypertension

Hepatopulmonary syndrome	**Portopulmonary hypertension**
Intrapulmonary vasodilatation	Intrapulmonary vasoconstriction
Alveolar arterial gradient > 20 mmHg	Alveolar arterial gradient usually normal
Normal mean pulmonary artery pressure	Mean pulmonary artery pressure > 25 mmHg
Perform shunt fraction study	Perform right heart catheterization
Trial of 100% O_2	Vasodilator therapy trial
Often reversible with liver transplantation	May not reverse with liver transplant
Poor prognosis: pAO$_2$ < 300 mmHg on 100% O_2 > 45 mmHg	Poor prognosis: pulmonary artery pressure
Histology: pulmonary artery normal	Histology: pulmonary artery abnormal; concentric medial hypertrophy

---

Hepatorenal syndrome

- Diagnostic criteria
  - oliguria: urine output < 1 ml/kg per day
  - fractorial excretion sodium < 1%
  - urine-to-plasma creatinine ratio < 10
  - ↓ glomerular filtration rate, ↑ creatinine
  - absence of hypovolemia
  - other kidney pathology excluded
- Type 1 rapidly progressive with poor prognosis
- Type 2 less precipitous loss of renal function
- Mortality of > 90% with severe liver disease
- Reversed with liver transplantation

Causes of chronic liver disease in children

Onset in infancy
Structural
  Extrahepatic biliary atresia
  Alagille syndrome, biliary hypoplasia
  Choledochal cyst, tumours, stones
Storage/metabolic diseases
  Carbohydrate defects
      galactosaemia, fructosaemia, glycogen storage III and IV
  Amino acid defects
      tyrosinaemia, urea cycle disorders
  Metal storage defects
  Lipid storage diseases
      Gaucher disease, Niemann–Pick type C
  Fatty acid oxidation defects
  Peroxisomal disorders
  Zellweger syndrome
  Mitochondrial disorders
  Progressive familiar intrahepatic cholestasis syndrome
  Total parenteral nutrition-associated cholestasis
  Cystic fibrosis liver disease
Haematological
  Langerhans cell histiocytosis
Infection/inflammation
  Neonatal hepatitis
  Hepatitis B and hepatitis C

Onset in childhood
All of the above and
Autoimmune liver disease
  Autoimmune hepatitis
  Autoimmune sclerosing cholangitis
Sclerosing cholangitis
Drugs/toxins (e.g. chemotherapy-induced veno-occlusive disease)
Fibropolycystic disorders
Chronic hepatic venous outflow obstruction
  Hepatic vein thrombosis
  Budd–Chiari syndrome
  Veno-occlusive disease
  Cardiac cirrhosis

4.1 Autoimmune hepatitis

Autoimmune hepatitis has a 75% female preponderance. Other autoimmune disorders are present in 20% and 40% of first-degree relatives may also have autoimmune disease.

Clinical presentation is variable:

- Acute hepatitis
- Insidious onset
- Portal hypertension

Diagnostic criteria are based on:

- Serum non-organ-specific autoantibodies
- Type 1
  - Anti-nuclear antibody (ANA)
  - Anti-smooth muscle antibody (SMA)
- Type 2
  - Anti-liver-kidney microsomal (LKM-1)
  - Up to 20% may not have antibodies detectable at presentation
- Serum biochemistry
  - ↑ Aminotransferases
- Serum IgG
  - > 1.5× normal
- Liver histology
- Absence of
  - Markers of viral infection and metabolic disease
  - Excessive alcohol consumption
  - Use of hepatotoxic drugs

Treatment involves:

- Corticosteroids
- Azathioprine for poor response or as steroid sparing
- Liver transplant for fulminant hepatic failure or failure of medical therapy

Response to therapy (International Autoimmune Hepatitis Group) is defined as follows:

- Marked improvement of symptoms and return of serum AST/ALT, bilirubin and immunoglobulin levels to completely normal within 1 year and sustained for at least a further 6 months on maintenance therapy

  ±

- Liver biopsy specimen during this period showing minimal activity

  OR

- Marked improvement of symptoms together with at least 50% improvement of all liver test results during the first month of treatment, with AST/ALT levels continuing to fall to less than twice the upper limit of normal within 6 months during any reduction towards maintenance therapy

±
- Liver biopsy within 1 year showing minimal activity

Relapses are common (occurring in 40%).

IgG levels and autoantibody titres correlate with disease activity.

4.2 Chronic viral hepatitis

Hepatitis B and C viruses (HBV and HCV) are the top causative agents

Hepatitis B (a DNA hepadnavirus)

- World-wide prevalence of 5% (chronic carriers)
- Transmission
  - Perinatal — HbeAg-positive mothers have a 70–90% risk of transmission to their offspring
  - Horizontal — parenteral, sexual and environmental transmission
- Symptomatic acute hepatitis
  - Complete resolution occurs in 90%
  - Lifelong immunity
- Asymptomatic chronic infection (HbsAg-positive for at least 6 months)
  - 90% progress to chronic liver disease
  - Three stages — immune tolerance; immune clearance; and residual non-replicative infection
- Chronic infection may lead to cirrhosis and hepatocellular carcinoma

Serological markers of HBV

Host HBV status	ALT	HBV DNA	cAb	sAg	sAb	*eAg	eAb
Acute	↑	Detectable	IgM then IgG	+	–	+	–
Chronic							
Immune tolerance	N	High	IgG	+	–	+	–
Immune clearance	↑	Detectable	IgG	+	–	+	–
Non-replicative	N	Undetectable	IgG	+	–	–	+
Resolved	N	Undetectable	IgG	–	+	–	+

*eAg is absent in pre-core mutant.

Immunization

Maternal status			Anti–HBV	HBV vaccine
sAg	eAg	eAb	immunoglobulin 200 IU within 12 h	3 doses within 12 h, and at 1 and 6 months
+	+	–	Y	Y
+	–	+	N	Y
+	–	–	Y	Y

Treatment
- Immunomodulation — interferon-α, pegylated interferon
- Antivirals — lamivudine, famciclovir, adefovir
- Not much paediatric experience
- 50% of patients seroconvert with therapy (adult data)
- Liver transplantation for fulminant HBV disease, chronic liver disease, hepatocellular carcinoma

Hepatitis C infection (an RNA flavivirus)

- World-wide prevalence is 3%
- Transmission
  - From blood transfusion or plasma-pooled products
  - Vertical transmission (rare)
- Usually asymptomatic but leads to cirrhosis over years
- One of the commonest indications for liver transplant in adults
- Serology
  - Anti-HCV antibody positive
  - HCV RNA positive in two consecutive samples
- Treatment
  - Interferon-α monotherapy
  - Interferon-α/ribavarin combination therapy
  - Paediatric experience is minimal
  - 70% of patients seroconvert with therapy (adult data)

4.3 Liver transplantation

Indications for transplant
- Acute liver failure
- Decompensated chronic liver disease
- Liver-based metabolic diseases
- Liver tumours

Relative contraindications
- Severe systemic sepsis
- Malignant hepatic tumours with extrahepatic involvement

- Severe, irreversible extrahepatic disease (e.g. structural brain damage, severe cardiopulmonary disease not correctable with surgery)
- Severe systemic oxalosis with cardiac involvement (haemodynamic instability)
- Mitochondrial cytopathies with multisystem involvement
- Giant cell hepatitis with Coomb's positive haemolytic syndrome

Source of organ
- Deceased donor
- Living related donor

Type of graft
- Whole liver
- Segmental graft

Procedure
- Orthotopic
- Auxiliary

Lifelong immunosuppression is required
- Calcineurin inhibitors
  - Ciclosporine
  - Tacrolimus
- Renal sparing drugs
  - Mammalian target of rapamycin (mTOR) inhibitor
  - Sirolimus (mTOR inhibitor)
  - Mycophenolate mofetil
  - Azathiaprine
  - Interleukin-2 receptor antibodies — basiliximab, daclizumab
  - Others — anti-thymocyte globulin, OKT3
- Steroids

Post-operative complications
- Early
  - Graft failure (primary non-function)
  - Surgical (intra-abdominal haemorrhage, hepatic artery thrombosis, portal vein thrombosis
  - Drug side-effects (renal failure, hyperglycaemia, hypertension)
- After 1st week
  - Acute rejection
  - Biliary leaks and strictures
  - Persistent wound drainage
  - Sepsis
- Late
  - Epstein–Barr virus infection
  - Side-effects of immunosuppression (renal failure, hyperglycaemia, hyperlipi-daemia)
  - Post-transplant lymphoproliferative disease
  - Graft rejection
  - Late biliary strictures, hepatic artery thrombosis or portal vein thrombosis

- Recurrent disease (HBV infection, malignant hepatic tumours)
- De novo autoimmune hepatitis

Patient survival:

- 1-year — 80–90%
- 5-year — 70–80%
- 10-year — 70–75%

5. PORTAL HYPERTENSION

The portal vein contributes to two-thirds of the liver's blood supply. Portal venous pressure is a product of blood flow from the splanchnic circulation and vascular resistance within the liver.

- Portal hypertension is defined as a portal vein pressure > 5 mmHg or portal vein to hepatic vein gradient > 10 mmHg
- A rise in portal pressure leads to splenomegaly and development of portosystemic collaterals and varices
- A gradient of > 12 mmHg is associated with the development of oesophageal varices. The junction between the mucosal and submucosal varices in the lower 2–5 cm of the oesophagus is the usual site of variceal bleeding
- Not all portal hypertension is a result of intrinsic liver disease although chronic liver disease is the commonest overall cause. Portal vein occlusion is the most frequent extrahepatic cause of portal hypertension

Causes of portal hypertension

Pre-hepatic (portal vein occlusion)
General factors
    Developmental malformation
    Septicaemia
    Thrombophilia
        Myeloproliferative disorders
        Paroxysmal nocturnal haemoglobinuria
        Protein C deficiency
        Protein S deficiency
        Antithrombin III deficiency
        Factor V Lieden mutation
        Anti-phospholipid antibodies
        Factor II gene mutation (G20210A)
        Homocysteinaemia

Local factors
    Umbilical sepsis, catheterization, infusion of irritant solutions
    Intra-abdominal sepsis and portal pyaemia
    Abdominal trauma
    Structural lesions
    Cholangitis/choledochal cyst
    Pancreatitis
    Malignant disease/lymphadenopathy
    Splenectomy

Intrahepatic
Pre-sinusoidal
    Hepatoportal sclerosis
    Neoplasia
    Hepatic cyst
Sinusoidal
    Chronic liver disease and congenital hepatic fibrosis
Post-sinusoidal
    Veno-occlusive disease

Post-hepatic
Budd–Chiari syndrome
Chronic constrictive pericarditis
Right ventricular failure

- Presentation is typically with acute gastrointestinal haemorrhage, splenomegaly or as part of the manifestation of chronic liver disease
- In long-standing disease, varices around the common bile duct may cause portal hypertensive biliopathy resulting in bile duct dilatation and obstructive jaundice
- Rarely, pulmonary hypertension may coexist with portal hypertension, more often in children with chronic liver disease
- Anaemia, leukopenia and thrombocytopenia may result from hypersplenism
- Management
    - Portal hypertension associated with chronic liver disease
        - variceal banding or sclerotherapy
        - liver transplantation if variceal bleeding is uncontrolled with therapy
    - Extrahepatic portal hypertension
        - variceal banding or sclerotherapy
        - portocaval or mesoportal shunt
    - Pharmacotherapy is not proven in children

6. LIVER FUNCTION TEST

This reflects the severity of liver dysfunction but rarely provides diagnostic information on individual diseases.

Bilirubin

- Conjugated (direct) hyperbilirubinaemia
  - Specific to liver disease
  - Conjugated fraction > 20% of total bilirubin is indicative of hepatic dysfunction
- Unconjugated (indirect) hyperbilirubinaemia
- Normal bilirubin levels does not exclude liver cirrhosis

Aminotransferases

- Aspartate aminotransferase (AST) and alanine aminotransferase (ALT)
- Most common tests of liver cell dysfunction
- Intracellular enzymes
- Indicate hepatic necrosis
- AST is produced in the cytosol and mitochondria of the liver, heart, skeletal muscle, kidney, pancreas and red cells
- ALT is found in the cytosol of liver and muscle cells and so is more liver specific
- In isolated AST or ALT elevations, a normal creatine kinase level is helpful in ruling out muscle pathologies
- ALT : AST ratio > 1 is suggestive of fibrosis in some liver pathologies like steatohepatitis and chronic hepatitis C
- There is no correlation between the enzyme levels and the severity of disease
- Levels may be normal in compensated cirrhosis or end-stage liver disease

Alkaline phosphatase (ALP)

- Found in liver, kidney, bone, placenta and intestine
- Reflects biliary epithelial damage
- Children have higher ALP levels than adults (bone isoenzyme)
- Levels are low in zinc deficiency

Gamma-glutamyl transferase (GGT)

- Present in biliary epithelia, hepatocytes, renal tubules, pancreas, brain, breast and small intestine
- Reference range is age related. Normal levels in newborns are five to eight times higher than those of adults but reach adult values by 9 months
- Most sensitive test for hepatobiliary disease but cannot differentiate between extra- or intrahepatic biliary disease
- May be normal in familial intrahepatic cholestasis, bile acid synthesis disorders, ARC syndrome (arthrogryposis, renal and cholestasis) and very advanced liver disease

Albumin concentration

- Reflects the synthetic capacity of the liver
- Produced in the liver
- Long half-life, so is not decreased in acute liver injury
- Levels < 35 g/dl in chronic liver disease suggest decompensation

Prothrombin time (PT)

- Prolongation of PT > 3 s above normal or INR > 1.3 may indicate vitamin K deficiency
- Failure of INR to normalize after a parenteral dose of vitamin K (1 mg/year of age up to a maximum of 5 mg) suggests liver failure
- Reflects the decreased synthesis of factor VII and IX which have short half-lives
- Useful in monitoring progress of acute liver failure

Causes of hepatosplenomegaly

Cirrhosis (early)	biliary atresia, sclerosing cholangitis, congenital hepatic fibrosis
Haematological	thalassaemia, spherocytosis, sickle cell anaemia
Infection	infectious mononucleosis, TORCH, malaria, septicaemia
Immune	juvenile rheumatoid arthritis, systemic lupus erythematosus, immunodeficiency states
Metabolic	α1-antitrypsin deficiency, tyrosinaemia, cystic fibrosis
Proliferative	leukaemia, lymphoma, Langerhans cell histiocytosis
Storage diseases	Gaucher (long-term), Niemann–Pick, mucopolysaccharidoses

Causes of hepatomegaly — SHIRT

S — Structural

Extrahepatic biliary atresia, choledochol cyst, intrahepatic biliary hypoplasia, polycystic disease, congenital hepatic fibrosis

Storage/metabolic

Defective lipid metabolism — Gaucher disease, Niemann–Pick disease, hyperlipoproteinaemias, cholesteryl ester storage disease, carnitine deficiency, mucolipidoses
Defective carbohydrate metabolism — diabetes mellitus, glycosyltransferase deficiency (types 1, 3, 4 and 6), hereditary fructose intolerance, galactosaemia, Cushing syndrome, mucopolysaccharidoses
Defective amino acid/protein metabolism — tyrosinaemia (type 1), urea cycle enzyme disorders
Defective mineral metabolism — Wilson disease, juvenile haemochromatosis
Defective electrolyte transport — cystic fibrosis
Defective nutrition — protein calorie malnutrition, total parenteral nutrition
Deficiency of protease — α1-antitrypsin deficiency
Defective bile flow — progressive familial intrahepatic cholestasis syndrome

H — Haematological

Thalassaemia, sickle cell disease (chronic haemolysis and transfusion haemosiderosis), acute lymphoblastic, acute myeloid and chronic myelocytic leukaemias.

Heart/vascular

Congestive cardiac failure, constrictive pericarditis, obstructed inferior vena cava, Budd–Chiari syndrome

I — Infection

Viral infection — congenital rubella, CMV infection, coxsackievirus, echovirus, hepatitis A, B, C, D and E viruses, infectious mononucleosis

Bacterial infections — neonatal septicaemia, *Escherichia coli* urinary tract infection, tuberculosis, syphilis

Parasitic infections — hydatid disease, malaria, schistosomiasis, toxoplasmosis, visceral larva migrans

Fungal infection — coccidiomycosis

Inflammatory

Autoimmune liver disease

Inflammatory bowel disease associated liver disease

R — Reticuloendothelial

Non-Hodgkin lymphoma, Hodgkin disease, Langerhans cell histiocytosis

Rheumatological

Systemic juvenile chronic arthritis, systemic lupus erythematosus

T — Tumour/hamartoma

Primary hepatic neoplasms — hepatoblastomas, hepatocellular carcinoma (hepatoma)
Secondary deposits — neuroblastoma, Wilm's tumour, gonadal tumours
Vascular malformation/benign neoplasm — infantile haemangioendothelioma, cavernous haemangioma

Trauma

Hepatic haematoma

7. THE PANCREAS

7.1 Acute pancreatitis

- Defined clinically as the sudden onset of abdominal pain associated with a rise in amylase or lipase of at least three times the upper limit in the blood or urine
- Rare in children
- Involves premature activation of trypsinogen
- Presents with epigastric or back pain. May have prominent nausea and vomiting. Less commonly there may be fever, tachycardia, hypotension, jaundice, and abdominal signs such as guarding, rebound tenderness and a decrease in bowel sounds

Causes of acute pancreatitis
Idiopathic
Pancreatitis associated with systemic illness
Trauma
Structural abnormalities of pancreas, pancreatic or common bile duct
Medications (valproate, L-asparaginase, prednisolone, azathioprine, 6-mercaptopurine, frusemide, phenytoin)
Infections (mainly viral, e.g. mumps, enterovirus, Epstein–Barr virus, hepatitis A, CMV, rubella, cosackievirus, rubeola, measles, influenza)
Gallstones
Familial (*PRSS1*, *SPINK1* or *CFTR* mutation)
Post-endoscopic retrograde cholangiopancreatography
Metabolic
    Diabetic ketoacidosis
    Hypercalcaemia
    Hypertriglyceridaemia
Cystic fibrosis

- Recurrent acute pancreatitis is seen in 10% of children after a first episode of acute pancreatitis and is commonly associated with structural abnormalities, idiopathic or familial pancreatitis
- Commonest cause of familial pancreatitis
  - Mutations in cationic trypsinogen gene (e.g. *PRSS1*) enhance trypsin activation
  - Mutations in the *SPINK1* (serine protease inhibitor Kazal type 1) gene result in an abnormal pancreatic secretory trypsin inhibitor
  - Mutations of the *CFTR* (cystic fibrosis transmembrane conductance regulator) gene, which reduces the pancreatic fluid secretion capacity, increase the risk of keeping activated trypsin in the pancreas for a longer period of time
- The mainstay of current treatment is analgesia, intravenous fluids, pancreatic rest, and monitoring for complications
- Acute pancreatitis scoring system for children that predicts severity of disease and mortality include the following parameters
  - Age (< 7 years)
  - Weight (< 23 kg)
  - Admission white blood cell count ($> 18.5 \times 10^9$/litre)
  - Admission lactate dehydrogenase (> 2000 IU/litre)
  - 48-hour fluid sequestration (> 75 m/kg per 48 h)
  - 48-hour rise in urea (> 5 mg/dl)
  - Each criterion is assigned a value of 1 point, cumulative score predicts the outcome of patients
  - 0 to 2 points — 8.6% severe, 1.4% death
  - 2 to 4 points — 38.5% severe, 5.8% death
  - 5 to 7 points — 80% severe, 10% death
- Surgical management is limited to debridment of infected necrotic pancreas or cholecystectomy or endoscopic sphincterotomy in the presence of gallstones

- Antibiotics are usually not necessary unless in severe pancreatic necrosis
- Octreotide infusions may reduce pancreatic secretions in those with pancreatic fluid sequestration

Complications of pancreatitis

Local	Systemic
Oedema	Shock
Inflammation	Pulmonary oedema
Fat necrosis	Pleural effusions
Phlegmon	Acute renal failure, coagulopathy
Pancreatic necrosis	Haemoconcentration
Sterile	Bacteraemia, sepsis
Infected	Distant fat necrosis
Abscess	Vascular leak syndrome
Haemorrhage	Multiorgan system failure
Fluid collections	Hypermetabolic state
Pseudocysts	Hypocalcaemia
Duct rupture and strictures	Hyperglycaemia
Extension to nearby organs	

7.2 Chronic pancreatitis

- Defined as a complex process beginning with acute pancreatitis and progressing to end-stage fibrosis as the result of recurrent and chronic inflammatory processes
- It is the final common pathologic pathway of a variety of pancreatic disorders
- Usually associated with genetic conditions like cystic fibrosis or hereditary pancreatitis or is idiopathic
- Cystic fibrosis is the most important cause of chronic pancreatitis in children. *CFTR* mutation-associated pancreatitis can be divided into four mechanistic subtypes, where $CFTR_{sev}$ is severe CFTR mutation phenotype and $CFTR_{m-v}$ is mild or variable *CFTR* mutation phenotype
  - Type 1 — $CFTR_{sev}/CFTR_{sev}$ genotype
  - Type 2 — $CFTR_{sev}/CFTR_{m-v}$ genotype
  - Type 3 — $CFTR_{sev}$ or $CFTR_{m-v}$ plus a second pancreatitis modifier or susceptibility gene (e.g. $CFTR_{sev}/SPINK1$)
  - Type 4 — $CFTR_{sev}$ or $CFTR_{m-v}$ plus a strong environmental risk factor such as alcohol
- Pancreatic insufficiency is a sign of chronic pancreatitis but is not diagnostic. The pancreas has marked functional reserve and has to be severely damaged before functional loss can be clinically recognized
- Faecal elastase < 150 µg/g is quite specific for exocrine pancreas insufficiency
- Invasive pancreatic stimulation tests are the standard for assessment of pancreatic insufficiency but are not usually indicated

- Chronic pancreatitis with calcifications can be identified on abdominal radiography or by transabdominal ultrasonography. When present, the diagnosis of chronic pancreatitis can be made with 90% confidence
- Other abdominal imaging methods used include computed tomography, endoscopic retrograde cholangiopancreatogram, endoscopic ultrasonography, and magnetic resonance imaging or MRCP (magnetic resonance cholangio pancreatography)
- Genetic testing for *PRSS1*, *SPINK1*, *CFTR* and other mutations can be performed if there is history of recurrent acute pancreatitis, unexplained chronic pancreatitis or presence of a positive family history of hereditary pancreatitis

8. FURTHER READING

American Academy of Pediatrics. 2004. Management of hyperbilirubinemia in the newborn infant 35 or more weeks of gestation. American Academy of Pediatrics clinical practice guidelines. *Pediatrics*; 114:1, 297–316.

Decker BC. 2004. *Pediatric Gastrointestinal Disease*, 4th edn. Ontario, Canada: BC Decker Inc.

Dhawan A, Cheeseman P, Mieli-Vergani G. 2004. Approaches to acute liver failure in children. *Pediatric Transplantation* 8, 584–588.

Kelly, D (Ed). 2004. *Diseases of the Liver and Biliary System in Children*, 2nd edition. Oxford: Blackwell Publishing.

North American Society for Pediatric Gastroenterology, Hepatology and Nutrition 2004. Guideline for the evaluation of cholestatic jaundice in infants: recommendations of the North American Society for Pediatric Gastroenterology, Hepatology and Nutrition. *Journal of Paediatric Gastroenterology and Nutrition* 39, 115–128.

Chapter 13

Immunology

Waseem Qasim and Bobby Gaspar

CONTENTS

Immunology

1. INTRODUCTION

Immunity against specific infectious agents is brought about by a complicated set of interactions between host and pathogen which, under normal circumstances, maintains an adequate balance between the two. From early in life humans come into contact with a wide variety of infectious agents including bacteria, fungi and viruses. Some of these become commensals, some cause troublesome infections in the neonatal period, some are pathogenic throughout childhood, while others remain significant pathogens throughout life. Increased susceptibility to infectious diseases occurs in individuals with a wide variety of abnormalities including anatomical, metabolic, haematological, oncological and immunological abnormalities.

The immune system can be divided into specific and non-specific components. Non-specific immunity refers to the first-line of defence against pathogens which, if breached, leads to the specific or adaptive immune response being activated. This first-line of defence consists of a variety of components including mechanical barriers (e.g. skin), secretions (e.g. tears), mucus in the respiratory tract and gut, bile and enzymes in the gastrointestinal tract, acidity of urine and gastric acid fluid and the normal commensals of the skin and gut which prevent colonization with pathogenic organisms. Second-line, non-specific mechanisms include complement components which bind to phagocytic receptors found on cells, and particularly neutrophils and macrophages, which may interact with antigens in a non-specific way.

Specific immunity is divided into humoral and cellular responses. Humoral immunity refers to the production of antibody specific for an invading pathogen or antigen, while cellular immunity is mediated via cells of the immune system. Lymphocytes are central to both arms of the specific immune system. B lymphocytes produce antibodies and present antigens to T lymphocytes. T lymphocytes themselves may act as cytotoxic cells killing virally infected cells, or as helper cells providing help or suppression to other cells involved or recruited into the specific immune response.

The crucial difference between the specific and non-specific arms of the immune system is the ability of the specific arm to develop memory. This immunological memory allows the rapid mobilization of specific immune mechanisms on the second and subsequent challenges with a particular antigen such as a virus. This response may be mediated via the humoral (antibody) or cellular (T-cell) system. Either way, the consequence of memory is the protection from recurrent infection with the same antigen. Memory is learnt during the development of the immune system and explains the difference in frequency between infections in adults and children.

The immune system is a complicated structure/organ made up of many parts that have, with time, evolved and become increasingly sophisticated. Different aspects of the immune system are discussed below.

2. THE IMMUNE SYSTEM

2.1 Haematopoietic stem cells

- Multipotent cells capable of giving rise to the entire haematopoietic system
- Capable of self-renewal
- Characterized by the presence of CD34 surface antigen
- CD34 does not identify stem cells alone but also more committed progenitor cells
- Present at 1% in the bone marrow
- Found at very low frequency in the periphery but can be mobilized into periphery by the use of granulocyte colony-stimulating factor (G-CSF)
- Can be selected, purified and used in bone marrow transplantation

2.2 T- and B-cell development

Both T and B lymphocytes arise from a common lymphoid progenitor cell.

- B-cell development occurs predominantly in the bone marrow
- B-cell development requires a functional pre-B-cell and B-cell receptor
- *VDJ* (variable, diversity and joining) immunoglobulin gene rearrangement is necessary for functional receptor complexes to be assembled
- Immature B cells migrate to the periphery
- On meeting antigen, B-cell receptors then undergo antigen-mediated somatic hypermutation to develop high-affinity immunoglobulin receptors
- Cells develop into antibody-secreting plasma cells or become memory cells ready for further antigenic encounter
- T-cell development occurs in the thymus
- Early pro-thymocytes express both CD4 **and** CD8 markers (double-positive cells)
- During thymopoiesis cells rearrange the T-cell receptor (TCR) by VDJ recombination as for B cells
- Thymic epithelium expresses self-antigen, allowing elimination of T cells bearing receptors that recognize self
- Single positive CD4+ or CD8+ cells exit the thymus
- T cells recognize antigen presented by professional antigen-presenting cells

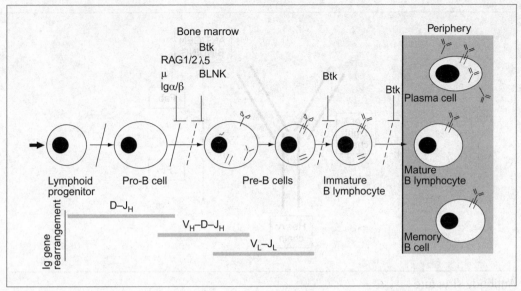

B-cell development

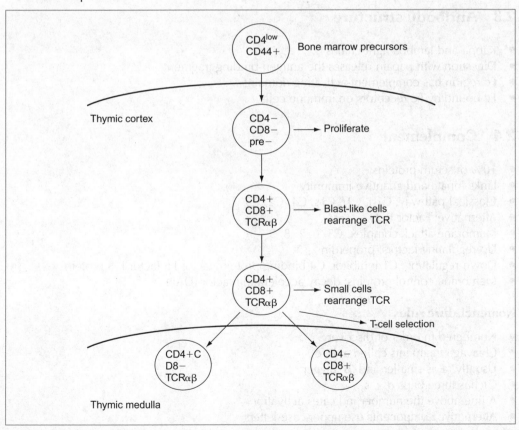

T-cell development

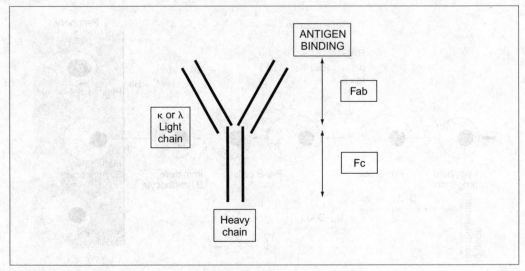

Antibody structure

2.3 Antibody structure

- Kappa and lambda light chains
- Digestion with papain releases the antigen-binding fragment
- Fc region has complement-activating domains
- Fc bound by Fc receptors on immune cells

2.4 Complement

- 10% of serum proteins
- Links innate and adaptive immunity
- Classical pathway: C1q, C1r, C1s, C4, C2, C3
- Alternative: Factor B, D
- Membrane attack complex: C5, 6, 7, 8, 9
- Up-regulating factors: properdin
- Down-regulating: C1 inhibitor, C4 binding protein, factor H, factor I, S protein
- Membrane control proteins: decay accelerating factor (DAF)

Nomenclature rules

- Numbered in order of discovery
- Cleavage fragments called a, b, c
- Usually 'a' is smaller and 'b' bigger
- C1 has three parts q, r, s
- A line above the number indicates activation
- Alternative components use upper-case letters

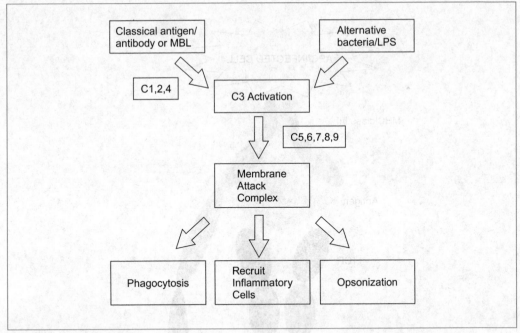

Complement pathway

2.5   Recognition of antigens

Substances that induce an immune response are called **antigens**. The specific region of an antigen that is recognized by an immune receptor is termed an **epitope**. Antibody and antigen binding is non-covalent and is dependent on complementary molecular structures. The strength of this interaction defines antibody **affinity**, and the likelihood of cross-reactivity with similar epitopes on alternative antigens dictates the antibody **specificity**.

TCR recognize short linear peptides when they are presented in association with major histocompatibility complex (MHC) molecules on the surface of antigen-presenting cells. The α T-cell receptor on **helper** T cells uses the CD4 co-receptor to interact with the MHC class II and peptide complex. **Cytotoxic** T cells use the CD8 co-receptor to stabilize interactions with peptide presented by MHC class I molecules.

Professional antigen-presenting cells, such as dendritic cells, ingest and degrade proteins by endocytosis, and have the intracellular machinery to load short peptide sequences into the groove between the two chains of MHC class II molecules before expressing the complex on their surface.

Most cells employ proteosomes to degrade proteins and traffic selected peptides into the endoplasmic reticulum to be loaded onto class I MHC molecules. The process relies on transporter molecules encoded by the *TAPI* and *TAPII* genes, and mutations of these genes leading to immunodeficiency have been described.

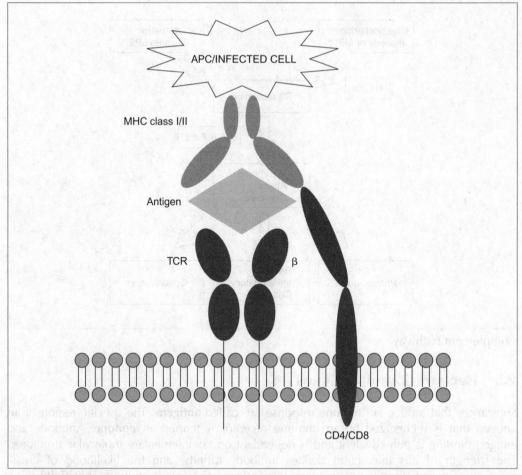

MHC class I/II

Antigen

TCR β

APC/INFECTED CELL

CD4/CD8

Antigen presentation

A number of polysaccharide and polymerized flagellin antigens carry numerous repeating epitopes that can stimulate B cells without assistance from T cells (**T-independent**). They usually give rise to low-affinity immunoglobulin M (IgM) antibodies because of limited class-switching potential, and do not generate memory B cells. Most antigens are **T-dependent** because B cells process and present the antigen to CD4 T cells in association with MHC class II molecules. Once activated, T cells express the CD40 ligand on their surface, which in turn binds CD40 on the B cell, and induces processes of somatic hypermutation and immunoglobulin class switching. Defects of CD40 ligand result in immunodeficiency associated with increased serum levels of IgM.

2.6 Cytokines

Cytokines are soluble factors that mediate signalling between immune cells. They may act in an autocrine, paracrine or endocrine manner.

Cytokine	Origin	Action
Interleukin-1 (IL-1)	Macrophages	Fever, cachexia, angiogenesis; activates immune cells
IL-2	T_{H1} cells	Proliferation Immune cell activation
IL-4	T_{H2} cells	B-cell class-switching Proliferation
IL-5	T_{H2}	IgA class-switching Proliferation
IL-10	T_{H2} cells, macrophages	Inhibits T_{H1} cells
IL-12	T_{H1} B cells, macrophages	Promotes cytotoxicity
IL-15	Natural killer (NK) cells	NK growth and survival
Tumour necrosis factor-α	Macrophages, T cells, B cells, Kupffer cells, astrocytes	Inflammation; Role in rheumatoid arthritis, Crohn disease, multiple sclerosis; activates macrophages and other immune cells. Cytotoxic for tumours; sometimes promotes tumour growth; angiogenesis
Interferon-γ	T cells and NK cells	Antiviral

3. INVESTIGATION OF A CHILD WITH PRIMARY IMMUNODEFICIENCY

The usual rules of careful history taking, examination and logical investigations apply.

3.1 History

- Recurrent infections at different sites
- Regular courses of antibiotics
- Infections at multiple sites or infections that persist and do not clear easily with antibiotics
- Infection with atypical or unusual organisms
- Prolonged separation of the umbilical cord may be linked to leukocyte adhesion deficiency (LAD)
- Family history of early infant deaths; take careful X-linked history because a number of conditions are X-linked
- Consanguineous family history

3.2 Examination

- Faltering growth and falling off centile charts after 4–6 months (i.e. after protection from maternal immunoglobulin has waned)
- Absence of lymphoid tissue, especially tonsils and lymph nodes
- Dysmorphism (e.g. Di George syndrome)
- Eczema +/− petechiae in Wiskott–Aldrich syndrome
- Evidence of chronic organ disease (e.g. in lungs or liver)
- Evidence of scar tissue or granuloma formation may be indicative of LAD or chronic granulomatous disease (CGD)
- Gingivitis is associated with LAD
- Ataxic gait and evidence of telangiectasia

3.3 Investigations

These need to be directed by accurate history and examination. Initial investigations would include the following:

- Full blood count and differential
- Serum IgG, IgA and IgM (must be compared with age-related normals)
- IgG subclasses
- Antigen-specific antibodies (e.g. diphtheria, tetanus, *Haemophilus influenzae* type b (Hib)) (reference values for a normal response are available in specialist laboratories)
- Lymphocyte subsets
- T-cell stimulation (response to phytohaemagglutinin, Candida antigen, tetanus or tuberculin)
- Nitroblue tetrazolium test (NBT) if history is suggestive of CGD
- Total haemolytic complement (THC), C3, C4 (if history is suggestive of complement defect, i.e. recurrent meningitis)
- Human immunodeficiency virus (HIV) testing (if clinically appropriate)

(Always check that patient has not received blood products or intravenous immunoglobulin (IVIG) before interpreting immunoglobulin levels — if the patient has received such products, it is necessary to wait approximately 3 months before reassessment.)

Lymphocyte markers

- CD3 — T cell
- CD4 — helper T cell
- CD8 — memory/cytotoxic T cell
- CD19/20 — B cell
- CD14 — monocyte
- CD16/CD56 — natural killer (NK) cell
- CD34 — haematopoietic stem cells

Normal numbers and percentages of lymphocyte subsets vary with age and with clinical state, i.e. viral infection may lead to a relative CD8 lymphocytosis.

More specialized tests include testing for specific defects, e.g. adenosine deaminase (ADA) metabolites in ADA deficiency or expression of Bruton tyrosine kinase for diagnosis of X-linked agammaglobulinaemia. These can be carried out in specialist laboratories.

4.   IMMUNOGLOBULINS AND B-CELL DEFICIENCIES

- Newborns rely on maternal IgG for 6 months
- Production of IgG1 and IgG3 is greater than that of IgG2 and IgG4
- Adult levels by 7–12 years
- Detect IgM by 1 week of age; adult levels by 12 months
- IgA detectable by 2 weeks; adult levels by 7 years
- Poor response to polysaccharide antigen until > 2 years

	IgG	IgM	IgA	IgD	IgE
Size (kDa)	150	950	160	175	190
Cross placenta	Yes	No	No	No	No
Complement	Classical	Classical	Alternative	No	No
Normal levels mg/ml (adult)	13	1.5	3.5	0.03	0.0001

Causes of low immunoglobulins

- **Prematurity**: under 36 weeks' gestation, transfer of maternal antibody is low
- **Excessive losses**: nephrotic syndrome, enteropathy, burns
- **Transient hypogammaglobulinaemia of infancy**: as the name suggests, this is a maturational problem which resolves as patients get older. Protection with immunoglobulin may be necessary during this period
- **Drug-induced**: antimalarials, captopril, carbamazepine, phenytoin, gold salts, sulphasalazine
- **Infections**: HIV, Epstein–Barr virus, congenital cytomegalovirus, congenital toxoplasmosis
- **Others**: malignancy, systemic lupus erythematosus

4.1   X-linked agammaglobulinemia

- Primary defect of B cells with < 2% CD19+ B cells
- Defect in B-cell development with arrest at the pre-B-cell stage
- Mutations in the Bruton tyrosine kinase (*Btk*) gene, on the X chromosome (Xq22); Btk being a molecule involved in B-cell signalling
- *Streptococcus pneumoniae* and *H. influenzae* infections of the upper and lower respiratory tract, sinuses and middle ear
- Particular susceptibility to *Mycoplasma* infections and central nervous system infection with enteroviruses

- Severe cases present before the age of two, milder cases may not diagnosed until school age
- Poor or no responses to vaccines and low levels of isohaemagglutinins are found
- In some atypical forms there is a small number of circulating B cells and some make immunoglobulin
- Patients respond well to IVIG therapy

4.2   Autosomal recessive congenital agammaglobulinaemia

- Other defects giving rise to abnormal B-cell development have been found
- These include components of the pre-B-cell receptor which are essential for B-cell development: μ heavy chain, λ surrogate light chain, Igα accessory molecule

4.3   IgA deficiency

- Produced and secreted at mucosal surfaces
- Two subclasses
- Serum IgA produced by B cells in lymph nodes
- Activates alternative complement pathway
- Most common form of primary immunodeficiency
- 1 : 600–1 : 300 incidence of deficiency; usually asymptomatic
- Increased risk of atopy, infections of lungs, gastrointestinal tract
- Association with IgG2 deficiency
- Associations: autoimmunity, ulcerative colitis, Crohn disease, coeliac disease, malignancy
- 40% have antibodies to IgA; risk of transfusion/IVIG anaphylaxis

4.4   Common variable immunodeficiency (CVID)

- Catch-all term to describe heterogeneous group of poorly characterized immunodeficiencies
- Molecular basis being defined in some families e.g. ICOS (inducible costimulatory molecules) deficiency
- History of recurrent infections, often of the respiratory tract and involving a range of pathogens
- A subgroup of patients have granulomatous disease affecting the gastrointestinal tract, lungs and skin; normally responsive to steroids
- Autoimmune diseases occur in over half the patients and there is an increased risk of malignancy
- May be reduced T-cell numbers, though the majority of patients have normal numbers of B cells
- Diagnosis is usually made in patients older than 2 years with reduced serum immunoglobulins, absent isohaemagglutinins and poor vaccine responses

The patients with persistently low immunoglobulin levels benefit from supplemental IVIG infusions. Prophylactic antibiotics are given to those with recurrent infection despite IVIG. Severe cases may require bone marrow transplantation.

5. COMBINED IMMUNODEFICIENCIES

5.1 Severe combined immunodeficiency (SCID)

- SCID arises from severe defects in both cellular and humoral immunity
- Same phenotype arises from different molecular defects
- Both X-linked and autosomal recessive forms of SCID exist
- Characterized by recurrent infections, often severe, involving opportunistic pathogens
- Overall prognosis for SCID without effective management is very poor
- Only curative option is bone marrow transplantation; but for certain types of SCID other treatments such as gene therapy (presently for X-linked SCID) and enzyme replacement therapy (for ADA SCID) are available (see below)

Incidence

- Rare
- Estimated at 1 : 50,000 to 1 : 500,000 for all forms of SCID
- Males affected more than females because of X-linked inheritance in one specific type of SCID

Clinical manifestations

- Mean age of presentation is approximately 6–7 months
- **Respiratory complications** — interstitial pneumonitis caused by *Pneumocystis carinii*, respiratory syncytial virus, cytomegalovirus, adenovirus, influenza and parainfluenza infections. Bacterial and fungal pneumonias are also described
- **Diarrhoea and faltering growth** — there may be a viral aetiology (rotavirus, adenovirus) but in many cases no cause is defined. Faltering growth as a result of diarrhoea or recurrent infection is seen in nearly all patients.
- **Skin rash** — may be the result of a viral infection but an erythrodermic macular rash is often indicative of maternal T-cell engraftment or Omenn syndrome

HIV infection can also present as faltering growth with a similar spectrum of infectious pathogens, and may need to be formally excluded (see Section 7.1, Chapter 14).

Immunological phenotype

- SCID is characterized by both humoral and cellular defects
- Abnormality in T-cell development with variable defects in B-cell and NK-cell development
- IgG present early on because of maternal transfer, but IgM and IgA production impaired
- SCID is categorized by the pattern of T/B/NK-cell development and this can be indicative of the underlying molecular defect

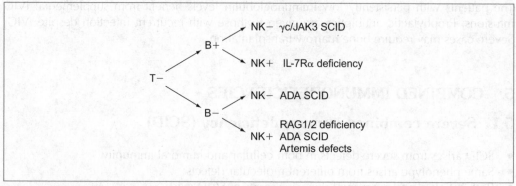

Pattern of T/B/NK-cell development

Exceptions to the above scheme include:

- **Maternal engraftment**: maternal T cells are present but these are non-functional CD8+ cells
- **Omenn syndrome (OS)**: characteristic immunological profile with activated non-functional CD8+ cells, lack of B cells, increased IgE and eosinophilia
- **Atypical variants**: for many of the defined forms there have been reports of less severe phenotypes where there may be small but not normal numbers of T/B or NK cells present

Genetic diagnosis

- The molecular basis of the known SCID types is shown in the table on p. 484.
- Diagnosis is made on the basis of pedigree, immunological phenotype and genetic analysis

Management

- Prophylactic – septrin for prevention of *P. carinii* pneumonitis, immunoglobulin replacement, aciclovir for antiviral prophylaxis and itraconazole/fluconazole for antifungal prophylaxis
- Supportive — nutrition, skin care, genetic counselling for family
- Specific treatment of infectious complications

Bone marrow transplantation (BMT) (see Section 9)

- BMT is the only treatment option for the majority of SCID cases
- Best results are available following a genotypically matched donor transplant (> 90% success rates). In most SCID cases such transplants can be undertaken without prior chemotherapy conditioning.
- If no genotypically identical donor is present, BMT from a matched family donor, volunteer unrelated donor or parental haplo-identical donor can be undertaken. Results following such procedures are less good, with haplotransplants having the worst outcome.

PEG-ADA (for treatment of ADA-SCID)

- Exogenous enzyme replacement therapy using a bovine form of ADA conjugated to polyethylene glycol (PEG-ADA or Pegademase) has been used in patients who lack a good bone marrow donor
- PEG-ADA can be used indefinitely, or to stabilize the condition until a donor for BMT can be found
- Side-effects such as autoimmune haemolytic anaemia and thrombocytosis have been reported

Gene therapy

- Gene therapy has been used to treat X-linked SCID and ADA deficiency
- The patient's own bone marrow is harvested and stem cells are collected
- In the laboratory, a modified retrovirus, incapable of replication, is used to deliver a corrected copy of the defective gene
- The retrovirus stably integrates into the genome of the stem cells
- The gene-modified stem cells are then infused back to the patient
- Immune reconstitution follows over a period of several months
- Although this approach has been shown to be potentially curative, there have been some serious complications, with the development of leukaemic changes in some patients
- It is thought that the retrovirus may activate oncogenes in some situations
- This approach is currently offered if no matched donors are available for transplant

5.2   Combined immunodeficiency (CID)

- CID refers to a genetically undefined group of immunodeficiencies in which there are variable defects in T- and B-cell function
- CID patients present at a later stage with less severe infections
- Over time, immune function deteriorates leading to recurrent infection and resulting in chronic damage especially to liver and lungs
- Principles of management are the same as for SCID
- BMT is less successful in CID because of underlying chronic organ damage and increased age at time of transplant

Major types of SCID and their genetic defect

Disorder	Chromosomal location	Gene	Function/defect	Diagnostic tests other than direct mutation analysis
X-linked severe combined immunodeficiency	Xq13	**Common γ chain (γ$_c$)**	Component of interleukin (IL) 2,4,7,9,15 cytokine receptors; T- and NK-cell development, T- and B-cell function	γ$_c$ Expression by FACS (flow cytometric) analysis
Adenosine deaminase (ADA) deficiency	20q12–13	**Adenosine deaminase**	Enzyme in purine salvage pathway; accumulation of toxic metabolites	Red cell ADA levels and metabolites
Recombinase activating gene (*RAG1/2*) deficiency Omenn syndrome	11p13	***RAG1* and *RAG2***	Defective DNA recombination affecting immunoglobulin and T-cell receptor gene rearrangements	
Artemis gene defect	10p	**Artemis**	Defective DNA recombination affecting immunoglobulin and T-cell receptor gene rearrangements	
T-cell receptor deficiencies	11q23	***CD3$_γ$/CD3$_ε$***	T-cell receptor function and signalling	CD3 fluorescence intensity; mutation analysis
Zap70 deficiency	2q12	**ZAP-70**	T-cell function — selection of CD8+ cells during thymocyte development	ZAP-70 expression
JAK3 deficiency	19p13	**JAK3**	IL-2, -4, -7, -9, -15 receptor signalling, T- and NK-cell development, T- and B-cell function	JAK3 expression/ signalling
IL-7 receptor deficiency	5p13	**IL-7 receptor-α**	Essential role in T-cell development and function	IL-7 receptor α expression

6. MISCELLANEOUS IMMUNODEFICIENCY SYNDROMES

6.1 Wiskott–Aldrich syndrome

- X-linked inheritance pattern
- Approximately 1 : 1,000,000 live male births
- Classical clinical features include thrombocytopenia, combined immunodeficiency and eczema
- Patients are susceptible to lymphoproliferative disease in later life
- Autoimmune features with peripheral and large-vessel vasculitis are seen in older patients
- Considerable clinical heterogeneity with some patients having thrombocytopenia alone
- Arises from mutations in the *WASP* (Wiskott–Aldrich syndrome protein) gene
- *WASP* expressed in all haematopoietic tissues
- *WASP* involved in organization of cytoskeleton and defects affect immune-cell motility

Thrombocytopenia is the most consistent clinical feature and patients also have small fragmented platelets ($< 70,000$ platelets/mm³) and a reduced mean platelet volume.

Immune defects include decreased IgM levels, decrease in T-cell numbers and function with time and impaired responses to polysaccharide antigens. Extent of eczema is variable.

Diagnosis

Diagnosis is made on clinical phenotype, platelet count morphology, x-linked pedigree and mutation analysis of the *WASP* gene.

Management

Management is orientated to the different clinical problems.

- Topical care of eczema
- Thrombocytopenia sometimes responds to high-dose immunoglobulin (2 g/kg) and steroids
- In most cases splenectomy is successful in improving the platelet count
- Immune defect is treated by prophylactic antibiotics, IVIG and aggressive management of active infection
- Only curative option is BMT which can be difficult if a fully matched donor is unavailable
- BMT after 5 years of age is associated with worse prognosis

6.2 Di George syndrome

- Now usually diagnosed in infants with cardiac malformations undergoing genetic analysis for detection of microdeletions of chromosome 22q11.2
- Defects of the fourth branchial arch and third and fourth pharyngeal pouches
- Aortic arch and conotruncal anomalies (truncus arteriosus, tetralogy of Fallot, interrupted aortic arch or aberrant right subclavian) are associated with significant neonatal mortality

- Parathyroid hypoplasia may lead to hypocalcaemic tetany, and thymic hypoplasia may lead to profound cellular immunodeficiency (less than 500/mm^3 CD3 T cells)
- Dysmorphic features include lateral displacement of the inner canthi, short philtrum, micrognathia and ear abnormalities. Learning difficulties are common
- Increased likelihood of autoimmune phenomena in older children
- Usually confirmed by the detection of the 22q11.2 deletion by fluorescent in situ hybridization
- Attempts to correct T-cell deficiency by thymic transplantation have been unsuccessful

Management

Includes the use of irradiated blood products before surgery and then management of specific syndromic problems. Management of immunodeficiency is dependent on the severity of immune compromise and varies from prophylactic antibiotics to BMT.

6.3   CD40 ligand deficiency (X-linked hyper-IgM syndrome)

- Presents before the age of 2 years with a history of recurrent infections, usually of the sinuses or middle ear
- Increased susceptibility to *P. carinii* pneumonitis, viral infections and mycobacterial organisms
- *Cryptosporidium* infection often leads to chronic diarrhoea and sclerosing cholangitis
- Liver disease is the major cause of death in older patients
- Predisposition to haematological malignancy and autoimmune diseases
- Maps to Xq26.3–7 and results from mutations in the gene for CD40 ligand — resulting in defects in immunoglobulin class-switching
- Associated with anaemia and neutropenia but T- and B-cell numbers are often normal
- Serum levels of IgM are usually elevated but can be normal, with reduced IgG and IgA levels
- Diagnosis by immunoglobulin profile, flow cytometric analysis for the absence of CD40 ligand on T cells and by genetic analysis
- Treat with regular IVIG infusions and antibiotic prophylaxis. Patients are screened, treated for *Cryptosporidium* infection and regularly monitored for liver disease (including cholangiography and liver biopsy in some cases)
- BMT offers the possibility of cure, but in the absence of matched donors carries high risks of morbidity and mortality

6.4   X-linked lymphoproliferative syndrome (Duncan syndrome)

Affected boys are well until they contract EBV infection when they can exhibit a variety of clinical manifestations:

- Fulminant infectious mononucleosis (FIM) (58%)
- Lymphoma (31%)
- Dysgammaglobulinaemia (30%)
- Aplastic anaemia (3%)

- Phenotypes can exist together or evolve from one to another
- EBV is not always the trigger for these dysregulatory phenomena and a significant number of boys are EBV-negative
- FIM has the poorest outcome, with > 90% mortality. Major cause of death is hepatic necrosis
- Diagnosis difficult because of clinical variability
- No specific immunological defect in affected boys before the onset of severe symptoms
- After infection, a variety of immunological defects are seen including reversed CD4/CD8 ratio and dysgammaglobulinaemia
- Gene identified as *SAP* which plays a critical role in the regulation of T-cell stimulation
- Identification of mutations in *SAP* can provide unambiguous diagnosis

Treatment

- Is difficult
- In affected boys identified by family history, prophylactic IVIG and antibiotics do not provide protection from severe EBV infection
- Retuximab (anti-CD20) is used to treat EBV by eliminating B cells
- BMT offers only curative option but is difficult to perform if child is in acute phase

6.5   Purine nucleoside phosphorylase (PNP) deficiency

- Autosomal recessive inheritance
- Lack of expression of PNP and defect in purine salvage pathway
- Triad of immune deficiency, neurological manifestations and autoimmune phenomena
- Two-thirds have neurological problems ranging from spasticity to global developmental delay
- One-third develop autoimmune disease including autoimmune haemolytic anaemia and immune thrombocytopenia
- Infective complications are the most common presenting complaint. Infections as for other forms of SCID/CID but presentation is generally at a later age than most SCID types
- BMT offers the only cure. Increased risks are associated with non-HLA identical transplant
- BMT reported anecdotally to correct/halt neurological deterioration, although other reports contradict this

6.6   Ataxia telangiectasia

- Early onset of progressive neurological impairment: cerebellar ataxia and choreoathetosis
- Oculocutaneous telangiectasia in those aged 2 years and above
- Immunodeficiency, leading to recurrent sinopulmonary infection
- Increased risk of developing lymphoid malignancies
- Associations include growth retardation, diabetes and liver dysfunction
- *ATM* (ataxia telangiectasia mutated) gene maps to chromosome 11q22–23

- Usually the clinical diagnosis is supported by genetic analysis
- IgA levels are reduced and serum α-fetoprotein is raised
- Cultured cells exhibit increased radiation-induced chromosomal breakage

6.7 Chronic mucocutaneous candidiasis

- Presents in childhood with extensive *Candida* infections of the skin, nails and mucous membranes
- May be associated with endocrine abnormalities such as hypoparathyroidism and Addison disease
- Pathogenesis of this disease is poorly understood
- The mainstay of therapy is prophylactic, systemic antifungal therapy

7. DEFECTS OF NEUTROPHILS

Neutrophil immunodeficiency may arise because of reduced numbers of circulating neutrophils, a failure of neutrophil precursor maturation or defective neutrophil function.

7.1 Congenital neutropenia

- Recurrent bacterial infections (often *Staphylococcus aureus*) in the first year of life leading to abscesses, cellulitis and meningitis
- There is a failure of myeloid-cell maturation, but the condition responds to treatment with G-CSF
- There are a variety of underlying molecular defects, including stem-cell receptor defects, and some patients may later develop myelodysplastic syndromes

7.2 Schwachman–Diamond syndrome

- Combination of pancreatic exocrine insufficiency, skeletal abnormalities and recurrent infections of lungs, bones and skin
- Most patients have neutropenia and up to 25% may develop pancytopenia
- The risks of myelodysplasia and leukaemia are increased
- BMT may be curative

7.3 Cyclical neutropenia

- Patients recurrently become neutropenic for between 3 and 6 days, and may develop stomatitis, mouth ulcers or bacterial infections
- There is usually a 21-day cyclical pattern, but this can range between 14 and 36 days
- The condition is autosomal dominant and has been linked to mutations in the elastase gene, *ELA2*

7.4 Leukocyte-adhesion deficiency

History of delayed umbilical separation, periodontitis, recurrent orogenital infections. Pathogens include *S. aureus*, *Aspergillus*, *Candida* and Gram-negative enteric bacteria.

- **Type 1** — autosomal recessive defect of δ_2-integrin adhesion molecules (CD18) on neutrophils, resulting in defective aggregation and a paradoxical leukocytosis. There is no expression of CD18 on neutrophils and early death occurs without BMT in the most severe forms. CD18 is expressed in milder forms and patients can survive to adulthood
- **Type 2** — defective carbohydrate fucosylation. Associated dysmorphic features and growth and developmental retardation.

7.5 Chronic granulomatous disease

X-linked form of CGD accounts for two-thirds of cases and usually presents earlier and with more severe disease than patients with autosomal recessive forms.

- Faltering growth, severe bacterial infections, abscesses or osteomyelitis within the first year of life are common
- Pneumonia and lymphadenitis caused by *S. aureus* or *Aspergillus* infections are the most common infections
- Granulomas may result in intrathoracic, gastrointestinal or urinary obstruction
- X-linked CGD is the result of mutations in the gene for the phagocyte oxidase cytochrome glycoprotein *gp91phox*
- Defects of *p47phox* account for the majority of recessive cases, and mutations of *p22phox* and *p67phox* are uncommon
- These mutations result in defects of NADPH oxidase and the generation of hydrogen peroxide, resulting in defective intracellular killing of pathogens
- Diagnosis is usually made by demonstrating an impaired neutrophil respiratory burst using the nitroblue tetrazolium test (NBT) or flow cytometric analysis of hydrogen peroxide production using fluorescent detector dyes. Immunoblot analysis or flow cytometry using antibodies to the various NADPH oxidase subunits may help to define the particular subtype of CGD.
- Treatment usually involves prophylactic antibiotics and the use of steroids to treat granulomatous disease. Aggressive use of antifungal agents and granulocyte infusions along with interferon-γ may be required to manage severe fungal infections. BMT has been used successfully in those who have a matched sibling donor. Gene therapy has been attempted and longer term outcome is awaited

7.6 Chédiak–Higashi syndrome

- Rare autosomal recessive disorder of lysosomal granule-containing cells of the immune and nervous systems caused by mutations of the *LYST* gene.
- Features include peripheral neuropathy, albinism, giant inclusions in hair
- Ocular albinism may result in severe visual defects

- Diagnosis by identification of giant lysosomal granules in neutrophils on peripheral blood film and clinical features of albinism
- Neutrophils respond poorly to infections and patients may develop T-cell and monocytic infiltration of tissues (so-called accelerated phase) which is often fatal
- BMT is the treatment of choice. If a matched donor is available this should be undertaken before the onset of the accelerated phase.

7.7 Rac deficiency

Rare inhibitory mutation of *Rac2* causing neutrophil immunodeficiency, clinically similar to leukocyte adhesion deficiency, with abnormal neutrophil chemotaxis and superoxide production.

8. DEFECTS OF THE INTERFERON-γ/INTERLEUKIN-12 AXIS

- Intracellular pathogens normally trigger interleukin-12 (IL-12) production by antigen-presenting cells, and this in turn binds specific receptors on T cells to induce interferon-γ (IFN-γ) production which enhances phagocyte-mediated killing through tumour-necrosis factor (TNF) release
- Defects of the IFN-γ receptor, IL-12 or IL-12 receptor lead to increased susceptibility to intracellular organisms such as *Mycobacterium* and *Salmonella*
- Inheritance of autosomal recessive cases of IFN-γ receptor defects occurs in consanguineous Maltese populations
- Infants may present with disseminated BCG and atypical mycobacterial infection and are usually unable to form granulomas
- Milder cases may respond to high-dose infusions of IFN-γ

Major types of non-SCID immunodeficiencies and their genetic defects

Disorder	Chromosomal	Gene location	Function/defect	Diagnostic tests
X-linked chronic granulomatous disease	Xp21	*gp91phox*	Component of phagocyte NADPH oxidase-phagocytic respiratory burst	Nitroblue tetrazolium test *gp91phox* by immunoblotting mutation analysis
X-linked agammaglobulinaemia	Xq22	Bruton tyrosine kinase (*Btk*)	Intracellular signalling pathways essential for pre-B-cell maturation	*Btk* by immunoblotting or FACS analysis and mutation analysis
X-linked hyper-IgM syndrome (CD40 ligand deficiency)	Xq26	CD40 ligand (*CD154*)	Isotype switching, T-cell function	CD154 expression on activated T cells by FACS analysis mutation analysis
Wiskott–Aldrich syndrome	Xp11	*WASP*	Cytoskeletal architecture formation, immune-cell motility and trafficking	*WASP* expression by immunoblotting mutation analysis
X-linked lymphoproliferative syndrome	Xq25	*SAP*	Regulation of T-cell responses to EBV and other viral infections	Mutation analysis *SAP* expression — under development
Properdin deficiency Leukocyte-adhesion deficiency type 1	Xp21 21q22	properdin CD11/CD18	Terminal complement component. Defective leukocyte adhesion and migration	Properdin levels CD11/CD18 expression by FACS analysis; mutation analysis
Chronic granulomatous disease	7q11 1q25 16p24	*p47phox p67phox p22phox*	Defective respiratory burst and phagocytic intracellular killing	*p47phox, p67phox, p22phox*, expression by immunoblotting; mutation analysis
Chédiak–Higashi syndrome	1q42	*LYST*	Abnormalities in microtubule-mediated lysosomal protein trafficking	Giant inclusions in granulocytes; mutation analysis
MHC class II deficiency	16p13 19p12 1q21 13q13	*CIITA (MHX2TA)* RFXANK RFC5 RFXAP	Defective transcriptional regulation of MHC II molecule expression	HLA-DR expression; mutation analysis
Autoimmune lymphoproliferative syndrome (ALPS)	10q24	*APT1* (Fas)	Defective apoptosis of lymphocytes	Fas expression; apoptosis assays; mutation analysis
Ataxia telangiectasia	11q22	ATM	Cell-cycle control and DNA damage responses	DNA radiation sensitivity; mutation analysis
Inherited mycobacterial susceptibility	6q23 5q31 19p13	**Interferon-γ receptor** IL-12 p40 IL-12 receptor β1	Defective IFN-γ production and signalling function	Interferon-γ receptor expression; IL-12 expression; IL-12 receptor expression; mutation analysis

9. BONE MARROW/HAEMATOPOIETIC STEM-CELL TRANSPLANTATION (BMT/HSCT)

BMT/HSCT offers a curative option for haematological malignancies/congenital immunodeficiencies/haemoglobinopathies/inherited metabolic defects and recently for autoimmune conditions. Bone marrow is a rich source of haematopoietic stem cells (HSC) but also contains mature T, B and NK cells. HSC can also be harvested by leukophoresis after giving the donor a course of G-CSF.

Autologous transplants are used for treatment of malignancies especially solid tumours and autoimmune conditions. HSC are collected from the patient, usually before intensive chemotherapy/radiotherapy for malignancy, and then re-infused to rescue the haematopoietic system.

Allogeneic transplants are from another person who is ideally HLA-matched. Parents are usually haplo-identical. Indications in childhood include relapsed leukaemias, primary immune deficiencies, haematological disorders (Fanconi syndrome, thalassaemia, sickle-cell disease) or metabolic conditions (adrenoleukodystropy, Hurler syndrome, osteopetrosis).

Umbilical cord blood: is also rich in HSC and can be used for transplants. Is associated with less graft-versus-host disease (GvHD) (see below) and faster immune reconstitution. However, the number of cells that can be obtained from a cord collection limits the applicability of this source.

Recipients usually require **pre-conditioning** with chemotherapy/radiotherapy to remove the existing immune cells (unless they are non-functional as in X-linked SCID).

Cytotoxic agents can have significant side-effects: e.g. cyclophosphamide (haemorrhagic cystitis, infertility), busulphan (pulmonary fibrosis).

T cells in the graft may cause **graft-versus-host disease** (GvHD) and this may be managed by T-cell depleting grafts and/or immunosuppression using cyclosporin and steroids.

GvHD is graded I to IV on the basis of skin rash, liver impairment and gastrointestinal involvement.

T cells also mediate a **graft-versus-leukaemia** effect which helps eradicate tumour cells.

Early post-transplant complications

These include: raft rejection or failure; infection (bacterial, cytomegalovirus, Epstein–Barr virus (EBV), adenovirus, fungal); GvHD; and veno-occlusive disease.

Late complications

These include: incomplete immune reconstitution; chronic GvHD; growth retardation and endocrine problems; and cognitive impairment in some patients.

10. ROUTINE VACCINATION IN THE IMMUNOSUPPRESSED

- All live vaccines are contraindicated in SCID and only poor responses are obtained to killed vaccines
- In the UK the new five in one immunization contains inactivated vaccines and is safe to give, though responses may be poor
- Bacillus Calmette–Guérin (BCG) is contraindicated in all primary immunodeficiencies; chemotherapy patients; and patients on significant steroids or immunosuppressants
- HIV patients in UK should not be given BCG; other live vaccines can be given if asymptomatic
- No specific contraindications for complement deficiencies

11. COMPLEMENT DEFICIENCY STATES

Component	Deficiency
C1q,r,s C4, C2	Infection (pneumococcal), systemic lupus erythematosus, glomerulonephritis
C5,6,7,8	Infection (*Neisseria*)
Mannose-binding lectin	Recurrent infections
Factor D	Infection (meningococcal)
Properdin	Infection (meningococcal)
C1 inhibitor	Hereditary angioedema
DAF, protectin	Paroxysmal nocturnal haemaglobinuria
C3 receptor	Infections

12. HYPERSENSITIVITY REACTIONS

Type	Type 1	Type 2	Type 3	Type 4
Immune mediator	IgE	IgG, IgM	IgG	T cells
Antigen	Soluble	Cell surface	Soluble	Soluble or cellular
Mechanism	Mast-cell degranulation	Altered signalling complement activation	Immune complexes	T_{H1} (IL-2, IFN-γ) T_{H2} (IL-4, IL-5) Cytotoxic T cells
Clinical conditions	Asthma; Food allergy; Disease of hayfever Anaphylaxis	Haemolytic Arthus reaction Newborn penicillin allergy	Serum sickness dermatitis Erythema nodosum	Contact conditions Tuberculin Chronic asthma

13. IMMUNOSUPPRESSANTS AND IMMUNE-MODULATING AGENTS

T–cell immunosuppressants

Drug	Indications	Major side–effects
Prednisolone	Prevent rejection Prevent GvHD Immunosuppression for many indications	Hypertension, thin skin, truncal obesity, proximal myopathy
Cyclosporin	Prevent rejection Prevent GvHD Suppress autoimmune disease	Nephrotoxicity, hirsutism, hypertension
Tacrolimus	Prevent rejection	Nephrotoxicity, neurotoxic cardiomyopathy
Mycophenolate mofetil (MMF)	Prevent rejection	Leukopenia, marrow suppression
Azathioprine	Prevent rejection Suppress autoimmune disease	Marrow suppression, hepatotoxic

Clinically used monoclonal antibodies/fusion proteins

Drug	Target	Indication
Rituximab	CD20 on B cells	B-cell lymphoma Lymphoproliferative disease
Dacluzimab	Anti-CD25	Inflammation caused by activated T cells
Infliximab	TNF-α	Rheumatoid arthritis, juvenile idiopathic arthritis, Crohn's disease
Etanercept	TNF-α receptor	Juvenile idiopathic arthritis; rheumatoid arthritis,
Anti-thymocyte globulin (ATG)	T cells	T-cell depletion
OKT3	T cells	T-cell depletion
Campath	CD52 on human T and B cells	T-cell depletion in BMT and for certain lymphomas

Interferons

Drug	Possible indications	Side-effects/comments
IFN-α	Myeloma Renal carcinoma Melanoma	Flu-like illness, fever Myelosuppression Depression
IFN-2α	Hepatitis C	Given with ribavirin
IFN-β	Multiple sclerosis	Fever, flu-like illness
IFN-γ	Mycobacterial infection Chronic granulomatous disease	Fever, flu-like illness

14. FURTHER READING

Fischer A, Cavazzana-Calvo M, De Saint Basile G, *et al.* 1997. Naturally occurring primary deficiencies of the immune system. *Annual Review of Immunology* 15, 93–124.

Ochs M, Smith C, Puck J. 1999. *Primary Immunodeficiency Disease.* Oxford University Press.

Steihm ER (Ed.). 1995. *Immunologic Disorders in Children and Infants*, 4th edn. WB Saunders.

Vergani D, Peakman M. 2000. *Basic and Clinical Immunology*. Churchill Livingstone.

Gaspar, HB, Gilmour, KC. 2001. Severe combined immunodeficiency — molecular pathogenesis and diagnosis. *Archives of Diseases in Childhood* 84, 169–73.

Chapter 14

Infectious Diseases

Katy Fidler, Nigel Klein and Karyn Moshal

CONTENTS

Infectious Diseases

1. NOTIFICATION OF INFECTIOUS DISEASES

Doctors in England and Wales have a statutory duty to notify the local authority, usually the CCDC (Consultant in Communicable Disease Control), of cases of certain infections: this is done via the notification book in each hospital.

Notifications of infectious diseases, some of which are microbiologically confirmed, prompt local investigation and action to control the diseases.

Notifiable diseases

Acute encephalitis	Measles	Malaria
Meningitis	Mumps	Yellow fever
– meningococcal	Rubella	Typhoid fever
– pneumococcal	Whooping cough	Paratyphoid fever
– *Haemophilus influenzae*	Viral hepatitis	Relapsing fever
– viral	– hepatitis A	Leptospirosis
– other specified	– hepatitis B	Viral haemorrhagic fever
– unspecified	– hepatitis C	Typhus fever
Meningococcal septicaemia	– other	Plague
(without meningitis)	Smallpox	Rabies
Tetanus	Acute poliomyelitis	Dysentery
Tuberculosis		Food poisoning
Scarlet fever		
Ophthalmia neonatorum		
Anthrax		
Cholera		
Diphtheria		

2. PATHOGENESIS OF INFECTION

The course and outcome of any infectious disease is a function of the interaction between the pathogen and host.

The pathogens

Human infections are caused by bacteria, viruses, fungi and parasites. However, despite the vast array of potential pathogens, only a minority have the capacity to cause infection in a human host. Many factors determine an individual organism's ability to initiate disease, but successful organisms have three essential characteristics: the ability to invade a host; the ability to travel to an environment within the host which is conducive to their propagation; and the ability to survive the host's defence mechanisms. Increasing understanding of the molecular mechanisms underlying these pathogenic events should enable the development of new treatment strategies.

Bacterial properties important in the pathogenesis of infections

Bacterial characteristic	Function
Pili	Aid adhesion to host targets
Capsular polysaccharide	Inhibit phagocytosis
Enzyme production	Inactivate antibody, degrade host tissue
Toxin production	Lyse circulating cells
Antigen variation	Evade host defences

The host

The essential elements of all components of the immune system are present at birth. Initially, however, the baby's circulating immunoglobulin is derived predominantly from the mother. It is only after encountering a wide range of potential pathogens that defences fully mature to provide adequate protection in later life. Meanwhile, these children are particularly susceptible to infections.

The importance of acquiring a fully competent host defence system is illustrated clinically by the problems encountered in immunodefective individuals, e.g. primary immunodeficiencies, acquired immunodeficiency syndrome (AIDS) and those receiving chemotherapy and radiotherapy. These patients suffer not only from severe and persistent infections caused by common organisms, but are also vulnerable to a range of unusual or opportunistic pathogens. The role played by each component of the host defence system can be deduced from the nature of infections associated with specific immunological defects, many of which present in childhood.

Immune deficiency and susceptibility to infection

Immune defect	Infectious susceptibility	
Antibody	Bacteria	*Staphylococcus, Streptococcus* spp., *Haemophilus influenzae, Moraxella (Branhamella) catarrhalis*
	Viruses	Enteroviruses
	Protozoa	*Giardia*
Cellular immunity	Bacteria	*Mycobacterium, Listeria* spp.
	Viruses	Cytomegalovirus (CMV), herpesvirus, measles, respiratory syncytial virus, adenovirus
	Fungi	*Candida, Aspergillus* spp.
	Protozoa	*Pneumocystis* spp.
Neutrophils	Bacteria	Gram +ve, Gram −ve
	Fungi	*Aspergillus, Candida* spp.
Complement	Bacteria	*Neisseria, Staphylococcus* spp.

3. FEVER WITH FOCUS

3.1 Central nervous system (CNS) infections

Meningitis and encephalitis

Encephalitis is predominantly viral in origin.

Common viral causes include:

- Enteroviruses
- Herpes simplex virus (HSV)-1 and HSV-2
- Varicella zoster
- Measles
- Mumps
- Influenza

Rare causes include:

- Adenoviruses, rubella virus, Epstein–Barr virus (EBV), arenaviruses (e.g. Japanese B encephalitis), rabies virus and *Mycoplasma* spp.

Herpes simplex virus causes a predominantly encephalitic illness. Aciclovir dramatically reduces mortality if given early in HSV disease.

The peak incidence of viral encephalitis is in the first 6 months of life with one or two cases per 1,000 children. In about 50% of cases a mild lymphocellular pleocytosis is seen.

The commonest cause of viral meningitis is enterovirus and these infections peak in summer.

Bacterial meningitis

- *Neisseria meningitidis* is the commonest cause of community-acquired bacterial meningitis in the UK, with most cases being *N. meningitidis* B since the introduction of the conjugate meningococcal C vaccine.
- *Streptococcus pneumoniae* is the second most common cause
- The incidence of *Haemophilus influenzae* type B (Hib) meningitis has dropped from around 2,500 cases per year to less than 40 per year since the introduction of the Hib vaccine
- A rare, but serious, form of bacterial meningitis is caused by *Mycobacterium tuberculosis*. This organism can affect patients of all ages and should be considered in any atypical presentation of meningitis, particularly in patients presenting with an insidious illness

Neonatal meningitis

In the neonatal period, group B streptococcus is the predominant meningeal pathogen, followed by Gram-negative bacilli, *Strep. pneumoniae* and *Listeria monocytogenes*.

Diagnosis of bacterial meningitis

If meningitis is suspected, the diagnosis should be confirmed by lumbar puncture and examination of cerebrospinal fluid (CSF).

Specific contraindications to lumbar puncture include:

- Signs of raised intracranial pressure with changing level of consciousness, focal neurological signs or severe mental impairment
- Cardiovascular compromise with impaired peripheral perfusion or hypotension
- Respiratory compromise with tachypnoea, an abnormal breathing pattern or hypoxia
- Thrombocytopenia or a coagulopathy
- A lumbar puncture should also be avoided if it causes a significant delay in treatment

Very high white cell counts of more than $1,000/mm^3$ can be seen in bacterial meningitis. There is a broad correlation between a predominance of polymorphonuclear leukocytes in the CSF and bacterial meningitis. However, lymphocytes may predominate in early or partially treated bacterial meningitis, in tuberculous meningitis and in neonates.

In bacterial meningitis, the CSF glucose level is usually low with a CSF/blood ratio less than 0.5, and the protein level is frequently raised to > 0.4 g/l. Numerous studies have now shown that, even after the administration of intravenous antibiotics, the diagnostic cellular and biochemical changes in the CSF may persist for at least 48 hours.

Treatment — Antibiotics for bacterial meningitis

In infants up to 3 months of age a combination of ampicillin and cefotaxime is a logical choice: cefotaxime provides cover for both neonatal and infant pathogens, and ampicillin is effective against *L. monocytogenes*.

Penicillin-resistant meningococci are emerging world-wide, as are chloramphenicol-resistant strains, but these have not yet resulted in treatment failures. Fortunately, almost all strains in the UK remain sensitive to the third-generation cephalosporins. At the moment, the routine use of vancomycin for community-acquired meningitis is not justified in the UK.

- If the cause of meningoencephalitis is unclear it is usual to start empirical treatment with aciclovir, erythromycin and cefotaxime/ceftriaxone to cover HSV, *Mycoplasma* and bacteria, respectively

Treatment — The role of corticosteroids

Several studies of patients with Hib meningitis have demonstrated some improvement in morbidity (deafness or neurological deficit) if corticosteroids were given either before antibiotic administration or at the same time. Data supporting the use of steroids in pneumococcal and meningococcal meningitis are lacking.

Complications

- Convulsions occur in 20–30% of children, usually within 72 h of presentation
- Subdural collections of fluid are common, particularly during infancy. They are usually sterile and rarely require aspiration
- The commonest long-term complication of meningitis is sensorineural deafness. The overall rate of deafness following meningitis is less than 5%. Hearing impairment is higher in cases of pneumococcal meningitis than in meningococcal infections

Prevention

Conjugate vaccines against Hib and group C *N. meningitidis* are now routinely given in the UK as part of the primary course of immunization at 2, 3 and 4 months of age. Conjugated pneumococcal vaccines are available, but are not yet part of the routine vaccination schedule. They are recommended for children with conditions which predispose them to pneumococcal infections.

3.2 Respiratory infections

See Chapter 21 — Respiratory.

3.3 Bone and joint infections

Bacterial infections of bones (osteomyelitis) and of joints (septic arthritis) should be suspected in infants of children who present with:

- Fever
- Unexplained limp and/or abnormal posture/gait and/or reluctance to use the limb
- Musculoskeletal pain, especially in the presence of local bone or joint tenderness, swelling, erythema and complete or partial limitation of movement
- Osteomyelitis and septic arthritis may occur separately or together and may affect one or many joints, often depending on the organism and host immunity

Osteomyelitis

This is either **haematogenous** (most common), resulting from bacterial seeding to the bone secondary to a bacteraemia, or **non-haematogenous**, which is secondary to trauma resulting in compromised bone tissue which then becomes infected. Long bones, followed by vertebrae, are the most common sites of infection.

- Most common in those under 1-year-old or 3–10 years of age
- More frequent in boys than girls
- Mild (often unnoticed) trauma causes bone compromise, allowing bacterial seeding during transient bacteraemic events and subsequent osteomyelitis
- Destruction of the growth plates can occur in neonates, but not in older children

Acute haematogenous osteomyelitis presents as an acute bacteraemic illness with fever and localized bone symptoms within a week.

Subacute haematogenous osteomyelitis has an insidious onset, over 1–4 weeks, with fewer systemic features and more pronounced localized bone signs.

Chronic osteomyelitis lasts for months, often as the result of an infection that has spread from a contiguous site, e.g. a fracture, or an infection with an unusual organism e.g mycobacteria.

Organisms

Staphylococcus aureus is the most common organism causing osteomyelitis in the normal host, followed by streptococci. Consider *Mycobacterium tuberculosis* in patients who present with chronic or atypical osteomyelitis, as well as *Kingella kingae*, a more recently recognized pathogen.

Organisms involved in acute haematogenous osteomyelitis

Age	Expected organism	Comments
Neonate (0–2 months)	Group B streptococcus *Staph. aureus* *Escherichia coli*	Usually affects femur or humerus Multifocal in 20–40%, Usually associated with septic arthritis
Infant (2–24 months)	*Staph. aureus,* *Strep. pneumoniae* Hib Group B streptococcus Group A streptococcus *K. kingae*	Single long-bone metaphysis affected, usually femur now rare Following varicella infection
Child	*Staph. aureus* Streptococci *E. coli* *K. kingae* Salmonella	As for infant

Sickle-cell anaemia	Salmonella	
	Strep. pneumoniae	Diaphysis rather than
	Staph. aureus	metaphysis affected
	Gram-negative bacilli	

Diagnosis

- Increased white cell count (inconsistent) with neutrophilia, increased erythrocyte sedimentation rate (ESR) and C-reactive protein (CRP) — present in 92–98% of cases, but is non-specific
- Blood cultures positive in only 40–60% of cases
- Needle aspiration of periosteal space or bone or arthrocentesis if associated septic arthritis
- Tuberculin skin test if tuberculosis is suspected
- Characteristic X-ray changes occur after 10–14 days with periosteal elevation and radiolucent metaphyseal lesions
- Technetium bone scan is positive within 24–48 h of infection
- Magnetic resonance imaging detects changes early in the disease

Differential diagnosis

Malignant and benign bone tumours, e.g. Ewing sarcoma, osteosarcomas, leukaemia with bony infiltrates and bone infarcts, e.g. sickle-cell disease.

Treatment

- 4–6 weeks of intravenous antibiotics depending on the organism. The commonest cause is *Staph. aureus* and should be treated with an anti-staphylococcal penicillin. Some authorities also add fusidic acid. A definitive diagnosis from bone culture at debridement is optimal. Positive blood cultures or joint fluid cultures provide useful information
- Surgery is required if dead or necrotic bone is present
- Associated septic arthritis (especially the hip) requires incision and drainage
- Subacute or chronic infections, or disease caused by atypical organisms e.g mycobacteria, require longer courses of antibiotics

Complications

Serious damage to the growth plate can cause differential limb length and a limp (if leg is involved).

Septic arthritis

- Serious pyogenic infection of the joint space
- Slightly more common than osteomyelitis
- Secondary to bacteraemia — caused by haematogenous spread
- Most common in children less than 3 years old and in sexually active young women
- Usually monoarticular, except in neonates when it is often multifocal

Clinical presentation
Characterized by fever and a swollen, painful joint. Similar to haematogenous osteomyelitis. Neonates often present with crying when changing their nappy because of the movement of the hip joint.

Organism

- Depends on age and immune status of the child
- Infectious arthritis may be caused by viral, fungal (very rare in immunologically normal hosts, but is well documented in the premature neonatal population) or bacterial agents
- Septic arthritis implies pyogenic arthritis secondary to bacterial infections, including *Mycobacterium tuberculosis*
- Organisms are similar to those in osteomyelitis with *Staph. aureus* being the most common. Group A streptococci are also often implicated. *Neisseria* spp. should be considered
- *N. meningitidis* infection may present with acute or occasionally chronic arthritis
- *N. gonorrhoeae* infection is not uncommon in sexually active teenagers who have polyarticular septic arthritis
- *Brucella* spp. may cause chronic septic arthritis

Differential diagnosis

- Viral infections such as rubella, mumps, parvovirus B19 and hepatitis B
- Post-infectious, reactive and immune-complex arthritides
- Intermittent polyarticular arthritis of *Borrelia burgdorferi* (Lyme disease)
- Migrating arthritis of rheumatic fever
- Connective tissue diseases
- 'Irritable hip' – a transient synovitis of the hip in children < 5 years old following an upper respiratory tract infection; there is mild fever and limp with minimal systemic features, a normal ESR and white cell count and an almost full range of movement of the affected limb

Diagnosis — Clinical

- Ultrasound scan and aspiration of joint fluid for Gram staining and microbiological culture
- Look for associated osteomyelitis
- Technetium bone scan
- Computerized tomography and magnetic resonance imaging can provide useful information early in the disease
- Blood cultures will be positive in 50% of cases

Treatment

- Antibiotic treatment depending on the organism for at least 2 weeks
- Open surgical drainage is indicated for recurrent joint effusions and for **any** case of septic arthritis of the **hip** at the time of presentation
- Needle aspiration of fluid in other joints +/– washout of the joint

Septic arthritis of the hip in a child is an emergency. Immediate open drainage reduces the intra-articular pressure and avoids aseptic necrosis of the femoral head. The femoral metaphysis can be drilled during this procedure if osteomyelitis is suspected.

3.4 Gastrointestinal infections

See Chapter 9 — Gastroenterology and Nutrition, Section 11

3.5 Urogenital infections

See Chapter 17, Nephrology, Section 12

4. FEVER WITH NO FOCUS/PROLONGED FEVER

4.1 Bacteraemia/septicaemia

Definitions

- **SIRS** (systemic inflammatory response syndrome) is defined by the presence of two or more abnormalities in temperature, heart rate, respiratory rate and white blood count. SIRS can follow any severe insult including infection, trauma, major surgery, burns or pancreatitis
- **Sepsis** is used to describe SIRS in the context of bacterial infection
- **Severe sepsis** is used to describe a state characterized by hypoperfusion, hypotension and organ dysfunction
- **Septic shock** is restricted to patients with persistent hypotension despite adequate fluid resuscitation, and/or hypoperfusion even following adequate inotrope or pressor support

Microbial aetiology of sepsis

- The commonest organisms in childhood are:
  - *Strep. pneumoniae*
  - *N. meningitidis*
  - Hib (drastically reduced in countries with a vaccination programme)
- Rarer causes of sepsis in healthy children include:
  - *Staph. aureus*
  - Group A streptococcus
  - *Salmonella* spp.
- these may be associated with wound and skin infections, varicella or a history of diarrhoea, respectively.
- In neonates the usual causes of sepsis are:
  - Group B streptococcus
  - *E. coli* and other Gram-negative bacteria
  - *L. monocytogenes*
- In immunocompromised patients:

509

- Gram-negative organisms, such as *Pseudomonas aeruginosa*
- Fungi
- In patients with indwelling catheters:
  - Coagulase-negative staphylococci
  - Enterococci

Some viruses, including herpesviruses, enteroviruses and adenoviruses, can produce diseases that may be indistinguishable clinically from bacterial sepsis, particularly in neonates and infants. Children with chronic diseases are more susceptible to infection with specific organisms, e.g cystic fibrosis and pseudomonal infections and sickle cell disease and salmonella infections.

Pathophysiology of sepsis

Lipopolysaccharides from Gram-negative bacteria and a variety of other microbial products have the capacity to stimulate the production of mediators from many cells within the human host.

Tumour necrosis factor, interleukin-1 and interleukin-6 are just a few of the many inflammatory mediators reported to be present at high levels in patients with sepsis. Recently, a family of receptors has been identified capable of transducing cellular signals in response to bacteria. These are known as human Toll-like receptors.

It is the cytokines and inflammatory mediators which are produced in response to microbial stimuli that stimulate neutrophils, endothelial cells and monocytes and influence the function of vital organs, including the heart, liver, brain and kidneys.

The net effect of excessive inflammatory activity is to cause the constellation of pathophysiological events seen in patients with sepsis and septic shock.

Treatment

Successful treatment involves the administration of appropriate antibiotics, intensive care with particular emphasis on volume replacement and inotropic and respiratory support. A number of adjuvant therapies have been investigated, but, at present, none are used routinely.

4.2 Kawasaki disease

- In 1967, Tomisaku Kawasaki described 50 Japanese children with an illness characterized by fever, rash, conjunctival injection, erythema and swelling of the hands and feet and cervical lymphadenopathy
- Kawasaki disease (KD) is associated with the development of systemic vasculitis (multisystem disease affecting medium-sized muscular arteries) complicated by coronary and peripheral arterial aneurysms, and myocardial infarction in some patients
- It is the commonest cause of acquired heart disease in children in the UK and the USA
- KD is commonest in Japan, where more than 125,000 cases have been reported. The disease is also commoner in Japanese and other Oriental children living abroad.
- Children aged between 6 months and 5 years are most susceptible, with peak incidence

in children aged 9–11 months. Seasonal variation in the disease incidence has been reported, with the peak occurrence during the winter and spring months.
- Slight male predominance (1.6 : 1)

Diagnosis of KD

- There is no diagnostic test for KD, therefore diagnosis is based on clinical criteria
- The differential diagnosis includes toxic-shock syndrome (streptococcal and staphylococcal), staphylococcal scalded-skin syndrome, scarlet fever and infection with enterovirus, adenovirus, measles virus, parvovirus, Epstein–Barr virus, CMV, *Mycoplasma pneumoniae*, rickettsiae and *Leptospira* spp.

Diagnostic criteria

- Fever of 5 days' duration plus four of the five following criteria:
  - Conjunctival injection
  - Lymphadenopathy
  - Rash
  - Changes in lips or oral mucosa
  - Changes in extremities
- **or:** the presence of fever and coronary artery aneurysms with three additional criteria is required for the diagnosis of 'complete' cases
- 'Incomplete' cases comprise those with fewer than the prerequisite number of criteria. Irritability is an important sign — which, although virtually universally present, is not included as one of the diagnostic criteria
- Other relatively common clinical findings in KD include arthritis, aseptic meningitis, pneumonitis, uveitis, gastroenteritis, meatitis and dysuria as well as otitis. Relatively uncommon abnormalities include hydrops of the gallbladder, gastrointestinal ischaemia, jaundice, petechial rash, febrile convulsions and encephalopathy or ataxia. Cardiac complications other than coronary arterial abnormalities include cardiac tamponade, cardiac failure, myocarditis, endocardial disease and pericarditis
- Acute-phase proteins, neutrophils and the ESR are usually elevated. Thrombocytosis occurs towards the end of the second week of the illness and therefore may not be helpful diagnostically. Liver function may be deranged. Sterile pyuria is occasionally observed, and also CSF pleocytosis (predominantly lymphocytes) representing aseptic meningitis

Treatment of KD

Treatment of KD is aimed at reducing inflammation and preventing the occurrence of coronary artery aneurysms and arterial thrombosis. Patients receive aspirin and intravenous immunoglobulin, 2 g/kg as a single dose infused intravenously.

An echocardiogram is performed at 10–14 days, 6 weeks, 6 months and then at further times if an abnormality is detected.

Cardiac complications of KD

- 20–40% of untreated KD patients develop coronary artery abnormalities
- 50% of these lesions regress within 5 years, and regression occurs within 2 years in most cases of mild coronary artery aneurysms (3–4 mm)
- The risk of these complications is markedly reduced with the use of intravenous immunoglobulins

In 1993, a report from the British Paediatric Surveillance Unit (BPSU) indicated a mortality rate of 3.7% in the UK for KD. Current mortality rates reported from Japan are much lower at 0.14%.

4.3 Infective endocarditis

- Usually occurs as a complication of congenital or rheumatic heart disease or of prosthetic valves, but it can occur in children without cardiac malformations
- There is an increased risk with central lines and intravenous drug use
- Highest risk lesions are those associated with high-velocity blood flow, e.g. ventricular septal defects, left-sided valvular lesions and systemic–pulmonary arterial communications. Uncommon with atrial septal defects
- Vegetations occur at the site of endocardial erosion from turbulent flow

Organisms

Most common organisms

- Native valve:
  - *Streptococcus viridans* group (*Strep. mutans, Strep. sanguis, Strep. mitis*)
  - *Staph. aureus*
  - Enterococcus (e.g. *Strep. faecalis, Strep. bovis*)
- Prosthetic valves:
  - *Staph. epidermidis*
  - *Staph. aureus*
  - *Strep. viridans*

Uncommon organisms

- *Strep. pneumoniae, H. influenzae, Coxiella burnetii* (Q fever), *Chlamydia psittaci, Chlamydia trachomatis* and *Chlamydia pneumoniae, Legionella* spp., fungi and the HACEK organisms (*Haemophilus* spp. (*H. parainfluenzae, H. aphrophilus, H. paraphrophilus*), *Actinobacillus actinomycetem comitans, Cardiobacterium hominis, Eikenella corrodens* and *K. kingae*)

Clinical presentation

- Acute: fever and septicaemia
- Non-acute: more common — prolonged fever, non-specific symptoms, e.g. fatigue, myalgia, arthralgia, weight loss, or no symptoms at all
- New murmurs or changes in known murmurs, splenomegaly, neurological

manifestations, e.g. emboli, cerebral abscesses (usually *Staph. aureus*), mycotic aneurysms and haemorrhage
- Cardiac failure from valve destruction
- The classic skin lesions occur late in the disease and are now rarely seen, e.g. Osler's nodes (tender nodules in pads of the fingers and toes), Janeway lesions (painless haemorrhagic lesions on soles and palms) and splinter haemorrhages (linear lesions below nails). These are caused by circulating antigen–antibody complexes

Investigations

- At least three separate blood cultures taken from different sites and at different times over 2 days, cultured on enriched media for > 7 days. This increases the likelihood of a positive yield, as does an increased volume of blood inoculum in each blood culture bottle.
- Look for raised white cell count, high ESR, microscopic haematuria
- Echocardiography — the presence of vegetations or valvular abnormalities

Treatment

- Broad-spectrum intravenous (iv) antibiotics, e.g. penicillin and gentamicin or vancomycin and gentamicin (depending on the most likely organism), at high bactericidal levels should be started as soon as possible after the blood cultures have been taken, because delay causes progressive endocardial damage
- Treatment duration is usually 4–6 weeks, but may be shorter for fully sensitive organisms
- Surgical intervention may be required

Prevention

- Antibiotic prophylaxis before and after various procedures, e.g. dental extraction in high-risk patients
- Proper dental care and oral hygiene. The teeth and gums are an important source of bacteria and poor dental hygiene significantly increases the risk of bacteraemic and septicaemic episodes

4.4   Toxic-shock syndrome

- Syndrome of high fever, conjunctivitis, diarrhoea, vomiting, confusion, myalgia, pharyngitis and rash with rapid progression to severe, intractable shock in some cases
- Caused by exotoxins produced by *Staph. aureus*, e.g. staphylococcal enterotoxin B or C (SEB, SEC) or toxic-shock syndrome toxin-1 (TSST-1) or group A streptococcus, e.g. streptococcal pyrogenic exotoxin A (SPEA)
- In staphylococcal toxic shock the focus of infection is often minor, e.g. skin abrasion
- Classically occurred in the past in females using tampons
- In streptococcal toxic shock the focus is usually severe and deep-seated, e.g. fasciitis and myositis

- Superantigen-mediated, i.e. causes massive, non-major histocompatibility complex-restricted, T-cell response

Diagnostic criteria

- Fever > 38.8°C
- Diffuse macular erythroderma
- Desquamation 1–2 weeks after onset, especially on palms and soles
- Hypotension
- Involvement of three or more organs – gastrointestinal tract, renal, hepatic, muscle, CNS; mucositis, disseminated intravascular coagulation

Diagnosis

- Clinical
- Identification of toxin or antibodies to toxin

Treatment

- Supportive
- Intravenous antibiotics
- Intravenous immunoglobulin

4.5 Brucellosis

- *Brucella* species (e.g. *B. abortus*, *B. melitensis*) are non-motile Gram-negative bacilli
- Zoonotic disease, transmitted to humans by ingestion of unpasteurized milk or by direct inoculation to abraded skin
- Incubation period 1–4 weeks
- Disease is often mild in children

Acute brucellosis

- Fever, night-sweats, headaches, malaise, anorexia, weight loss, myalgia, abdominal pain, arthritis, lymphadenopathy, hepatosplenomegaly
- Complications include meningitis, endocarditis, osteomyelitis

Chronic brucellosis

- Fevers, malaise, depression, splenomegaly

Diagnosis

- Prolonged culture of blood, bone marrow or other tissue, paired serology

Treatment

- Co-trimoxazole at high dose for 4–6 weeks

4.6 Lyme disease

- Disease occurs on the east coast of the United States and in parts of Europe and the UK
- Caused by spirochaete *Borrelia burgdorferi*, transmitted by *Ixodes* ticks
- Incubation from tick bite to erythema migrans is 3–31 days

Clinical manifestations

There are three stages:

- **Early localized** — distinctive rash (bull's eye lesion) — erythema migrans — red macule/papule at site of tick bite, which expands over days/weeks to large annular erythematous lesion with partial clearing, approximately 15 cm in diameter. Associated with fever, malaise, headache, neck stiffness
- **Early disseminated** — 3–5 weeks post bite — multiple erythema migrans, cranial nerve palsies especially the VIIth cranial nerve, meningitis, conjunctivitis, arthralgia, myalgia, headache, malaise, rarely carditis
- **Late disease** — recurrent arthritis, pauciarticular, large joints, neuropathy, encephalopathy

Diagnosis

- Clinical
- Serology and immunoblotting to detect production of antibodies to *B. burgdorferi* can be problematic because they are negative in early disease and, once present, persist beyond resolution of disease
- Polymerase chain reaction (PCR) amplification — is currently a research tool only

Treatment

- Doxycycline for child > 8 years (avoid sun exposure), or amoxacillin if < 8 years for 14–21 days if early disease, 21–28 days if disseminated or late disease
- Intravenous ceftriaxone or iv penicillin if meningitis, encephalitis, carditis or recurrent arthritis

4.7 Listeriosis

- Caused by *Listeria monocytogenes*, a Gram-positive bacillus
- Variable incubation of 3–70 days
- Isolated from a range of raw foods, including vegetables and uncooked meats, as well as processed foods and soft cheeses and meat-based patés
- The majority of cases are believed to be food-borne. Some cases are the result of direct contact with animals. Mother to fetus transmission in utero or during birth or via person-to-person spread between infants shortly after delivery
- Unborn infants, neonates, immunocompromised individuals, pregnant women and the elderly are at high risk

Clinical manifestations

- Influenza-like illness or meningoencephalitis/septicaemia; spontaneous abortion
- Maternal infections can be asymptomatic

Treatment

- Ampicillin

4.8 Leptospirosis

- This is a spirochaetal disease caused by *Leptospira* spp.
- Many wild and domestic animals, e.g. rats, dogs and livestock, harbour and excrete *Leptospira* spp. in their urine
- Transmission is by direct contact of mucosal surfaces or abraded skin with urine or carcasses of infected animals; or by indirect contact, e.g. swimming in water contaminated by infected urine
- Incubation period is 1–2 weeks

Clinical manifestations

- This is an acute febrile illness which can be biphasic. The initial phase is septicaemic in nature and varies in severity from a mild self-limited illness to life-threatening disease. The initial illness lasts 3–7 days. Clinically, there is abrupt onset with fevers, rigors, headaches, myalgia, malaise and conjunctival injection
- Recovery can then be followed, a few days later, by an immune-mediated disease. Clinical presentation includes fever, aseptic meningitis, uveitis, myalgias, lymphadenopathy and vasculitis rashes
- 90% will be anicteric; however, 10% will be severely unwell with jaundice, renal dysfunction, respiratory, cardiac and CNS disease. There is a case fatality rate of 5–40% in this group

Diagnosis

- Blood and CSF culture in the first 10 days of illness and urine after 1 week. Yield is low, the incubation period is prolonged and special culture media are required
- Serology, although retrospective, is the most reliable diagnostic tool
- PCR is available in a few laboratories but for research purposes only

Treatment

- Penicillin iv for severe disease
- Oral doxycycline (if child is > 8 years old) or oral amoxicillin for < 8 years old for mild disease

4.9   Cat-scratch disease

- Caused by *Bartonella henselae* — a fastidious Gram-negative bacterium
- Organism transmitted between cats by the cat flea. Humans are incidental hosts. There is no person-to-person spread
- More than 90% of patients have a history of contact with cats (usually kittens)

Clinical manifestations

- Fever and mild systemic symptoms occur in 30% of patients
- A skin papule is often found at the site of presumed bacterial inoculation
- Predominant sign is regional lymphadenopathy, involving the nodes that drain the site of inoculation
- In up to 30% of cases the lymph node will suppurate spontaneously

Complications

- Encephalitis, aseptic meningitis, neuroretinitis, hepatosplenic microabscesses and chronic systemic disease occur occasionally but are more common in the immunocompromised patient

Diagnosis

- Immunofluorescence antibody assays are the most useful diagnostic tests
- PCR is available in some laboratories but is not recommended
- Histology of the lymph node and staining with Warthin–Starry silver stain may show characteristic necrotizing granulomata and/or the causative organism

Treatment

- Most disease is self-limiting so treatment is symptomatic
- For those who are severely unwell and for immunocompromised patients, antibiotics such as ciprofloxacin, rifampicin, azithromycin and iv gentamicin are used

5.   MYCOBACTERIAL INFECTIONS

5.1   Tuberculosis (TB)

- Disease caused by infection with *Mycobacterium tuberculosis*, an acid-fast bacillus
- Incubation period, i.e. infection to development of positive tuberculin skin test, is 2–12 weeks (usually 3–4 weeks)
- Incidence is increasing again in the UK (especially in immigrant patients and those with human immunodeficiency virus (HIV))
- Host (immune status, age, nutrition) and bacterial (load, virulence) factors determine whether infection progresses to disease. Defects in interferon-γ and interleukin-12 pathways predispose to infection

- Children usually have primary TB, adults may have either new infections or reactivation disease
- Children are rarely infectious
- Children are usually infected by an adult with 'open', i.e sputum-positive pulmonary TB, therefore notification and contact tracing are essential
- Approximately 30% of healthy people closely exposed to TB will become infected, of whom only 5–10% will go on to develop active disease. Young children exposed to TB are more likely to develop disease than healthy adults
- Risk of disease is highest in the first 6 months after infection

TB exposure:	Patient exposed to person with contagious pulmonary TB
	Clinical examination, chest X-ray and Mantoux-negative
	Some will have early infection, not yet apparent
TB infection:	Positive Mantoux test
	Asymptomatic with normal clinical examination
	Chest X-ray normal
	Treat with chemoprophylaxis
TB disease:	Positive Mantoux test
	Clinical symptoms/signs of TB, and/or
	Chest X-ray signs consistent with TB
	Treat with chemotherapy

Pathogenesis

- Majority of infections are acquired via the respiratory route, occasionally ingested
- Organisms multiply in periphery of the lung and spread to regional lymph nodes, which may cause hilar lymphadenopathy
- Pulmonary macrophages ingest bacteria and mount a cellular immune response
- In the majority of children, this primary pulmonary infection is controlled by the immune system over 6–10 weeks. Healing of the pulmonary foci occurs, which later calcifies (Ghon focus). Any surviving bacilli remain dormant but may reactivate later in life and cause tuberculous disease which can be smear positive and contagious

Clinical symptoms/signs

TB infection — usually asymptomatic, may develop fever, malaise, cough or hypersensitivity reactions — erythema nodosum or phlyctenular conjunctivitis.

Clinical signs = disease

- Progressive primary pulmonary TB — foci of infection not controlled but enlarge to involve whole middle and/or lower lobes, often with cavitation (look for immunodeficiency) — fever, cough, dyspnoea, malaise, weight loss

- Dissemination to other organs (especially in children < 4 years of age)
  - Miliary TB — acutely unwell, fever, weight loss, hepatosplenomegaly, choroidal tubercules in retina, miliary picture on chest X-ray
  - TB meningitis (see Section 3.1, this chapter)
  - TB pericarditis — fever, chest pain, signs of constrictive pericarditis
  - Bone and joint infection
  - Urogenital infection (very rare in childhood)
  - Gastrointestinal tract — abdominal pain, malabsorption, obstruction, perforation, fistula, haemorrhage, 'doughy' abdomen (usually ingested rather than disseminated)

Congenital TB

(See Section 11, this chapter)

Neonatal contact for mother with TB

Infant is at high risk of acquiring TB. Evaluate mother and child (with clinical examination and chest X-ray)

- If mother is 'smear positive' or has an abnormal chest X-ray, separate neonate and mother until both are on adequate medication and mother is non-contagious
- If congenital TB is excluded, give 3 months of prophylactic isoniazid
- At 3 months, perform a Mantoux test:
  - If this is negative and a repeat chest X-ray is negative then give BCG and stop chemoprophylaxis
  - If it is positive reassess for TB disease — if there is no disease continue isoniazid for another 3 months; if disease is present then treatment with triple or quadruple therapy is required

Diagnosis

Tuberculin tests
Tuberculin tests involve an intradermal test of delayed hypersensitivity to tuberculin purified-protein derivative.

- **Heaf test** — used for mass screening, if positive refer to TB clinic. Positive is grade 2–4 if no previous BCG, grade 3 or 4 if BCG received previously. This is not an appropriate test for contact tracing
- **Mantoux test** — dose in UK is 0.1 ml of 1 : 1,000, i.e. 10 tuberculin units (use 1 : 10,000 if risk of hypersensitivity, e.g. erythema nodosum or phlyctenular conjunctivitis). Mantoux tests are more accurate than Heaf tests and should be used for all patients where disease is suspected and for contact tracing. Measure induration, not erythema, at 48–72 h. Interpretation is difficult but test is positive if:
  - > 15 mm induration in anyone (equivalent to Heaf 3–4)
  - > 5–14 mm induration (equivalent to Heaf 2) if not had BCG and at high risk, e.g. found at contact or new immigrant screening, or in child< 4 years old
  - NB — A negative Mantoux test does **not** exclude a positive diagnosis — the test may be negative if it was incorrectly inserted; if anergy is present (in 10% of the normal population and also occurs in the very young), if there is overwhelming disseminated TB and in some viral infections, e.g. HIV, measles, influenza

Microbiological tests

- Ziehl–Neelsen stain for acid-fast bacilli, and culture for 4–8 weeks of sputum, gastric washings, bronchoalveolar lavage fluid, CSF, biopsy specimens (culture is required because it will provide details of type and sensitivities)
- All have low yield in children because there are lower numbers of bacteria

Other

- **Histology** — caseating granuloma and acid-fast bacilli
- **PCR** — poor sensitivity and specificity at present
- **Chest X-ray** — typical changes of hilar lymphadenopathy +/– parenchymal changes

Treatment

Chemoprophylaxis

Chemoprophylaxis is required:

- For those with TB infection (i.e. a positive Mantoux test, well child, normal chest X-ray) to prevent progression to disease
- For close contacts of smear-positive TB patients if they are HIV-positive or immunosuppressed patients because they may not develop a positive Mantoux response

Options for chemoprophylaxis are:

- Isoniazid for 6 months (+ pyridoxine for breast-fed infants and malnourished)
- **or** isoniazid and rifampicin for 3 months

A repeat chest X-ray at the end of treatment is not required if there has been good compliance and the child is asymptomatic.

Chemotherapy

For those with signs of disease four drugs are used in the initial 2 months of treatment because of the increase in isoniazid resistance (now 6% in London, UK). The fourth drug (usually ethambutol/streptomycin) can be **omitted** if there is a **low** risk of isoniazid resistance, i.e. previously untreated, Caucasian, proven or suspected HIV-negative patients, or those who have had **no** contact with a TB patient with drug resistance.

- Pulmonary and non-pulmonary disease (except meningitis) — isoniazid and rifampicin for 6 months with pyrazinamide and a fourth drug for the first 2 months
- Meningitis — 12 months' total therapy with isoniazid and rifampicin with pyrazinamide and a fourth drug for the first 2 months
- Multidrug-resistant TB — seek expert advice
- **NB** Directly observed therapy is recommended if there is any chance of non-compliance
- Corticosteroids should be used for 6–8 weeks if there is TB meningitis, pericarditis, miliary TB and endobronchial disease with obstruction, but only **with** anti-TB therapy

Prevention

- Improvement of social conditions and general health
- BCG vaccination (live attenuated strain of *M. bovis*) gives approximately 50% protection. It is effective in the prevention of extra-pulmonary disease in the < 4-year age group. In the UK, BCG given at birth to high-risk groups and at 12–14 years of age to tuberculin test-negative children

Complications of BCG vaccination

Include subcutaneous abscess, suppurative lymphadenitis and disseminated disease in severely immunocompromised children.

5.2   Atypical mycobacteria

- Infections caused by non-tuberculous mycobacteria, e.g. *M. avium* complex, *M. scrofulaceum, M. kansasii*
- Ubiquitous organisms — found in soil, food, water and animals
- Found world-wide
- Acquired via ingestion, inoculation, or inhalation of organism
- Many people exposed, but only a small number have infection or disease
- May cause disseminated disease in immunodeficient patients, e.g. HIV-positive

Clinical presentations

- Lymphadenitis (usually cervical), pulmonary infections, cutaneous infections and occasionally, osteomyelitis

Diagnosis

- Isolation and identification by culture (PCR in some laboratories)
- May have weakly positive Mantoux test (with no signs of TB)

Treatment

- For non-tuberculous mycobacterial lymphadenitis — surgical excision alone
- If excision is incomplete, or other site is involved, medical treatment with at least two drugs for 3–6 months is required

NB For differential diagnosis of persistent cervical lymphadenopathy see Section 12.2.

6.   FUNGAL INFECTIONS

- Many fungi are ubiquitous, growing in soil, decaying vegetation and animals
- Infection is acquired by inhalation, ingestion and inoculation from direct contact
- Often produce spores
- Superficial infections are common

- Invasive disease occurs almost exclusively in immunocompromised people, mainly those with neutrophil defects or neutropenia. Consider if a neutropenic patient is not responding to antibacterial therapy after 48 h of illness

6.1 Cutaneous fungal infections

Tinea versicolor or pityriasis versicolor

- Caused by *Malassezia furfur* (*Pityrosporum orbiculare*)
- Oval, macular lesions on neck, upper chest, back, arms; may be hypo- or hyperpigmented
- Diagnosis by microscopy of skin scrapings
- Treatment with topical antifungals and salicylic acid preparations

Ringworm (dermatophytoses)

These are caused by filamentous fungi belonging to three main genera — *Trichophyton*, *Microsporum* and *Epidermophyton*, diagnosed by skin scrapings.

Tinea capitis (ringworm of scalp)

- Causes patchy dandruff-like scaling with hair loss, discrete pustules or kerion — boggy, inflammatory mass +/− fever and local lymphadenopathy
- Treat with oral antifungals, e.g. griseofulvin, terbinafine. Topical agents not effective

Tinea corporis (ringworm of body)

- Usually dry, erythematous annular lesion with central clearing, on face, trunk and limbs
- Treat with topical antifungals for 4 weeks, if no response use oral antifungals

Tinea cruris (Jock itch!)

- Infection of groin and upper thighs causing itchy erythematous, scaly skin
- Treat as tinea corporis

Tinea pedis (athlete's foot)

- Infection in interdigital spaces, may involve the whole foot. Fungi are common in damp areas, e.g. swimming pools. Treat as tinea corporis

6.2 Candidiasis (thrush, moniliasis)

- Usually caused by *Candida albicans*
- Present on skin, in the mouth, and in the gastrointestinal tract and vagina of healthy individuals
- Person-to-person transmission occurs
- Use of antibiotics may promote overgrowth of yeasts

Clinical manifestations

Mild mucocutaneous infection

- Oral thrush and/or nappy-area dermatitis are common in infants
- Vulvovaginal candidiasis occurs in adolescents
- Intertriginous lesions, e.g. in neck, groin, axilla

Chronic mucocutaneous candidiasis

- Associated with endocrine disease and progressive T-cell immunodeficiencies

Invasive disease

- Disseminated disease to almost any organ, especially in very low-birth-weight newborns and those who are immunocompromised

Diagnosis

- Microscopy showing pseudohyphae or germ-tube formation (*C. albicans* only)
- Culture

Treatment

- For minor mucocutaneous disease — use oral nystatin or topical nystatin/clotrimazole/miconazole
- For severe or chronic mucocutaneous disease — use an oral azole, e.g. fluconazole
- For invasive disease — treat as for *Aspergillus* infection (see below)

6.3   Aspergillosis

- Caused by *Aspergillus fumigatus*, *A. niger*, *A. flavus* and, rarely, others
- No person-to-person transmission

Clinical manifestations

- Allergic bronchopulmonary aspergillosis — episodic wheezing, low-grade fever, brown sputum, eosinophilia, transient pulmonary infiltrates. Usually in children with cystic fibrosis or asthma. Treat with steroids
- Sinusitis and otomycosis of external ear canal — usually benign in immunocompetent patients
- Aspergilloma — fungal balls that grow in pre-existing cavities or bronchogenic cysts — non-invasive
- Invasive aspergillosis — extremely serious
  - May cause peripheral patchy bronchopneumonia with clinical manifestations of acute pneumonia
  - Often disseminates to brain, heart, liver, spleen, eye, bone and other organs in the immunocompromised patient population

Diagnosis

- High clinical index of suspicion
- Microscopy shows branched and septate hyphae
- Culture

Treatment

- For invasive disease treat with liposomal amphotericin in high dose +/– a second antifungal, e.g. caspofungin, an azole or flucytosine depending on culture results
- Surgical excision of localized lesion

7. VIRAL INFECTIONS

7.1 Human immunodeficiency virus (HIV)

- HIV is a retrovirus, i.e. it contains the enzyme reverse transcriptase, which allows its viral RNA to be incorporated into host-cell DNA
- Two main types are known: HIV-1 (widespread) and HIV-2 (West Africa)
- Mainly infects CD4 helper T cells, causing reduction of these cells and acquired immunodeficiency

Transmission

- Vertical (most common mode of transmission in children)
    - Prenatal
    - Intrapartum (most common)
    - Postnatally via breast milk
- Blood or blood products, e.g.
    - Haemophiliacs (of historical interest only in the UK now)
    - Unsterile needle use
- Via mucous membranes, e.g.
    - Sexual intercourse, **NB** sexual abuse

Diagnosis

- Virus detection by PCR (rapid, sensitive, specific)
- Detection of immunoglobulin G (IgG) antibody to viral envelope proteins (gp120 and subunits)

Diagnosis of HIV infection if:

- HIV antibody-positive after 18 months old if born to an infected mother, or at any age if mother is not infected – on two occasions
- PCR positive on two separate specimens taken at different times

Babies of HIV-positive mother:

- Start zidovudine (AZT, azidothymidine) orally for baby within 12 h of birth. This is continued for four weeks
    - 24–48 h — HIV PCR (50% true-positive by 1 week, 90% by 2 weeks)
    - 6 weeks — repeat HIV PCR, start septrin prophylaxis
    - 3–4 months — repeat HIV PCR
- If all 3 PCRs are negative then > 95% chance baby is **not** infected
- Stop septrin
- Follow-up until HIV antibody (vertically acquired from mother) is negative
- **NB**. Still HIV affected, ie. many issues re infection in family

Follow-up of HIV-positive babies/children:

- Every 3–6 months depending on health
- History and examination for signs of persistent or unusual infections and growth/puberty
- Psychological and social support, issues re awareness of diagnosis
- Full blood count, T-cell subsets/CD4 count, HIV viral load
- Hepatitis B and C viruses, CMV, *Toxoplasma* status if indicated
- Immunization information
- Septrin prophylaxis is continued for the first year of life in all HIV-positive children regardless of CD4 count
    - All infants under the age of 18 months with a CD4 count < 20% require antiretroviral treatment
    - All children over 18 months, with a CD4 count < 15% require antiretroviral treatment
    - Children who fulfil the clinical criteria for treatment should be given antiretroviral treatment regardless of their CD4 counts

Clinical manifestations

These include AIDS-defining and non-defining illnesses.

Clinical categories for children < 13 years with HIV infection. CDC Classification to be used in conjunction with the CDC Immunological classification

Category N	Not symptomatic	Children who have no signs or symptoms considered to be the result of HIV infection, or those who have only one of the conditions listed in Category A
Category A	Mildly symptomatic	Children with two or more of: lymphadenopathy; hepatomegaly; splenomegaly; dermatitis; parotitis; recurrent or persistent upper respiratory infection, sinusitis or chronic otitis media

Category B	Moderately symptomatic	Anaemia, neutropenia or thrombocytopenia; single episode of bacterial meningitis, pneumonia, or sepsis; persistent oropharyngeal candidiasis; cardiomyopathy; chronic diarrhoea; hepatitis; recurrent HSV stomatitis; herpes zoster (shingles); leiomyosarcoma; lymphoid interstitial pneumonia; nephropathy; nocardiosis; persistent fever (lasting > 1 month); toxoplasmosis; disseminated varicella
Category C	Severely symptomatic (AIDS-defining)	1. Serious bacterial infections, multiple or recurrent 2. Opportunistic infections: candidiasis (oesophageal or pulmonary), coccidioidomycosis, cryptococcosis, cryptosporidiosis or isosporiasis with diarrhoea persisting > 1 month; CMV disease with onset of symptoms at age > 1 month; HSV bronchitis, pneumonitis, or oesophagitis; histoplasmosis; *Mycobacterium tuberculosis*, disseminated or extrapulmonary; *M. avium* complex or *M. kansasii*, disseminated; *Pneumocystis carinii* pneumonia; progressive multifocal leukoencephalopathy; toxoplasmosis of the brain 3. Encephalopathy 4. Wasting syndrome 5. Malignancy, e.g. Kaposi sarcoma, lymphoma

- 1997 — 20% of vertically infected children developed AIDS in infancy, most common AIDS-defining illness was *P. carinii* pneumonia
- 2001 — improved antenatal detection and prophylaxis, therefore fewer AIDS-defining illnesses in infancy
- Approximately 5% of children with HIV develop AIDS per year

Recurrent bacterial infections

- B-cell dysregulation occurs, despite often high immunoglobulin levels, because of poor CD4 (T-helper cell) function
- Recurrent serious bacterial infections, such as pneumonia, meningitis, septicaemia and osteomyelitis, may occur. The commonest organisms are those which are normally pathogenic, *Strep. pneumoniae*, *H. influenzae*, coliforms and Salmonella.
- Treatment depends on clinical condition and probable infective organism

Faltering growth

This is frequently multifactorial, e.g.:

- Reduced nutrient and fluid intake — psychosocial reasons or oral and oesophageal thrush
- Increased nutrient and fluid requirement with chronic disease (30–50%)
- Increased fluid loss with diarrhoea – look for gut pathogens, microsporidiosis, cryptosporidiosis, *Giardia*, atypical *Mycobacteria* and viruses
- **Treatment**: improve immune function with highly active antiretroviral therapy (HAART); treat specific infections; provide dietary supplements

Lymphocytic interstitial pneumonitis

- Caused by diffuse infiltration of pulmonary interstitium with CD8 (cytotoxic) lymphocytes and plasma cells
- Often diagnosed from a chest X-ray in an otherwise asymptomatic child
- May cause progressive cough, hypoxaemia and clubbing
- Is associated with parotitis
- Superimposed bacterial infections and bronchiectasis may occur
- May have element of reversible bronchoconstriction
- **Treatment**: symptomatic; HAART may help; if severe use oral prednisolone

HIV encephalopathy

- May present with regression of milestones, behavioural difficulties, acquired microcephaly, motor signs, e.g. spastic diplegia, ataxia, pseudobulbar palsy
- Exclude CNS infections and lymphoma
- **Treatment**: HAART

Thrombocytopenia

- Not associated with other indicators of disease progression
- **Treatment**: only if symptomatic or platelet count persistently $< 20,000/mm^3$. Options include intravenous immunoglobulin, steroids, HAART, or last-resort splenectomy (not recommended because it further increases the risk of sepsis)

Opportunistic infections

Protozoa

- *P. carinii* pneumonia +/– CMV pneumonitis:
  - Most common at 3–6 months of age; presents with persistent non-productive cough, hypoxaemia, dyspnoea, minimal chest signs on auscultation
  - Chest X-ray shows bilateral perihilar 'butterfly' shadowing; diagnosis by bronchoalveolar lavage; ensure no concurrent CMV infection
  - **Treatment**: supportive, may need to be treated in paediatric intensive care unit. High-dose co-trimoxazole (septrin) for 21 days in conjunction with steroids. Ganciclovir iv if there is concurrent CMV disease. Once stable, commence HAART. Prophylactic low-dose septrin following treatment

- Cerebral toxoplasmosis
  - Rare in childhood HIV infection; may present with focal signs +/– fits
  - Computerized tomography shows multiple intraparenchymal ring-enhancing lesions. Positive toxoplasmosis serology
  - **Treatment**: 6 weeks of pyrimethamine and sulfadiazine with folinic acid and HAART
- Cryptosporidosis
  - *Cryptosporidium parvum* causes severe secretory diarrhoea, abdominal pain and sometimes sclerosing cholangitis
  - Diagnosis by stool microscopy +/– small-bowel biopsy
  - **Treatment**: supportive, paromomycin

Fungi

- *Candida albicans* — oropharyngeal, oesophageal, vulvovaginal, disseminated (rare)
  - **Treatment**: chronic antifungal therapy, e.g. fluconazole, voriconazole, iv liposomal amphotericin B if severe
- *Cryptococcus neoformans* — meningitis (insidious onset), pneumonia
  - Diagnosis by CSF examination (Indian ink stain, antigen, culture), serum culture, antigen
  - **Treatment**: fluconazole. In severe disease, two antifungal agents should be used

Viruses

- CMV — retinitis, colitis, pneumonitis, hepatitis, pancreatitis
  - Diagnosis by serum PCR, immunofluorescence in relevant sample and characteristic retinal changes if present; differentiate disease from carriage
  - **Treatment**: iv ganciclovir; HAART
- Herpes simplex virus
  - Types 1 and 2 – extensive oral ulceration
  - **Treatment**: iv aciclovir, oral prophylaxis if recurrent and severe; HAART may help
- Measles, varicella zoster virus, respiratory syncytial virus, adenovirus — all may cause severe disease in HIV-infected children, especially pneumonitis

TB and atypical TB

- Increased risk of TB and atypical TB, especially disseminated *M. avium* complex
- See Section 5

Tumours

These are rare in children.

Kaposi sarcoma — tumour of vascular endothelial cells, associated with human herpesvirus-8 (HHV–8); involves skin, gut, lung and lymphatics
- **Treatment**: HAART, local radiotherapy, chemotherapy if disseminated
Lymphoma — non-Hodgkin B-cell primary CNS lymphoma
- Focal neurological signs +/– fits; computerized tomography shows single lesion
- Definitive diagnosis by brain biopsy
- **Treatment**: radio/chemotherapy; poor prognosis

HIV treatment

Highly active antiretroviral therapy (HAART).

- When to start treatment in children differs in each country
- In the UK, start treatment if there are an AIDS-defining illness, many B-category symptoms and rapidly decreasing CD4 count (< 20% in children under 2 years of age, and < 15% in older children)
- Three-drug therapy is the gold-standard. This reduces resistance and suppresses viral load to undetectable levels
- Standard HAART regime comprises a backbone of two nucleoside reverse transcriptase inhibitor (NRTIs) and **either** a non-NRTI **or** a protease inhibitor. Liaise with tertiary centre
- Monitor for efficacy (viral load and CD4 count) and side-effects

P. carinii prophylaxis

- For first 12 months of life if vertically infected
- If CD4 count < 15%

Reduction of vertical transmission

With breast-feeding and no intervention vertical transmission rate is 15–30%.

Interventions:
- No breast-feeding (where safe alternative is possible) transmission rate is 15%
- + Antiretrovirals to mother and baby, e.g. ACTG 076 trial — reduces rate to 5%
- + elective Caesarean section — reduces transmission to 2% (or less if very low maternal viral load)

To allow intervention, women need to be diagnosed before giving birth. National targets and objectives were set in 1999 that involve the offer and recommendation of an HIV test to all pregnant women throughout the UK. By 2001 80% of maternity units in the UK offered this service, with an uptake of approximately 70%

NB If vaginal delivery — avoid invasive fetal procedures, e.g. fetal blood sampling

Major side-effects of antiretroviral drugs used in children

Drug	Side-effect
Nucleoside reverse transcriptase inhibitors	
AZT – zidovudine	Nausea, bone marrow suppression, myopathy
DDI – didanosine	Peripheral neuropathy, pancreatitis
D4T – stavudine	Peripheral neuropathy, pancreatitis, elevation of liver function test
3TC – lamivudine	Rare – peripheral neuropathy, pancreatitis
Abacavir	Life-threatening hypersensitivity reactions – usually present as rash and fever

Non-nucleoside reverse transcriptase inhibitors

Efavirenz	Rash, sleep disturbances, hallucinations (rare in children)
Nevirapine	Rash, hepatitis

Protease inhibitors

Ritonavir	Gastrointestinal side-effects common in first 4 weeks, paraesthesia
Kaletra (Lopinavir boosted with ritonavir)	Raised transaminases
Nelfinavir	Diarrhoea

NB Protease inhibitors and D4T are associated with lipodystrophy

7.2 Hepatitis

(See Chapter 12 — Hepatology)

7.3 Epstein–Barr virus (EBV)

This causes infectious mononucleosis (glandular fever). EBV infects pharyngeal epithelial cells and then B lymphocytes. These disseminate and proliferate until checked by activated T cells.

- **Transmission**: saliva, aerosol
- **Incubation**: 30–50 days
- **Clinical presentation**:
  - Fever, sore throat, lymphadenopathy, palatal petechiae and malaise
  - Splenomegaly (50%), hepatomegaly (30%), hepatitis (80%), clinical jaundice (5%), thrombocytopenia, haemolytic anaemia
  - Maculopapular rash (5–15%), 90% if given ampicillin
- **Complications**:
  - Meningitis, encephalitis, Guillain–Barré, syndrome, myocarditis, splenic rupture, airway obstruction from pharyngotonsillar swelling
  - Chronic fatigue-like syndrome
  - Disseminated disease with B-cell proliferation in those with T-cell immunodeficiencies
- **Diagnosis**: atypical lymphocytosis, positive Paul–Bunnell (often negative in young children) or Monospot test, serology, heterophile antibodies, PCR
- **Treatment**: supportive, steroids for severe inflammatory processes

7.4 Cytomegalovirus (CMV)

- **Transmission**: close contact, blood, organ transplant
- **Clinical presentation**:
  - In normal hosts — often asymptomatic or glandular fever-like picture
  - In immunocompromised patients — severe disease may occur with pneumonitis, retinitis, encephalitis, hepatitis and gastrointestinal disturbance
  - CMV is the most common congenital infection
- **Diagnosis**: immunofluorescence, intranuclear inclusions in biopsy specimens, culture, detection of early antigen fluorescence foci (DEAFF) test, PCR
- **Treatment**: symptomatic, iv ganciclovir and/or iv foscarnet if immunosuppressed

7.5 Herpes simplex virus (HSV)

Infection:
- Two types recognized: HSV-1 (usually infects skin and mucous membranes) and HSV-2 (usually genital)
- Primary infections — 85% subclinical
- Recurrent infections — reactivation of latent infection

Incubation: 2–12 days

Transmission: direct contact. Congenital infections occur in approximately 1 : 10,000 live births in the UK. They can present as localized infection, disseminated infection or neonatal encephalitis

Clinical presentation:
- Acute herpetic gingivostomatitis — primary infection — acute painful mouth ulcers and fever, most common between 1 and 3 years of age, self-limiting, lasts 4–9 days (may be asymptomatic)
- Recurrent stomatitis — localized vesicular lesions in nasolabial folds, 'cold sores'
- Keratoconjunctivitis and corneal ulcers
- Meningoencephalitis (peak incidence in the neonatal group and in adolescence)
- Eczema herpeticum — widespread infection of eczematous skin with HSV vesicles — may be very severe
- Genital lesions — usually in sexually active adolescents, **NB** child abuse
- Neonatal HSV — usually from vaginal secretions at delivery — high morbidity and mortality

Diagnosis:
- Clinical, electron microscopy of vesicular fluid (very fast), PCR, culture (this is a fast-growing virus and cultures can be positive within 2–5 days)

Treatment:
- Aciclovir — iv if severe disease, immunocompromised, neonate or eczema herpeticum
- Oral, topical, eye drops

7.6 Varicella zoster virus (VZV)

This produces chickenpox (varicella) as a primary infection. Shingles (herpes zoster) is caused by reactivation of dormant VZV from dorsal root or cranial ganglia. You can catch chickenpox from contact with chickenpox **or** shingles. You cannot 'catch' shingles.

Chickenpox

- **Incubation**: chickenpox: 11–24 days
- **Transmission**: direct contact, droplet, airborne; infectious from 24 h before rash appears until all spots have crusted over (approx. 7–8 days)
- **Clinical presentation**: prodrome of fever and malaise for 24 h; rash appears in crops, papular then vesicular and itchy, usually start on trunk and spread centripetally; crops continue to appear for 3–4 days and each crusts after 24–48 h. Household contacts, who receive a higher viral inoculum, tend to have more severe disease
- **Complications**:
  - Secondary bacterial infection often with group A streptococcus
  - Thrombocytopenia with haemorrhage into skin
  - Pneumonia
  - Purpura fulminans
  - Post-infectious encephalitis
  - Immunocompromised patients — severe disseminated haemorrhagic disease
- **Diagnosis**: clinical, viral culture, serology and immunofluorescence assay, PCR
- **Treatment**: supportive; intravenous aciclovir for immunosuppressed or severely unwell patient
- **Prophylaxis**: zoster immunoglobulin (ZIG) if high risk (e.g. immunodeficiency, immunosuppressive treatment). **NB** If mother develops chickenpox within 5 days' pre- to 2 days' post-delivery give neonate ZIG. If baby develops chickenpox treat with iv aciclovir. **NB** The incubation period in children who have received ZIG is extended to 28 days

Herpes zoster

Increased incidence if immunosuppressed

- **Clinical presentation**:
  - Prodrome of pain and tenderness in affected dermatome with fever and malaise; within a few days the same rash as varicella appears in distribution of one (sometimes 2 or 3) unilateral dermatomes
  - If infection of Vth cranial nerve occurs, it may affect the cornea (ophthalmic branch)
  - If VIIth nerve is involved, may develop paralysis of facial nerve and vesicles in external ear (Ramsey–Hunt syndrome)
- **Complications**: dissemination in immunocompromised; post-herpetic pain rare in children

- **Treatment**: supportive; iv aciclovir if severe and patient is immunocompromised

NB VZV vaccine now available routinely in the USA, and for at-risk patients in the UK

7.7 Parvovirus B19 (erythema infectiosum, 'slapped cheek' or fifth disease)

This virus affects red cell precursors and reticulocytes in the bone marrow.

- **Incubation**: approx. 1 week
- **Transmission**: respiratory secretions, blood; not infectious once rash has appeared
- **Clinical presentation**:
  - Very erythematous cheeks, then erythematous macular papular rash on trunk and extremities, which fades with central clearing giving the characteristic lacy or reticular appearance
  - Rash lasts 2–30 days
- **Complications**:
  - Aplastic crisis in chronic haemolytic diseases, e.g. sickle-cell disease, thalassaemia
  - Aplastic anaemia
  - Arthritis, myalgia more common in older children/adults
  - Congenital infection with anaemia and hydrops (see Section 11)
- **Diagnosis**: clinical, serology, PCR
- **Treatment**: supportive

7.8 Roseola infantum (exanthem subitum or HHV-6)

- **Transmission**: respiratory secretions
- **Clinical presentation**: characteristic — sudden onset of high fever (up to 41°C) with absence of clinical localizing signs; at day 3–4 fever abruptly stops and macular/papular rash appears which lasts from < 24 h to a few days
  - This is one of the commonest causes of febrile convulsions in the 6- to 18-month age group. Febrile convulsions typically occur on the first day of illness
  - This virus is ubiquitous in the population and can occur either sub-clinically or as a non-specific febrile illness without focus
- **Diagnosis:** Diagnostic tests are not well established. PCR is available on a research basis and serological tests are available but differentiating primary disease from reactivation is problematic
- **Treatment**: antipyretics

7.9 Measles

- **Incubation**: 7–14 days
- **Transmission**: respiratory droplets; infectious from 7 days after exposure, i.e. from pre-rash to 5 days after rash starts

- **Clinical presentation**:
  - Prodrome: 3–5 days, low fever, brassy cough, coryza, conjunctivitis, Koplik spots (pathognomonic white spots opposite lower molars)
  - Eruptive stage: abrupt rise in temperature to 40°C associated with macular rash which starts behind ears and along hairline, becomes maculopapular and spreads sequentially to face, upper arms, chest, abdomen, back, legs; lasts approximately 4 days
- **Complications**:
  - Otitis media, laryngitis, bronchitis
  - Interstitial pneumonitis, secondary bacterial bronchopneumonia, myocarditis
  - Encephalomyelitis: mainly post-infectious, demyelinating (1 : 1,000 cases)
  - Subacute sclerosing panencephalitis (see Chapter 18 — Neurology)
  - Temporary immunosuppression for up to 6 weeks post-infection, causing increased susceptibility to secondary bacterial infections
- **Diagnosis**: clinical, viral culture, immunofluorescence, serology
- **Treatment**: symptomatic; human pooled immunoglobulin < 5 days of exposure to high-risk patients only. Vitamin A in children who are malnourished or who have severe measles. Ribavirin has been used in immunocompromised children, but no controlled studies demonstrating efficacy have been performed
- **Prophylaxis**: immunization — measles, mumps, rubella (MMR)

7.10 Mumps

- **Incubation**: 14–21 days
- **Transmission**: respiratory droplets, infectious 24 h pre- to 3 days post-parotid swelling
- **Clinical presentation**: mild prodrome of fever, anorexia, headache; painful bilateral (may be unilateral) salivary +/− submandibular gland swelling
- **Complications**: occur as a result of viraemia early in the infection:
  - Meningoencephalitis clinically 10% (subclinically 65%):
    - Infectious — symptoms same time as parotitis
    - Post-infectious — symptoms approx. 10 days post-parotitis
  - Orchitis/epididymitis:
    - Rare in childhood, 14–35% in adolescents/adults
    - Occurs within 8 days of parotitis, abrupt onset of fever and tender, swollen testes
    - Approx. 30–40% of affected testes atrophy; may cause subfertility
  - Pancreatitis, nephritis, myocarditis, arthritis, deafness, thyroiditis
- **Diagnosis**: viral culture, serology
- **Treatment**: supportive
- **Prophylaxis**: vaccination (MMR) to ensure 'herd immunity'

7.11 Rubella (German measles)

- **Incubation**: 14–21 days
- **Transmission**: respiratory droplets; transplacental
- **Clinical presentation**:
  - Mild coryza, palatal petechiae
  - Characteristic tender, retroauricular, posterior cervical and suboccipital adenopathy 24 h before rash appears, lasting 1 week
  - Rash is an erythematous maculopapular generalized rash which begins on face, spreading quickly to trunk.
- **Complications**: arthritis, encephalitis, congenital rubella syndrome (see Section 11)
- **Diagnosis**: clinical, serology
- **Treatment**: supportive
- **Prophylaxis**: although a mild illness, vaccination of all children prevents childbearing women contracting rubella

7.12 Adenovirus

- **Transmission**: respiratory droplets, contact, fomites, very contagious, strict infection control policy
- **Incubation**: 2–14 days
- **Clinical presentation**:
  - Upper respiratory tract infection
  - Conjunctivitis +/– pharyngitis
  - Gastroenteritis – more common in those < 4 years old
- **Complications**: severe pneumonia (more common in infants); disseminated disease in immunocompromised patients
- **Diagnosis**: viral culture, PCR
- **Treatment**: supportive, Ribavirin has been used with limited success in immunocompromised patients

7.13 Enteroviruses

These include polioviruses: types 1–3; coxsackieviruses: A and B and echoviruses.

- **Transmission**: faecal/oral and respiratory droplets, infections peak during summer and early autumn
- **Clinical presentation**:
  - Non-specific febrile illness: abrupt onset of fever and malaise +/– headache and myalgia, lasts 3–4 days
  - Respiratory manifestations: pharyngitis, tonsillitis, nasopharyngitis, lasts 3–6 days
  - Gastrointestinal manifestations: diarrhoea, vomiting, abdominal pain

- Skin manifestations: 'hand, foot and mouth' — usually coxsackievirus A16 and enterovirus 71; intraoral ulcerative lesions, vesicular lesions on hands and feet 3–7 mm; rash clears within 1 week
  - Pericarditis and myocarditis: usually coxsackie B viruses
  - Neurological manifestations: aseptic meningitis (esp. coxsackie virus B5), encephalitis (esp. echovirus 9), cerebellar ataxia and Guillain–Barré, syndrome
  - Although some clinical entities are more closely associated with specific enterovirus species, any of the enteroviruses can cause any of the clinical syndromes
- **Diagnosis**: viral culture, PCR. There is no place for the use of serology in the diagnosis of enteroviral infections
- **Treatment**: supportive
- **Prophylaxis**: Nil for coxsackie- and echoviruses. Polio vaccine for prevention of polio. The WHO are aiming for worldwide eradication.

7.14 Molluscum

- **Incubation**: 2–8 weeks
- **Transmission**: direct contact with infected person or fomites or autoinoculation
- **Clinical presentation**: discrete, pearly papules 1–5 mm, face, neck, axillae and thighs
- **Diagnosis**: clinical, microscopy
- **Treatment**:
  - Self-limiting but may last months–years
  - Need to treat in immunodeficient patients or it will become widespread, e.g. remove with liquid nitrogen

8. PARASITIC INFECTIONS

8.1 Toxoplasmosis

- Caused by *Toxoplasma gondii*
- World-wide distribution and infects most warm-blooded animals
- Cat is the definitive host and excretes oocysts in stools
- Intermediate hosts include sheep, pigs and cattle who have viable cysts in their tissues
- Human infection is by eating undercooked meat containing cysts or by ingestion of oocysts from soil; may also be acquired from blood transfusion or bone marrow transplantation
- Congenital infection (See Section 11)

Clinical manifestations

- Often asymptomatic, or non-specific fever, malaise, myalgia, sore throat
- May also have lymphadenopathy or mononucleosis-like illness
- Complications rarely include myocarditis, pericarditis and pneumonitis, encephalitis

- Isolated ocular toxoplasmosis is usually a result of reactivation of congenital infection, but may be acquired
- Immunodeficient patients may have more serious/disseminated disease

Diagnosis

- By serology (PCR in special cases)
- Isolation of *T. gondii* is difficult and is not performed routinely.
- Atypical lymphocytosis, eosinophilia and inversion of CD4 : CD8 ratio

Treatment

- Supportive if mild
- Pyrimethamine (and folinic acid) and sulfadiazine if symptomatic. If sulfadiazine is not tolerated, clindamycin can be used instead. A prolonged course of treatment, up to 1 year, is usual but the optimal length of treatment is not established

8.2   Head lice (Pediculosis capitis)

- Caused by lice – *Pediculus humanus capitis*
- Itching is the most common complaint
- Adult lice or eggs (nits) may be seen in the hair
- Very common in school-aged children

Transmission

- Occurs by direct contact with hair of infested individuals

Diagnosis

- Clinical, can confirm by microscopy

Treatment

- Two applications, 1 week apart, of a parasiticidal lotion, left on overnight, e.g. permethrin and malathion. Resistance is developing, so if the treatment fails try another insecticide for the next course. Many people use mechanical means of louse control, e.g. 'nit comb'. **Remember** to treat the whole family (+/– school class) at the same time.

Malaria (See Section 9.1)

Leishmaniasis (See Section 9.9)

Schistosomiasis (See Section 9.10)

Pneumocystis (See Section 7.1)

9. TROPICAL AND GEOGRAPHICALLY CIRCUMSCRIBED INFECTIONS

Travel is increasing, with people travelling to ever more exotic regions of the world, and a mobile population brings immigrants to our shores. This presents a challenge when confronted with unusual patterns of illness. There are a number of infections which are endemic to very specific regions of the world, and others which are endemic to large swathes of the globe.

Always obtain a travel history because imported infections in returning travellers, those from abroad holidaying in the UK and recent immigrants are part of the differential diagnosis of fever.

In the last decade, 100 people of all ages have died in the UK from malaria contracted in malarious areas. Only one of these people was taking full doses of what would currently be considered an adequate antimalarial. Of these 100 cases, 94 were contracted in Africa and six in the countries of South Asia. Four African countries accounted for 67% of all the fatal cases (Kenya 25%, Nigeria 17%, the Gambia 14% and Ghana 11%).

However, it is not just in the developing world and in the tropics that diseases unknown in the UK occur. There are a number of diseases, endemic to the Americas, that need to be considered in travellers returning from those regions. Babesiosis and Lyme disease are found on the east coast of the United States, Rocky Mountain Spotted Fever (a rickettsial infection) and Ehrlichiosis occur in the south and south-west of the country, as does coccidiomycosis, a fungal respiratory infection. Outbreaks of Hantavirus infections have occurred in Texas and Arizona and also in Eastern Europe, where tularaemia can also be found. Leishmaniasis occurs in the Mediterranean as well as in Africa, and should be considered in patients returning from European holidays with symptoms. The list continues. However, a good travel and contact history can point to the possibility of an imported infection in a timely fashion, even if the precise nature of the infection is initially elusive.

9.1 Malaria

- Caused by *Plasmodium* spp. (*P. vivax*, *P. malariae*, *P. ovale* and *P. falciparum*) invading erythrocytes
- Endemic in the tropical world, especially sub-Saharan Africa and parts of South-East Asia
- Transmitted by bite of the female *Anopheles* mosquito
- Congenital infection and blood transfusion-acquired infection may also occur
- *P. vivax* and *P. ovale* have hepatic stages and may cause relapses of infection
- Recrudescence of *P. falciparum* and *P. malariae* occurs from persistent low levels of parasitaemia
- *P. falciparum* malaria is the most severe and potentially fatal disease. This is the predominent species in Africa

Clinical manifestations

Symptoms appear 8–15 days after infection, with high fevers, chills, rigors and sweats, which classically occur in a cyclical pattern depending on the type of *Plasmodium* spp. involved. Patients can present with malaria up to 3 months after returning from an endemic area and a high index of suspicion is the key to making the diagnosis

- Headaches, abdominal pain, arthralgia, diarrhoea and vomiting are common
- Pallor and jaundice occur secondary to haemolysis
- Hepatosplenomegaly is more common in chronic infections
- Nephrotic syndrome may occur with *P. malariae*, because of immune-complex deposition in the kidney
- *P. falciparum* may present as a febrile or flu-like illness with no localizing signs, or as one of the following clinical syndromes:
  - Cerebral malaria — with confusion, fits, decreased level of consciousness, coma
  - Severe anaemia with signs of haemolysis
  - Hypoglycaemia from disease (metabolic requirements of parasites) and also quinine treatment
  - Pulmonary oedema (rare in children)
  - Renal failure with acute tubular necrosis, or 'blackwater fever' as a result of haemaglobinuria resulting from severe, acute intravascular haemolysis (rare in children)

Diagnosis

- Thick blood films allow the detection of parasites, thin films allow species identification and determination of parasitaemia (% of erythrocytes harbouring parasites)
- Need at least three negative films at 12- to 24-h intervals to be confident of negative result if there is a high index of clinical suspicion
- New tests being evaluated include PCR and malarial ribosomal RNA (urine dipstix are in use in the developing world)
- **NB** In hyperendemic areas, low-level parasitaemia, indicating a semi-immune state in childeren over the age of 4 years, is common and malaria is not necessarily the cause of the symptoms. However, people who move from these endemic areas do not retain their semi-immune status and any parasitaemia does become significant

Treatment

- Look for and treat hypoglycaemia

Chemotherapy is based on the infecting species, possible drug resistance and disease severity

P. falciparum malaria

- In the UK, we assume that all cases of *P. falciparum* malaria are chloroquine-resistant and treat with quinine, orally if possible, or iv if severely unwell for 3–7 days (monitor glucose and ECG if iv regimen used). One dose of pyrimethamine–sulfadoxine (Fansidar) is given on the last day of quinine therapy, or, increasingly, a 3-day course of Atovaquone/proguanil (Malarone) because fansidar resistance is on the increase in Africa
- Exchange transfusion may be warranted if parasitaemia exceeds 10%
- Monitor sequential blood smears

P. malariae malaria

- Treat with chloroquine (if no resistance)

P. vivax and *P. ovale* malaria

- Treat with chloroquine then primaquine to eradicate the liver stage and prevent relapses. Quinine can also be used, and is increasingly the drug of choice, as chloroquine resistance is increasing on the Indian subcontinent. Check that the patient is not glucose 6-phosphate dehydrogenase (G6PD)-deficient before giving primaquine

Prophylaxis

- From dusk to dawn (because the *Anopheles* are night-biters) use protective clothing, mosquito repellents, bed nets impregnated with insecticide
- Prescribe chemoprophylaxis from 1 week before departure until 4 weeks after return:
  - Chloroquine-sensitive area — chloroquine once a week **or** proguanil daily
  - Chloroquine-resistant areas — mefloquine once a week **or** doxycycline daily

9.2   Enteric (typhoid/paratyphoid) fever

- Caused by *Salmonella typhi*, *S. paratyphi* — Gram-negative bacilli in family Enterobacteriacae
- *S. typhi* found only in humans, transmitted by faecal–oral route
- Onset of illness is gradual with fever, headache, malaise, constipation (initially), diarrhoea (2nd week), abdominal pain, hepato/splenomegaly, rose spots. Infants may present with Gram-negative septicaemia. Within a week, fever becomes unremitting, delirium and disorientation may occur. The paradoxical relationship between high fever and low pulse rate is uncommon in children.

Complications

- Intestinal perforation occurs in 0.5–3%, severe haemorrhage occurs in 1–10% of children
- Focal infections, e.g. meningitis, osteomyelitis, endocarditis, pyelonephritis more common in the immunocompromised host
- Osteomyelitis and septic arthritis in children with haemoglobinopathies

- Chronic carriage — local multiplication in the wall of the gallbladder produces large numbers of Salmonellae, which are then discharged into the intestine and may cause chronic carriage and shedding (in 5% of adults but much less in children)

Diagnosis

- Perform bacterial cultures on blood, stool, bone marrow or rose spot aspirate
- Microscopy of stool reveals many leukocytes, mainly mononuclear
- Blood leukocyte count is at the low end of normal. Frank neutropenia can occur

Treatment

Drug choice and route of administration depend on susceptibility of organism, host response and site of infection – includes:

- Ampicillin, ceftriaxone, cefotaxime, chloramphenicol; in view of resistance, a fluoroquinolone is now frequently used as first-line therapy for 14 days
- For osteomyelitis — as above for 4–6 weeks
- For meningitis – ceftriaxone or cefotaxime for 4 weeks
- To eradicate carriage — high-dose ampicillin or amoxicillin or cholecystectomy

Prophylaxis

- Personal hygiene and proper sanitation for food processing and sewage disposal
- Vaccine is available, but only 17–66% effective depending on type

9.3   Dengue fever

- Caused by an arbovirus (i.e. arthropod borne); 570 arboviruses have been identified with more than 30 being human pathogens
- Dengue fever is caused by the genus Flavivirus (which also cause Japanese encephalitis and yellow fever)
- Transmitted by the mosquito *Aedes aegypti* — a day-biting mosquito
- Dengue fever is now endemic in South-East Asia, Central and South America and the Caribbean

Clinical manifestations

- Include fever for 1–7 days, frontal or retro-orbital headaches, back pain, myalgia and arthralgia ('breakbone' fever), nausea and vomiting
- 1–2 days after defervescence a generalized morbilliform rash occurs lasting 1–5 days. As this rash fades the fluctuating temperature reappears, producing the biphasic temperature curve

Complications

- Dengue haemorrhagic fever (DHF) – fever, haemorrhage, including epistaxis and bleeding of the gums and capillary fragility and fluid leakage. Complications include hepatitis, pneumonia, encephalopathy and cardiomyopathy. DHF occurs with the second infection with the arbovirus and there is an immunological component which causes augmentation of the disease and an increased severity of the clinical presentation. Rare in childhood

Diagnosis

- PCR, serology, isolation of virus (**NB** Prior yellow-fever vaccination will give positive dengue IgG)

Treatment

- None is specific, supportive only. Aggressive fluid resuscitaton in DHF markedly decreases mortality

9.4 Viral haemorrhagic fevers

- Many different viruses are found in different parts of world, so an accurate travel history is necessary, e.g. Lassa fever caused by lassa virus (an arenavirus) or Ebola haemorrhagic fever caused by Ebola virus
- These diseases range from mild infections to severe acute febrile illnesses with cardiovascular collapse. Fever, headaches, myalgia, conjunctival suffusion and abdominal pain are early symptoms. Mucosal bleeding occurs with vascular damage and thrombocytopenia and may cause life-threatening haemorrhage. Shock develops 7–10 days after the onset of illness
- Elevated alanine aminotransferase (ALT) is a poor prognostic factor in Lassa fever. Transmission is by inhalation or by contact of broken skin with the urine or saliva of infected rodents

Diagnosis

- Serology

Treatment

- Intravenous ribavirin for Lassa fever, especially in the first week of illness, reduces mortality

Prevention

- Strict isolation of patient and contacts. **These infections are highly contagious**.
- For suspected cases — examine a malarial film only (labelled 'Very high risk' for laboratory staff awareness). If negative, i.e. diagnosis is NOT malaria, then contact local microbiologist/public health laboratory service urgently for transfer of the patient to the designated unit.

9.5 Hantaviruses

- These are bunyaviruses and cause two different clinical syndromes. Rodents are the definitive hosts and are asymptomatic carriers that shed virus in their saliva and excreta. Disease is contracted through contact with infected rodents and their excreta
- Old World hantaviruses cause **haemorrhagic fever with renal syndrome**. Found throughout Asia and Eastern and Western Europe. Cause up to 100,000 cases a year
- New World hantaviruses, which occur in the southwest states of the USA and in the Andes region of South America, cause **hantavirus pulmonary syndrome**
- Both have an incubation period of 1–6 weeks and present with a prodrome of a non-specific flu-like illness

Clinical presentation

Haemorrhagic fever with renal syndrome (Old World)

- Prodrome characterized by vascular instability followed by renal failure presenting with oliguria followed by polyuria, hypotension, bleeding and shock
- The European disease is milder and presents most commonly as non-specific flu-like symptoms and proteinuria. Acute severe renal failure is rare

Pulmonary syndrome (New world)

- Non-specific flu-like prodrome followed by the abrupt onset of progressive pulmonary oedema, hypoxaemia and hypotension. This is the result of diffuse pulmonary leakage and is most likely immune mediated
- After 2–4 days, there is onset of diuresis with rapid improvement and resolution of pulmonary disease

Diagnosis

- Serology
- Characteristic full blood count abnormalities in pulmonary syndrome which include: haemoconcentration, thrombocytopenia and neutrophilia with the presence of immunoblasts on blood film

Treatment

- Supportive and symptomatic as required. Intubation and ventilation in pulmonary syndrome. Dialysis is rarely required in haemorrhagic fever. Meticulous fluid management
- Ribavirin has been used and thought anecdotally to be useful, but evidence for efficacy is lacking

9.6   Giardia

- Caused by *Giardia lamblia*, a protozoan that produces infectious cysts
- Faecal–oral transmission
- Infection limited to small intestine and/or biliary tract
- Worldwide distribution, some animals and humans infected, may infect water supply

Clinical manifestations

- Very varied
- Acute watery diarrhoea with abdominal pain, or foul-smelling stools and flatulence with abdominal distension and anorexia

Diagnosis

- Stool microscopy, rarely by duodenal biopsy

Treatment

- Metronidazole

9.7   Amoebiasis

- Caused by *Entamoeba histolytica*, a protozoan, excreted as cysts or trophozoites in stool of infected patients
- Faecal–oral transmission of cysts
- World-wide distribution, with infection rates as high as 20–50% in the tropics

Clinical manifestations

- Intestinal disease — asymptomatic or mild symptoms, e.g. abdominal distension, flatulence, constipation, loose stools
- Acute amoebic colitis (dysentery) — abdominal cramps, tenesmus, diarrhoea with blood and mucus — complications include toxic megacolon, fulminant colitis, ulceration and, rarely, perforation

Extraintestinal disease

- Liver abscess — acute fever, abdominal pain and liver tenderness, or subacute with weight loss and vague abdominal symptoms; rupture of the abscess into the abdomen or chest may occur
- Rarely, abscesses in the lung, pericardium, brain and genitourinary tract

Diagnosis

- Microscopy of stool, biopsy specimens and aspirates, serology if extraintestinal disease

Treatment

- To eliminate the tissue-invading trophozoites as well as cysts
- Metronidazole followed by a luminal amoebicide, e.g. paromomycin

9.8 Hookworm

- Caused by *Ancylostoma duodenale* and *Necator americanus*
- Prominent in rural, tropical areas where soil may be contaminated with human faeces
- Humans are the major reservoir
- Infection is by infectious larvae penetrating the skin, usually the soles of feet

Clinical manifestations

- May be asymptomatic
- May develop pruritis and papulovesicular rash for 1–2 weeks after initial infection
- Pneumonitis associated with migrating larvae in this phase is uncommon and usually mild

Diagnosis

- Stool microscopy

Treatment

- Antihelminthic drug, e.g. mebendazole. (**NB** Also treat any associated iron-deficiency anaemia)

9.9 Leishmaniasis

- *Leishmania* species are obligate intracellular parasites of monocytes/macrophages
- Variety of hosts including canines and rodents
- Vector is the sandfly
- Incubation period is usually days–months, but may even be years
- Three major clinical syndromes:
    - Cutaneous leishmaniasis — shallow ulcer at site of sandfly bite; lesions commonly on exposed skin, i.e. face and extremities; may have satellite lesions and regional lymphadenopathy
    - Mucosal leishmaniasis — initial cutaneous infection disseminates to midline facial structures, e.g. oral and nasopharyngeal mucosa
    - Visceral leishmaniasis (kala-azar) — parasites spread throughout the reticular endothelial system and are concentrated in the liver, spleen and bone marrow. Presents with fevers, weight loss, splenomegaly (may be massive), hepatomegaly, lymphadenopathy, anaemia, leukopenia, thrombocytopenia and hypergammaglobulinaemia

Diagnosis

- Microscopic identification of intracellular leishmanial organisms from skin or splenic biopsy, or bone marrow
- Serology may be helpful

Treatment

- Sodium stiboglutonate or amphotericin B. Liposomal amphotericin is particularly effective and is the treatment of choice in the developed world

9.10 Schistosomiasis

- Caused by the trematodes (flukes) *Schistosoma mansoni*, *Schistosoma japonicum*, *Schistosoma haematobium* and others
- Humans are the principal host, snail is intermediate host
- Eggs are excreted in urine or stool into fresh water, hatch and infect snails; after further development, cercariae emerge and penetrate human skin

Clinical manifestations

- Usually infection is asymptomatic
- May have initial transient pruritic, papular rash
- May have acute infection — Katayama fever: 4–8 weeks after infection an acute illness with fever, malaise, cough, rash, abdominal pain, diarrhoea, arthralgia, lymphadenopathy and eosinophilia
- Chronic infection with *Schistosoma mansoni* and *Schistosoma japonicum* may cause diarrhoea, tender hepatomegaly, chronic fibrosis, hepatosplenomegaly and portal hypertension
- Chronic infection with *Schistosoma haematobium* may cause dysuria, terminal microscopic haematuria, gross haematuria, frequency and obstructive uropathy
- Haematogenous spread to the lungs, liver and central nervous system may occur

Diagnosis

- Identification of the eggs in stool/urine, respectively
- Bladder biopsy
- Serology

Treatment

- Praziquantel

9.11 Travellers' diarrhoea

- Travellers' diarrhoea (TD) is a syndrome characterized by a two-fold or greater increase in the frequency of unformed bowel movements
- Food- and water-borne diseases are the number one cause of illness in travellers

- TD can be caused by viruses, bacteria or parasites, which can contaminate food or water
- The most important determinant of risk is the destination of the traveller
- Attack rates of 20–50% are commonly reported

Clinical manifestations

- Diarrhoea, abdominal cramps, nausea, bloating, urgency, and malaise; sometimes vomiting also occurs
- Nature of stool may indicate particular organism
- TD usually lasts from 3 to 7 days, but is rarely life-threatening

Enteric bacterial pathogens

- Enterotoxigenic *E. coli* (ETEC) are among the most common causative agents; ETEC produce a watery diarrhoea associated with cramps and a low-grade or no fever
- Salmonella gastroenteritis is usually caused by non-typhoidal *Salmonella* spp. which cause dysentery characterized by small-volume stools containing bloody mucus
- Shigella bacillary dysentery is seen in up to 20% of travellers to developing countries
- *Campylobacter jejuni* causes a small percentage of the reported cases of TD, some with bloody diarrhoea
- *Vibrio parahaemolyticus* is associated with the ingestion of raw or poorly cooked seafood

Less common bacterial pathogens include other diarrhoeagenic *E. coli*, *Yersinia enterocolitica*, *Vibrio cholerae* 01 and 0139, non-01 *V. cholerae*, *Vibrio fluvialis* and possibly *Aeromonas hydrophila* and *Plesiomonas shigelloides*.

Viral enteric pathogens

- Rotaviruses and Norwalk-like virus may cause TD

Parasitic enteric pathogens

- These include *Giardia intestinalis*, *Entamoeba histolytica*, *Cryptosporidium parvum* and *Cyclospora cayetanensis*. The likelihood of a parasitic aetiology is higher when diarrhoeal illness is prolonged. *Entamoeba histolytica* should be considered when the patient has dysentery or invasive diarrhoea (bloody stools)

Treatment

- Antimotility agents should NOT be used in children. Occasionally in adolescents, like adults, they may be used to provide prompt symptomatic but temporary relief of uncomplicated TD. However, they should **not** be used by people with high fever or with blood in their stools
- Oral rehydration solutions and plenty of fluids should be drunk to prevent dehydration
- Antibiotics should be reserved for: those with severe diarrhoea that does not resolve within several days; if there is blood or mucus, or both, in the stools; if fever occurs with shaking chills

Prevention

- Treatment of water:
  - Boiling for at least 5 minutes is the most reliable method to make water safe to drink
  - Chemical disinfection can be achieved with either iodine or chlorine, with iodine providing greater disinfection in a wider set of circumstances
- Food:
  - Any raw food can be contaminated, particularly in areas of poor sanitation
  - Foods of particular concern include salads, uncooked vegetables and fruit, unpasteurized milk and milk products, raw meat and shellfish
  - Some fish are not guaranteed to be safe even when cooked because of the presence of toxins in their flesh. Tropical reef fish, red snapper, amber jack, grouper and sea bass can occasionally be toxic at unpredictable times if they are caught on tropical reefs

10. NEW AND EMERGING INFECTIONS

10.1 Severe acute respiratory syndrome (SARS)

- New infectious disease. Restricted to China, Hong Kong and Vietnam and visitors to those regions and their contacts, resulting in outbreaks in Toronto and Singapore. Probably originated in the animal populations and crossed over into humans. Disease restricted to a single outbreak
- **Aetiology**: novel coronavirus
- **Incubation period**: 2–10 days. More severe cases present earlier
- **Clinical presentation**: non-specific flu-like prodrome followed by fever, shortness of breath and diffuse pneumonia and acute respiratory distress syndrome. Associated diarrhoea in some patients. Less severe in children and few cases < 15 years. 10% mortality rate
- **Diagnosis**: PCR of nasopharyngeal aspirate, stool and urine. Serology is useful for epidemiological purposes only
- **Treatment**: No effective treatment. Ribavirin has been used and also steroids in the more severe patients, with limited success. Intensive care with mechanical ventilation required for a large percentage of infected patients

10.2 West Nile virus

- West Nile virus is a flavivirus. Widely distributed throughout Africa, the Middle East, Asia, Australia and parts of Europe. First detected in the USA in 1999 and is now widespread throughout the continent. Primary hosts are birds and the vectors are mosquitos. Peak infection is late summer, but sporadic cases occur
- **Clinical presentation**: Most patients present with a self-limiting febrile flu-like infection, characterized by headaches, myalgias, malaise, back pain and loss of appetite. Vomiting, diarrhoea, abdominal pain and pharyngitis are common, and disease lasts 3–10 days

- Mortality in this group is approximately 2%
- Neurological complications occur in < 1% of patients, and the elderly and immunocompromised are more at risk. This presents typically as an encephalitis with muscle weakness, and in some cases a flaccid paralysis. Parkinsonian-like features can also occur
- **Diagnosis**: serology
- **Treatment**: supportive

10.3   Avian influenza virus

- The H5N1 strain of avian influenza virus is endemic in the bird population in South-East Asia, with sporadic human spread, and culling of domestic birds has been necessary to prevent further spread. Pigs are an important reservoir that could facilitate mutation of the virus
- Concern that close proximity of birds, swine and humans in South-East Asia will facilitate mutation and, although no cases have been reported outside this region, there is widespread concern that mutation and spread to the human population will cause a severe influenza pandemic world-wide
- > 90 cases in humans in 2004–2005. Mortality rate of 68%. Predominance in children and young adults
- Treatment: Oseltamivir

11.   CONGENITAL INFECTIONS

Congenital infections are acquired in utero, usually transplacentally, during maternal infection.

Manifestations are most severe if acquired in the first trimester.

Suspect if:

- Small for gestational age
- Microcephaly or hydrocephalus
- Ocular defects
- Hepatosplenomegaly
- Thrombocytopenia
- Developmental delay/fits

11.1   Diseases

CMV, congenital rubella syndrome, toxoplasmosis

- Approximately two-thirds of pregnancies complicated by rubella during the first 8 weeks of gestation will result in fetal death or severe abnormality
- There is a 40% risk of toxoplasmosis transmission from mother to fetus

- In CMV and toxoplasmosis, approximately 10% of infected infants are clinically affected at birth, although symptoms will often become apparent during childhood

Characteristic features of CMV, rubella and toxoplasmosis infection

Abnormality	Rubella	CMV	Toxoplasmosis
Neurological:			
Sensorineural hearing loss	+++	++	+
Microcephaly	+	++	+
Hydrocephalus	–	–	++
Calcification	–	++ (peri-ventricular)	++ (widespread)
Eyes:			
Micro-ophthalmia	+	–	+
Cataracts	+++	–	+
Chorioretinitis	+	++	+++
Growth retardation:	++	+++	+
Hepatosplenomegaly	+++	+++	++
Petechiae ('blueberry muffin' rash)	++	++	+
Cardiac malformations	++	–	–
Pneumonitis	+	++	+
Bony involvement	++	–	

Parvovirus B19

- Women who become infected with parvovirus B19 during first 20 weeks of pregnancy have a 9% fetal loss
- Hydrops fetalis occurs in approximately 3% if the mother is infected between 9 and 20 weeks' gestation

Congenital varicella

- Infection during the first or second trimester may rarely cause congenital varicella syndrome (0.5–2%)
- Skin scarring, limb malformation/shortening, cataracts, chorioretinitis, micro-ophthalmia, microcephaly, hydrocephalus

Herpes simplex virus

- Vast majority of infants are infected peripartum, only 5% transplacentally
- Cutaneous scars or vesicles
- Choreoretinitis, keratoconjunctivitis, micro-ophthalmia
- Microcephaly, intracranial calcifications
- Hepatosplenomegaly
- Developmental delay

Syphilis

- High transmission rate, 40% mortality if left untreated
- 'Snuffles', congenital nephrotic syndrome, chorioretinitis, glaucoma
- Osteochondritis, periostitis
- Hepatosplenomegaly, lymphadenopathy
- Rash — maculopapular, desquamative, bullous, condylomas

Mycobacterium tuberculosis

- Very rare, high mortality
- Presents as disseminated disease with fevers and often respiratory distress
- Needs Mantoux testing, chest X-ray, lumbar puncture, quadruple therapy + steroids if meningitis is confirmed

Diagnosis

- 'TORCH screen' — **T**oxoplasmosis, '**O**ther', **R**ubella, **C**MV and **H**erpes-specific IgM in neonates < 4 weeks old implies congenital infection
- Screen for specific infection based on clinical findings in neonate and mother, rather than requesting a TORCH screen
- **NB** Look at specific antibody responses in mother's booking-visit blood samples and post-delivery blood samples to see rise/fall in titres depending on time of infection acquisition
- PCR can be useful in some infections
- Ophthalmological examination — characteristic retinal changes

Treatment

- Prevention through vaccination is the only way to reduce the risk of congenital rubella
- Spiramycin may be used for toxoplasmosis in pregnancy to reduce transmission to the fetus. Affected infants are treated with pyrimethamine and sulfadiazine after birth
- Ganciclovir may be used in cases of congenital CMV, aciclovir for herpes simplex, penicillin for syphilis
- Highly active antiretroviral therapy (HAART) used for HIV infection
- Anti-TB treatment

12. MISCELLANEOUS

12.1 Differential diagnosis of prolonged fever

Systemic bacterial disease:	Viral disease:
Salmonellosis	CMV
Mycobacterial infection	Hepatitis viruses
Brucellosis	EBV
Leptospirosis	Human herpesvirus-6
Spirochaete infections	

Focal bacterial infections:	Parasitic infections:	Other infections
Abscesses	Malaria	Chlamydia
Sinusitis	Toxoplasmosis	Rickettsia
Osteomyelitis	Leishmaniasis	Fungi
Endocarditis		
Urinary sepsis		

Non-infectious diseases:

Collagen vascular diseases: systemic lupus erythematosus (SLE), juvenile inflammatory arthritis (JIA)	Inflammatory bowel disease
	Malignancies
	Drugs
Familial Mediterranean fever	Haemophagocytic
Kawasaki disease	lymphohistiocytosis
Sarcoidosis	Autonomic/CNS abnormalities

12.2 Differential diagnosis of cervical lymphadenopathy

Differential diagnosis of cervical lymphadenopathy

- Cervical abscess
- Tuberculosis (usually atypical)
- Cat-scratch fever (caused by Gram-negative organism *Bartonella henselae*)
- Mumps
- Malignancy
- Infectious mononucleosis
- Toxoplasmosis
- Brucellosis
- Salivary stone

12.3 Infections commonly associated with atypical lymphocytosis

- EBV
- CMV
- Toxoplasmosis
- Mumps

- Tuberculosis
- Malaria

12.4   Diseases associated with eosinophilia

An increase above 0.4×10^9/l is seen with:

- Allergic disease, e.g. asthma, eczema
- Parasitic disease, e.g. hookworm, amoebiasis, ascariasis, tapeworm infestation, filariasis, schistosomiasis
- Recovery from acute infection
- Skin disease, e.g. psoriasis, pemphigus
- Hodgkin disease
- Polyarteritis nodosa
- Drug sensitivity
- Hyper-eosinophilia syndrome
- Eosinophilic leukaemia (very rare)

12.5   Causes of hydrops fetalis

10–15% 'immune' aetiology

- Fetal anaemia caused by anti-D, anti-Kell and anti-C antibodies

85–90% non-immune cause

- Human parvovirus B19 infection (most common), CMV, toxoplasmosis, syphilis, leptospirosis
- Aneuploidy
- Cardiac cause, e.g. supraventricular tachycardia and congenital complete heart block
- Primary hydrothorax
- Cystic hygroma
- Twin–twin transfusion syndrome
- Massive transplacental haemorrhage
- Fetal akinesia and muscular dystrophy

12.6   Oxazolidinones: a new class of antibiotics

Linezolid

- Active against methicillin-resistant *Staphylococcus aureus* (MRSA) and vancomycin-resistant enterococci
  - Bacteriostatic agent
  - Good CNS penetration
- Does not have good activity against Gram-negative organisms
- Reserve for those with infections resistant to other antibacterial agents
- Side-effects include myelosuppression — monitor blood count weekly

553

12.7   Echinocandins: a new class of antifungals

- Active against *Aspergillus* and candidal species. Fungistatic in aspergillosis, but fungicidal in candidal disease. Useful as adjunctive therapy together with either Ambisome or voriconazole in severe fungal infections
- Widely distributed in all tissues and has good CNS penetration when disease is present
- IV preparation only
- Adverse effects: raised transaminases, headaches and gastrointestinal disturbances

12.8   Erythema multiforme (EM)

- Characteristic target lesions; also macules, papules, wheals, vesicles and bullae
- Systemic symptoms common — fever, malaise, arthralgia
- Stevens–Johnson syndrome – severe EM with mucosal bullae in mouth, anogenital region and conjunctiva

Causes

- Idiopathic (> 50%)
- Herpes simplex
- Mycoplasma
- Viruses — enterovirus spp.
- Drugs — sulphonamides, penicillins, barbiturates

Treatment

- Treat underlying cause; supportive; steroids in severe EM (early)

12.9   Erythema nodosum

Inflammatory disease of skin and subcutaneous tissues characterized by tender, red nodules predominantly pretibial (also arms and other areas)

- Streptococcal upper respiratory tract infection
- Sarcoid
- Primary tuberculosis
- Ulcerative colitis
- Drugs (sulphonamides, contraceptive pills, bromides)
- Other — leprosy, histoplasmosis, psittacosis, lymphogranuloma venereum, coccidiomycosis

Treatment

- Antimicrobials specific to the infection
- Steroids: systemic most effective

12.10 Anthrax

- Caused by the Gram-positive organism *Bacillus anthracis*
- Wild and domestic animals in Asia, Africa and parts of Europe carry the bacterium
- The bacterium can exist as a spore, which allows the bacterium to survive in the environment (e.g. in the soil)

Cutaneous anthrax (95% of cases)

- Caught by direct contact with the skin or tissues of infected animals. A lesion appears on the skin, often on the head, forearms or hands, and develops into a characteristic ulcer with a necrotic centre. It is rarely painful. Untreated, the infection can spread to cause bacteraemia, which can be fatal in 5–20% of cases

Inhalation anthrax

- Much less common. Caused by breathing in anthrax spores. Symptoms begin with a flu-like illness, followed by respiratory difficulties and shock after 2–6 days. High fatality rate

Intestinal anthrax

- Very rare form of food poisoning, which results in severe gut disease, fever and septicaemia. Mortality of up to 50%
- Vaccine — available for very high-risk groups only
- Post-exposure prophylaxis with antibiotics can be very effective in preventing disease, providing it is given early enough

Treatment

- High-dose penicillin and doxycycline or ciprofloxacin

12.11 Botulism

- Botulism is caused by a botulinum toxin, produced by the bacterium *Clostridium botulinum*
- The bacterium is anaerobic and common in the soil in the form of spores
- Food-borne botulism occurs when the spores of *C. botulinum* have germinated and the bacteria have reproduced in an environment (usually food) outside the body and produced toxin. The toxin is consumed when the food is eaten
- The toxin is destroyed by normal cooking processes

Clinical manifestations

Botulism is a neuroparalytic disorder that can be classified into three categories:

- Foodborne:
  - Onset of symptoms is usually abrupt, within 12–36 h of exposure

555

- Symmetrical, descending, flaccid paralysis occurs, typically involving the bulbar musculature initially
- Sometimes diarrhoea and vomiting occur
- Most cases recover, but the recovery period can be many months; the disease can be fatal in 5–10% of cases
- Infant botulism:
  - Extremely rare, but occurs when spores are ingested that germinate, multiply and release toxin in the intestine; not related to food ingestion in this population; more common in breast-fed babies and in certain regions of the world
  - Incubation period is much longer, 3–30 days
  - Presents with 'floppy infant' with poor feeding, weak cry, generalized hypotonia, constipation
- Wound botulism:
  - Same symptoms as other forms, but occurs when the organisms get into an open wound and are able to reproduce in an 'anaerobic' environment

Diagnosis

- Enriched selective media are used to culture *C. botulinum* from stools and food
- A toxin neutralization assay can identify botulinum toxin in serum, stool or food
- Electromyography has characteristic appearances

Treatment

- Supportive care, especially respiratory (e.g. ventilation) and nutritional
- Antitoxin
- Concerns about the effectiveness and side-effects of the vaccine against botulism; it is not widely used
- Immunity to botulism toxin does not develop, even with severe disease

Prevention

Education regarding food preparation.

Therapeutics

Botulinum A toxin, in small doses, is used therapeutically to prevent excessive muscular activity, e.g. in torticollis, cerebral palsy, and recently in cosmetics to reduce wrinkles.

12.12 Bovine spongiform encephalopathy (BSE) and new variant Creutzfeldt–Jakob disease (nv-CJD)

- Transmissible spongiform encephalopathies (TSEs) are caused by proteinaceous infectious particles or prions. These are abnormal isoforms of a cell-surface glycoprotein designated PrP
- Disease is caused when a disease-specific isoform, PrP^{Sc}, interacts with PrP producing conversion to PrP^{Sc}. This protein is not readily digested by proteases and therefore accumulates, causing a rapidly progressive and fatal encephalopathy

- PrP^{Sc} is very resistant to standard methods of sterilization and disinfection. The genotype of polymorphic codon 129 of the human *PrP* gene appears to influence susceptibility to infection and disease phenotype. 37% of Caucasians are methionine-homozygous (MM), 12% are valine homozygous (VV) and 51% are heterozygous (MV). Cases of new variant-CJD have been found in MM individuals

Creutzfeldt–Jakob disease (CJD)

The principal human spongiform encephalopathy. Features include a progressive dementia, movement disorder and death in a median of 4 months. The incidence is between 0.5 and 1 case per million. Most cases present between 55 and 75 years of age. Most cases have no known cause; 15% have a hereditary predisposition to CJD, with recognized mutations of the human *PrP* gene on chromosome 20. A small number of iatrogenic cases have occurred following the use of contaminated growth hormone.

Kuru

A disease of motor incoordination, it was endemic in Papua New Guinea in the 1950s and 1960s. Kuru was a TSE spread by the ritual cannibalism of deceased relatives. Cannibalism ceased in the late 1950s, but there are still a few cases in older adults indicating a long incubation period.

New variant CJD (nv-CJD)

This was first reported with 10 cases in 1996. The source appeared to be BSE, acquired following the ingestion of infected cattle. The disease starts as a psychiatric illness followed by ataxia, myoclonus, akinetic mutism and death after about 12 months. There are now more than 100 cases. The incubation period may be very long and therefore the total number of cases is difficult to predict.

13. FURTHER READING

Behrman, R. E., 2004. *Nelson Textbook of Paediatrics*, 17th edn. WB Saunders.

British National Formulary, March 2005.

British Thoracic Society. 1998. Chemotherapy and management of tuberculosis in the United Kingdom: recommendations: Joint Tuberculosis Committee of the British Thoracic Society BTS guidelines. *Thorax* 53, 536–48.

Feigin R. and Cherry J. 1998. *Textbook of Paediatric Infectious Diseases*, 4th edn. WB Saunders.

Georges P. 2003. *Report of the Committee on Infectious Diseases*. American Academy of Paediatrics, Red Book.

Hull D. 1999. *Medicines for Children*. British Paediatric Association.

Public Health Laboratory Services (PHLS) and Centres for Disease Control (CDC) websites.

Chapter 15

Metabolic Medicine

Michael P Champion

CONTENTS

Metabolic Medicine

1. BASIC METABOLISM

1.1 Carbohydrate metabolism

Glucose has three metabolic fates in the body: oxidation for energy, storage as glycogen, and conversion to amino acids and triglycerides.

A steady supply of adenosine triphosphate (ATP) is needed to power each cell's essential processes. This ATP is usually supplied from the oxidation of glucose provided in the diet and from glycogen stores. In the fasted state, the hormone-mediated response is to draw on the body's reserves — fat and protein (catabolism) — to make up the fuel shortfall to generate ATP.

The diet rarely contains glucose as the only carbohydrate source, other carbohydrates, e.g. fructose, galactose, lactose etc., need to be converted to glucose first before they can be used for energy.

Glycolysis

Glycolysis takes place in the cytoplasm of all cells and describes the break down of one molecule of glucose to produce two molecules of pyruvate. It can occur under aerobic (large energy production via the tricarboxylic acid (TCA) cycle and oxidative phosphorylation) or under anaerobic conditions (small energy production via lactate). Glycolysis provides an emergency mechanism for energy production when oxygen is limited, i.e. in red cells (which have no mitochondria, thus glycolysis is their only means of energy production) or in skeletal muscle during exercise. Glycolysis also provides intermediates for other metabolic pathways, e.g. pentoses for DNA synthesis. The three enzyme steps are irreversible.

Pyruvate metabolism

Pyruvate, produced by glycolysis and other metabolic pathways, can be converted to oxaloacetate (by pyruvate carboxylase) for entry into the TCA cycle, or acetyl-CoA (by pyruvate dehydrogenase) which has a number of potential fates. These being:

- Oxidation in TCA cycle
- Fatty acid synthesis
- Ketone body synthesis
- Steroid synthesis

Tricarboxylic acid (TCA) cycle

This cycle is present in all cells with mitochondria (not red cells) and provides the final common pathway for glucose, fatty acids and amino acid oxidation via acetyl-CoA or other TCA cycle intermediates. The cycle's main function is the provision of reduced cofactors (NADH, FADH$_2$) which donate electrons to the respiratory chain for ATP production (see Section 7). The cycle also provides metabolic intermediates for other synthetic pathways, e.g. amino acid synthesis. It also has a key regulatory role in metabolism.

Glycogen metabolism

Glycogen is a branched glucose polymer stored in liver, kidney and muscle for the rapid release of glucose when needed. Liver glycogen is a store to release glucose to the rest of the body, whereas muscle glycogen supports muscle glycolysis only.

Glycogen synthesis is promoted by insulin and involves :

- UDP glucose synthesis (glucose donor) from glucose-1-phosphate
- Elongation of glycogen (glucose linked to existent glycogen strand (α-1,4 glycosidic bond)
- Branch formation (α-1,6 glycosidic bond)

Glycogenolysis is promoted by adrenaline and glucagon and involves:

- Shortening of chain to release glucose-1-phosphate
- Sequential removal until the branch point is reached
- Removal of branch point

1.2 Protein metabolism

Proteins are assembled from amino acids which are composed of an amino group metabolized to urea via ammonia, and a carbon skeleton which has a number of potential metabolic fates: acetyl-CoA, pyruvate and ketone bodies.

Amino acids may be used for protein synthesis, or may be converted to other non-essential amino acids (transamination) or oxidized via the TCA cycle. Essential amino acids cannot be synthesized in the body. There is a continual turnover of the body's protein as amino acids in the body's amino acids pool are used for protein synthesis and then broken down back to amino acids. Protein cannot be stored and therefore any amino acids not used are catabolized, and hence to remain in neutral nitrogen balance, protein is an essential constituent of a healthy diet.

Gluconeogenesis is the de novo synthesis of glucose from non-carbohydrate sources such as amino acids, lactate and glycerol. This usually occurs in the liver but also occurs in the kidney in prolonged starvation. Gluconeogenesis is promoted by glucagon, cortisol and adrenocorticotrophic hormone (ACTH).

1.3 Fat metabolism

Fat has the highest caloric value and therefore is an essential energy source. Triglycerides comprise three fatty acid molecules and one glycerol molecule which are broken down by lipase (**lipolysis**). The released glycerol is converted to glyceraldehyde-3-phosphate in the liver, a key intermediate of both **glycolysis** and **gluconeogenesis**. The fatty acids undergo β-oxidation (see Section 6) within mitochondria which shortens the fatty acid by two carbons per cycle releasing acetyl-CoA for entry to the TCA cycle or for the production of ketone bodies.

Fatty acids can be synthesized from acetyl-CoA by adding two carbons sequentially to the elongating fatty acid chain (**lipogenesis**). This occurs mainly in the liver, adipose tissue, lactating mammary gland and, to a minor degree, in the kidney. Essential fatty acids cannot be synthesized by the body because the enzyme required to form double bonds beyond nine carbons in length is not present. The principal essential fatty acids are linoleic (C18:2) and α-linolenic (C18:3) acids.

1.4 Vitamins

Vitamins are organic compounds needed in very small quantities in the body.

- **Fat-soluble vitamins** A, D, E and K are stored in the liver and can be toxic in excess, especially vitamins A and D.
- **Water-soluble vitamins** are the B group vitamins and vitamin C. They are required regularly in the diet because the body does not store them in significant quantities.

Vitamin sources and vitamin deficiency states

Vitamin	Sources	Deficiency state	Symptoms
A retinol	Milk, butter, eggs, liver	Xerophthalmia	Night blindness, dry eyes
B_1 thiamin	Whole grain, liver, pork, cereals	Beri beri	Heart failure (wet), neuropathy (dry)
B_2 riboflavin	Milk, eggs, liver, green vegetables, nuts		Angular stomatitis, cataracts, glossitis
B_6 pyridoxine	Meat, fish, poultry, whole grain, nuts, legumes		Dermatitis, seizures, anaemia
B_{12} cobalamin	Liver, meat, dairy (animal only)		anaemia, cognitive Decline, neuropathy
C ascorbate	Fruit (especially citrus), green vegetables	Scurvy	Bleeding gums, loose teeth, anaemia

Vitamin	Sources	Deficiency state	Symptoms
D cholecalciferol	Fish endogenous synthesis	Rickets	Petaechiae
E tocopherol	Vegetable oils, margarine, nuts, green vegetables	Very rare only seen in premature infants and abetalipo-proteinaemia	Myopathy, ataxia, neuropathy, retinopathy
K	Green vegetables, eggs, liver, cereal, fruit, gut flora	Haemorrhagic disease of the newborn	Coagulopathy
Niacin	Cereals, meat, fish, legumes	Pellagra	Dermatitis, diarrhoea, cognitive function
Folate	Green vegetables, liver, cereals	Megaloblastic anaemia	Anaemia, neural tube defects (in utero)
Pantothenic acid	Meat, fish, cereals, legumes	Rare	
Biotin	Offal, yeast, nuts, liver, eggs		Rash, hair loss, neurology

2. APPROACH TO THE METABOLIC CASE

2.1 Inheritance

Inborn errors of metabolism are individually rare but collectively they have an incidence of about 1 per 3,000 to 4,000 births. Autosomal recessive inheritance is commonest. Exceptions include:

- **X-linked recessive** — Lesch–Nyhan syndrome; Hunter syndrome; ornithine transcarbamylase (OTC) deficiency; Fabry disease; adrenoleukodystrophy
- **Autosomal dominant** — Porphyrias (some recessive)
- **Matrilineal** — Mitochondrial DNA mutations

2.2 Presentation

Presentation is notoriously non-specific, therefore clues should be sought in the history. The commonest misdiagnosis is sepsis.

Clues from history

- Consanguineous parents
- Previous sudden infant death (especially late, i.e. > 6 months)
- Ethnicity (for certain conditions only)
- Previous multiple miscarriages (indicating non-viable fetuses)
- Maternal illness during pregnancy, e.g.:
  - Acute Fatty Liver of Pregnancy (AFLP) and Haemolysis, Elevated Liver enzymes, Low Platelets (HELLP) syndrome association with carrying fetus with long-chain fat oxidation defect
  - Increased fetal movements (in utero fits)
- Faddy eating (avoidance of foods that provoke feeling unwell)
- Previous encephalopathic or tachypnoeic episodes (latter implies acidosis)

Inborn errors of metabolism present at times of metabolic stress, e.g.:

- Neonatal period
- Weaning (increased oral intake, new challenges, e.g. fructose)
- End of first year (slowing in growth rate, therefore more protein catabolized as less used for growth. May exceed metabolic capacity of defective pathway)
- Intercurrent infections
- Puberty

Neonatal presentation can be divided into three groups for diagnostic purposes.

- Failure to make or break complex molecules
- Intoxication
- Energy insufficiency

Failure to make or break complex molecules

These are usually dysmorphic syndromes at birth because of the absence of structural molecules that are important for embryogenesis (failure to make complex molecules). Many storage disorders appear normal at birth and become progressively more obvious with time as storage accumulates (failure to break down complex molecules).

- Smith–Lemli–Opitz syndrome (cholesterol synthesis defect)
- Zellweger syndrome (peroxisomal disorder)
- Congenital disorders of glycosylation (glycosylation defects)

Intoxication

Key feature is a symptom-free period before decompensation whilst the toxic metabolites build up, i.e. once feeds are established and the neonate no longer relies on the placenta for clearance. Classical presentation is collapse on day 3 of life. Differential diagnosis includes sepsis and duct-dependent cardiac problems.

- Aminoacidopathies: tyrosinaemia, maple syrup urine disease (MSUD)
- Urea cycle defects (UCDs)
- Organic acidaemias (OAs)
- Sugar intolerances: galactosaemia

Energy insufficiency

Absence of symptom-free period with immediate onset of symptoms in congenital lactic acidosis. There is a spectrum of severity and some may take longer to decompensate. The group includes conditions that only present if there is a delay in fuel provision, e.g. fat oxidation defects, and glycogenolysis and gluconeogenesis defects; these may not present for some months or longer.

- Respiratory chain defects
- Pyruvate metabolism defects (pyruvate dehydrogenase, pyruvate carboxylase)
- Fat oxidation defects — medium-chain acyl-CoA dehydrogenase (MCAD), long-chain hydroxyacyl-CoA dehydrogenase (LCHAD), very-long-chain acyl-CoA dehydrogenase (VLCAD)
- Glycogen storage disease (GSD) types I and III
- Defects of gluconeogenesis — fructose bisphosphatase deficiency

2.3 Examination

Clinical examination may reveal few clues in many disorders of intermediary metabolism. Dysmorphic features may suggest certain diagnoses. Odours are usually unhelpful and rarely significant (exceptions include MSUD, in which the nappies smell sweet, and isovaleric acidaemia, in which there is a pungent sweaty odour). Eyes should be carefully examined for corneal clouding (mucopolysaccharidoses, cystinosis), cataracts (galactosaemia, peroxisomal, mitochondrial), pigmentary retinopathy (fat oxidation, mitochondrial) and cherry-red spot (Tay–Sachs, Niemann–Pick, Sandhoff, G_{M1}). Organomegaly is a key revealing sign. Hepatosplenomegaly is a feature of storage disorders. Massive hepatomegaly in the absence of splenomegaly suggests glycogen storage disease because glycogen is not stored in the spleen. More prominent splenomegaly is suggestive of Gaucher disease.

2.4 Investigation

Perform investigations at the time of decompensation when diagnostic metabolites are most likely to be present and avoid the need for stress tests at a later date.

Key initial metabolic investigations

- Blood gas (venous, capillary or arterial)
- Glucose
- Lactate
- Ammonia
- Amino acids (blood)
- Organic acids (urine)
- Acylcarnitines
- Ketones (urinary dipstick)

Acid–base status

Anion gap $= Na^+ + K^+ - (Cl^- + HCO_3^-)$

A normal anion gap (10–18 mmol/l) in the presence of metabolic acidosis signifies bicarbonate loss rather than an excess of acid, e.g. renal or gut. Marked ketosis is unusual in the neonate and is therefore highly suggestive of an underlying metabolic disorder. Urea cycle defects may initially present with a mild respiratory alkalosis because ammonia acts directly on the brainstem as a respiratory stimulant.

Characteristics of metabolic and respiratory acidosis and alkalosis

Metabolic acidosis (low pH, low CO_2)	Metabolic alkalosis (high pH, high CO_2)
Increased acid load	Increased alkali load
Organic acids (OAs)	Drugs/poisoning
lactate hypotension, hypoxia	Loss of unbuffered acid
mitochondrial, OAs	gastrointestinal
ketosis diabetic ketoacidosis,	gastric aspiration
OAs	pyloric stenosis
Drugs/poisoning	chloride-losing diarrhoea
Reduced acid excretion	renal
distal renal tubular acidosis	mineralocorticoid excess
renal failure	(Cushing, Conn)
	diuretics
Bicarbonate loss	correction of chronic raised CO_2
gastrointestinal	
severe diarrhoea	
total villus atrophy	
renal loss	
proximal renal tubular acidosis	

Respiratory acidosis (low pH, high CO_2)	Respiratory alkalosis (high pH, low CO_2)

Hypoventilation
    encephalopathy (includes metabolic,
        drugs, anoxia, trauma, raised
        intracranial pressure, etc.)
    neural/neuromuscular
    thoracic restriction
        dysostosis multiplex
        kyphoscoliosis
    lung compression
        pleural effusion
        pneumothorax
    lung disease
        airway obstruction
        pneumonia etc
	Hyperventilation
	    hyperammonaemia
	    drugs, e.g. salicylate
	    mechanical ventilation/overbagging
	    pain/anxiety

Hypoglycaemia

Hypoglycaemia is defined as a blood glucose concentration of ≤ 2.6 mmol/l, and should always be confirmed in the laboratory. The key additional investigation is the presence or absence of ketosis. Hypoketotic hypoglycaemia has a limited differential diagnosis that can usually be resolved on history and examination:

- Hyperinsulinism (endogenous or exogenous)
- Fat oxidation defects (e.g. MCAD)
- Liver failure

Hyperinsulinism is suggested by a persistently increased glucose demand > 10 mg/kg per min

Glucose requirement (mg/kg per min) = (ml/h $\times$ % dextrose) / ($6 \times$ weight (kg))

Lactate

Lactate is a weak acid which can be used directly as a fuel for the brain and is readily produced during anaerobic respiration. Secondary causes of lactate level anomalies (e.g. hypoxia, sepsis, shock, liver failure, poor sampling, etc.) are much more common than primary metabolic causes. Ketosis is usually present in primary metabolic disease, unlike in secondary causes, with the exception of pyruvate dehydrogenase deficiency, GSD type I and fat oxidation defects. The level of lactate is unhelpful in distinguishing the cause, and the lactate : pyruvate ratio usually adds little. A low ratio (< 10) may indicate pyruvate dehydrogenase deficiency. Exacerbation when a patient is fasted is a feature of gluconeogenesis defects, of GSD type I compared to GSD type III and of respiratory chain disorders in which lactate may increase post-prandially. The markedly raised lactate in decompensated fructose bisphosphatase deficiency characteristically rapidly resolves on treating the hypoglycaemia.

Cerebrospinal fluid (CSF) lactate is raised in mitochondrial disorders, central nervous system (CNS) sepsis and seizures.

Ammonia

Hyperammonaemia may result from poor sampling (squeezed sample) and/or delays in processing. The level of ammonia may prove discriminatory as to the cause.

Diagnosis from ammonia concentration

Ammonia concentration (µmol/l)	Differential diagnosis
< 40	Normal
40 to < 150	Sick patient, fat oxidation defect, OA, liver failure, UCD
150 to < 250	Fat oxidation defect, OA, liver failure, UCD
250 to < 450	OA, liver failure, UCD
450 to > 2000	Liver failure, UCD, (OA rarely)

OA, organic acidaemia; UCD, urea cycle defect.

Transient hyperammonaemia of the newborn (THAN) is characterized by very early onset, usually in the first 36 hours before feeding is truly established. It is associated with low glutamine. THAN is managed as other urea cycle defects but has an excellent prognosis if treated early as the hyperammonaemia is secondary to blood bypassing the liver (e.g. patent ductus venosus), rather than a block in the urea cycle.

Amino acids

Amino acids are measured in both blood and urine. The latter reflects renal threshold, e.g. generalized aminoaciduria of a proximal renal tubulopathy or the specific transporter defect of cystinuria (**C**ystine, **O**rnithine, **A**rginine, **L**ysine). An increase in the serum levels of a specific amino acid may be missed if only a urine sample is analysed and the renal threshold has yet to be breached. Plasma amino acids are useful in the work up of a number of metabolic disorders, and are essential in monitoring some metabolic disorders.

- ↑Leucine, isoleucine and valine — maple syrup urine disease (MSUD)
- ↑Glutamine, ↓ arginine (+/– ↑ citrulline) — ↑ UCDs
- ↑Alanine — lactic acidosis
- ↑Glycine — non-ketotic hyperglycinaemia, OAs
- ↑Phenylalanine — phenylketonuria
- ↑Tyrosine — tyrosinaemia

Organic acids

These are measured in urine only and are diagnostic in many organic acidaemias, e.g. increased propionate in propionic acidaemia, increased isovalerate in isovaleric acidaemia, etc. but are also essential in the diagnosis of other disorders.

- ↑Orotic acid — UCDs, mitochondrial, benign hereditary

- ↑Succinylacetone — tyrosinaemia type I
- ↑Dicarboxylic acids — fat oxidation defects, medium-chain triglyceride feeds, mitochondrial

Acylcarnitines

Carnitine conjugates with acyl-CoA intermediates proximal to the block in fat oxidation defects. The chain length of the acylcarnitines formed is diagnostic of where the block lies, e.g. medium-chain (MCAD), very long-chain (VLCAD), etc. Likewise, conjugation with organic acids allows diagnosis of organic acidaemias, e.g. propionylcarnitine. Total and free carnitine levels can be measured at the same time.

Urate

Urate is the end product of the breakdown of purines. Raised levels in plasma may indicate increased production (eg Lesch–Nyhan syndrome, GSD type I, rhabdomyolysis) or decreased excretion (familial juvenile hyperuricaemic nephropathy, FJHN). It is essential to measure a concurrent urinary urate because urate clearance in children is so efficient that plasma levels may be in the upper normal range in Lesch–Nyhan syndrome, whereas urinary levels are grossly elevated. In FJHN the reverse is true with high plasma urate, but low urinary urate. Low plasma urate is seen in molybdenum cofactor deficiency as a result of a block in the conversion of purine bases to urate.

Acute patient screening

Specific metabolites are used to screen acute patients for specific disorders or groups of disorders.

Specific metabolite screens

Metabolite	Disorder
Very-long-chain fatty acids	Peroxisomal disorders, e.g. Zellweger syndrome, adrenoleukodystrophy
Transferrin isoelectric focusing	Congenital disorders of glycosylation
Urate	Purine disorders
7-Dehydrocholesterol	Smith–Lemli–Opitz syndrome
Biotinidase	Biotinidase deficiency
Urinary glycosaminoglycans and oligosaccharides	Mucopolysaccharidoses and mucolipidoses
Urinary reducing substances	Galactosaemia
Urinary sulphites	Sulphite oxidase deficiency, molybdenum cofactor deficiency
Urinary purine and pyrimidine metabolites	Purine and pyrimidine disorders

Secondary investigations include:

- Neuroimaging — basal ganglia signal change in mitochondrial disorders
- Neurophysiology — mitochondrial, peroxisomal
- Echocardiogaraphy — especially hypertrophic cardiomyopathy, mitochondrial, fat oxidation, Pompe (GSD type II), storage disorders
- ECG — fat oxidation, mitochondrial
- EEG — metabolic encephalopathy, e.g. MSUD, hyperammonaemia

Enzymology

Definitive diagnosis is confirmed on enzymology. The sample requirement depends on which tissues express the enzyme, e.g. galactosaemia (blood), OTC deficiency (liver), mitochondrial (muscle). Genotype has superseded invasive biopsy in some conditions, e.g. GSD type I (glucose 6-phosphatase deficiency).

White cell enzymes are often requested in patients with potential neurodegenerative or storage disorders. Laboratories usually undertake different lysosomal assays for different presentations. The neurodegeneration panel includes Tay–Sachs, Sandhoff, Sly mucopoly-saccharidosis (MPS VII) and mannosidosis in plasma; G_{M1} gangliosidosis, arylsulphatase A deficiency, Krabbe and fucosidosis in white cells. The organomegaly panel includes Sly (MPS VII), and mannosidosis in plasma, G_{M1} gangliosidosis, Gaucher, Niemann–Pick A and B, mannosidosis, fucosidosis and Wolman disease in white cells.

2.5 Acute management

- Stop feeds
- Promote anabolism — give 10% dextrose with appropriate electrolyte additives (add insulin rather than reduce % dextrose if hyperglycaemic). NB High-concentration glucose can exacerbate the lactic acidosis of pyruvate and respiratory chain defects, therefore 5% dextrose should be used if primary lactic acidosis is suspected
- Correct biochemical disturbance along standard guidelines, e.g. hypernatraemia, low phosphate, etc.
- Clear toxic metabolites
  - Dialysis — lactate, organic acids, ammonia, leucine
  - Drugs — UCDs: phenylbutyrate, sodium benzoate; OAs: carnitine, glycine
- Supplement enzyme cofactors — e.g. biotin, thiamine, riboflavin
- Specific treatment
  - Dietary restriction
  - Drugs, e.g. nitisinone in tyrosinaemia
  - Enzyme replacement therapy in Gaucher, Fabry, Pompe, Hurler, and Hunter syndromes
  - Substrate deprivation therapy in Niemann Pick C and Gaucher
  - Transplantation (liver, bone marrow)
  - Hepatocyte transfer (future)
  - Gene therapy (future)

- Genetic counselling (+/− future prenatal counselling)
- Screen siblings if indicated

In defects of intermediary metabolism feeds are stopped during intercurrent infections to reduce the metabolic load and glucose polymer drinks are substituted to avoid catabolism. Failure to tolerate the emergency regimen requires admission for intravenous therapy.

3. DISORDERS OF AMINO ACID METABOLISM

3.1 Phenylketonuria (PKU)

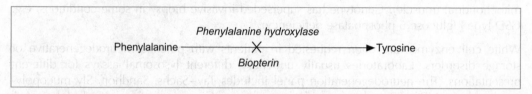

This is the commonest inborn error of metabolism in the UK with an incidence of 1 : 10,000 and a carrier rate of 1 : 50. Untreated classical PKU (phenylalanine > 1,000 µmol/l) presents with developmental delay in the first year. Characteristic features include mental retardation, behavioural problems, decreased pigmentation and eczema. There is considerable variation in phenotype and genotype; 1–2% of cases result from defects in biopterin, which is the essential cofactor for phenylalanine hydroxylase and neurotransmitter synthesis.

Diagnosis

Detection of a raised phenylalanine level on neonatal screening; confirmed on plasma amino acids and exclusion of biopterin defects.

Management

Phenylalanine is an essential amino acid and therefore cannot be totally excluded from the diet. The developing brain is most vulnerable to the deleterious effects of high phenylalanine; however, evidence is increasing that dietary restrictions should be continued for life. Patients with milder elevations of phenylalanine have hyperphenylalaninaemia and may or may not require treatment dependent on how elevated their levels are.

- Phenylalanine restriction (given as exchanges of natural protein titrated against phenylalanine levels monitored on home fingerprick blood tests)
- Amino acid supplement (no phenylalanine)
- Special PKU products (minimal or no phenylalanine)
- Free foods (negligible phenylalanine)
- Neurotransmitter replacement in biopterin defects (+/− folinic acid)

Biopterin is currently being evaluated as a treatment for hyperphenylalaninaemia because some patients are responsive and can then give up the restrictive diet. This is currently very expensive.

3.2   Tyrosinaemia (type 1)

Tyrosinaemia type 1 results from a block in the catabolism of tyrosine, producing by-products which damage the liver and kidney.

Clinical features of tyrosinaemia

- Early onset (severe) liver disease with coagulopathy, proximal renal tubulopathy
- Late onset: Faltering growth and rickets (secondary to renal Fanconi)
- Development of hepatocellular carcinoma in late childhood/adolescence

Diagnosis

Tyrosine is raised in the plasma and the presence of succinylacetone in urine is pathognomonic. Coagulation is almost always deranged even in the minimally symptomatic patient and should be actively sought in a patient with renal tubulopathy. Confirm by liver enzymology (fumarylacetoacetase).

Management

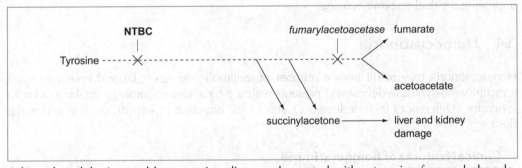

A low phenylalanine and low tyrosine diet supplemented with a tyrosine-free and phenylalanine-free amino acid supplement has been the mainstay of management; improving both liver and renal function but failing to prevent the development of hepatocarcinoma. Nitisinone has revolutionized the management by blocking the catabolic pathway proximal to the production of the damaging metabolites. Nitisinone is a derivative of the bottle-brush plant originally developed as a weed-killer. Dietary restriction remains but it is hoped that the risk of tumours is greatly reduced. Liver transplantation is reserved for patients failing to respond to nitisinone, or who develop tumours or progressive cirrhotic liver disease. Tumour surveillance includes interval hepatic MRI and monitoring of α-fetoprotein.

3.3   Maple syrup urine disease (MSUD)

MSUD results from a block in the degradation of the branch-chain amino acids leucine, isoleucine and valine. MSUD also belongs to the family of organic acidaemias.

Clinical features

The severe neonatal form presents as a classic intoxication with encephalopathy and seizures. Biochemical disturbance, i.e. acidosis, ketosis, may be minimal and therefore the diagnosis is often delayed with the illness often being attributed to sepsis. The neonate has a sweet odour, hence the name. Intermittent forms may present at a later age, patients appearing entirely symptom-free between bouts. Cerebral oedema is a well-recognized complication during acute episodes.

Diagnosis

- Elevated branch-chain amino acids plus alloisoleucine
- Elevated branch-chain oxo-acids on urinary organic acids
- Enzymology on fibroblasts

Management

Long-term management centres on controlling leucine levels with a low-protein diet supplemented with an amino acid supplement that is free of branch-chain amino acids. Valine and isoleucine may require additional supplementation because levels may fall too low while controlling leucine. The enzyme cofactor thiamine is given in the hope of improving residual enzyme activity.

3.4   Homocystinuria

Homocystinuria may result from a number of metabolic defects. Classical homocystinuria (cystathione-β-synthase deficiency) presents with a typical dysmorphology similar to Marfan syndrome. Differences include lower IQ, stiff joints, direction of lens dislocation and malar flush.

Clinical features of homocystinuria

- Marfanoid habitus (span greater than height), high arched palate, arachnodactyly
- Restricted joint movements
- Ectopia lentis (classically downward, but may be sideways!)
- Developmental delay/retardation (variable severity)
- Thrombosis (deep vein thrombosis and pulmonary embolus commonest)
- Osteoporosis

Diagnosis

Measurement of total plasma homocysteine is becoming the method of choice, superseding free homocysteine plasma levels. In classical homocystinuria, the plasma methionine is elevated. Definitive diagnosis is based on enzymology in fibroblasts.

Management

Treatment aims to reduce plasma total homocysteine to reduce the risks of thrombosis and lens dislocation. Protein restriction is used in patients diagnosed on screening, but is particularly difficult to institute in the cases who present later. Fifty per cent of patients respond to cofactor supplementation (pyridoxine). Folate should also be supplemented as depletion affects response. Betaine is effective at lowering homocysteine by remethylation and is particularly useful in the pyridoxine non-responsive patient.

3.5   Non-ketotic hyperglycinaemia

Defective glycine cleavage produces this early-onset convulsive disorder. Glycine is a neurotransmitter; excitatory centrally and inhibitory peripherally. In the absence of birth asphyxia, metabolic causes of neonatal seizures include non-ketotic hyperglycinaemia, pyridoxine and pyridoxal phosphate-dependent seizures, biotinidase deficiency, sulphite oxidase deficiency and molybdenum cofactor deficiency.

Clinical features of non-ketotic hyperglycinaemia

- Increased fetal movements (in utero seizures)
- Hiccups, hypotonia
- Progressive apnoeas/encephalopathy
- Seizures
- Marked developmental delay/psychomotor retardation

Diagnosis

The first clue is usually elevated glycine on urinary or plasma amino acids. The diagnosis is confirmed by measuring simultaneously the CSF : plasma glycine ratio (> 0.09). Enzymology is traditionally assessed in the liver, but a new assay using lymphocytes is now available.

Management

Glycine is reduced with sodium benzoate but has little effect on neurological outcome. Dextromethorphan (a partial N-methyl-D-aspartate (NMDA)) receptor antagonist helps block the central action of glycine and has helped reduce fits in some patients compared to conventional anticonvulsants. Prognosis remains poor for development. Newer NMDA receptor blockers are currently under investigation. Prenatal testing is available.

4. ORGANIC ACIDAEMIAS

Defects in the catabolism of amino acids result in the accumulation of organic acids which are detected in urine. Propionic acidaemia (PA) and methylmalonic aciduria (MMA) result from blocks in branched-chain amino acid degradation, isovaleric acidaemia (IVA) is the result of a block in leucine catabolism and glutaric aciduria type 1 (GA-1) results from a block in lysine and tryptophan metabolism.

4.1 Propionic, methylmalonic and isovaleric acidaemias

Clinical features of organic acidaemias

- Acute neonatal encephalopathy (intoxication), or chronic intermittent forms
- Dehydration
- Marked acidosis (↑ anion gap), ketosis
- Neutropenia +/– thrombocytopenia (acute marrow suppression)
- Progressive extrapyramidal syndrome (MMA, PA) basal ganglia necrosis
- Renal insufficiency (MMA)
- Pancreatitis
- Acute-onset cardiomyopathy (PA, MMA)

Diagnosis

Marked acidosis with ketosis is a key feature. Lactate and ammonia are invariably raised. Blood glucose may be low, normal or raised. Propionate is partly produced by gut organisms, therefore decompensation in PA and MMA may be precipitated by constipation. Neutropenia is another useful clue to the diagnosis. The key metabolites are detected on urinary organic acids, and enzyme deficiency is confirmed on enzymology.

Management

Long-term management is based on dietary protein restriction. Carnitine supplementation helps eliminate organic acids via conjugation and renal excretion. Glycine is used similarly in IVA. Some forms of MMA are vitamin B_{12} responsive. Metronidazole is used in MMA and PA to alter the gut flora to reduce propionate production and help avoid constipation. Liver transplantation is gaining acceptance as a definitive treatment in PA in view of the high risk of subsequent neurological decompensation; however the procedure does not eliminate the risk of neurological deterioration in MMA.

4.2 Glutaric aciduria type 1 (GA-1)

Before decompensation precipitated by an intercurrent infection, usually occurring towards the end of the first year, there may be little clue as to the underlying disorder except macrocephaly.

Diagnosis

The diagnosis must be actively sought in children with large heads and no other explanation, in an effort to prevent metabolic decompensation and subsequent severe neurology.

GA-1 may mimic non-accidental injury with encephalopathy and bilateral subdurals. Diagnosis is made on urinary organic acid metabolites and acylcarnitine analysis (low free carnitine and raised glutaryl-carnitine). A minority of cases are non-excretors, therefore fibroblasts are required for definitive enzymology in cases that have a strongly suggestive clinical picture but negative organic acids.

Clinical features of glutaric aciduria type 1

- Macrocephaly
- Normal development before catastrophic decompensation (usually <1 year)
- Choreoathetosis and dystonia (basal ganglia involvement)
- Magnetic resonance imaging features: bifrontotemporal atrophy, subdural haematomas, basal ganglia decreased signal

Management

In the absence of screening, the diagnosis is usually only made post-decompensation. In prospectively treated siblings, protein restriction in conjunction with aggressive treatment of infections and hyperalimentation has improved the prognosis; however, there is a broad spectrum of phenotypes and some children still decompensate in spite of treatment.

5. UREA CYCLE DEFECTS

The urea cycle is the pathway by which waste nitrogen is converted to urea for disposal. Urea cycle defects (UCDs) are inherited in an autosomal recessive manner except ornithine transcarbamylase (OTC) deficiency which is X-linked recessive. Girls may present symptomatically if during lyonization enough good genes are switched off in the liver.

Clinical features of urea cycle defects

- Vomiting (may be a cause of cyclical vomiting)
- Encephalopathy (intoxication following symptom-free period in neonate)
- Tachypnoea (ammonia is a respiratory stimulant acting centrally)
- Progressive spastic diplegia and developmental delay (arginase deficiency)
- Arginase deficiency rarely presents with classical hyperammonaemia

Diagnosis

UCDs are suggested by the presence of a respiratory alkalosis in the child with encephalopathy. Indication of the exact level of the enzyme block depends on plasma amino acids and urinary organic acids for the presence or absence of orotic acid. Orotic aciduria indicates a block at the level of OTC or beyond. Final confirmation of the diagnosis requires enzymology.

Characteristics of urea cycle defects

Urea cycle defect	Enzyme deficiency	Amino acids	Orotic acid
NAGS deficiency	*N*-acetyl glutamate synthase	Glu ↑, Arg ↓ Cit ↓	**Normal**
CPS deficiency	Carbamyl phosphate synthase	Glu ↑, Arg ↓ Cit ↓	**Normal**
OTC deficiency	Ornithine transcarbamylase	Glu ↑, Arg ↓ Cit ↓	↑↑↑
Citrullinaemia	Argininosuccinic synthase	Glu ↑, Arg ↓ **Cit ↑↑↑**	↑
Argininosuccinic aciduria	Argininosuccinic lyase	Glu ↑, Arg ↓ Cit ↑ **Argininosuccinate ↑**	↑
Argininaemia	Arginase	Glu ↑, **Arg ↑↑↑**	↑

Glu, glutamine; Arg, arginine; Cit, citrulline.

Management

Treatment follows the basic principles as detailed at the beginning of this chapter. Elimination of ammonia is accelerated by dialysis because earlier reduction in ammonia improves the long-term neurological outcome. Sodium benzoate and sodium phenylbutyrate conjugate with glycine and glutamine, respectively, to produce water-soluble products that can be excreted by the kidney, therefore bypassing the urea cycle and reducing the nitrogen load on the liver. Arginine becomes an essential amino acid in UCDs (except argininaemia) and is supplemented. Long-term protein is restricted and medicines are adjusted according to growth, amino acids and ammonia.

Liver transplantation has been used successfully in patients with brittle control; however, numbers are small and follow-up is limited.

6. FAT OXIDATION DISORDERS

The fat oxidation defects form a large group of conditions which commonly present with hepatic, cardiac or muscle symptoms. Fatty acids are a major fuel source in the fasted state and are oxidized by most tissues except the brain, which is reliant on hepatic fatty acid β-oxidation for ketone production. Fatty acids are the preferred substrate for cardiac muscle, and during prolonged exercise they are a vital energy source for skeletal muscle.

6.1 Medium-chain acyl-CoA dehydrogenase (MCAD) deficiency

MCAD deficiency is the commonest fat oxidation disorder with an incidence of 1 in 10,000 in the UK (as common as PKU). Peak presentation occurs in autumn and winter precipitated by intercurrent infections.

Clinical features of MCAD deficiency

- Hypoketotic hypoglycaemia
- Encephalopathy
- Reye-like syndrome: hepatomegaly, deranged liver function
- Mean age at presentation 15 months, commonest precipitant is diarrhoea
- Sudden infant death (consider in older infant > 6 months)
- Common *G985* mutation

Diagnosis

Detection requires a strong clinical suspicion to ensure that appropriate investigations are performed at the time. The presence or absence of ketosis should be sought in all cases of hypoglycaemia. Plasma-free fatty acids are raised, while ketone formation is impaired. Urinary organic acids reveal a characteristic dicarboxylic aciduria in the acute state, but may be normal between episodes. Acylcarnitines detect an elevated octanoyl carnitine, and genotyping is used for confirmation. The *G985* common mutation accounts for > 90% of allelles in clinically presenting cases in the UK. It is therefore a useful tool with which to assess at-risk siblings. A newborn screening pilot study began in the UK in 2004 (see Section 14.2).

Management

Prevention is better than cure. Mortality is 25% on first presentation, and 33% of survivors have neurological sequelae. Once the diagnosis is known, further decompensations can be avoided by employing an emergency regimen of glucose polymer drinks during intercurrent illnesses or admission for a 10% dextrose infusion if the drinks are not tolerated. In the at-risk neonate born to a family with a previously affected sibling, feeds should be frequent with intervals no longer than 3 hours, and top-up feeds established if needed while acylcarnitine results are awaited. Neonatal deaths have been reported.

6.2 Long-chain defects

The long-chain fat oxidation defects, very long-chain acyl-CoA (VLCAD) and long-chain hydroxyacyl-CoA (LCHAD) dehydrogenase are more severe, presenting at an earlier age and requiring meticulous dietary management to ensure normoglycaemia and to reduce long-term complications. Liver dysfunction may occur in the carrier mother during pregnancy: AFLP or HELLP syndrome.

Clinical features of long-chain defects

- Hypoketotic hypoglycaemia
- Myopathy
- Hypertrophic cardiomyopathy
- Pigmentary retinopathy (LCHAD)
- Peripheral neuropathy (LCHAD)
- Maternal hepatic symptoms in pregnancy

Diagnosis

Characteristic dicarboxylic aciduria is noted in acute episodes on urinary organic acids. Creatine kinase may rise acutely and frank rhabdomyolysis can occur. Acylcarnitines form the mainstay of diagnosis with confirmation on fibroblast flux studies. There is a common LCHAD mutation. Urine and blood samples from infants born to mothers with AFLP or HELLP should be screened post-delivery.

Management

Long-chain fat intake is severely restricted and the diet is supplemented with medium-chain fat and essential fatty acids. Normoglycaemia is maintained with frequent bolus feeds during the day, and overnight nasogastric or gastrostomy feeds in infancy. Uncooked cornstarch can be introduced from 2 years of age to smooth and prolong glycaemic control. An emergency regimen is used during intercurrent infections with admission for intravenous therapy if not tolerated. Carnitine supplementation is used to correct acute depletion, secondary to increased excretion of carnitine–fatty acid conjugates in the urine.

7. MITOCHONDRIAL CYTOPATHIES

Mitochondria are the power stations of the cell, producing ATP to drive cellular functions. The respiratory chain, the site of oxidative phosphorylation, is embedded in the inner mitochondrial membrane and consists of five complexes. Electrons are donated from reduced cofactors and passed along the chain, ultimately reducing oxygen to water, while the energy so produced pumps hydrogen ions from the mitochondrial matrix into the intermembrane space. Discharge of this electrochemical gradient through complex V (ATP synthase) generates ATP.

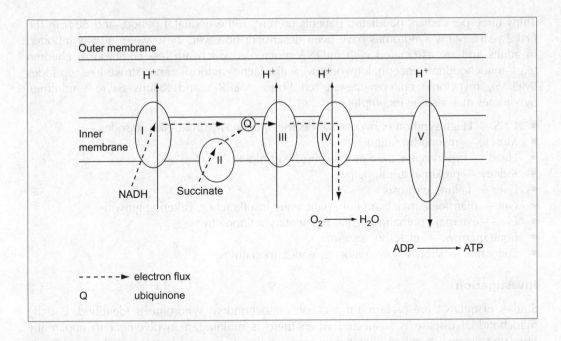

7.1 Mitochondrial genetics

Mitochondria are unique in containing their own DNA (mtDNA), contained within a circular double-stranded molecule. The mtDNA is inherited solely from the maternal egg, the sperm's mitochondria being left outside within the tail at fertilization. Inheritance of mtDNA mutations is therefore matrilineal; only being handed on by females. However, the mitochondrion is not self-sufficient but relies on nuclear genes for many essential proteins, including respiratory chain subunits. All complex II subunits are encoded within the nucleus. If a nuclear gene is at fault then normal Mendelian inheritance applies. Autosomal recessive inheritance is probably the commonest mode of inheritance for paediatric practice.

Mitochondria also contain more than one copy of mtDNA, and each cell may contain many mitochondria. It is possible to have mutant mtDNA and wild-type present in the same cell (heteroplasmy). The accumulation of mutant mtDNA will result in symptoms when a threshold is breached. As a result of heteroplasmy, symptoms may be patchy within and between organ systems. In rapidly dividing cells, such as the bone marrow and gut, wild-type cells may have a reproduction advantage and therefore symptoms in these organ systems may improve compared to the progressive brain and muscle involvement. Unless a nuclear defect is identified, prenatal diagnosis is not available.

7.2 Clinical features

As mitochondria are present in all cells except erythrocytes, any organ system can be involved at any time with any inheritance. High-energy-demand tissues are more commonly involved, particularly brain, muscle, kidney and liver, but any system can be involved.

581

Thirty-three per cent of paediatric patients present in the neonatal period, and 80% in the first 2 years. Many syndromes have been described; however, these were initially reported in adults and are associated with mtDNA mutations which are less common in children (e.g. mitochondrial encephalomyopathy with lactic acidosis and stroke-like episodes (MELAS), myoclonic epilepsy-ragged red fibres (MERRF) and Kearns–Sayre syndrome). Syndromes may also be incomplete.

- CNS — Leigh syndrome, hypotonia, deafness, epilepsy, stroke-like episodes
- Muscle — myopathy, fatigue
- Heart — hypertrophic cardiomyopathy, heart block
- Kidney — proximal tubulopathy
- Liver — failure, cirrhosis
- Gut — diarrhoea, malabsorption, pancreatic insufficiency, Faltering growth
- Eye — external ophthalmoplegia, pigmentary retinopathy
- Bone marrow — refractory anaemia
- Endocrine — short stature, diabetes, endocrinopathies

Investigation

Studies of mtDNA are preferred if a classic mitochondrial syndrome is identified. Usually mitochondrial disease is suspected when there is multiorgan involvement in apparently unrelated organs: so-called 'illegitimate associations'. Peripheral lactate may be persistently elevated. Further organ involvement may be sought before muscle biopsy for histochemistry (staining for complex II and IV), and respiratory chain enzymology (complexes I–IV).

- CNS — magnetic resonance imaging, brainstem auditory evoked potentials, CSF lactate
- Heart — echocardiography, electrocardiogram (ECG)
- Kidney — proximal tubular proteins, tubular resorption of phosphate
- Liver — biopsy, enzymology
- Gut — stool elastase
- Eye — fundoscopy, electroretinogram, visual evoked responses
- Marrow — full blood count, aspirate
- Endocrine — electrolytes

Management

Management remains supportive. A variety of antioxidants and respiratory-chain pick-me-ups have been described with success in only a handful of cases, e.g. ubiquinone, riboflavin. Dichloroacetate resolves the raised lactate but does not appear to improve outcome.

8. DISORDERS OF CARBOHYDRATE METABOLISM

8.1 Glycogen storage disease

Glucose is stored in the liver and muscles as glycogen. Glycogen storage disorders (GSDs) result from defects of glycogen breakdown. Hepatic forms present with hepatomegaly and hypoglycaemia, the muscle forms present with weakness and fatigue.

GSD Ia (glucose 6-phosphatase deficiency — von Gierke disease)

The enzyme deficiency fails to remove the phosphate from glucose 6-phosphate, therefore export of glucose from the liver from glycogenolysis and gluconeogenesis is blocked. Fasting tolerance is therefore limited, usually 1–4 h. Infants usually present at around 3 months when feeds are spread further apart. Massive hepatomegaly in the absence of splenomegaly is strongly suggestive of a hepatic GSD because glycogen is not stored in the spleen (unlike the material in lysosomal storage disorders). Nephromegaly is common. Abnormal fat distribution results in 'doll-like' faces and thin limbs. Bruising is a feature of poor control. Long-term complications include renal insufficiency, liver adenomas with potential for malignant change, gout, osteopenia and polycystic ovaries.

Investigations show raised plasma lactate levels, hyperuricaemia and hyperlipidaemia. Lactate levels fall on glucose loading. Genotyping has superseded liver enzymology for confirmation.

Treatment consists of frequent feeds during the day with continuous feed overnight. From age 2, uncooked corn starch is introduced as a slow-release form of glucose, prolonging the gap between feeds. Allopurinol controls the uric acid level in the blood. Liver transplantation is reserved for patients with malignant change in an adenoma or failure to respond to dietary treatment.

GSD Ib (glucose 6-phosphate translocase deficiency)

The translocase deficiency shares the above phenotype with the addition of neutrophil dysfunction with associated recurrent skin sepsis, large mouth ulcers and inflammatory bowel disease. Management is as above with the addition of prophylactic septrin for severe recurrent mouth ulcers, or granulocyte colony-stimulating factor (GCSF) in resistant cases.

GSD II (Pompe disease)

GSD II, acid maltase deficiency, is really a lysosomal storage disorder with accumulation of glycogen in lysosomes. The infantile form presents with severe hypotonia, weakness, hyporeflexia and a large tongue. ECG reveals giant QRS complexes. Vacuolated lymphocytes are seen on the blood film. Confirmatory enzymology is performed on fibroblasts. Death is usual within the first year; however, enzyme replacement therapy trials have shown encouraging results. Milder forms with mainly myopathy exist.

GSD III (debrancher enzyme)

Type IIIa affects liver and muscle, whereas **type IIIb** is purely hepatic. Type III may be clinically indistinguishable from type I; however, fasting tolerance is longer because gluconeogenesis is not blocked, and glycogen can be pruned to near the branch points. Nephromegaly is not a feature. Myopathy is notable and may be progressive in type IIIa. Cardiomyopathy is a rare complication. Adenomas, liver fibrosis and cirrhosis are rare.

Lactate level rises, unlike in type I, on glucose loading. The diagnosis may be confirmed on white cell enzymology. Dietary management is similar to but not as intensive as for type I. A high protein diet has been suggested for the type IIIa.

GSD IV (branching enzyme)

This form is very rare and presents with hepatomegaly and progressive liver disease. The diagnosis is usually made on liver histology and enzymology. Liver transplantation is the treatment for progressive disease.

GSD VI (liver phosphorylase deficiency) and GSD IX (phosphorylase-b-kinase deficiency)

Hypoglycaemia is rarely a problem. Hepatomegaly may be an incidental finding. GSD IX enzymology is assayed in red cells but may be normal in the isolated liver form. Treatment consists of uncooked corn starch once or twice a day to aid growth. Inheritance is X-linked or recessive depending on subgroup.

Muscle GSDs

GSD V (muscle phosphorylase deficiency) McArdle disease and GSD VII (phosphofructo-kinase deficiency)

Weakness and fatigue with post-exercise stiffness are the presenting features. Serum creatine kinase is usually elevated along with uric acid. On exercise, lactate fails to rise with excessive increases in uric acid and ammonia. After a brief rest, exercise can be restarted ('second-wind') as fatty acids slowly become available as an alternative fuel. Protein in the diet may be beneficial. Glucose is of benefit in McArdle disease because glycolysis is still intact. Extreme exercise should be avoided but regular gentle exercise is probably of benefit.

8.2   Galactosaemia

Clinical features of galactosaemia

- Neonatal onset — jaundice, hepatomegaly, coagulopathy and oil-drop cataracts, usually at the end of the first week
- Later presentation with Faltering growth, proximal tubulopathy and rickets at a few months
- Association with *Escherichia coli* sepsis

Diagnosis

Diagnosis is based on the clinical picture, the presence of reducing substances in the urine and enzymology for galactose 1-phosphate uridyltransferase (Gal 1-Put) in red cells. If the child has already received a transfusion, the parents should be screened for carrier-level activity instead. Even in the absence of obvious major liver involvement, the clotting is nearly always slightly prolonged. Galactosaemia should be considered in all cases of severe early-onset jaundice.

Management

This consists of a strict lactose/galactose-free diet for life. Milk is replaced with a soya-based formula. Long-term complications, in spite of good control, include developmental delay, particularly involving speech, feeding problems and infertility in girls.

8.3 Hereditary fructose intolerance

The key to diagnosis is the linking of symptoms with the exposure to fructose which usually occurs at weaning.

Clinical features of hereditary fructose intolerance

- Acute — vomiting and symptomatic hypoglycaemia
- Chronic exposure — Faltering growth, hepatomegaly, ascites, jaundice and proximal renal tubulopathy
- Milder cases — learn to avoid sugary foods
- Exacerbations may occur following exposure to fructose contained in medicines

Diagnosis

Lactic acidosis and hyperuricaemia are common features. Confirmation is by exposure to fructose and measurement of aldolase b activity in liver. Genotyping is used when liver biopsy is contraindicated because of coagulopathy.

Management

Lifelong avoidance of fructose.

9. HYPERLIPIDAEMIAS

Cholesterol and triglycerides are transported in the circulation bound to lipoproteins.

The four major classes are:

- **Chylomicrons** — carry dietary lipids, mainly triglycerides, from the gut to the liver. Lipoprotein lipase releases free fatty acids from chylomicrons in the portal circulation
- **Very low-density lipoprotein** (VLDL) — carries predominantly triglycerides and some cholesterol synthesized in the liver to the peripheries. Lipoprotein lipase releases the free fatty acids leaving IDL (**intermediate-density lipoprotein**)
- **Low-density lipoprotein** (LDL) — transports cholesterol and some triglyceride from the liver to the peripheries. Direct uptake by cells via the LDL receptor

- High-density lipoprotein (HDL) — carries cholesterol from the peripheries to the liver. Inverse association with ischaemic heart disease ('good cholesterol')

9.1 Hypertriglyceridaemias

- Defective chylomicron removal — lipoprotein lipase deficiency, apolipoprotein C-II deficiency
- Overproduction of VLDL — familial hypertriglyceridaemia

Hypertriglyceridaemias are rare. Clinical features include colic, hepatosplenomegaly, eruptive xanthomas and creamy plasma. Complications include abdominal pain and pancreatitis but rarely develop in patients until the triglyceride level exceeds 20 mmol/l. Secondary causes of elevated triglycerides include obesity, chronic renal failure, diabetes mellitus and liver disease. Treatment comprises a very low-fat diet supplemented with essential fatty acids. Drugs used to lower triglycerides include fibric acid derivatives, niacin or statins. Fibrate drugs reduce hepatic triglyceride synthesis and enhance peripheral triglyceride clearance, statins reduce triglycerides, probably by reducing VLDL synthesis.

9.2 Hypercholesterolaemias

- Defective LDL removal — familial hypercholesterolaemia
- Familial combined hyperlipidaemia

Familial hypercholesterolaemia is a monogenic disorder with a heterozygote incidence of 1 : 500, and homozygote 1 : 1,000,000. It is the commonest hyperlipidaemia, resulting from LDL-receptor gene mutations. Patients are picked up through premature ischaemic heart disease, or through screening for hypercholesterolaemia following diagnosis in a relative. Family history is an important risk factor for ischaemic heart disease, particularly at a young age and especially in females. In homozygotes, xanthomas may appear in the first decade, and angina before the age of 20.

In children, diet and exercise are the mainstay of treatment. These were previously supplemented with binding resins, e.g. cholestyramine and colestipol, which bind cholesterol and bile acids in the gut, increasing their loss in the faeces, and were preferred in paediatrics because they are not systemically absorbed. However, taking the sachets can be likened to drinking wet sand and so compliance was low. The new cholesterol-lowering margarines containing plant sterols are a more palatable alternative, reducing cholesterol absorption in the gut, but are expensive and have to be paid for by the families. Smoking is strongly discouraged. Increasingly, statins are being used in the over-10s as more safety data becomes available. However, theoretical concerns remain over their safety in this age group, particularly with regard to puberty. Statins are teratogenic. Liver function and creatine kinase are regularly monitored for adverse-effects. Their mechanism of action is the competitive inhibition of 3-hydroxy-3-methylglutaryl-CoA reductase, the rate-limiting step of cholesterol synthesis. Liver transplantation, or plasma apheresis, is the treatment of choice for homozygotes.

10. PEROXISOMAL DISORDERS

Peroxisomes harbour many vital cellular functions, including the synthesis of plasmalogens, (essential constituents of cell walls), cholesterol and bile acids, and the β-oxidation of very-long-chain fatty acids and breakdown of phytanic acid (vitamin A) and glyoxylate. Disorders are biochemically characterized by the number of functions impaired.

- Multiple enzymes affected (peroxisomal biogenesis defects) — Zellweger syndrome (ZS), neonatal adrenoleukodystrophy (NALD), infantile refsum disease (IRD)
- Several enzymes involved — rhizomelic chondrodysplasia punctata (RCDP)
- Single enzyme block — X-linked adrenoleukodystrophy (XALD), Refsum disease, hyperoxaluria

Inheritance is autosomal recessive with the exception of the XALD. The first-line investigation is very-long-chain fatty acids which are elevated in ZS and XALD but normal in RCDP. In this group, plasmalogens are the first screen. Further investigation requires fibroblast studies.

10.1 Zellweger syndrome

ZS is the classic peroxisomal biogenesis disorder with distinctive dysmorphic features. There is clinical overlap with NALD and IRD, which are milder with better prognosis.

Clinical features of Zellweger syndrome

- Dysmorphic faces — prominent forehead, hypertelorism, large fontanelle
- Severe neurological involvement including hypotonia, seizures and psychomotor retardation
- Sensorineural deafness
- Ocular abnormalities — retinopathy, cataracts
- Hepatomegaly and liver dysfunction
- Calcific stippling (especially knees and shoulders)
- Faltering growth

Diagnosis

Loss of all peroxisomal functions — raised very-long-chain fatty acids, phytanate and bile acid intermediates and decreased plasmalogens. Confirmatory enzymology on fibroblasts.

Treatment

Management is supportive. Docosahexaenoic acid supplementation has been tried but no clear benefit has been demonstrated. Death usually occurs within the first year.

10.2 X-linked adrenoleukodystrophy (XALD)

The paediatric cerebral form presents with severe neurological degeneration, usually between 5 and 10 years, progressing to a vegetative state and death within a few years. Brothers in the same family may present at different ages.

Clinical features of XALD

- School failure, behaviour problems
- Visual impairment
- Quadriplegia
- Seizures (late sign)
- Adrenal insufficiency

Adrenal involvement may precede or follow neurological symptoms by years. Some only develop neurological symptoms, and others just have adrenal insufficiency. All males developing adrenal failure should have very-long-chain fatty acid measurements taken to ensure that the diagnosis is not missed. Neurological symptoms may occur for the first time in adults (adrenomyeloneuropathy) resembling a cord syndrome with spastic gait and bladder involvement. Female carriers may develop multiple sclerosis-like symptoms in adulthood.

Diagnosis

Elevated very-long-chain fatty acids, blunted synacthen response or frank hypoglycaemia. Neuroimaging shows bilateral, predominantly posterior, white-matter involvement. The differential diagnosis for neurodegeneration in the school-age child includes:

- Subacute sclerosing panencephalitis
- Batten disease
- Wilson disease
- Niemann–Pick C disease.

Management

Lorenzo's oil (oleic and erucic acid) normalizes the very-long-chain fatty acids but fails to prevent progression. Bone marrow transplantation is the mainstay of therapy in patients before neurodegeneration, i.e. prospectively diagnosed siblings, and those diagnosed after presentation with adrenal insufficiency or other problems. Serial psychometry and neuroimaging are used to detect the first signs of neurological deterioration — the stimulus for transplantation. Adrenal function should be closely monitored, and steroid replacement therapy should be given once it is indicated.

11. MUCOPOLYSACCHARIDOSES (MPS)

Mucopolysaccharides (glycosaminoglycans) are structural molecules integral to connective tissues such as cartilage. Degradation occurs within lysosomes, requiring specific enzymes.

Patients with MPS appear normal at birth and usually present with developmental delay in the first year. The features of storage become more obvious with time.

11.1 Classification

Type	Disorder	Inheritance	Corneal clouding	Skeleton	Hepato-splenomegaly	Mental retardation
I	Hurler	AR	+	+++	+++	+++
II	Hunter	X-linked	–	+++	+++	+++
III	Sanfillipo	AR	+	+	+	+++
IV	Morquio	AR	+	+++	+	–
VI	Maroteaux–Lamy	AR	+	+++	+++	–
VII	Sly	AR	+	+++	+++	+++

AR, autosomal recessive.

Hurler syndrome is the classical MPS with storage affecting the body and CNS. Sanfillipo syndrome predominantly affects the CNS and Morquio and Maroteaux–Lamy syndromes affect the body. Atlantoaxial instability is common in the latter two, often necessitating prophylactic cervical spinal fusion in the first 2–3 years. Hunter syndrome is phenotypically similar to Hurler syndrome, however there is no corneal clouding and scapular nodules are seen.

11.2 Hurler syndrome

Hurler syndrome typifies the MPS group and their associated clinical problems. The enzyme deficiency is α-iduronidase, a deficiency shared with Scheie disease, the milder variant.

Clinical features of Hurler syndrome

- Coarse faces, macroglossia, hirsutism, corneal clouding
- Airway/ear, nose, throat problems, secretory otitis media
- Dysostosis multiplex
- Cardiomyopathy, valvular disease
- Hepatosplenomegaly
- Hernias — umbilical, inguinal, femoral
- Stiff joints
- Developmental delay and retardation

Diagnosis

Urinary screen for glycosaminoglycans (raised dermatan and heparan sulphate). Enzymology confirmed on white cells.

Management

Treatment depends on early recognition to allow early bone marrow transplantation, which significantly modifies the phenotype. Enzyme replacement clinical trials are currently underway. Supportive care is the mainstay of untransplanted patients, with particular regard to the chest and airway requiring 3-monthly sleep studies.

12. SPHINGOLIPIDOSES

Sphingolipids are complex membrane lipids. They are all derived from ceramide and can be divided into three groups: cerebrosides, sphingomyelins and gangliosides. Lysosomal hydrolases break these molecules down; deficiencies result in progressive storage and disease. Typical features include psychomotor retardation, neurological degeneration including epilepsy, ataxia and spasticity, with or without hepatosplenomegaly.

12.1 Tay–Sachs disease

Clinical features of Tay–Sachs disease

- Developmental regression within first year
- Macrocephaly
- Hyperacusis
- Cherry-red spot
- Spastic quadriplegia
- Death within 2–4 years
- No hepatosplenomegaly compared to Sandhoff syndrome

Diagnosis

The presence of vacuolated lymphocytes on the blood film is a further clue. Hexosaminidase A deficiency is confirmed on white cell enzymology.

Management

Currently, management is supportive. However, research into substrate-deprivation therapy, thereby avoiding accumulation in the first place, is under investigation.

12.2 Gaucher disease

Glucocerebrosidase deficiency results in the accumulation of cerebroside in the visceral organs +/– the brain depending on the type.

Clinical features of Gaucher disease

- Type 1
  - Non-neuronopathic (commonest)
  - Splenomegaly > hepatomegaly
  - Anaemia, bleeding tendency
  - Skeletal pain, deformities, osteopenia
  - Abdominal pain (splenic infarcts)
- Type 2
  - Acute neuronopathic
  - Severe CNS involvement (especially bulbar), rapidly progressive
  - Convergent squinting and horizontal gaze palsy
  - Hepatosplenomegaly
- Type 3
  - Sub-acute neuronopathic
  - Convergent squint and horizontal gaze palsy (early sign)
  - Splenomegaly > hepatomegaly
  - Slow neurological deterioration

Diagnosis

Elevated angiotensin-converting enzyme (ACE) and acid phosphatase are markers for the disease. Bone marrow aspiration may reveal Gaucher cells (crumpled tissue-paper cytoplasm). White cell enzymes for glucocerebrosidase give the definitive diagnosis. The enzyme chitotriosidase is markedly elevated and may be used to follow disease activity.

Management

Enzyme replacement therapy is effective in visceral disease in types 1 and 3. Bone marrow transplant has been used in the past, and may have benefit for cerebral involvement in type 3. Splenectomy has been used to correct thrombocytopenia and anaemia and relieve mechanical problems but may accelerate disease elsewhere. There is no effective treatment for type 2.

12.3   Niemann–Pick disease

Niemann–Pick is the eponymous name for the sphingomyelinoses; however, types A and B are biochemically and genetically distinct from C and D.

Type 1 (sphingomyelinase deficiency)

Clinical features of type 1

- Type A (infantile)
  - Feeding difficulties
  - Hepatomegaly > splenomegaly
  - Cherry-red spot
  - Lung infiltrates
  - Neurological decline, deaf, blind, spasticity
  - Death within 3 years
- Type B (visceral involvement)
  - Milder course, no neurological involvement
  - Hepatosplenomegaly
  - Pulmonary infiltrates
  - Ataxia
  - Hypercholesterolaemia

Diagnosis

Bone marrow aspirate for Niemann–Pick cells. White cell enzymes. Genotyping may help distinguish between the two types before the onset of neurological signs.

Management

Supportive.

Type 2 (lysosomal cholesterol-export defect, secondary sphingomyelin accumulation)

Clinical features of type 2

- Type C
  - Conjugated hyperbilirubinaemia (earliest sign)
  - Hepatosplenomegaly
  - Neurological deterioration (variable age of onset)
  - Dystonia
  - Cherry-red spot
  - Vertical ophthalmoplegia
- Type D (Nova Scotia variant)
  - As above, single mutation (founder effect)

Diagnosis

Niemann–Pick cells on bone marrow aspirate; however, white cell enzymes show normal or mildly decreased sphingomyelinase deficiency. Definitive diagnosis requires cholesterol studies on fibroblasts.

Management

Supportive. Prognosis is guided by age of onset.

12.4 Fabry disease

An α-galactosidase deficiency results in the storage of glycolipids in blood vessel walls, heart, kidney and autonomic spinal ganglia. It is X-linked recessive. Increasingly, female carriers with symptoms are being recognized.

Clinical features of Fabry disease

- Severe pain in extremities (acroparaesthesia)
- Angiokeratoma (bathing-trunk area)
- Corneal opacities
- Cardiac disease
- Cerebrovascular disease
- Nephropathy
- Normal intelligence

Diagnosis

Maltese crosses (bi-refringent lipid deposits) in urine under microscope. White cell enzymes.

Management

Analgesia, dialysis and renal transplantation are the established therapies. Enzyme replacement therapy has now been licensed for the treatment of Fabry disease in adults, with clinical trials in children underway.

13. MISCELLANEOUS

13.1 Porphyria

Porphyrias are a group of disorders of haem biosynthesis that may be classified as acute (neuropsychiatric), cutaneous or mixed. Symptoms in children are extremely rare. Inheritance is autosomal dominant except in congenital δ-aminolaevulinic acid dehydratase deficiency, erythropoietic porphyria and hepatoerythropoietic porphyria.

Clinical features of porphyria

- Acute (acute intermittent porphyria, aminolaevulinic acid dehydratase)
  - Abdominal pain, vomiting
  - Polyneuropathy (muscular weakness)
  - Neuropsychiatric disturbance
  - Postural hypotension/hypertension
- Cutaneous (erythropoietic protoporphyria, porphyria cutanea tarda, congenital erythropoietic porphyria, hepatoerythropoietic porphyria)
  - Photosensitive skin lesions
  - Liver damage
- Mixed (variegate porphyria, hereditary coproporphyria)

Diagnosis

- Acute attacks
  - Raised urinary aminolaevulinic acid and porphobilinogen during attacks (fresh urine)
  - Faecal porphyrin analysis to distinguish type
- Cutaneous forms
  - Total plasma porphyrins (raised if active lesions)
  - Total faecal porphyrins
  - Erythrocyte porphyrins

Management

Cutaneous forms are managed by avoidance of precipitants, especially sunlight, and good skin care. Acute attacks are managed with glucose and haem arginate, reducing synthesis of aminolaevulinic acid by negative feedback. Many drugs precipitate attacks, therefore only those known to be safe should be used during an attack.

Drugs used:

- Pain — opiates
- Psychosis — chlorpromazine
- Tachycardia, hypertension — β-blockers
- Seizures — gabapentin, vigabatrin

13.2   Smith–Lemli–Opitz syndrome

Smith–Lemli–Opitz (SLO) is the commonest sterol biosynthesis defect; a group of disorders characterized by limb defects, major organ dysplasia and skin abnormalities.

Clinical features of Smith–Lemli–Opitz syndrome

- Dysmorphic faces — microcephaly, narrow frontal area, upturned nose, ptosis
- Genital anomalies
- Syndactyly second and third toes
- Mental retardation
- Renal anomalies
- Faltering growth

Diagnosis

SLO is the result of a block in the penultimate step of cholesterol biosynthesis, therefore cholesterol is low with a raised 7-dehydrocholesterol level, the immediate precursor.

Management

At present, management is supportive. However, trials are underway evaluating the use of statins to block the build-up of precursors. Cholesterol supplementation has not shown convincing benefit.

13.3 Congenital disorders of glycosylation (CDG)

This group of disorders result from defects in the synthesis of the carbohydrate moiety of glycoproteins. Group I contains defects in oligosaccharide chain synthesis and in transfer to the protein, and group II have defects in the further processing of the protein-bound oligosaccharide chain. The two commonest disorders are CDG Ia (phosphomannomutase deficiency), and CDG Ib (phosphomannose isomerase deficiency).

CDG are multiorgan disorders affecting particularly the brain, except CDG Ib which is mainly a hepatogastrointestinal disorder. CDG Ia has typical dysmorphology.

Clinical features of CDG 1a

- Dysmorphic features — inverted nipples, fat pads
- Muscular hypotonia
- Faltering growth
- Cerebellar hypoplasia

Diagnosis

Transferrin isoelectric focusing is used to screen for CDG syndromes. Enzymology is performed on white cells and fibroblasts.

Management

CDG Ib is effectively managed with mannose supplementation. The other types are treated symptomatically.

13.4   Lesch–Nyhan syndrome

This is an X-linked disorder of purine metabolism caused by hypoxanthine guanine phosphoribosyltransferase (HGPRT) deficiency.

Clinical features of Lesch–Nyhan syndrome

- Motor disorder
    - Hypotonia initially, evolving dystonia or choreoathetosis + spasticity
    - Bulbar disorder — speech and feeding difficulties
- Growth faltering
- Hyperuricaemia — stones, nephropathy, gout
- Compulsive self injury
- Cognitive impairment

Diagnosis

Elevated urate and hypoxanthine in urine. Plasma urate may be normal because of the excellent renal clearance in childhood and so a urinary urate must also be measured. Enzymology red cells or fibroblast studies.

Management

Allopurinol and liberal fluids are used to reduce the risk of renal complications. Seating and positioning are essential to aid development and avoid self injury in conjunction with relaxation techniques and communication skills. A full multi-disciplinary team is essential. A low-purine diet is often undertaken but the evidence base for its use is limited.

13.5   Menkes syndrome

An X-linked membrane copper-transporter defect. Copper uptake by cells is normal, however export from the cell is blocked and the copper-requiring enzymes do not receive the necessary copper for normal function.

Clinical features of Menkes syndrome

- Hypothermia
- Epilepsy
- Hypotonia
- Prominent cheeks
- Pili torti
- Retardation
- Connective tissue problems
- Early death

Diagnosis

Low serum copper and caeruloplasmin, although these may be normal in the neonatal period. Confirmed on copper-flux studies in fibroblasts, and ultimately by genotyping.

Management

Daily copper–histidine injections have proven effective in altering the neurological outcome if the diagnosis is made early and treatment is not delayed. The connective tissue complications subsequently dominate the clinical picture in treated patients.

14.   SCREENING

14.1   Principles of screening

Screening for defined disorders aims to prevent avoidable morbidity and mortality. The sensitivity of a screening test is the rate of true-positives, and its specificity is the rate of true-negatives. The aim is not to miss any cases with the minimum of false-positives. The necessary requirements for including a condition in a screening programme are:

- Important health problem
- Accepted treatment
- Facilities available for diagnosis and treatment
- Latent or asymptomatic disease
- Suitable test
- Natural history understood
- Agreed case definition
- Early treatment improves prognosis
- Economic
- Case-finding may need to be continuous

The UK National Screening Committee added a further requirement; randomized controlled trial evidence to support introduction of new screens.

14.2   UK neonatal screening programme

Neonatal blood spots are collected on day 5–8 with the aim of commencing treatment by day 21 for hypothyroidism and PKU. Laboratories still using the Guthrie test for PKU, which relies on phenylalanine-dependent bacterial growth, may give false-negatives if the baby is receiving antibiotics. This information is requested on the card in those regions. The feeding status is also requested to ensure adequate protein intake, but newer techniques are able to detect PKU reliably on day 1 (routine screening day in the USA).

Current UK programme

- Universal
  - Congenital hypothyroidism (thyroid-stimulating hormone)
  - Phenylketonuria (phenylalanine)
  - Haemoglobinopathies (sickle-cell disease and thalassaemia)
- Some regions
  - MCAD
  - Cystic fibrosis (to become universal)
  - Galactosaemia
  - Homocystinuria
  - Duchenne muscular dystrophy

Haemoglobinopathies and cystic fibrosis have now been agreed for inclusion in the national screening programme. MCAD screening commenced in March 2004 in six laboratories screening half of the UK (300,000 births each year) to compare outcomes between the screened and unscreened populations with the aim of subsequent roll out nationally at the end of the study.

Duchenne muscular dystrophy is an example of a condition not fulfilling the criteria (being ultimately incurable); however, the public and professional support for the programme has grown with time. An 'important health problem' has been interpreted on an individual rather than a population basis. Potential benefits include 'avoidance of the diagnostic odyssey', with all its associated emotional and financial expense before the correct diagnosis is made, influences on reproductive choice in the parents (at a time before subsequent pregnancies) and the hope that earlier identification may lead to positive interventions to influence outcome and better research.

Newer screening technologies, such as tandem mass spectrometry, further challenge the established criteria because it is now much easier to diagnose a whole number of not only inborn errors of metabolism, but also liver disease, haemaglobinopathies, etc. Although additional screening costs may be minimal because the current system of blood-spot collection can be utilized, there is a large burden placed on diagnostic and support services dealing with the new caseload. Rarity may no longer preclude screening a whole population when there is an effective treatment available, e.g. biotinidase deficiency cured with biotin supplementation.

The number of conditions screened for has been massively increase in some countries. The US is expanding to 30 conditions; however, for many of these disorders the natural history is poorly understood and the diagnostic test does not always clearly decide who will develop symptoms. Concerns remain that individuals will be given a diagnostic label on the basis of a raised marker or mutation, but will never develop symptoms. The so-called 'un-patient'. Considering MCAD screening, many new mutations have been detected since the introduction of screening, many of which have never previously been found in clinically presenting cases.

15. FURTHER READING

McIntosh N, Helms P, Smyth R (Eds). 2003. *Forfar and Arneil's Textbook of Pediatrics*, 6th edn, Chapter 24, *Inborn Errors of Metabolism*. London: Churchill Livingstone.

Campbell NP, Smith AD, Peters TJ. 2005. *Biochemistry illustrated*, 5th edn. London: Churchill Livingstone.

Fernandes J, Saudubray J-M, van den Berghe G, Walter J (Eds). 2006. *Inborn Metabolic Diseases: Diagnosis and Treatment*, 4th edn. Berlin: Springer-Verlag.

Scriver CR, Beaudet AL, Sly WS, Valle D (Eds). 2001. *The Metabolic and Molecular Basis of Inherited Disease*, 8th edn. New York, NY, USA: McGraw Hill 2001.

Chapter 16

Neonatology

Grenville F Fox

CONTENTS

Neonatology

1. EMBRYOLOGY, OBSTETRICS AND FETAL MEDICINE

1.1 Embryology of the cardiovascular system

- The heart develops initially as a tube from yolk sac mesoderm. It begins to beat from about 3 weeks' gestation
- In the fourth week the primitive heart loops to form four chambers. Septation between the four chambers and the aorta and pulmonary trunk occurs in the fifth week. The septum primum grows down from the upper part of the primitive atrium and then fuses with the endocardial cushions (septum intermedium) in the atrioventricular canal
- Bulbotruncal septation divides the common arterial trunk into the aorta and pulmonary trunk as spiral ridges develop in the caudal end of the heart. Completion of ventricular septation occurs as these fuse with the septum intermedium
- Blood is pumped caudally from the embryonic heart by six pairs of pharyngeal arch arteries to the paired dorsal aortas. Some of this system regresses and the third arch arteries form the carotid vessels. The right fourth arch artery forms the right subclavian artery with that of the left forming the aortic arch. The left sixth arch artery forms the ductus arteriosus with branch pulmonary arteries forming from the right

1.2 Embryology and post-natal development of the respiratory system

- Embryonic phase (3–5 weeks' gestation) — the lung bud begins as an endodermal outgrowth of foregut. This branches into the surrounding mesoderm to form the main bronchi
- Pseudoglandular phase (6–16 weeks) — airways branch further to terminal bronchioles (preacinar airways). Cartilage, lymphatics and cilia form. Main pulmonary artery forms from sixth left branchial arch
- Canalicular phase (17–24 weeks) — airways lengthen, epithelium becomes cuboidal, pulmonary circulation develops. The acinar structures (gas-exchanging units) begin to develop and surfactant production begins by 24 weeks' gestation as type 1 and 2 pneumocytes become distinguishable. Lungs fill with amniotic fluid, which facilitates further lung growth
- Terminal sac phase (24–40 weeks) — further development of the acinar structures (respiratory bronchioles, alveolar ducts and terminal sacs (alveoli)) occurs and increasing amounts of surfactant are produced. Type 1 pneumocytes eventually cover approximately 95% of the alveolar surface and facilitate gas exchange. The surfactant-producing type 2

cells cover only about 5%. Development of the pulmonary circulation continues and results in a thicker intra-arteriolar smooth muscle layer by term, which may respond to intrauterine hypoxia by vasoconstriction. This regresses rapidly after birth

- Post-natal lung development — the number and size of alveoli increases rapidly during the first 2 years (approximately 150 million at term to 400 million by 4 years). The conducting airways also increase in size
- Diaphragm development — arises as a sheet of mesodermal tissue, the septum transversum. It begins close to the third, fourth and fifth cervical segments and therefore its nerve supply, the phrenic nerve, is derived from this area. The primitive septum transversum migrates caudally to form the pleural space and the two posterolateral canals in which the lung buds develop fuse. Failure to do this results in a Bochdalek hernia. Failure of the retrosternal part of the septum transversum to form causes a Morgagni-type diaphragmatic hernia. The diaphragm is completed as primitive muscle cells migrate from the body wall. If this fails eventration of the diaphragm results

1.3 Embryology of the gastrointestinal system

- The endodermal lining of the yolk sac forms the primitive gut
- The midgut lengthens and protrudes into the yolk sac via the vitelline duct. Meckel's diverticulum is the remnant of this
- The extra-abdominal gut rotates 270 degrees anticlockwise around the mesentery which contains the superior mesenteric artery. Failure to complete this results in malrotation
- The gut returns to the abdominal cavity by the end of the 12th week. Exomphalos is the result of this not occurring
- Gastroschisis is a failure of closure of the anterior abdominal wall

1.4 Embryology of the central nervous system

- The neural plate develops from ectoderm and forms the neural tube by 3 weeks' gestation. The neural groove closes in a cranial to caudal direction by the end of the fourth week
- Three swellings evolve from the caudal end of the neural tube — the prosencephalon (forebrain) forms the cerebral hemispheres, the mesencephalon forms the midbrain and the rhombencephalon (hind brain) forms the pons, medulla and cerebellum
- Neuroblasts migrate from the centre of the brain to further develop the cerebral hemispheres
- Myelination from Schwann cells occurs from 12 weeks' gestation
- Neural crest cells form the meninges, peripheral nerves, chromaffin cells, melanocytes and adrenal medulla

1.5   Embryology of the genitourinary system

- The genitourinary systems develop from mesoderm on the posterior abdominal wall and drain into the urogenital sinus of the cloaca
- The pronephros is the primitive kidney resulting from this and is replaced initially by the mesonephros. The ureteric bud appears at the start of week 5 of embryogenesis as a small branch of the mesonephric duct. The mesonephric (Wolffian) ducts drain urine from primitive tubules into the urogenital sinus. Repeated branching from week 6 onwards gives rise to the calyces, papillary ducts and collecting tubules by week 12
- Differentiation of the metanephros into nephrons — glomeruli, tubules and loop of Henlé occurs from 4 weeks. These structures then join with the lower Wolffian ducts to form the collecting systems. Branching and new nephron induction continues until week 36
- The metanephros develops from the most caudal part of the mesodermal ridge, but the kidney eventually becomes extrapelvic because of the growth of surrounding areas
- The Y chromosome (*SRY* gene) influences development of primitive gonads to form testes after 6 weeks. Testes 'secrete' Müllerian inhibition factor (MIF) which results in regression of Müllerian structures (uterus, Fallopian tubes and vagina)
- Testosterone influences the development of Wolffian structures (prostate, seminiferous tubules and vas deferens) as well as later masculinization

1.6   Maternal conditions affecting the fetus and newborn

- **Diabetes**
  - Three-fold increased risk of congenital malformations (congenital heart disease, sacral agenesis, microcolon, neural tube defects)
  - Small for gestational age (SGA) three times the normal rate because of small-vessel disease
  - Macrosomia as a result of increased fetal insulin
  - Hypoglycaemia
  - Hypocalcaemia
  - Hypomagnesaemia
  - Surfactant deficiency
  - Transient hypertrophic cardiomyopathy (septal)
  - Polycythaemia and jaundice
- **Hypertension** and pre-eclampsia — SGA, polycythaemia, neutropenia, thrombocytopenia, hypoglycaemia
- **Maternal thyroid disease**
  - Neonatal thyrotoxicosis can be caused by transplacental thyroid-stimulating antibodies (i.e. long-acting thyroid stimulator) with maternal Graves disease
  - Rare — only 1 : 70 mothers with thyrotoxicosis
  - May present with fetal tachycardia or within 1–2 days of birth, but sometimes delayed if mother is taking antithyroid drugs
  - Usually causes goitre

- Only severe cases require treatment with β-blockers and antithyroid drugs because it resolves spontaneously as antibody levels fall over the first few months

Neonatal hypothyroidism may be caused by maternal antithyroid drugs taken during pregnancy.

Systemic lupus erythematosus (SLE)

Maternal SLE is associated with:

- Increased risk of miscarriage. Recurrent miscarriage is associated with antiphospholipid antibody
- Increased risk of SGA babies. Risk is higher with maternal hypertension and renal disease
- Congenital complete heart block — associated with presence of anti-Ro and anti-La antibodies
- Butterfly rash — transient because of transplacental passage of SLE antibodies

Thrombocytopenia

Transplacental passage of maternal antiplatelet antibodies causes neonatal thrombocytopenia. If the mother is also thrombocytopenic the cause is likely to be maternal idiopathic thrombocytopenia (also associated with maternal SLE).

- Platelet count proportional to that of mother
- Rarely causes very low neonatal platelet counts or symptoms
- Risk of intracranial haemorrhage if platelet count $< 50 \times 10^9$/l (may occur antenatally, therefore Caesarean section not always protective)
- Treatment: intravenous immunoglobulin G (IgG) and platelet transfusion

Alloimmune thrombocytopenia occurs following maternal sensitization if mother is PL^{A1} antigen-negative.

- Approximately 3% of White people are PL^{A1} antigen-negative
- First pregnancies may be affected; severity is usually greater in subsequent pregnancies
- Antenatal intracranial haemorrhage is common (20–50%)
- Treatment — washed irradiated maternal platelets or intravenous IgG and random donor platelets

See Chapter 11 — Haematology and Oncology

Myasthenia gravis

Babies of mothers with myasthenia gravis have a 10% risk of a transient neonatal form of the disease.

- Usually the result of transplacental passage of anti-acetylcholinesterase receptor antibodies but baby may produce own antibodies
- Risk is increased if a previous baby was affected
- Maternal disease severity does not correlate with that of baby; a range of symptoms from mild hypotonia to ventilator-dependent respiratory failure may occur

- Diagnosis — antibody assay, electromyography and edrophonium or neostigmine test (also used as treatment)
- Babies of mothers with myasthenia gravis should be monitored for several days after birth
- Usually presents soon after birth and resolves by 2 months. Physiotherapy may be required to prevent/relieve contractures
- Congenital myasthenia gravis should be considered if antibodies are absent or if symptoms persist or recur

Fetal alcohol syndrome

Although more than three or four alcohol units per day during pregnancy are thought to be necessary to cause fetal alcohol syndrome, even moderate alcohol intake may reduce birth weight.

Features of fetal alcohol syndrome include:

- Small for gestational age
- Dysmorphic face with mid-face hypoplasia — short palpebral fissures, epicanthic folds, flat nasal bridge (resulting in small upturned nose), long philtrum, thin upper lip, micrognathia and ear abnormalities
- Microcephaly with subsequent intellectual impairment
- Congenital heart disease
- Post-natal growth failure

Maternal smoking

- Reduces birth weight by 10% on average
- Increases risk of sudden infant death syndrome

Maternal drugs

Teratogenic drugs include:

- Phenytoin (fetal hydantoin syndrome) — dysmorphic face (broad nasal bridge, hypertelorism, ptosis, ear abnormalities)
- Valproate — neural tube defects, fused metopic suture, mid-face hypoplasia, congenital heart disease, hypospadias, talipes, global developmental delay
- Retinoids (isotretinoin) and large doses of vitamin A — dysmorphic face (including cleft palate), hydrocephalus, congenital heart disease
- Cocaine — SGA, prune belly and renal tract abnormalities, gut, cardiac, skeletal and eye malformations
- Other teratogenic drugs include thalidomide (limb defects), lithium, carbamazepine, chloramphenicol and warfarin

Maternal opiate abuse

- Causes SGA infants
- Results in withdrawal symptoms or neonatal abstinence syndrome — onset usually

within 1–2 days of birth but may be delayed until 7–10 days and continue for several months; onset is later and symptoms persist for longer with methadone

Symptoms are:

- **W**akefulness
- **I**rritability
- **T**remors, temperature instability, tachypnoea
- **H**igh-pitched cry, hyperactivity, hypertonia
- **D**iarrhoea, disorganized suck
- **R**espiratory distress, rhinorrhoea
- **A**pnoea
- **W**eight loss
- **A**utonomic dysfunction
- **L**acrimation

Also — seizures, myoclonic jerks, hiccups, sneezing, yawning

- Surfactant deficiency is less common
- Sudden infant death syndrome is more common
- Management — monitor using withdrawal score chart. Less than 50% require pharmacological intervention. Indications for this are severe withdrawal symptoms or seizures. Oral morphine is the usual treatment of choice. Methadone, phenobarbital, benzodiazepines and chlorpromazine have also been used

1.7 Placental physiology, fetal growth and wellbeing

The fertilized ovum divides to form a blastocyst which attaches itself to the inside wall of the uterus. The outer cells of the blastocyst, the trophoblasts, eat their way into the endometrium and these and surrounding endometrial cells form the placenta and membranes. The trophoblasts are therefore the source of nutrition for the early embryo in the first 12 weeks.

In the second and third trimesters, maternal blood flows into the placental sinuses which surround the placental villi. Active transport of amino acids and other nutrients occurs across the chorionic epithelium into the villi, early in pregnancy, but this becomes less after the first trimester. Oxygen and nutrients diffuse into the fetal blood supply via the villi. Diffusion of oxygen occurs because maternal $p(O_2)$ is approximately 7 kPa, compared to 4 kPa in the fetus.

Oestrogen

- Initially produced by the corpus luteum and then in increasing amounts by the placenta as pregnancy progresses
- Causes the uterine smooth muscle to proliferate
- Enhances development of the uterine blood supply
- Changes pelvic musculature and ligaments to facilitate birth
- Causes breast development by increasing proliferation of glandular and fatty tissue

Progesterone

- Limited amounts produced by the corpus luteum in the early part of pregnancy — much larger amounts produced by the placenta after the first trimester
- Causes endometrial cells to store nutrients in first trimester
- Relaxes uterine smooth muscle; decrease in secretion of progesterone in the final few weeks of pregnancy coincides with onset of labour
- Facilitates glandular development of breasts

Human chorionic gonadotrophin

- Secreted by trophoblasts
- Prevents degeneration of corpus luteum
- Peak concentration at around 10 weeks, falls rapidly to low levels by 20 weeks' gestation

Human placental lactogen

- Secreted by placenta in increasing amounts throughout pregnancy
- Has growth hormone-like effect on fetus
- Has prolactin-like effect on breasts, facilitating milk production

Oxytocin

- Produced by the hypothalamic–posterior pituitary axis
- Release is stimulated by irritation of the cervix
- Oxytocin causes contraction of uterine smooth muscle
- Causes milk secretion — stimulation via the hypothalamus

Prolactin

- Produced by the hypothalamic–anterior pituitary axis
- Production is inhibited during pregnancy by high levels of oestrogen and progesterone produced by the placenta; the sudden decrease in these after delivery of the placenta increases prolactin release
- Prolactin causes secretion of milk from the breasts
- Hypothalamic production of a prolactin inhibitory factor increases if the breasts are engorged with milk and decreases as the baby breast-feeds
- Prolactin inhibits follicle-stimulating hormone immediately post-partum, thereby preventing ovulation

Identifying fetal compromise

- Kick charts
- Symphysis–fundus height — to estimate fetal size/growth
- Ultrasound scan measurement — to estimate fetal size/growth
- Amniotic fluid volume (see below)
- Umbilical artery Doppler studies — reflect placental blood flow
- Fetal Doppler scans — reflect hypoxia if abnormal

- Biophysical profile — fetal movement, posture and tone, breathing, amniotic fluid volume and cardiotachograph assessed

1.8 Amniotic fluid, oligohydramnios and polyhydramnios

- Amniotic fluid is produced by the amnion, fetal urine and fetal lung secretions
- Diagnosed on ultrasound scan if clinically suspected
- Deepest pool of amniotic fluid normally 3–8 cm. The amniotic fluid index (AFI) is the sum of the depth of the deepest pool in each quadrant
- Oligohydramnios (decreased AFI) may be caused by:
  - Placental insufficiency (intrauterine growth retardation (IUGR) is usually also present)
  - Fetal urinary tract abnormalities
  - Prolonged rupture of membranes (PROM)
- Polyhydramnios (increased AFI) may be the result of:
  - Maternal diabetes
  - Karyotype abnormalities
  - Twin-to-twin transfusion syndrome (sometimes called polyhydramnios–oligohydramnios sequence)
  - Neuromuscular disorders such as:
    - Congenital myotonic dystrophy
    - Spinal muscular atrophy (types 1 or 0 – type 0 is antenatal presentation of the disease)
    - Congenital myopathies
    - Moebius syndrome
- Oesophageal atresia
- Congenital diaphragmatic hernia
- Idiopathic/unexplained (a cause is more likely to be found in severe cases)

1.9 Body composition at birth

- There is a gradual decrease in extracellular fluid with increasing gestation (approx. 65% of weight at 26 weeks, 40% at 40 weeks)
- Early post-natal diuresis occurs within 1–2 days because of further loss of extracellular (interstitial) fluid and partly accounts for up to 10% of the weight loss — this may be delayed in babies with respiratory failure
- Surface area to weight ratio is high in newborn babies (more so in pre-term) so that the heat loss to heat production ratio is also high
- Newborn babies are able to generate heat as a response to cold stress using brown adipose tissue (non-shivering thermogenesis). Peripheral vasoconstriction may also help maintain body temperature. These mechanisms may be impaired in pre-term or sick babies and are also limited during the first few hours of post-natal life

1.10   Hydrops fetalis

Definition — subcutaneous oedema and fluid in at least two of: pleural effusions, ascites, pericardial effusion.

Causes

Immune cause is usually Rhesus disease.

Non-immune causes include:

- Anaemia:
  - Twin-to-twin transfusion
  - Fetomaternal haemorrhage
  - Homozygous α-thalassaemia
- Heart failure:
  - Arrhythmias (supraventricular tachycardia, complete heart block)
  - Structural (cardiomyopathy, hypoplastic left and right heart, etc.)
  - High-output (arteriovenous malformations, angiomas)
- Chromosomal abnormalities (Turner syndrome, trisomy 21 and other trisomies)
- Congenital malformations:
  - Congenital cystic adenomatoid malformation
  - Diaphragmatic hernia
  - Cystic hygroma
  - Chylothorax and pulmonary lymphangiectasia
  - Osteogenesis imperfecta
  - Asphyxiating thoracic dystrophy
- Infection:
  - Parvovirus B19
  - Cytomegalovirus (CMV)
  - Toxoplasmosis
  - Syphilis
  - Chagas disease (a South American parasite infection)
- Congenital nephrotic syndrome
- Idiopathic — 15–20% cases

1.11   Fetal circulation, adaptation at birth and persistent pulmonary hypertension of the newborn

Fetal haemoglobin (HbF)

- Four globin chains are $\alpha_2\gamma_2$ (adult is predominantly $\alpha_2\beta_2$)
- The γ-chains have reduced binding to 2,3-diphosphoglycerate (2,3-DPG)
- The reduced 2,3-DPG in HbF causes the oxyhaemoglobin dissociation curve to be shifted to the left — i.e. there is a higher saturation for a given PO_2 or p_{50} decreases (the PO_2) at which half the haemoglobin is saturated). Fetal red blood cells therefore have a higher affinity for oxygen, making it easier to unload from the maternal circulation. Delivery of oxygen to the fetal tissues is facilitated by the steep oxyhaemoglobin

dissociation curve of HbF, but the lower p_{50} leads to a decreased rate of unloading to tissues. Levels of 2,3-DPG rise rapidly in the first few days to meet the increased metabolic requirements that occur after birth. Pre-term infants have lower 2,3-DPG levels and therefore have a limited ability for oxygen to be unloaded from red blood cells

- Approximately 80% of haemoglobin is HbF at term. This falls to < 10% by 1 year
- The following also shift the oxyhaemoglobin dissociation curve to the left:
  - Alkalosis
  - Hypocarbia
  - Hypothermia

Circulatory changes at birth

- Functional closure of the ductus venosus occurs within hours of birth, with anatomical closure completed within 3 weeks.
- Ductus arteriosus patency is maintained in fetal life by prostaglandin E_2 and prostaglandin I_2. Functional closure of the ductus arteriosus usually occurs within 15 hours of birth and is facilitated by:
  - Reduced sensitivity of the ductus to prostaglandins and increased breakdown of prostaglandin E_2 occurring in the lungs towards the end of pregnancy
  - Increased PO_2 after the onset of breathing
  - Reduced pulmonary vascular resistance
- Before birth only about 10% of cardiac output goes to the lungs because pulmonary vascular resistance is higher than systemic
- Chemosensitivity of the pulmonary arteriolar bed increases with advancing gestation
- Increased PO_2 and lung expansion immediately after birth along with increased release of vasodilator substances (prostaglandins, bradykinin and nitric oxide) lead to a fall in pulmonary vascular resistance after birth
- Pulmonary artery pressure falls to half the pre-birth levels within 24 hours and pulmonary blood flow doubles as a result
- After birth, the left atrial pressure increases as a result of increased pulmonary blood flow and right atrial pressure falls because of the absence of placental blood from the umbilical vein. This results in a functional closure of the foramen ovale within a few minutes of birth. Anatomical closure may take weeks

Persistent pulmonary hypertension of the newborn

- Normal circulatory changes after birth are delayed either because of increased muscularization of the pulmonary arterioles or as a response to hypoxia
- Treatment includes ventilation with hyperoxia, induced metabolic alkalosis and the use of pulmonary vasodilators such as nitric oxide

Nitric oxide

- Free radical
- Synthesized in endothelial cells from L-arginine by the enzyme nitric oxide synthase — also known as endothelium-derived relaxing factor
- In vascular smooth muscle — nitric oxide activates guanylate cyclase to increase

intracellular cyclic guanosine monophosphate (cGMP). This leads to smooth muscle relaxation and vasodilatation by stimulating cGMP-dependent protein kinase which reduces intracellular calcium

2. PREMATURITY — DEFINITIONS AND STATISTICS

2.1 Mortality — definitions

- **Stillbirth** — in utero death after 24 weeks' gestation (28 weeks in most other European countries, 20 weeks in USA, 12 weeks in Japan)
- **Perinatal mortality rate** — stillbirths and deaths within 6 days of birth per 1,000 live and stillbirths (perinatal mortality rate for England and Wales in 2004 = 8.2)
- **Neonatal mortality rate** — deaths of liveborn infants < 28 days old per 1,000 live births (neonatal mortality rate for England and Wales in 2004 = 3.5). **NB** This includes infants born at less than 24 weeks' gestation if liveborn

2.2 Incidence and causes/associations of pre-term birth

Approximate UK incidences (live births) are:

- Pre-term birth (i.e. before 37 completed weeks' gestation)   7%
- Low birth weight (< 2500 g)   7%
- Very low birth weight (< 1500 g)   1.2%
- Extremely low birth weight (< 1000 g)   0.5%

All of these incidences are higher in developing countries but lower in some other European countries.

The incidence of pre-term birth appears to be increasing both in the UK and in other countries and this is probably the result of:

- Increased number of multiple births because of assisted conception
- Increased obstetric intervention
- Increased use of gestational age assessments (which tends to decrease estimates of gestational age)
- An increase in the registration of live births at very low gestation

The following are associated with an increased risk for spontaneous pre-term birth:

- Social/demographic factors:
  - Maternal country of birth Africa or Caribbean
  - Low socioeconomic class
  - Age < 20 or > 40 years

- Past obstetric or medical history
    - Previous pre-term birth
    - Uterine abnormalities
    - Cervical abnormalities
- Current pregnancy
    - Multiple pregnancy
    - Poor nutrition
    - Low pre-pregnancy weight
    - Poor pre- and antenatal care
    - Anaemia
    - Smoking
    - Bacteriuria
    - Genital tract colonization (particularly group B streptococcus)
    - Cervical dilatation > 1 cm
    - Pre-term PROM

2.3 Outcome after pre-term birth

The only national study of survival and long-term follow-up after extreme pre-term birth published so far is the EPICure study. This documented outcome after birth between 20 and 25 weeks' gestation in 1,289 live births in the UK and Republic of Ireland in 1995.

Survival to discharge from hospital was as follows:

- 22 weeks   1%
- 23 weeks   11%
- 24 weeks   26%
- 25 weeks   44%

Neurodevelopmental follow-up of survivors at 30 months showed:

- No disability   49%
- Severe disability   23%
- Mild to moderate disability   25%
- Died after hospital discharge   2%
- Not followed up   1%

Outcome for pre-term SGA infants is less well documented but there is some evidence that outcome is marginally better than that expected in an appropriately grown infant of the same birth weight — i.e. a baby born at 28 weeks weighing 750 g (below the third centile) would be expected to have the same outcome as a 25-week gestation infant of the same weight (50th centile).

The ethics of resuscitation of extremely pre-term infants are controversial and any decisions in individual cases should be made by the most senior paediatrician available at the time, with parents' views taken into consideration when possible. It seems reasonable to actively resuscitate most appropriately grown (i.e. > approximately 500 g) infants greater than 23 weeks' gestation who have reasonable signs of life after birth.

2.4   Small-for-gestational-age babies

- The definition of SGA varies between birth weight less than the third centile to a birth weight < 10th centile. Over 50% of babies with birth weight < 10th centile are constitutionally small; the rest have IUGR
- There are many causes of SGA infants including maternal (hypertension, diabetes, lupus, smoking, altitude), fetal (multiple gestations, malformations, infections) and placental

Fetal/neonatal complications of IUGR

- In utero death/stillbirth
- Fetal hypoxia/acidosis (associated with neonatal encephalopathy/birth depression)
- Polycythaemia, neutropenia (and increased infection risk), thrombocytopenia
- Hypothermia
- Hypoglycaemia
- Necrotizing enterocolitis

Long-term complications of IUGR

- Increased risk of neurodevelopmental problems
- Hypertension
- Diabetes
- Hyperlipidaemias

3.   RESPIRATORY PROBLEMS

3.1   Surfactant deficiency

Endogenous surfactant is produced by type 2 pneumocytes, which line 5–10% of the alveolar surface. Surfactant-containing osmiophilic granular inclusion bodies cause these to appear different from the thinner and more numerous type 1 pneumocytes, which are responsible for gas exchange.

Composition of endogenous surfactant

Phospholipids — 85%

- The main surface-active components which lower surface tension at the air–alveolar interface preventing alveolar collapse
- Dipalmitoylphosphatidylcholine (DPPC) — 45–70% — is the major constituent of all exogenous surfactant preparations
- Other phospholipids include:
  - Phosphatidylcholine
  - Phosphatidylglycerol
  - Phosphatidylinositol
  - Phosphatidylethanolamine

- Phosphatidylserine
- Sphingomyelin

Neutral lipids — 10%

Apolipoproteins — 5%

- Facilitate adsorption, spreading and recycling of surfactant and have immunoregulatory properties

Surfactant-associated proteins

- Surfactant protein A
  - Mainly immune function but also has a role in spreading and recycling of surfactant
  - Has been shown to increase microbial killing by alveolar macrophages
  - Increases resistance to inhibitors of surface activity which occurs in sepsis
- Surfactant protein B
  - Major role in adsorption, spreading and recycling of surfactant
  - Case reports suggest that congenital deficiency of surfactant protein B is a lethal, autosomal recessive condition
- Surfactant protein C
  - Similar function to surfactant protein B
- Surfactant protein D
  - Immune function

Platelet activating factor (PAF) — may increase surfactant secretion

Exogenous surfactants

	Contains	Onset	Mortality	Air leak	CLD/BPD
Synthetic	DPPC Hexadecanol	Hours	↓	↓	↓
Tyloxapol Animal Surf. proteins B+C	Lipids (inc. DPPC)	Minutes	↓↓	↓↓	↓↓

CLD/BPD, chronic lung disease/bronchopulmonary dysplasia

Estimated incidence of surfactant deficiency by gestational age (without maternal steroids)

Gestation (completed weeks)	Incidence of surfactant deficiency (%)
26	90
27	85
28	80
29	75
30	70
31	60
32	55
33	40
34	25
35	20
36	12
37	6
38	3
39	2
40	<1–2

Increased incidence of surfactant deficiency in:

- Prematurity
- Male sex
- Sepsis
- Maternal diabetes
- Second twin
- Elective Caesarean section
- Strong family history

Surfactant deficiency is decreased in:

- Female sex
- PROM
- Maternal opiate use
- IUGR
- Antenatal glucocorticoids
- Prophylactic surfactant

Amniotic fluid (or gastric aspirate) lecithin : sphingomyelin (L : S) ratios

- <1.5   = immature   — 70% risk of surfactant deficiency
- 1.5–1.9 = borderline   — 40% risk of surfactant deficiency
- 2.0–2.5 = mature   — very small risk unless mother is diabetic
- >2.5   = safe

Management of surfactant deficiency

There is currently no evidence that routine high-frequency oscillation is of any long-term benefit in pre-term infants with surfactant deficiency, although this mode of ventilation may be used as a 'rescue' in severe cases. Routine paralysis is not used in most neonatal units, although this sedation with opiates and various modes of trigger ventilation may help reduce the incidence of pneumothoraces. Exogenous surfactant considerably reduces mortality and incidence of pneumothoraces and chronic lung disease. Early treatment with surfactant and use of animal rather than synthetic surfactants enhance these outcomes.

3.2   Chronic lung disease — (bronchopulmonary dysplasia)

Definition — respiratory support with supplementary oxygen +/– mechanical ventilation for >28 days with typical chest X-ray changes (see below). In very-low-birth-weight (VLBW) infants an alternative definition has been suggested — requiring oxygen +/– mechanical ventilation >36 weeks' corrected gestational age and typical chest X-ray changes.

Risk factors for chronic lung disease

*   Prematurity
*   Prolonged mechanical ventilation with high pressures and high functional inspired oxygen (FiO_2)
*   Baro- (volume) trauma
*   Pulmonary air leak (pneumothoraces or pulmonary interstitial emphysema)
*   Gastro-oesophageal reflux
*   Patent ductus arteriosus (PDA)
*   Pulmonary infection (particularly *Ureaplasma urealyticum*)

Radiological stages

*   Stage 1   1st few days   indistinguishable from surfactant deficiency
*   Stage 2   2nd week   generalized opacity of lung fields
*   Stage 3   2–4 weeks   streaky infiltrates
*   Stage 4   >4 weeks   hyperinflation, cysts, areas of collapse/consolidation, cardiomegaly

Management of chronic lung disease

*   Ventilatory support as required
*   Supplementary oxygen to maintain oxygen saturations 94–96% or $p(O_2)$ >7 kPa (to reduce risk of pulmonary hypertension and cor pulmonale)
*   Good nutrition is of paramount importance; increased alveolar growth accompanies general growth — particularly in the first 1–2 years
*   Treatment of underlying exacerbating factors — infection, gastro-oesophageal reflux, fits, cardiac problems, etc.
*   Dexamethasone — the only proven benefit is to facilitate weaning off mechanical ventilation but concern has been raised over short- and long-term side-effects, particularly adverse neurodevelopmental outcome

- Inhaled steroids — only proven benefit is to reduce the need for systemic steroids
- Bronchodilators
- Diuretics — only likely to be of benefit in the presence of PDA, cor pulmonale or excessive weight gain
- Respiratory syncytial virus (RSV) prophylaxis with monoclonal antibodies (Palivizumab) has been shown to reduce hospitalization in high risk cases, but use is controversial because of the high cost of the drug and the need for monthly intramuscular injections throughout the RSV season

Outcome of babies with chronic lung disease

- Most are weaned off supplementary oxygen before discharge home
- Few require home oxygen
- Most babies discharged on home oxygen are weaned off before 1–2 years
- High risk of readmission to hospital with viral respiratory infections in the first 1–2 years of life
- Increased risk of recurrent cough and wheeze in pre-school age group but most outgrow this tendency and have normal exercise tolerance in childhood

3.3 Meconium aspiration syndrome (MAS)

Risk factors

- Term or post-term (incidence much higher in births after 42 weeks)
- Small for gestational age
- Perinatal asphyxia

Rare in pre-term but said to occur with congenital listeriosis (more likely to be pus than meconium). The passage of meconium in fetal distress may be the result of increased secretion of motilin. Meconium may be inhaled antenatally or post-natally. Antenatal inhalation is more likely in fetal distress because of abnormal fetal breathing (equivalent to gasping) that occurs with hypoxia and acidosis.

Major effects of MAS on lung function

- Airway blockage
  - Increased airways resistance with ball-valve mechanism and gas trapping
  - High risk of pneumothorax
- Chemical pneumonitis
- Increased risk of infection
  - Even though meconium is sterile
  - *Escherichia coli* is the most common infective agent
- Surfactant deficiency
  - Lipid content of meconium displaces surfactant from alveolar surface
  - Persistent pulmonary hypertension of the newborn

MAS changes on chest X-rays include initial patchy infiltration and hyperinflation. Pneumothoraces are common at this stage. A more homogeneous opacification of the lung fields may develop over the next 48 hours as chemical pneumonitis becomes more of a problem. In severe cases, changes similar to chronic lung disease may develop over the following weeks.

Uncontrolled trials of vigorous airway suction immediately after delivery suggest that it is possible to reduce the incidence of MAS. Intubation for lower airway suction is only needed if meconium can be seen below the vocal cords. Thoracic compression and routine bronchial lavage have no proven benefit. Intermittent positive-pressure ventilation with a relatively long expiratory time to prevent further gas trapping may be required in moderate to severe MAS. Surfactant replacement therapy in infants with MAS has proven benefit, but large doses may be required. Extracorporeal membrane oxygenation (ECMO) may be used in the most severe cases.

3.4 Pneumonia

Pneumonia can be congenital, intrapartum or nosocomial.

Congenital

Onset is usually within 6 hours of birth.

- **Bacterial**
  - Streptococci (group B streptococcus)
  - Coliforms (*E. coli, Klebsiella, Serratia, Shigella, Pseudomonas*, etc.)
  - Pneumococci
  - *Listeria*
- **Viral**
  - CMV
  - Rubella virus
  - Herpes simplex virus
  - Coxsackievirus
- **Other**
  - Toxoplasmosis
  - *Chlamydia*
  - *Ureaplasma urealyticum*
  - *Candida*

Intrapartum

Onset is usually within 48 hours.

- **Bacterial**
  - Group B streptococci
  - Coliforms (as above)
  - *Haemophilus*
  - Staphylococci

- Pneumococci
- *Listeria*
- **Viral**
  - Herpes simplex virus
  - Varicella zoster virus

Nosocomial

Onset is after 48 hours.

- **Bacterial**
  - Staphylococci
  - Streptococci
  - *Pseudomonas*
  - · *Klebsiella*
  - Pertussis
- **Viral**
  - RSV
  - Adenovirus
  - Influenza viruses
  - Parainfluenza viruses
  - Common cold viruses
- **Other**
  - *Pneumocystis carinii*

3.5 Pulmonary air leak

Pneumothorax

- Occurs in up to 1% of otherwise healthy term infants (it is usually asymptomatic)
- Overdistension of alveoli is more likely to occur in immature lungs because of a decreased number of pores of Kohn, which redistribute pressure between alveoli. Air ruptures through overdistended alveolar walls and moves towards the hilum where it enters the pleural or mediastinal space
- More common in surfactant deficiency, MAS, pneumonia and pulmonary hypoplasia.
- Risk is reduced by lower ventilator pressures to avoid overdistension, faster rate ventilation with shorter inspiratory times, paralysis of infants fighting the ventilator and surfactant replacement therapy.

Pulmonary interstitial emphysema

- May occur in up to 25% of VLBW infants, usually confined to those with the worst surfactant deficiency
- May be more common in chorioamnionitis
- Alveolar rupture results in small cysts in the pulmonary interstitium
- Ventilation is difficult and mortality and incidence of chronic lung disease are high

Pneumomediastinum

- May complicate surfactant deficiency or other forms of neonatal lung disease, when it may coexist with pneumothorax or may be iatrogenic following tracheal rupture secondary to intubation
- No symptoms may occur in isolated pneumomediastinum, but respiratory and cardiovascular compromise are more likely to occur if pneumothorax is also present

3.6 Congenital lung problems

Pulmonary hypoplasia

Primary pulmonary hypoplasia is rare but may present with persistent tachypnoea which resolves with lung growth several months after birth

Secondary pulmonary hypoplasia may be the result of:

- Reduced amniotic fluid volume — Potter syndrome (renal agenesis) or other severe congenital renal abnormalities resulting in markedly decreased urine volume (infantile (autosomal recessive) polycystic kidney disease, severe bilateral renal dysplasia, posterior urethral valves)
- Pre-term rupture of membranes — only occurs if membranes ruptured before 26 weeks; 23% of pregnancies with rupture of membranes before 20 weeks are unaffected; outcome with rupture of membranes before 24 weeks is usually poor
- Amniocentesis — mild to moderate respiratory symptoms are more likely to occur in the neonatal period and incidence of respiratory symptoms in the first year of life is increased
- Lung compression — pulmonary hypoplasia is common in small-chest syndromes including asphyxiating thoracic dystrophy and thanatophoric dwarfism, diaphragmatic hernia, congenital cystic adenomatoid malformation and pleural effusions
- Reduced fetal movements — pulmonary hypoplasia occurs in congenital myotonic dystrophy, spinal muscular atrophy and other congenital myopathies

Outcome with pulmonary hypoplasia depends on the severity and the underlying cause.

Congenital diaphragmatic hernia

- Commonest congenital abnormality of the respiratory system — incidence is 1 in 2,500–3,500 births
- Twice as common in males
- Other congenital malformations are common: 30% have karyotype abnormalities and 17% have other lethal abnormalities; 39% have abnormalities in other systems — malrotation occurs in 20%; those with other congenital abnormalities have double the mortality rate
- 90% are Bochdalek or posterolateral hernias
- 85–90% are left-sided
- Bilateral pulmonary hypoplasia occurs — ipsilateral >contralateral
- Usually diagnosed on routine antenatal ultrasound. May present with polyhydramnios. Those that have a normal routine antenatal ultrasound scan are likely to have a better

outcome because the hernia usually occurs later, allowing for reasonable lung growth. In utero repair and tracheal plugging have been attempted but with variable outcomes
- Respiratory distress (usually severe), heart sounds on the right side of the chest, bowel sounds on the left side, a scaphoid abdomen and vomiting may be found at birth. Less severe cases may not present initially but develop increasing respiratory distress over the first 24 hours as the gut becomes more air-filled. Differential diagnosis is congenital cystic adenomatoid malformation (or even pneumothorax)

During resuscitation

- Bag and mask positive-pressure ventilation should be avoided
- Wide-bore nasogastric tube should be placed as soon as possible to deflate gut and to confirm diagnosis, and therefore distinguish between differential diagnoses of congenital cystic adenomatoid malformation or pneumothorax on subsequent chest X-ray
- Consider paralysing baby to avoid air swallowing and to reduce the risk of pneumothorax

Surgical management

- There is some evidence to suggest that stabilizing the baby before surgery improves outcome
- Malrotation is corrected if present; the diaphragmatic defect is usually closed with a synthetic patch

Post-operative care

- High-frequency oscillation, nitric oxide or ECMO may be of benefit, but evidence for routine use of these is lacking
- Mortality overall is approximately 50–60%
- Survivors may have problems associated with underlying pulmonary hypoplasia

Congenital cystic adenomatoid malformation (CCAM)

- Rare, abnormal proliferation of bronchial epithelium, containing cystic and adenomatoid portions
- Lower lobes affected more frequently
- May disappear or become smaller spontaneously before or after birth
- Differential diagnosis is congenital diaphragmatic hernia
- Prognosis worse with associated hydrops, pre-term birth and with type 3 lesions
- Recurrent infection and malignant change have been described
- There are three types

Type 1 CCAM

- Single or small number of large cysts
- Commonest type (50% cases)
- May cause symptoms by compression or may be asymptomatic initially
- Good prognosis after surgery

Type 2 CCAM

- Multiple small cysts
- Usually cause symptoms by compression of surrounding normal lung
- Prognosis variable

Type 3 CCAM

- Airless mass of very small cysts giving the appearance of a solid mass
- Worst prognosis

Congenital lobar emphysema

- Affected lobe is overinflated
- Left upper lobe is most commonly affected (also right middle and upper lobes); rare in lower lobes
- More common in males
- Associated with congenital heart disease in 1 : 6 cases (usually as a result of compression of airways by aberrant vessels)
- Unaffected lobes in affected lung are compressed
- Mediastinal shift and compression of the contralateral lung may also occur
- Presents with signs of respiratory distress, wheezing, chest asymmetry and hyperresonance
- Chest X-ray shows hyperlucent affected lobe +/− compression of other lobes
- Reduced ventilation and perfusion of the affected lobe is seen on a ventilation/perfusion scan in more severe cases
- Surgical correction of underlying vascular abnormalities or resection of the affected lobe may be required but symptoms and signs may resolve following bronchoscopy

Chylothorax

- Effusion of lymph into the pleural space as a result of either:
  - Underlying congenital abnormality of the pulmonary lymphatics
  - Iatrogenic following cardiothoracic surgery
- Diagnosis by antenatal ultrasound scan allows antenatal drainage by insertion of intercostal drains, which may reduce the risk of pulmonary hypoplasia and facilitate resuscitation after birth
- Ventilatory support may be required post-natally, along with intermittent intercostal drainage
- Volume of chyle can be reduced by using a medium-chain triglyceride milk formula or avoiding enteral feeds for up to several weeks as the underlying abnormality resolves with time; protein and lymphocyte depletion may complicate this
- Surgical treatment is needed for the small number of cases that do not resolve spontaneously

3.7 Chest wall abnormalities

Asphyxiating thoracic dystrophy

- Autosomal recessive
- Variable severity
- Short ribs with bell-shaped chest
- May have polydactyly and other skeletal abnormalities also
- Long-term prognosis good in infants who survive >1 year

Ellis van Crefeld syndrome

- Autosomal recessive
- Short ribs, polydactyly, congenital heart disease, cleft lip and palate
- Pulmonary hypoplasia is usually not severe and symptoms improve later

Short-rib polydactyly syndromes

- Four variants — all autosomal recessive
- Death from severe respiratory insufficiency occurs in the neonatal period

Thanatophoric dysplasia

- Usually sporadic
- Very short limbs — femur X-ray described as 'telephone handle' shape
- Very small, pear-shaped chest
- Death from lung/chest hypoplasia occurs in the neonatal period

Camptomelic dysplasia

- Autosomal recessive
- Very bowed, shortened long bones
- Death from respiratory insufficiency usually occurs in childhood

3.8 Upper airway obstruction

Neonates are obligate nasal breathers.

Choanal atresia

- Incidence is 1 : 8,000
- More common in females
- Occurs as a result of a failure of breakdown of bucconasal membrane
- May be unilateral or bilateral, bony or membranous
- 60% associated with other congenital abnormalities including the CHARGE association:
  C = colobomata, H = heart defects, A = atresia of choanae, R = retarded growth and
  development, G = genital hypoplasia in males, E = ear deformities

- Presents at birth with respiratory distress and difficulty passing a nasal catheter. Oral airway insertion relieves respiratory difficulties. Diagnosis confirmed by contrast study or CT scan
- Surgical correction by perforating or drilling the atresia requires post-operative nasal stents

Pierre Robin sequence

- Consists of protruding tongue, small mouth and jaw, and cleft palate
- Incidence 1 : 2,000
- Problems include obstructive apnoea, difficulty with intubation and aspiration
- To maintain airway patency and prevent obstructive apnoea, prone position should be used initially; if this fails an oral airway should be inserted; intubation may be needed in severe cases which may eventually require tracheostomy
- Glossopexy and other surgical procedures have been attempted with some degree of success
- Gradual resolution of airway problems occurs as partial mandibular catch-up growth occurs during the first few years of life

Laryngomalacia

- Commonest cause of stridor in the first year of life
- Inspiratory stridor increases with supine position, activity, crying and upper respiratory tract infections
- Usually resolves during the second year of life
- Upper airway endoscopy is merited if persistent accessory muscle use occurs, with recurrent apnoea or faltering growth

Subglottic stenosis

- May be congenital but usually acquired.

Risk factors for acquired subglottic stenosis

- Prematurity
- Recurrent reintubation
- Prolonged intubation
- Traumatic intubation
- Inappropriately large or small endotracheal tube
- Black babies (keloid scar formation)
- Oral as opposed to nasal intubation (this is a theoretical but unproven factor)
- Gastro-oesophageal reflux
- Infection

Systemic steroids may facilitate extubation in mild to moderately severe subglottic stenosis. Laser or cryotherapy to granulomatous tissue seen on upper airway endoscopy may also be of benefit in these cases. Severely affected babies require surgery — anterior cricoid split or tracheostomy.

Tracheomalacia

- Causes expiratory stridor
- Usually caused from extrinsic compression — most commonly as a result of vascular rings
- Also associated with tracheo-oesophageal fistula
- Surgical treatment of underlying pathology usually leads to resolution, but tracheostomy and positive-pressure ventilation may be required

3.9 Principles of mechanical ventilation in neonates

- Aims are:
    - To ensure adequate oxygenation
    - To adequately remove carbon dioxide to prevent respiratory acidosis
    - To minimize the risk of lung injury
- Pressure-limited, time-cycled ventilation is used most commonly via either an oral or a nasal endotracheal tube. Patient-trigger modes may improve synchronicity with the baby's own respiratory efforts thus improving oxygenation, reducing the risk of air leak and facilitating weaning from the ventilator
- Volume cycle ventilation is being used more recently because of advances in ventilator technology, and may reduce the time taken to wean off the ventilator
- High-frequency oscillation may be used initially for any cause of neonatal respiratory failure, but is usually used as 'rescue' in severe cases where conventional ventilation has failed
- Nasal continuous positive airway pressure is often used in pre-term babies once extubated. This maintains functional residual capacity and reduces the work of breathing

3.10 Extracorporeal membrane oxygenation (ECMO)

A membrane 'lung' is used to rest the lungs and allow them to recover in severe respiratory failure. ECMO may be:

- Venoarterial (VA) — blood removed from right atrium (usually via right internal jugular vein) and returned via a common carotid artery
- Venovenous (VV) — a double-lumen, right atrial cannula is used

ECMO should be considered in severe neonatal respiratory failure if:

- Lung disease is reversible
- Infant is > 35 weeks' gestation
- Weight > 2 kg
- Cranial ultrasound scan shows no intraventricular haemorrhage > grade 1
- No clotting abnormality

- Oxygenation index > 40 (see below)

Oxygenation index (OI) is used to quantify the degree of respiratory failure.

It is measured as

$$OI = (\text{mean airway pressure} \times FiO_2 \times 100) \div p(O_2)$$

where mean airway pressure is in cmH_2O, FiO_2 (fractional inspired oxygen) is a fraction and PO_2 is in mmHg.

- OI > 25 indicates severe respiratory failure
- OI > 40 indicates very severe respiratory failure with a predicted mortality of $>80\%$ with conventional treatment — therefore consideration to refer for ECMO is appropriate

Other measures of the degree of respiratory failure that can be used include:

- **Alveolar–arterial oxygen difference** $(A–aDO_2)$
  - $A–aDO_2 = (716 \times FiO_2) – (PCO_2/0.8) – PO_2$
  - A normal $A–aDO_2$ is < 50 mmHg.
  - If > 600 mmHg for successive blood gases over 6 hours then there is severe respiratory failure with predicted mortality of $> 80\%$ with conventional treatment
- **Ventilation index** (VI) $= PCO_2 \times RR \times PIP/1,000$; where RR is the respiratory rate and PIP is the peak inspiratory pressure
  - VI > 70 indicates severe respiratory failure
  - VI > 90 indicates very severe respiratory failure — suitable for consideration of ECMO

4. CARDIOVASCULAR PROBLEMS

4.1 Patent ductus arteriosus (PDA)

- Uncommon in term infants after 1–2 days
- Often presents around third day of life in VLBW infants because left to right shunt increases as pulmonary vascular resistance falls; approximately 40% of VLBW infants with surfactant deficiency have clinically significant PDA on day 3 of life
- Clinical signs — systolic or continuous murmur, bounding pulses, wide pulse pressure, active precordium and possibly signs of cardiac failure and reduced lower body perfusion
- A clinically significant PDA in VLBW infants is associated with an increased risk of:
  - Pulmonary haemorrhage
  - Chronic lung disease
  - Intraventricular haemorrhage
  - Necrotizing enterocolitis
  - Mortality

- Early treatment of PDA with indomethacin has been shown to reduce necrotizing enterocolitis and chronic lung disease
    - Ibuprofen is likely to be equally effective in closing PDA but has fewer side-effects than indomethacin

4.2   Hypotension

Causes of hypotension in neonates

- Hypovolaemia
    - Antenatal acute blood loss
        - Placental abruption
        - Placenta praevia
        - Maternofetal haemorrhage
        - Twin-to-twin transfusion (usually not acute)
        - Vasa praevia
    - Postnatal acute blood loss
    - Internal
        - Intracranial haemorrhage
        - Intra-abdominal haemorrhage
        - Intrathoracic/pulmonary haemorrhage
        - Severe bruising
    - External
        - Dislodged vascular lines
- Excessive water loss
    - High urine output
    - High insensible losses — common in extreme prematurity
- Third spacing
    - Hydrops
    - Pleural effusions
    - Ascites
    - Post-operative
- Vasodilatation
    - Common in pre-term infants
    - Sepsis
    - Drug-induced (tolazoline, prostaglandins, prostacyclin)
- Cardiogenic
    - Myocardial dysfunction
        - Perinatal asphyxia
        - Metabolic acidosis
    - Congenital heart disease
        - Hypoplastic left heart
        - Other single-ventricle physiological conditions

- Arrhythmias
  - Supraventricular tachycardia
  - Complete heart block
- Reduced venous return
  - Pulmonary air leak
  - Pericardial effusion/tamponade
  - Lung hyperinflation (more common in high-frequency oscillation or with high positive end-expiratory pressure (PEEP))

4.3 Hypertension

Causes of hypertension in neonates

- Vascular
  - Renal artery thrombosis (associated with umbilical artery catheterization)
  - Aortic thrombosis (associated with umbilical artery catheterization)
  - Renal vein thrombosis (more common in infants of diabetic mothers)
  - Renal artery thrombosis
  - Coarctation of aorta
  - Middle aortic syndrome
- Renal
  - Obstructive uropathy
  - Dysplastic kidneys
  - Polycystic disease
  - Renal tumours
- Intracranial hypertension
- Endocrine
  - Congenital adrenal hyperplasia
  - Hyperthyroidism
  - Neuroblastoma
  - Phaeochromocytoma
- Drug-induced
  - Systemic steroids
  - Inotropes
  - Maternal cocaine

4.4 Cyanosis in the newborn

Causes of cyanosis in neonates

- Congenital cyanotic heart disease
  - Transposition of the great arteries
  - Pulmonary atresia
  - Critical pulmonary stenosis
  - Severe tetralogy of Fallot
  - Tricuspid atresia
  - Ebstein's anomaly
  - Truncus arteriosus
  - Total anomalous pulmonary venous drainage
  - Hypoplastic left heart syndrome
- Persistent pulmonary hypertension of the newborn
- Respiratory disease
- Methaemoglobinaemia
  - Arterial PO_2 is normal
  - Can be congenital:
    - NADH-methaemoglobin reductase deficiency (autosomal recessive)
    - Haemoglobin-M (autosomal dominant)
  - Can be iatrogenic:
    - Secondary to nitric oxide therapy
    - Nitrate or nitrite ingestion
  - Treat with i.v. methylene blue
  - Acrocyanosis and facial bruising also give the appearance of cyanosis

5. GASTROENTEROLOGY AND NUTRITION

5.1 Necrotizing enterocolitis (NEC)

Incidence varies — occurs in about 10% VLBW infants.

Risk factors

- Prematurity
- Antepartum haemorrhage
- Perinatal asphyxia
- Polycythaemia
- PDA
- PROM

Early enteral feeding has also been suggested as NEC rarely occurs in infants who have not been fed. However, randomized controlled trials suggest that early feeding with small amounts of breast milk is beneficial. The incidence of NEC in pre-term infants is 6–10 times higher in those fed formula milk compared to those given breast milk. There is some evidence that enteral vancomycin before initiating milk feeds reduces the incidence of NEC.

The severity of NEC can be classified using Bell's staging:

Stage 1 — suspected NEC

- General signs — temperature instability, lethargy, apnoea
- Increased gastric aspirates, vomiting, abdominal distension

Stage 2 — confirmed NEC

- Stage 1 signs, plus
- Upper or lower gastrointestinal bleeding
- Intramural gas (pneumatosis intestinalis) or portal vessel gas on abdominal X-ray

Stage 3 — severe NEC

- Stage 1 and 2 signs, plus
- Signs of shock, severe sepsis and/or severe gastrointestinal haemorrhage
- Bowel perforation

Complications

- Perforation occurs in 20–30% of confirmed NEC cases
- Overwhelming sepsis
- Disseminated intravascular coagulation (DIC)
- Strictures — occur in approximately 20% cases of confirmed NEC
- Recurrent NEC — occurs in < 5% cases (consider Hirschsprung disease)
- Short-bowel syndrome following extensive resection
- Lactose intolerance

Medical management

- Cardiorespiratory support as required
- Stop enteral feeds for 7–14 days (depending on the severity of illness)
- Nasogastric tube on free drainage
- Give intravenous fluids/total parenteral nutrition (TPN)
- Give intravenous antibiotics
- Treatment of thrombocytopenia, anaemia, DIC
- Serial abdominal X-rays (to exclude perforation)

Surgical management, may include

- Placement of peritoneal drain
- Early laparotomy — with resection of bowel +/– ileostomy/colostomy; indications for early surgery include perforation or failing medical management
- Late laparotomy +/– bowel resection; most common indication is stricture formation confirmed with contrast X-rays

5.2 Composition of infant milks

		Breast	Term formula	Pre-term formula	Cows' milk
Carbohydrate	(g/100 ml)	7.4	7.2	8.6	4.6
Protein	(g/100 ml)	1.1	1.5	2.0	3.4
Fat	(g/100 ml)	4.2	3.6	4.4	3.9
Sodium	(mmol/100 ml)	6.4	6.4	14	23
Potassium	(mmol/100 ml)	15	14	19	40
Calcium	(mmol/100 ml)	8.5	10.8	18	30
Phosphate	(mmol/100 ml)	5	10.6	13	32
Calories	(per 100 ml)	70	65	80	67

NB Cows' milk has an increased casein : lactalbumin ratio (4 : 1 compared with 2 : 3 in breast milk)

5.3 Breast-feeding

Physiology

- A surge in maternal prolactin (from the anterior pituitary) occurs immediately post-partum, which stimulates milk production
- Suckling stimulates prolactin receptors in the breast and oxytocin release (from the posterior pituitary). Oxytocin facilitates the 'let-down' reflex by contraction of breast myoepithelial cells
- Colostrum is produced over the first 2–4 days. Subsequent milk production is controlled mainly by the amount of suckling or expression

Benefits of breast-feeding

See Chapter 9 — Gastroenterology and Nutrition (Section 2.3 — Breast-feeding)

Contraindications to breast-feeding

See list of contraindicated maternal drugs below and Chapter 9 — Gastroenterology and Nutrition (Section 2.3 — Breast-feeding)

Complications

- Mother — breast engorgement, breast abscess, poor milk production
- Baby – poor weight gain/initial excessive weight loss, breast milk jaundice

Drugs contraindicated in breast-feeding mothers

- Amiodarone
- Antimetabolites (chemotherapy drugs)
- Atropine
- Chloramphenicol

- Dapsone
- Doxepin
- Ergotamine
- Gold
- Indomethacin
- Iodides
- Lithium
- Oestrogens (decrease lactation)
- Opiates (high dose should be avoided but weaning to a low dose may facilitate withdrawal in infant)
- Phenindione
- Vitamin D (risk of hypercalcaemia with high dose)

Maternal drugs that should be used with caution/monitoring if breast-feeding

- Some antidepressants
- Some antihistamines
- Carbamazepine
- Carbimazole
- Clonidine
- Co-trimoxazole
- Ethambutol
- Histamine antagonists
- Isoniazid
- Gentamicin
- Metronidazole (makes milk taste bitter)
- Oral contraceptives
- Phenytoin
- Primidone
- Theophylline
- Thiouracil

If in doubt refer to *British National Formulary* or discuss with pharmacist.

5.4 Fluid and nutritional requirements in neonates

Well term babies require little in the way of fluid and calorie intake during the first few days of life. Subsequently, over the next few months of life, there is an average fluid intake of approximately 150 ml/kg per 24 hours but this may vary considerably.

Sick or pre-term babies are likely to have reduced but variable fluid requirements, and initial fluid and electrolyte provision should facilitate post-natal weight loss with negative water and sodium balance. Failure to do this is likely to increase the risk of complications such as PDA, pulmonary haemorrhage, NEC and chronic lung disease. Close monitoring of fluid balance and individualized fluid and electrolyte prescription using daily weight, urine output, serum sodium and creatinine are essential, particularly in sick, extremely pre-term infants.

Daily nutritional requirements per kg for stable, growing preterm babies are approximately as follows:

- Protein — 3.0–3.8 g
- Energy — 110–120 kcal
- Carbohydrates — 3.8–11.8 g
- Fat — 5–20% of calories
- Sodium — 2–3 mmol
- Potassium — 2–3 mmol
- Calcium — 2–3 mmol
- Phosphate — 1.94–4.52 mmol
- + other minerals (iron, zinc, copper etc.), trace elements (selenium, manganese etc.) and vitamins

5.5 Parenteral nutrition

This may be partial, if the baby takes some enteral feeds, or it may be total parenteral nutrition (TPN). Indications for TPN include milk intolerance, poor gut motility (common in extreme prematurity), NEC, post-operative (congenital malformations, NEC etc.).

Parenteral nutrition consists of:

- Protein — up to 3.5 g/kg per day amino acids (mainly essential amino acids)
- Carbohydrates — up to 18 g/kg per day. Parenteral nutrition should be given via a central venous line if dextrose concentration > 12.5%
- Lipids — soya bean oil emulsions (e.g. Intralipid) provide essential fatty acids, a concentrated source of calories and a vehicle for delivering fat soluble vitamins; 20% Intralipid is tolerated better than 10%. Regular monitoring of plasma lipid levels is essential
- Water
- Minerals — sodium, potassium, calcium, phosphate, magnesium
- Trace elements — zinc, copper, manganese, selenium etc.
- Water-soluble vitamins
- Fat-soluble vitamins

Complications of parenteral nutrition in neonates include:

- Sepsis – mainly intravenous-line-related (bacterial/fungal)
- Intravenous line extravasation
- Venous thrombosis (line-related)
- Fluid/electrolyte imbalance
- Hyperlipidaemia
- Nutritional deficiencies
- Cholestatic jaundice

See also Chapter 9 — Gatroenterology and Nutrition, Section 3.3

5.6 Congenital abnormalities of the gastrointestinal system

Oesophageal atresia and tracheo-oesophageal fistula

- Occurs as a result of the failure of development of the primitive foregut
- Incidence is approximately 1 : 3,000
  - 85% — blind proximal oesophageal pouch with a distal oesophageal to tracheal fistula
  - 10% — oesophageal atresia without fistula
  - 5% — proximal +/– distal fistula

Clinical presentation

- Polyhydramnios
- Excessive salivation
- Early respiratory distress
- Abdominal distension
- Vomiting/choking on feeds
- Inability to pass nasogastric tube
- Absence of gas in gut on X-ray if no tracheo-oesophageal fistula
- Other anomalies in 30–50% — VACTERL (**V**ertebral, **A**nal, **C**ardiac, **T**racheo-oesophageal fistula, **E**ars, **R**enal, **L**imb), rib anomalies, duodenal atresia
- Prematurity common

Management

- Respiratory support as needed
- Riplogle tube (large-bore, double-lumen suction catheter) on continuous suction is placed in the proximal oesophageal pouch
- Surgical management includes early division of the fistula and early or delayed oesophageal anastomosis. This depends on the distance between the two ends of atretic oesophagus — for wide gaps, delayed anastomosis to allow growth may improve outcome. Cervical oesophagostomy or colonic transposition may also be used in this situation.

H-type tracheo-oesophageal fistula (tracheo-oesophageal fistula without oesophageal atresia) is much less common and is usually not associated with pre-term birth or other severe anomalies. It may present in the neonatal period or later with respiratory distress associated with feeding, or recurrent lower respiratory infections.

Duodenal atresia

- Approximately 70% are associated with other congenital anomalies (trisomy 21, congenital heart disease, malrotation, etc.)
- Often diagnosed antenatally with ultrasound 'double-bubble' or polyhydramnios
- Usually presents post-natally with bilious vomiting

Malrotation

- Occurs as a result of incomplete rotation of the midgut in fetal life resulting in intermittent and incomplete duodenal obstruction by Ladd's bands
- Associated with diaphragmatic hernia, duodenal and other bowel atresias and situs inversus
- Presents with bilious vomiting and some abdominal distension with sudden deterioration in the event of midgut volvulus
- Upper gastrointestinal contrast studies show the duodenal–jejunal flexure on the right of the abdomen with a high caecum

Meconium ileus

- Commonest presentation of cystic fibrosis in neonates (10–15% cases)
- > 90% of babies with meconium ileus have cystic fibrosis, therefore genetic testing for all common mutations and serum immune reactive trypsin must be used for confirmation
- May present with antenatal perforation, peritonitis and intra-abdominal calcification or post-natally with intestinal obstruction
- Water-soluble contrast enemas may lead to resolution of meconium ileus
- Important to distinguish between meconium ileus and meconium plug — with meconium plug, symptoms usually resolve after passage of plug and the problem is not associated with cystic fibrosis

Anorectal atresia

- May have other features of VACTERL association
- May be high or low with the puborectalis sling differentiating — more likely to be a low lesion in females
- Colostomy is needed for all high atresias
- Renal tract ultrasound scan, micturating cystogram +/– cystoscopy are needed to exclude rectovaginal, rectourethral or rectovesical fistula or other urinary tract anomaly
- High atresias often have problems with faecal incontinence, whereas those with intermediate/low lesions usually have good outcomes

Hirschsprung's disease

- Occurs as a result of an absence of ganglion cells in either the short or long segment of the bowel; the rectum and sigmoid colon are most often affected but cases extending to the upper gastrointestinal tract have been described
- May present with delayed passage of meconium (> 24 hours), bowel obstruction relieved by rectal examination (may be explosive!), enterocolitis or later constipation
- Diagnosis is made by rectal biopsy
- Regular rectal washouts are required before temporary colostomy formation (usually reversed at 6 months)

Exomphalos

- Results from failure of the gut to return into the abdominal cavity in the first trimester
- The defect is covered by peritoneum which may be ruptured at birth
- Approximately 75% cases have other congenital anomalies — trisomies, congenital heart disease, Beckwith–Wiedemann syndrome
- Primary or staged surgical closure is required

Gastroschisis

- Rarer than exomphalos and much less likely to be associated with other congenital anomalies
- Aetiology unknown but may be associated with teenage pregnancy
- Bowel is not covered by peritoneum and therefore becomes stuck together with adhesions; this leads to functional atresias and severe intestinal motility problems post-surgical repair of the abdominal wall defect
- Prognosis is mostly good

6. NEUROLOGICAL PROBLEMS

6.1 Peri-intraventricular haemorrhage (PIVH)

The germinal matrix or layer occurs in the caudothalamic notch of the floor of the lateral ventricles. It is the site of origin of migrating neuroblasts from the end of the first trimester onwards. By 24–26 weeks' gestation this area has become highly cellular and richly vascularized. This remains so until 34 weeks' gestation by which time it has rapidly involuted. The delicate network of capillaries in the germinal matrix is susceptible to haemorrhage, which is likely to occur with changes in cerebral blood flow. Preterm infants have decreased autoregulation of the cerebral blood flow, which contributes to the pathogenesis. In term infants PIVH may originate from the choroid plexus.

Risk factors for PIVH

- Prematurity (28% at 25 weeks; < 5% after 30 weeks)
- Lack of antenatal maternal steroids
- Sick and needing artificial ventilation
- Hypercapnia
- Metabolic acidosis
- Pneumothoraces (as a result of increased venous pressure or possibly related to surge in blood pressure when drained)
- Abnormal clotting
- Rapid volume infusions (particularly with hypertonic solutions) or increases in blood pressure with inotropes
- Perinatal asphyxia

- Hypotension
- PDA

Timing of PIVH

- ≥50% in first 24 hours
- Approx. 10–20% day 2–3
- Approx. 20–30% day 4–7
- Approx. 10% after the first week

Classification of PIVH

- Grade 1 — germinal matrix haemorrhage
- Grade 2 — intraventricular haemorrhage without ventricular dilatation
- Grade 3 — intraventricular haemorrhage with blood distending the lateral ventricle
- Grade 4 — echogenic intraparenchymal lesion associated with PIVH; previously this was thought to be an extension of bleeding from the lateral ventricles into the surrounding periventricular white matter but it is likely to be venous infarction

Several classification systems have been described. The most widely accepted is that of Papile (above). It may, however, be better to use a more descriptive classification.

Prevention of PIVH

The following have been shown to reduce the incidence of PIVH:

- Antenatal steroids
- Maternal vitamin K
- Indomethacin (but long-term neurodisability is not reduced)

The following have been evaluated but have no proven benefit:

- Vitamin E
- Ethamsylate
- Phenobarbital
- Fresh-frozen plasma (FFP)
- Nimodipine

Clinical presentation of PIVH

- Grades 1 and 2 PIVH present silently and are detected by routine ultrasonography
- Grade 3 PIVH occasionally presents with shock from blood volume depletion
- Grade 4 PIVH may present similarly and occasionally with neurological signs (seizures, hypotonia, bulging fontanelle)

Sequelae of PIVH

Death

- Mortality was 59% in one series of large grade 4 PIVH

Post-haemorrhagic ventricular dilatation (PHVD)

- Defined as lateral ventricle measurement > 4 mm above 97th centile following PIVH
- 30% of PIVH cases develop PHVD — risk is higher with more severe lesions
- Spontaneous resolution occurs in approximately 50% of cases of PHVD, the rest develop hydrocephalus (i.e. PHVD that requires drainage)
- As a sequel to PIVH, **communicating hydrocephalus** (as a result of malfunction of the arachnoid villi) is more common than **non-communicating hydrocephalus** (as a result of blockage of the cerebral aqueduct)
- Early, aggressive intervention with repeated lumbar puncture and/or ventricular taps has not been shown to be of benefit; drainage should probably be considered if the baby is symptomatic, cerebrospinal fluid (CSF) pressure is very high (> 12 mmHg or 15.6 cmCSF; normal CSF pressure is 5.25 mmHg or 6.8 cmCSF) or head circumference and/or ventricular measurement on ultrasound scan are increasing rapidly
- Timing of surgical intervention with CSF reservoir or ventriculoperitoneal shunt insertion is controversial
- Drug treatment with acetazolamide with or without diuretics has been shown to be ineffective
- Intraventricular fibrinolytic administration is experimental

Adverse neurodevelopment

- Cerebral palsy is the commonest adverse neurodevelopmental sequel but other and global problems may also arise
- Approximate risk of adverse outcome is as follows:
  - 4% in grades 1 and 2 PIVH if ventricles remain normal size
  - 50% in grade 2 with PHVD or grade 3 PIVH
  - 75% in PIVH requiring shunt
  - 89% with large, grade 4 lesions (difficult to quantify because pathology is varied)

6.2 Periventricular leukomalacia (PVL)

- PVL is haemorrhagic necrosis in the periventricular white matter which progresses to cystic degeneration and subsequent cerebral atrophy. It is often associated with infection and may be cytokine-mediated. Hypoxia and ischaemia may also play a role. On ultrasound scan, the initial necrosis appears as echogenicity within a few days of the causative insult. This sometimes resolves but it may become a multicystic area after 1–4 weeks. The long-term neurological effects are usually bilateral, although initial ultrasound appearances are often unilateral

- Long-term neurodevelopmental effects of cystic PVL are:
  - Spastic diplegia or tetraplegia (> 90%)
  - Learning difficulties
  - Seizures (including infantile spasms)
  - Blindness
- Worse outcomes are associated with subcortical PVL. Transient periventricular echodensities are associated with a risk of spastic diplegia of approximately 5–10% if they persist for more than 7–14 days

6.3   Neonatal encephalopathy

Neonatal encephalopathy is also known as hypoxic–ischaemic encephalopathy. The underlying cause is often unclear but it may originate antenatally, peripartum or post-natally, hence the term 'perinatal asphyxia'. Other evidence of organ dysfunction often occurs concurrently, especially if the insult occurs close to the time of birth. Placental insufficiency is a factor in the vast majority of cases.

Pathophysiology of neonatal encephalopathy

Primary and secondary neuronal injury have been described.

- **Primary neuronal injury** results from energy failure because of the inefficiency of anaerobic respiration to produce high-energy phosphocreatine and ATP. Glucose utilization increases and lactic acid accumulates. Energy failure and myocardial dysfunction further exacerbate this, leading to ion-pump failure ($Na^+ - K^+$-ATPase) and neuronal death as a result of cerebral oedema
- **Secondary** or **delayed neuronal injury** occurs because there are marked changes in cerebral blood flow with initial hypoperfusion and then reperfusion following resuscitation. This is associated with neutrophil activation and is exacerbated by prostaglandins, free radicals and other vasoactive substances. Excitatory amino acid neurotransmitters such as glutamate and *N*-methyl D-aspartate (NMDA) lead to excessive calcium influx and delayed neuronal death. The cellular mechanism for this may be necrosis or apoptosis (programmed cell death)

Clinical presentation

This can be staged according to the scheme suggested by Sarnat and Sarnat.

- Stage 1 — hyperalert, irritable; normal tone and reflexes; signs of sympathetic overactivity; poor suck; no seizures; symptoms usually resolve < 24 hours; good outcome in approximately 99%
- Stage 2 — Lethargic, obtunded, decreased tone and weak suck and Moro reflexes; seizures are common; approximately 75–80% have good outcomes; this is less likely if symptoms persist for > 5 days
- Stage 3 — Comatose with respiratory failure; severe hypotonia and absent suck and Moro reflexes; seizures less common but EEG abnormalities common — flat background or burst suppression; over 50% die and majority of survivors have major handicap

Management

Management is largely supportive but brain cooling may offer improved outcomes in the future.

6.4 Neonatal seizures

Causes of seizures in the newborn

- Neonatal encephalopathy
- Cerebral infarction:
  - Usually presents on day 1 or 2
  - Often presents with focal seizures
  - Aetiology uncertain but thrombosis secondary to hypercoagulation tendency is a possibility
  - Outcome good in approximately 50%; the other 50% may develop mono- or hemiplegia or long-term seizure disorder
- Intracranial haemorrhage (massive PIVH, subarachnoid or subdural haemorrhage)
- Birth trauma (head injury equivalent)
- Meningitis
- Other sepsis
- Congenital infection
- Neonatal drug withdrawal
- Fifth-day fits (onset day 3–5, unknown cause, resolve spontaneously)
- Hypoglycaemia
- Hypocalcaemia
- Hypo- or hypermagnesaemia
- Inborn errors of metabolism:
  - Non-ketotic hyperglycinaemia
  - Sulphite oxidase deficiency
  - Biotinidase deficiency
  - Maple-syrup urine disease
  - Pyridoxine dependence
  - Urea cycle defect
  - Organic acidaemias (e.g. methylmalonic acidaemia)
- Structural brain abnormalities (migration disorders, etc.)
- Hydrocephalus
- Polycythaemia
- Neonatal myoclonus – not a true seizure, benign and common in preterm infants

Management of neonatal seizures

- Investigate for, and treat, underlying condition
- Initial treatment with phenobarbital, followed by midazolam, other benzodiazepines and paraldehyde
- Currently no evidence that suppression of clinical or electrographic seizures improves outcome

6.5 Causes of hypotonia in the newborn

Central causes

- Neonatal encephalopathy
- Intracranial haemorrhage
- Infection — generalized sepsis, meningitis, encephalitis
- Chromosomal abnormalities — trisomy 21, 18 or 13
- Structural brain abnormalities — neuronal migration disorders, etc.
- Metabolic disease — amino and organic acidaemias, urea cycle defects, galactosaemia, non-ketotic hyperglycinaemia, peroxisomal disorders, mitochondrial disorders, congenital disorders of glycosylation, Menkes syndrome
- Drugs — opiates, barbiturates, benzodiazepines, etc.
- Prader–Willi syndrome
- Hypothyroidism
- Early kernicterus

Spinal cord lesions

- Trauma to the cervical spinal cord during delivery — usually involves traction and rotation with forceps
- Tumours, cysts and vascular malformations of spinal cord

Neuromuscular disease

- Spinal muscular atrophy
- Congenital myotonic dystrophy
- Congenital myopathies
- Myasthenia gravis

6.6 Retinopathy of prematurity (ROP)

- ROP consists of vascular proliferation secondary to retinal vasoconstriction. This may progress and lead to fibrosis and scarring
- Prematurity and hyperoxia are known associations, but other factors, including hypoxia, are also implicated
- Babies < 32 weeks' gestation at birth and < 1500 g birth weight should be screened by ophthalmological examination from 6 weeks of age
- ROP should be described by stage, location, extent and presence of additional disease

ROP stages

- Stage 1 — demarcation line
- Stage 2 — ridge
- Stage 3 — ridge with extraretinal fibrovascular proliferation
- Stage 4 — subtotal retinal detachment
- Stage 5 — total retinal detachment
- Stage 1 and 2 disease resolves without risk of visual impairment if there is no progression
- Stage 3 disease increases the risk of visual impairment
- Stages 4 and 5 always leads to visual impairment

ROP location

- Zone 1, 2 or 3 (where zone 1 is the most central (i.e. posterior) around the optic disc)
- The risk is greatest if zone 1 is affected

ROP extent is described in terms of the number of clock hours

Plus disease includes tortuosity of the retinal vessels, pupil rigidity and vitreous haze

Usually stage 3 plus disease should be treated with either cryotherapy or laser therapy, but location and extent of ROP also determines the need for treatment.

See also Chapter 19 — Ophthalmology.

7. GENITOURINARY PROBLEMS

7.1 Congenital abnormalities of the kidneys and urinary tract

Nephrogenesis (branching and new nephron induction) continues up to 36 weeks' gestation, but glomerular filtration rate is still < 5% of adult values at this stage. This increases rapidly in the 1st week and then more gradually over the next 2 years to adult values.

The renal function of a neonate is limited by:

- Renal blood flow
- Glomerular filtration rate
- Tubular concentrating and diluting ability
- Tubular excretion
- Urine output

More than 90% of neonates pass urine within 24 hours of birth. The collecting ducts have increased sensitivity to antidiuretic hormone (ADH) after birth and urine concentrating ability increases rapidly.

Preterm infants have immature tubular function leading to a high fractional excretion of sodium and high sodium intake requirements.

Antenatally, congenital renal abnormalities may present with:

- Oligohydramnios (Potter syndrome if severe)
- Urinary ascites — as a result of obstructive uropathy
- Other abnormalities seen on antenatal ultrasound scan include:
    - Obstructive uropathy — dilated renal tracts
    - Cystic dysplasia/polycystic disease

Obstructive uropathy

Posterior urethral valves

- Mucosal folds in posterior urethra of male infants leading to dilatation of renal tract proximal to obstruction
- Bladder is often hypertrophied
- Diagnosed by micturating cystourogram
- Suprapubic catheter is inserted initially, followed by surgical resection by cystoscopy or vesicostomy, followed by later resection

Pelviureteric junction (PUJ) obstruction

- Usually unilateral
- Diagnosed on antenatal ultrasound scan or presents with abdominal mass
- Gross hydronephrosis is associated with decreased renal function (confirmed with $^{99}Tc^m$ MAG-3 (mertiatide) renogram), nephrectomy is usually required. Ureteroplasty is carried out for milder cases

Mild renal pelvis dilatation

- Should be confirmed on post-natal ultrasound scan and investigated with micturating cystourogram to exclude reflux nephropathy, which is a risk for recurrent urinary tract infection and subsequent scarring

Prune-belly syndrome (megacystis-megaureter)

- Lax abdominal musculature, dilated bladder and ureters and undescended testes
- Neurogenic bladder
- Usually as a result of abnormalities of lumbosacral spine

Ureterocele

- Dilatation of distal ureter leading to obstruction

Urethral stricture

Tumours (neuroblastoma, Wilms' tumour)

See Chapter 11 — Haematology and Oncology, Sections 11.6 and 11.7.

7.2 Haematuria in the newborn

Causes of haematuria in the newborn

- Urinary tract infection
- Obstructive uropathy
- Acute tubular necrosis
- Renal artery or vein thrombosis
- Renal stones
- Trauma
- Tumours
- Cystic dysplasia and other malformations
- Abnormal clotting

7.3 Causes of acute renal failure in neonates

Pre-renal

- Hypotension
- Dehydration
- Indomethacin

Renal

- Cystic dysplasia and infant polycystic kidney disease
- Renal artery/vein thrombosis
- Congenital nephrotic syndrome
- DIC
- Nephrotoxins — gentamicin

Post-renal

- Obstructive nephropathy

7.4 Ambiguous genitalia

See Section 1.5 for embryology of sexual differentiation.

On examination, note the following:

- If gonads are palpable they are nearly always testes
- Length of phallus — if < 2.5 cm stretched length in a term baby it is unlikely that the baby can function as a male
- Severity of hypospadias and fusion of labia
- Other dysmorphic features/congenital abnormalities

The parents should be told that the child's sex is uncertain at this stage and that the genitalia are not normally/completely formed. Prompt diagnosis and appropriate management are essential to resolve this and to exclude or treat congenital adrenal hyperplasia before electrolyte imbalances occur. Also gonadal tumours may be a risk.

Differential diagnosis

- True hermaphroditism:
  - Testes and ovaries both present (rare)
- Male pseudohermaphroditism — underdevelopment ($\downarrow$ virilization) of male features
  - Androgen insensitivity (= testicular feminization) — most common
  - Defects in testosterone synthesis
  - Some forms of congenital adrenal hyperplasia
  - Panhypopituitarism (should be suspected if hypoglycaemia is also present)
  - Defects in testosterone metabolism (5α-reductase most common)
  - Defects in testicular differentiation (rare)
- Female pseudohermaphroditism — virilization of female
  - Congenital adrenal hyperplasia — commonest enzyme deficiency is 21-hydroxylase deficiency ($\uparrow$ 17α-hydroxyprogesterone)
- Chromosomal abnormalities
  - 45X/46XY mosaicism (rare)

Investigations

- Karyotype
- Daily electrolytes until diagnosis is established
- Blood pressure monitoring
- Blood sugar monitoring
- Abdominal ultrasound scan
- Serum hormone assay — 17α-hydroxyprogesterone, 11-deoxycortisol, testosterone, oestradiol, progesterone, luteinizing hormone, follicle-stimulating hormone
- Urine steroid profile
- Genitogram/micturating cystourogram

8. INFECTION

8.1 Bacterial infection

Group B streptococcus (GBS)

- Up to 20% of pregnant women have genital tract colonization with GBS
- Three serotypes have been identified
- Neonatal GBS infection may be early (within first few days, usually presenting by 24 hours) or late (after first week, usually at 3–4 weeks)
- Early disease often presents with septicaemia and respiratory distress (pneumonia or persistent pulmonary hypertension of the newborn)
- Late disease is usually septicaemia or meningitis — may be vertical or nosocomial

transmission; antibiotics given intrapartum or in first few days do not always prevent late GBS disease
- Serotype 3 is more common in late-onset GBS disease or meningitis if this is part of early-onset disease

Escherichia coli

- Usually causes vertical infections in neonates and is often associated with preterm birth; can also cause nosocomial infection
- K1 capsular antigen is commonest serotype
- Septicaemia and meningitis are commonest presentations if vertically transmitted; urinary tract infections and NEC have been noted in nosocomial *E. coli* sepsis in neonates

Coagulase-negative staphylococci

- Commonest nosocomial pathogen in neonatal intensive care units
- VLBW infants with indwelling catheters are most at risk
- Often resistant to flucloxacillin

Listeria monocytogenes

- Gram-positive rod
- Outbreaks have been caused by dairy products, coleslaw, paté and undercooked meat
- May present with a flu-like illness in pregnant women and then lead to stillbirth or severe neonatal septicaemia and meningitis
- Early- and late-onset disease have been noted, similar to GBS
- Early-onset disease is associated with preterm birth and 'meconium'-stained amniotic fluid (which is in fact often pus rather than meconium)
- A maculopapular or pustular rash is typical
- Amoxicillin and gentamicin is the antibiotic combination of choice

Other bacterial pathogens in neonates include

- *Haemophilus influenzae*
- *Klebsiella* spp.
- *Pseudomonas* spp.
- Pneumococcus

Risk factors for vertically acquired bacterial sepsis

- Pre-term rupture of membranes
- Prolonged rupture of membranes (> 12–24 hours)
- Maternal fever (> 8°C or other signs of chorioamnionitis — e.g. white cell count > 15 × 10^9/l)
- Maternal colonization with GBS
- Fetal tachycardia
- Lack of intrapartum antibiotics in the presence of above risk factors
- Foul-smelling amniotic fluid

- Pre-term birth/low birth weight
- Twin pregnancy
- Low Apgar scores

Risk factors for nosocomial sepsis

- Prematurity/low birth weight
- SGA infants
- Neutropenia
- Indwelling catheters
- TPN
- Surgery

8.2 Congenital viral infection

Cytomegalovirus (CMV)

- Member of the Herpesviridae family (DNA virus)
- Transmitted by close personal contact, blood products or breast-feeding. May also be sexually transmitted
- Causes mild symptoms in healthy adults or children
- Up to 1% of pregnancies are affected but symptoms occur in less than 10% of those infected
- Primary infection or reactivation may occur in affected pregnancies
- Symptoms in affected neonates include:
  - IUGR
  - Prematurity
  - Hepatosplenomegaly
  - Thrombocytopenia
  - Anaemia
  - Jaundice (raised conjugated and unconjugated bilirubin — often prolonged)
  - Pneumonitis
  - Microcephaly
  - Intracranial calcification
  - Choroidoretinitis
  - Osteitis
- Long-term neurodevelopmental sequelae are common and include cerebral palsy, learning disability, epilepsy, blindness and deafness

Diagnosis

- Rising specific IgG antibodies in mother or baby
- Specific IgM may be raised for up to 16 weeks after primary infection
- Virus can be isolated from urine or throat swab
- Detection of early-antigen fluorescent foci (DEAFF) is a newer technique used to detect viral antigen from urine and other body fluids

- Aciclovir has been used with some success in immunosuppressed adults but may be toxic in neonates and is not of proven efficacy

Rubella

First-trimester infection of the fetus results in congenital rubella syndrome. The most common features of this are:

- Congenital heart disease
- Cataracts
- Deafness

IUGR, microcephaly, hepatosplenomegaly, thrombocytopenia, choroidoretinitis and osteitis may also occur similar to congenital CMV infection. Vaccination of children has virtually eradicated congenital rubella in the UK.

Parvovirus

Parvovirus is a DNA virus. Serotype B19 causes epidemics of erythema infectiosum ('Slapped cheeks' syndrome or Fifth disease) in winter months. Fetal infection, particularly in the first trimester, leads to severely decreased red cell production and subsequent severe fetal anaemia, resulting in heart failure and non-immune hydrops. Fetal blood can be used to confirm the diagnosis by viral antigen detection with polymerase chain reactions. Fetal blood transfusions may reverse hydrops and improve outcome.

Neonatal human immunodeficiency virus (HIV)

Vertically transmitted HIV is the commonest cause of childhood AIDS. Approximately one-third of infections are transmitted across the placenta and two-thirds during birth. Babies of all HIV-positive mothers are also seropositive initially as IgG crosses the placenta. Non-infected infants become negative by 9 months. There is no evidence of HIV causing an embryopathy. Babies are usually initially asymptomatic but may present with hepatospleno-megaly and thrombocytopenia in the neonatal period. The following increase the risk of vertical transmission:

- Low maternal CD4 count
- High maternal viral load
- Presence of p24 antigen in the mother
- Pre-term birth
- Rupture of membranes > 4 hours
- Vaginal birth
- No maternal anti-retroviral treatment/poor compliance

Maternal zidovudine (AZT) during the third trimester and labour and given to the infant for 6 weeks post-natally reduces transmission rate from 25.5% to 8.3%. Other measures leading to avoidance of above risk factors have been shown to reduce risk further to well under 5%.

Vaccinations should be given routinely to infants of HIV-positive mothers with the following cautions:

- Give killed (Salk) rather than live (Sabin) polio vaccine
- Give BCG early

Hepatitis B virus

- Babies of women who are hepatitis B surface antigen (HbsAg)-positive or who have active hepatitis B during pregnancy should all receive hepatitis B vaccine in the neonatal period, and at 1 and 6 months
- Hepatitis B immunoglobulin should be given within 48 hours of birth to all babies of mothers who are HbsAg-positive apart from those with the hepatitis B e antibody
- Breast-feeding is not contraindicated

8.3   Fungal and protozoal infections

Candida albicans

Candida may cause superficial mucocutaneous infection or severe systemic sepsis, particularly in extremely pre-term infants. Amphotericin, flucytosine and fluconazole may be used to treat severe fungal infections.

Toxoplasmosis

- *Toxoplasma gondii* is a unicellular, protozoan parasite.
- Cats are the definitive hosts. Infection of humans occurs following ingestion of sporocysts after handling cat faeces, contaminated vegetables or undercooked meat.
- Toxoplasmosis is a mild illness in healthy adults
- Congenital infection is more likely with increasing gestation as the placenta provides less of a barrier with age. However, severe infection becomes less likely, falling from 75% in the first trimester to < 5% in the third.

Severe congenital toxoplasmosis causes:

- IUGR
- Pre-term birth
- Hydrocephalus and sequelae
- Choroidoretinitis
- Intracranial calcification
- Hepatitis
- Pneumonia
- Myocarditis

Babies born with no symptoms may go on to develop choroidoretinitis after months or even years. Serological diagnosis is made by specific IgG and IgM titres. Treatment of affected pregnant women with spiramycin reduces the rate of transmission to the fetus but does not reduce the severity of disease. Affected infants are treated with pyrimethamine and sulfadiazine for up to 1 year.

9. NEONATAL ENDOCRINE PROBLEMS

9.1 Neonatal hypoglycaemia

Definition — blood glucose ≤ 2.6 mmol/l

Normal term babies commonly have blood sugars < 2.6 mmol/l, particularly in the first 24 hours (especially if the baby is breast-fed), but are not at risk of any long-term sequelae because they can utilize alternative fuels (e.g. ketones, lactate). It is therefore unnecessary to perform blood glucose analysis on healthy term babies.

Infants at risk of clinically relevant hypoglycaemia include:

- Those with increased demand/decreased supply, i.e.
  - Pre-term
  - IUGR
  - Hypothermia
  - Infection
  - Asphyxia
  - Polycythaemia
- Hyperinsulinism
  - Infant of a diabetic mother
  - Haemolytic disease of the newborn
  - Transient neonatal hyperinsulinism
  - Beckwith–Wiedemann syndrome
  - Persistent hyperinsulinaemic hypoglycaemia of infancy (previously called nesidioblastosis)
  - Islet cell adenoma
- Endocrinopathies
  - Pituitary (e.g. growth hormone deficiency, septo-optic dysplasia)
  - Adrenal (e.g. congenital adrenal hyperplasia)
- Carbohydrate metabolism disorders
  - Glycogen storage disease
  - Galactosaemia
- Amino acidopathies
- Organic acidaemias
- Fat oxidation defects
  - Deficiencies of medium-chain and very-long-chain acyl-coenzyme A dehydrogenases (MCADD adn VLCAD), long-chain hydroxyacyl-coenzyme A dehydrogenase (LCHAD)

Babies at risk of clinically significant hypoglycaemia should be treated immediately with intravenous dextrose (2 ml/kg 10% dextrose followed by intravenous infusion) if blood glucose is < 1.5mmol/l.

9.2 Panhypopituitarism

Presents with:

- Persistent hypoglycaemia
- Poor feeding
- Micropenis
- Hyperbilirubinaemia (conjugated)
- Midline facial defects (cleft palate etc.)
- Optic atrophy
- Low growth hormone, cortisol (may cause hyponatraemia) and thyroid-stimulating hormone

9.3 Adrenal insufficiency

Causes include:

- Congenital adrenal hyperplasia
  - Commonest cause is 21α-hydroxylase deficiency (may or may not involve salt loss)
  - May be X-linked or autosomal recessive inheritance
- Smith–Lemli–Opitz syndrome
- Wolman syndrome (liposomal acid lipase deficiency)
- Adrenal haemorrhage
- Secondary causes:
  - Panhypopituitarism
  - Withdrawal from steroid treatment

Management of salt loss is an initial priority, followed by glucocorticoid (hydrocortisone) and mineralocorticoid (fludrocortisone) replacement.

10. NEONATAL JAUNDICE

10.1 Physiological jaundice

Jaundice becomes visible when serum bilirubin is greater than 80–100 mmol/l and up to 65% term infants become clinically jaundiced. However, only 1.2% become sufficiently jaundiced to require treatment (i.e. > 340 mmol/l). Physiological jaundice occurs as a result of:

- Increased haemolysis:
  - Bruising
  - Antibody-induced
  - Relative polycythaemia
  - Life span of red blood cells (in term infants — 70 days, in pre-term infants — 40 days)
- Immature hepatic enzyme systems
- 'Shunt' bilirubin from breakdown of non-red blood cell haem pigments

- Enterohepatic circulation

Breast-fed babies have higher maximum serum bilirubin levels and remain jaundiced for longer.

10.2   Causes of non-physiological jaundice

Jaundice is non-physiological if any of the following are present:

- Onset before 24 hours of age
- Serum bilirubin ≥ 270 mmol/l
- Lasting > 14 days (> 21 days in preterm infants)
- Associated pathological conditions that are known to cause jaundice

Causes of non-physiological jaundice (unconjugated hyperbilirubinaemia)

- Haemolysis
  - Isoimmunization (Rh, ABO, other)
  - Spherocytosis, etc.
  - Glucose-6-phosphate dehydrogenase or pyruvate kinase deficiency
  - Sepsis
  - α-Thalassaemia
- Polycythaemia
- Extravasated blood
- Increased enterohepatic circulation
- Endocrine/metabolic
- Rare liver enzyme deficiencies (Crigler–Najjar syndrome, etc.)

Haemolytic disease of the newborn

May be caused by Rhesus D (Rh) incompatibility (mother Rh D-negative, baby Rh D-positive) or by other antibodies (c, E, Kell, Duffy, etc.). Approximately 15% of the UK population are Rh D-negative. Sensitization occurs from previous pregnancy, antepartum haemorrhage, trauma or antenatal procedure.

Prevention of haemolytic disease is by the following:

- Intramuscular anti-D is given following any possible event leading to sensitization in Rh D-negative women
- Maternal serum screening for antibodies at booking with retesting between 28 and 36 weeks for Rh D-negative women with no antibodies
- Referral to a specialist fetal medicine centre for all those with significant levels of antibodies; initially antibody levels are measured but correlate poorly with the degree of fetal anaemia above a certain threshold; once this is reached, further monitoring is by ultrasound scanning to detect signs of hydrops, amniocentesis and spectrophotometric estimation of bilirubin in the amniotic fluid or fetal blood sampling to detect anaemia

- Serial fetal blood transfusions in severe cases
- Pre-term delivery

Causes of conjugated hyperbilirubinaemia:

- TPN cholestasis
- Viral hepatitis (hepatitis B virus, CMV, herpesvirus, rubella, HIV, coxsackievirus, adenovirus)
- Other infection (toxoplasmosis, syphilis, bacterial)
- Haemolytic disease (due to excessive bilirubin)
- Metabolic (α1-antitrypsin deficiency, cystic fibrosis, galactosaemia, tyrosinaemia, Gaucher disease and other storage diseases, Rotor syndrome, Dubin–Johnson syndrome)
- Biliary atresia
- Choledochal cyst
- Bile-duct obstruction from tumours, haemangiomas, etc.

10.3 Treatment of non-physiological unconjugated hyperbilirubinaemia

The aim of treatment is to reduce the risk of kernicterus. Treatment thresholds are controversial but most centres follow guidelines produced by the American Academy of Pediatrics. Treatment thresholds should be lower for babies who are sick, who are pre-term, who have evidence of haemolysis or who have rapidly rising serum bilirubin (> 100 µmol/l per 24 hours).

Phototherapy

This is used to treat moderately severe unconjugated hyperbilirubinaemia. Phototherapy photo-oxidizes and isomerizes bilirubin, facilitating increased excretion via urine and bile.

Complications of phototherapy are mainly minor and include:

- Diarrhoea
- Transcutaneous fluid loss
- Rashes

Exchange transfusion

This is used to treat severe unconjugated hyperbilirubinaemia, often with concomitant anaemia, most commonly as a result of haemolysis. The procedure dilutes bilirubin, removes sensitized red blood cells and corrects anaemia.

Usually a double-volume exchange transfusion is performed via arterial and central venous lines over 1–2 hours, replacing the baby's blood volume twice with donor blood.

Complications of exchange transfusion include:

- Infection and other line-related complications
- Fluid and electrolyte disturbance

- Thrombocytopenia and coagulopathy
- Transfusion reaction

11. NEONATAL HAEMATOLOGY/COAGULATION PROBLEMS

11.1 Polycythaemia

See also Chapter 11 – Haematology and Oncology, Section 10.2.

Definition — haematocrit > 65%.

Causes

- IUGR
- Maternal diabetes
- Delayed cord clamping
- Twin-to-twin transfusion
- Maternofetal transfusion
- Trisomies (13, 18, 21)
- Endocrine disorders (congenital adrenal hyperplasia, thyrotoxicosis, Beckwith syndrome)

Complications

- Hypoglycaemia
- Jaundice
- NEC
- Persistent pulmonary hypertension of the newborn
- Venous thromboses
- Stroke

Treatment

Treatment is recommended if the haematocrit is > 65% and the patient is symptomatic. A partial dilutional exchange transfusion should be carried out using normal saline.

11.2 Haemorrhagic disease of the newborn and vitamin K

- Results from relative deficiency of factors II, VII, IX and X and is prevented by vitamin K
- Breast milk contains inadequate amounts of vitamin K, therefore the recommendation in the UK is to give all babies either a single intramuscular injection of vitamin K at birth or an oral dose at birth followed by two further oral doses at 1–2 weeks and 6 weeks in those that are predominantly breast-fed
- May be exacerbated by perinatal asphyxia, liver dysfunction and maternal phenytoin or phenobarbital
- Usually presents between days 2 and 6 with gastrointestinal haemorrhage, umbilical stump bleeding, nose bleeds or intracranial haemorrhage

- Prothrombin time and activated partial thromboplastin are prolonged with normal thrombin time and fibrinogen
- Treat with fresh-frozen plasma and intravenous vitamin K +/− blood transfusion
- Late haemorrhagic disease may occur between 8 days and 6 months; intracranial haemorrhage is more common in these cases

11.3   Disseminated intravascular coagulation (DIC)

This may occur in any sick neonate, e,g. those with:

- Sepsis
- Placental abruption or other perinatal events
- NEC
- Meconium aspiration syndrome

Intravascular coagulation leads to thrombocytopenia and coagulopathy as a result of consumption of platelets, clotting factors and fibrinogen. Fibrinolysis is stimulated leading to accumulation of fibrin degradation products.

Management of DIC includes:

- Treatment of the underlying cause
- Platelet transfusion
- Transfusion of fresh-frozen plasma, cryoprecipitate may be used instead if fibrinogen is low

11.4   Haemophilia A

- Almost 40% of cases present in the neonatal period with intraventricular haemorrhage, cephalhaematoma or excessive bleeding elsewhere
- Antenatal diagnosis is possible by chorionic villous biopsy, if there is a family history
- Vaginal birth is safe if uncomplicated but ventouse delivery should be avoided
- Oral vitamin K (rather than intramuscular) should be given
- Bleeding should be treated with recombinant factor VIII, but prophylactic treatment is controversial

Clinical features of haemophilia B are similar to those of haemophilia B.

11.5   von Willebrand disease

- Two forms of von Willebrand disease may present in neonates
- Type 2b is autosomal dominant, presents with thrombocytopenia but rarely presents with bleeding
- Type 3 is autosomal recessive, presentation is similar to haemophilia A, but girls can be affected

12. NEONATAL ORTHOPAEDIC PROBLEMS

See Chapter 20 — Orthopaedics, Section 6.1.

13. FURTHER READING

American Academy of Pediatrics Committee on Drugs. 1998. Neonatal drug withdrawal. *Pediatrics,* 101:6, 1079–1088.

Costeloe K, Hennessy E, Gibson AT, Marlow N, Wilkinson AR. 2000. The EPICure study: outcomes to discharge from hospital for infants born at the threshold of viability. *Pediatrics,* 106:4, 659–671.

Findlay RD, Taeusch HW, Walther FJ. 1996. Surfactant replacement therapy for meconium aspiration syndrome. *Pediatrics,* 97, 48–52.

Greenough A, Robertson NRC, Milner AD (eds). 1996. *Neonatal Respiratory Disorders.* London: Arnold 1996.

Hansen TN, McIntosh N (eds). 1999. *Current Topics in Neonatology* Volume 3, pp. 43–61. London, W.B. Saunders.

Lucas A, Cole TJ. 1990. Breast milk and neonatal necrotising enterocolitis. *Lancet,* 336:8730, 1519–1523.

Lucas A, Brooke OG, Morley R, Cole TJ, Bamford MF. 1990. Early diet of preterm infants and development of allergic or atopic disease: randomised prospective study. *BMJ,* 300:6728, 837–840.

Lucas A, Morley R, Cole TJ, Lister G, Leeson-Payne C. 1992. Breast milk and subsequent intelligence quotient in children born preterm. *Lancet,* 339:8788, 261–264.

Polin RA, Fox WW (eds). 1998. *Fetal and Neonatal Physiology* 2nd edn. London: W.B. Saunders.

Rennie JM, Roberton NRC (eds). 1999. *Textbook of Neonatology,* 3rd edn, Chapter 44, pp. 1252–71, London: Churchill Livingstone.

UK Collaborative ECMO Trial Group. 1996. UK Collaborative randomised trial of neonatal ECMO. *Lancet,* 348, 75–82.

Wiseman LR, Bryson HM. 1994. A review of the therapeutic efficacy and clinical tolerability of a natural surfactant preparation (Curosurf) in Neonatal Respiratory distress syndrome. *Drugs,* 48, 386–403.

Wood NS, Marlow N, Costeloe K, Gibson AT, Wilkinson AR. EPICure Study Group. 2000. Neurologic and developmental disability after extremely preterm birth [see comments]. *New England Journal of Medicine,* 343:6, 378–384.

Yu VYH (ed.) 1995. Pulmonary problems in the new-born and their sequelae. *Balliere's Clinical Pediatrics,* 3, 1.

Chapter 17

Nephrology

Christopher J D Reid

CONTENTS

Nephrology

1. EMBRYOLOGY

- At the start of week 5 of embryogenesis, the **ureteric bud** appears
- A small branch of the mesonephric duct evolves into a tubular structure which elongates into the **primitive mesenchyme** of the **nephrogenic ridge**
- Ureteric bud forms the ureter, and from week 6 onwards repeated branching gives rise to the calyces, papillary ducts and collecting tubules by week 12
- The branching elements also induce the mesenchyme to develop into nephrons — proximal and distal tubules, and glomeruli
- Branching and new nephron induction continues until week 36
- Abnormalities in the signalling between branching ureteric bud elements and the primitive mesenchyme probably underlie important renal malformations including renal dysplasia
- There are on average 600,000 nephrons per kidney. Premature birth and low weight for gestational age may both be associated with reduced nephron numbers
- This in turn may underlie the later development of glomerular hyperfiltration, glomerular sclerosis and hypertension, and may explain the firmly established inverse association between birth weight and later adult-onset cardiovasular morbidity

2. FETAL AND NEONATAL RENAL FUNCTION

The placenta receives 50% of fetal cardiac output, and the fetal kidneys only 5% of cardiac output. By 36 weeks gestational age nephrogenesis is complete, but glomerular filtration rate (GFR) is < 5% of the adult value.

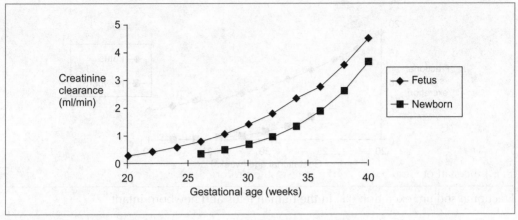

Creatinine clearance (ml/min) in the human fetus and newborn infant

The GFR of term infants at birth is approximately 25 ml/min/1.73 m^2, increasing by 50–100% during the first week, followed by a more gradual increase to adult values by the second year of life.

Fractional excretion of sodium (FENa) is:

$$\frac{\text{Urine Na (mmol/L)}}{\text{Urine creatinine (μmol/L)}} \times \frac{\text{Plasma creatinine (μmol/L)}}{\text{Plasma Na (mmol/L)}} \times 100\%$$

- Normal FENa in older children and adults is around 1%, and < 1% in sodium- and water-deprived states
- It is very high in the premature fetus, falling with increasing gestation; and it is significantly lower in the newborn (see figure below), as the kidney adapts to the demands of extrauterine life where renal tubular conservation of sodium and water is important

Premature neonates still have a relatively high FENa because of immmature renal tubular function, and require extra sodium supplementation to avoid hyponatraemia.

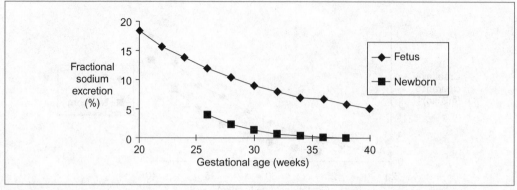

Fractional sodium excretion (%) in the human fetus and newborn infant

- Urine-concentrating capacity is low in the premature newborn and leads to susceptibility to dehydration. Fully mature urine-concentrating capacity is reached later in the first year of life
- The plasma bicarbonate concentration at which filtered bicarbonate appears in the urine (bicarbonate threshold) is low in the newborn (19–21 mmol/L), increasing to mature values of 24–26 mmol/L by 4 years. Hence plasma bicarbonate values are lower in infants

Abnormalities in fetal renal function and morphology are mainly inferred from:

- **Volume of amniotic fluid** — urinary tract obstruction and/or reduced production of urine by dysplastic kidneys, leads to oligohydramnios or anhydramnios
- **Appearance of kidneys on antenatal ultrasound** — bright echogenicity, lack of corticomedullary differentiation, cyst formation and hydronephrosis are all signs of fetal renal abnormality

Invasive assessment of fetal renal function includes sampling of fetal urine by fine-needle aspiration from the fetal bladder.

- Usually reserved for selected cases of fetal obstructive uropathy, classically caused by **posterior urethral valves** in male fetuses
- Analysis of fetal urinary electrolytes and amino acid composition may give further information about fetal renal function and prognosis for postnatal renal function
- Typical features of poor prognosis for renal function (in addition to oligohydramnios and abnormal ultrasound appearance as detailed above) include high urinary sodium and amino acid levels (implying tubular damage and failure to reabsorb these)
- Severe oligohydramnios may lead to pulmonary hypoplasia. This is the major determinant of whether newborns with congenital renal abnormalities live or die in the immediate postnatal period

3. COMMON UROLOGICAL ABNORMALITIES

3.1 Hydronephrosis

The main causes of hydronephrosis are:

- Vesicoureteric reflux (VUR) – see Section 12.1
- Pelviureteric junction obstruction
  - Usually detected on antenatal ultrasound
  - Occasionally detected during investigation of urinary tract infection (UTI) or abdominal pain
  - Main aspects of assessment are:
    - ultrasound — degree of renal pelvic dilatation measured in the anteroposterior diameter: 5–10 mm mild; 11–15 mm moderate; > 15 mm severe
    - MAG-3 renogram — findings that suggest significant obstruction are poor drainage despite frusemide given during scan and impaired function, e.g. < 40% on hydronephrotic side
    - surgical correction is by **pyeloplasty**; usual when MAG-3 indicates obstruction and/or ultrasound shows progressive increase in hydronephrosis: when dilatation is > 30 mm, surgery is likely
- Vesicoueretric junction obstruction
  - Usually detected in the same ways as for PUJ obstruction
  - Ultrasound shows renal pelvic and ureteric dilatation
  - Interventions include stenting the vesicoureteric junction (temporary measure); and surgical reimplantation

3.2 Duplex kidney

- Often detected on antenatal ultrasound or during investigation of UTI
- Two ureters drain from two separate pelvicalyceal systems; ureters sometimes join before common entry into bladder, but more commonly have separate entries, with upper pole ureter inserting below lower pole ureter
- Common complications associated with duplex systems are:
  - Obstructed hydronephrotic upper moiety and ureter, often poorly functioning, associated with bladder **ureterocoele**
    - dilatation and swelling of sub-mucosal portion of ureter just proximal to stenotic ureteric orifice can be seen on bladder ultrasound and as a filling defect on micturating cystogram (MCUG)
  - Ectopically inserted upper pole ureter, entering urethra or vagina; clue to this from history is true continual incontinence with no dry periods at all
  - VUR into lower pole ureter, sometimes causing infection and scarring of this pole

3.3 Multicystic dysplastic kidney

- Irregular cysts of variable size from small to several centimetres; no normal parenchyma
- Dysplastic atretic ureter

- No function on MAG-3 or dimercaptosuccinic acid (DMSA) scan
- 20–40% incidence of VUR into contralateral normal kidney

3.4 Polycystic kidneys

See Section 15.1.

3.5 Horseshoe kidney

- Two renal segments fused across midline at lower poles in 95%, upper poles in 5%
- Isthmus usually lies low, at the level of the fourth lumbar vertebra immediately below the origin of the inferior mesenteric artery
- Associations include Turner syndrome, Laurence–Moon–Biedl syndrome
- Usually asymptomatic but increased incidence of pelviureteric junction obstruction and VUR, so may develop UTI

3.6 Hypospadias

- Opening of urethral meatus is on ventral surface of penis, at any point from glans to base of penis or even perineum
- Meatus may be stenotic and require meatotomy as initial intervention
- Foreskin is absent ventrally; it is used in surgical reconstruction of a deficient urethra so circumcision should not be performed
- **Chordee** is the associated ventral curvature of the penis, seen especially during erection, and this requires surgical correction also; caused by fibrous tissue distal to the meatus along the ventral surface of penis

3.7 Bladder extrophy and epispadias

- More common in males
- Bladder mucosa is exposed (and with exposure and infection becomes friable), bladder muscle becomes fibrotic and non-compliant
- Anus anteriorly displaced
- Males — penis has epispadias (dorsal opening urethra) and dorsal groove on glans, with dorsal chordee and upturning; scrotum is shallow and testes are often undescended
- Girls — female epispadias with bifid clitoris, widely separated labia
- Pubic bones separated
- Requires surgical reconstruction; long-term urinary incontinence is common

4. PHYSIOLOGY

4.1 Glomerular filtration rate (GFR)

GFR is determined by:

- The transcapillary hydrostatic pressure gradient across the glomerular capillary bed (ΔP) favouring glomerular filtration
- The transcapillary oncotic pressure gradient ($\Delta \pi$) countering glomerular filtration
- The permeability coefficient of the glomerular capillary wall, k

Hence GFR = $k(\Delta P - \Delta \pi)$.

GFR is expressed as a function of body surface area. Absolute values for GFR in ml/min are corrected for surface area by the formula:

$$\text{Corrected GFR (ml/min/1.73m}^2) = \text{absolute GFR (ml/min)} \times 1.73/\text{surface area}$$

$1.73\ m^2$ is the surface area of an average adult male. Normal mature GFR values are 80–120 ml/min/1.73 m^2, and are reached during the second year of life

GFR can be estimated or measured.

It is **estimated from a calculated value** using the Schwartz formula:

$$\frac{\text{height (cm)}}{\text{plasma creat (μmol/L)}} \times 49\text{ml/min/1.73 m}^2$$

This method will tend to overestimate GFR in malnourished children with poor muscle mass

It is **measured** on a single injection plasma disappearance curve, using inulin, or a radio-isotope such as chromium-labelled EDTA. Following an intravenous injection of a known amount of one of these substances, a series of timed blood samples are taken over 3–5 h, and the slope of the curve generated by the falling plasma levels of the substance gives the GFR. This technique does **not** require any urine collection, thus making it suitable for routine clinical use.

NB: Creatinine clearance, based on a timed urine collection and paired plasma sample using the formula:

$$\frac{\text{Urine creatinine (μmol/L)} \times \text{urine flow rate (ml/min)}}{\text{Plasma creatinine (μmol/L)}}$$

Overestimates the true GFR because creatinine is secreted by the tubules.

4.2 Renal tubular physiology

The renal tubules play a fundamental role in:

- Maintaining extracellular fluid volume
- Maintaining electrolyte and acid–base homeostasis

These processes are energy demanding and render tubular cells most vulnerable to ischaemic damage and acute tubular necrosis. The proximal tubule and Loop of Henle are the sites of major reabsorption of most of the glomerular filtrate.

The distal tubule and collecting duct are where 'fine tuning' of the final composition of the urine occurs.

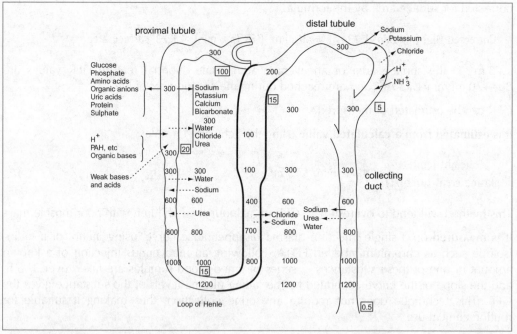

Diagram of tubular function, showing sites of active (solid arrows) and passive (broken arrows) transport. The boxed numbers indicate the percentage of glomerular filtrate remaining in the tubule, and the non-boxed numbers the osmolality of the tubular fluid under conditions of antidiuresis (reproduced from Godfrey and Baum, *Clinical Paediatric Physiology*, p. 368, Cambridge: Blackwell Scientific Publications, with permission)

Proximal tubule

The primary active transport system is the Na^+–K^+–ATPase enzyme, reabsorbing 50% of filtered Na^+. Secondary transport involves coupling to the Na^+–H^+ antiporter, which accounts for 90% of bicarbonate reabsorption with some Cl^-. In addition:

- **Glucose** is completely reabsorbed unless the plasma level is high, in which case glycosuria will occur

- **Amino acids** are completely reabsorbed, though premature and term neonates commonly show a transient aminoaciduria
- **Phosphate** is 80–90% reabsorbed under the influence of parathyroid hormone (PTH), which reduces reabsorption and enhances excretion of phosphate
- **Calcium** is 95% reabsorbed – 60% in proximal tubule; 20% in Loop of Henle; 10% in distal tubule; 5% in collecting duct
- A variety of organic solutes including creatinine and urate, and some drugs, including trimethoprim and most diuretics, are secreted in the proximal tubule

Loop of Henle

- A further 40% of filtered Na^+ is reabsorbed via the $Na^+-K^+-2Cl^-$ cotransporter in the thick ascending limb of the LoH
- The medullary concentration gradient is generated here because this segment is impermeable to water
- Loop diuretics block Cl^- binding sites on the cotransporter
- There is an inborn defect in Cl^- reabsorption at this same site in Bartter syndrome – see Section 7.2

Distal tubule

- A further 5% of filtered Na^+ is reabsorbed here, via a Na^+-Cl^- co-transporter
- Thiazide diuretics compete for these Cl-binding sites; and may have a powerful effect if combined with loop diuretics which increase NaCl and water to the distal tubule
- Aldosterone-sensitive channels (also present in the collecting duct) are involved in regulating K^+ secretion. K^+ secretion is proportional to:
  - Distal tubular urine flow rate
  - Distal tubular Na^+ delivery: so natriuresis is associated with increased K^+ secretion and hypokalaemia (e.g. Bartter syndrome; loop diuretics)
  - Aldosterone level — so conditions of elevated aldosterone are associated with hypokalaemia
  - $[pH]^{-1}$

Collecting duct

- A final 2% of filtered Na^+ is reabsorbed via aldosterone-sensitive Na^+ channels, in exchange for K^+
- Spironolactone binds to and blocks the aldosterone receptor, explaining its diuretic and K^+-sparing actions
- H^+ secreted into urine by H^+-ATPase
- Anti-diuretic hormone (ADH) opens water channels (aquaporins) to increase water reabsorption

4.3   Renin–angiotensin–aldosterone system

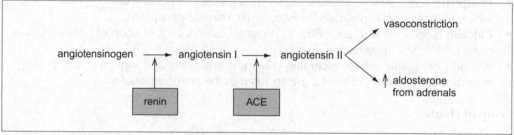

The renin–angiotensin–aldosterone system (ACE, acetylcholinesterase)

- Renin is released from the juxtaglomerular apparatus in response to decreased perfusion to the kidney, leading to increased angiotensin II levels (causing vasoconstriction); and increased aldosterone release (causing enhanced distal tubular sodium and water conservation and hence extracellular fluid (ECF) volume expansion)
- Abnormal renin release resulting in hypertension is associated with most forms of secondary renal hypertension, e.g. reflux nephropathy, renal artery stenosis

There are syndromes of **low-renin hypertension**, including:

- **Conn syndrome** — primary hyperaldosteronism: high aldosterone leading to ECF volume expansion, hypertension, hypokalaemia, and renin supression
- **Liddle syndrome** — constitutive activation of amiloride-sensitive distal tubular epithelial sodium channel: ECF volume expansion leading to renin and aldosterone suppression, and hypokalaemia

Pseudohypoaldosteronism is constitutive inactivation of the amiloride-sensitive distal tubular epithelial Na^+ channel, leading to excessive loss of salt and water with ECF volume depletion, and hyperkalaemia; renin and aldosterone levels are high secondary to the ECF volume depletion. There are transient and permanent forms.

4.4   Erythropoietin system

- Erythropoietin (EPO) is released by renal peritubular cells and stimulates marrow erythropoiesis
- Deficiency of EPO in renal disease is a major cause of the associated anaemia
- Recombinant human EPO is available for treatment and prevention of anaemia in renal failure

4.5   Vitamin D metabolism

- Vitamin D_3 (cholecalciferol) is mainly available from the action of ultraviolet light on its precursor in the skin
- In the liver it is hydroxylated to $25(OH)$-D_3

- Renal 1α-hydroxylase then leads to the production of 1,25(OH)$_2$-D$_3$, or calcitriol, the most biologically active vitamin D metabolite, in the kidney
- Hypocalcaemia leads to enhanced 1α-hydroxylase activity both directly, and indirectly by stimulating PTH secretion which also stimulates the enzyme. Other stimuli for increased 1α-hydroxylase activity include low serum phosphate and growth hormone
- Deficiency of renal production of calcitriol underlies the rickets of renal failure

5. INVESTIGATIONS

5.1 Urinalysis

Dipstick testing of urine is routinely used to detect blood, protein, glucose and pH. Multistix® can, in addition, detect **leukocyte esterase** (a marker of the presence of polymorphs) and **nitrite** (produced by the bacterial reduction of nitrate). If the urine appears clear to the naked eye and all panels on a Multistix® are negative, urine infection is almost certainly excluded.

NB: Urinary haemoglobin and myoglobin (from rhabdomyolysis) produce a false positive dipstick test for blood; microscopy of urine will not however reveal red blood cells.

5.2 Urine microscopy

A routine investigation for UTI, and in patients with dipstick haematuria. The finding of organisms and white blood cells on microscopy is strong supporting evidence for the presence UTI, before a culture result is available. Apart from infection, the major causes of haematuria in children are glomerular, rather than lower urinary tract. Glomerular red blood cells appear deformed or dysmorphic when examined by an experienced microscopist, helping to localize the site of haematuria to the kidneys.

Urinary casts usually signify renal pathology:

- Red cell casts — isolated renal haematuria; or glomerulonephritis
- Tubular cell casts — acute tubular necrosis
- White blood cell casts — pyelonephritis; acute tubular necrosis

5.3 Haematuria

The main causes are:

- UTI — other infections including tuberculosis and schistosomiasis
- Glomerulonephritis:
  - Often with proteinuria and urinary casts
  - Isolated haematuria with no other evidence of clinical renal disease may be the presenting feature of several important glomerulonephritides, including Alport syndrome and immunoglobulin A (IgA) nephropathy
- Trauma — usually a history

- Stones — usually painful
- Tumour
- Cystic kidney disease
- Bleeding disorders
- Vascular disorders, including renal vein thrombosis (especially neonates) and arteritis
- Sickle cell disease
- False positives — see Section 5.1
- Factitious — Munchausen syndrome; Munchausen syndrome by proxy

Other causes of red urine include beetroot consumption, haemoglobinuria and rifampicin.

5.4   Proteinuria

This is usually detected on dipstick testing. The minimum detectable concentration is 10–15 mg/dl, so in a patient producing a large volume of dilute urine the sticks may be negative even though the total amount of protein excreted per day may be significant.

In normal afebrile children, urine protein excretion should not exceed $60 \, \text{mg/m}^2/24 \, \text{h}$. Collection of an accurate 24-h urine collection is difficult in small children. Assessment of proteinuria may be made on a spot early morning urine sample by measuring urinary albumin (mg/L) and creatinine (mmol/L):

- Normal — < 3.5 mg/mmol
- Microalbuminuria — 3–30 mg/mmol
- Proteinuria — > 30 mg/mmol

Orthostatic proteinuria is detectable when the patient has been in an upright position for several hours but not when the patient is recumbent. It is important to assess protein excretion both when recumbent and when upright, because orthostatic proteinuria is a benign condition with a good prognosis, and does not warrant investigations such as renal biopsy.

5.5   Renal imaging

Ultrasound

This is a readily available non-invasive investigation that is operator-dependent for its interpretation. It is the standard for antenatal investigation, and in almost all renal conditions.

It gives good information about:

- Size, shape, symmetry and position of kidneys
- Hydronephrosis, ureteric dilatation
- Bladder distension, bladder emptying post-void, bladder wall thickness
- Stones — though small ureteric stones may not be seen
- Cystic disease, including autosomal dominant and recessive
- Tumours, including renal and adrenal tumours
- Gross cortical scarring
- Vascular perfusion using a Doppler technique

Ultrasound may not detect minor degrees of scarring. It is not sensitive or specific at detecting VUR. Doppler ultrasound may reveal renal artery stenosis, but there is a significant false-negative rate.

Micturating cystourethrogram

Used to look for VUR and the appearance of the bladder outline; also the urethra, specifically posterior urethral valves in males.

Nuclear medicine isotope scans

DMSA

- A **static** scan, i.e. isotope is filtered and retained in renal parenchyma
- Divided function and detecting cortical scars
- Main use is in investigation of UTI and hypertension
- Some perfusion defects seen when DMSA is performed during acute UTI may resolve; defects present 3 months after acute infection are permanent

DTPA (diethylenetriaminepenta-acetic acid), MAG-3

- **Dynamic** scans, i.e. isotope is filtered, and then excreted from kidney down ureters to bladder
- Divided function, and assessing drainage and obstruction
- Main use is in investigating upper tract dilatation seen on ultrasound; and for follow-up of surgery for obstructed kidneys or ureters
- **Indirect radioisotope reflux study** is a convenient way of assessing the presence of VUR in children old enough to co-operate with the scan — in practice > 3 years old. It avoids the need for a urethral catheter and has a lower radiation dose than MCUG

Intravenous urography

Little used now because the combination of ultrasound and isotope scans provides the required information in most cases, and avoids the risks of anaphylaxis and radiation dose that are involved with intravenous urography. Has a role in:

- Emergency evaluation of painful haematuria, if ultrasound is uninformative, when intravenous urography may reveal a ureteric stone
- Determining ureteric anatomy, course, and insertion if ectopic ureter is suspected

Renal arteriography

Used to diagnose renal artery stenosis. Approach is via femoral artery; usually requires general anaesthesia in children. Therapeutic approaches include balloon angioplasty of stenoses; and embolization of intrarenal arteriovenous aneurysms.

5.6 Renal biopsy

In general, the main indications for renal biopsy are:

- To make a diagnosis
- To guide therapy, and to assess response to therapy
- To assist in giving a prognosis

The commonest reasons for renal biopsy in children are:

- Steroid-resistant nephrotic syndrome
- Haematuria and/or proteinuria
- Unexplained acute nephritis/acute renal failure
- Assessment of renal transplant dysfunction

6. ACID–BASE, FLUID AND ELECTROLYTES

6.1 Metabolic acidosis

A primary decrease in plasma bicarbonate and a decrease in plasma pH as a result of:

- Bicarbonate loss, e.g.
  - Gastrointestinal loss in severe diarrhoea
  - Renal loss in proximal (type 2) renal tubular acidosis (RTA)
- Reduced hydrogen ion excretion, e.g.
  - Distal (type 1) RTA
  - Acute and chronic renal failure
- Increased hydrogen ion load, e.g.
  - ↑ endogenous load
    - inborn errors of metabolism, e.g. maple syrup urine disease, propionic acidaemia
    - lactic acidosis, e.g. cardiovascular shock
    - ketoacidosis, e.g. diabetic ketoacidosis (DKA)
  - ↑ exogenous load, e.g. salicylate poisoning

Anion gap

- A classification of metabolic acidosis involves assessing the **anion gap** — the 'gap' between anions and cations made up by unmeasured anions, e.g. ketoacids, lactic acid
- Measured as $[Na^+] - [HCO_3^- + Cl^-]$; thus normal anion gap is $[140] - [25 + 100] = 15$
- Acidosis may be a normal anion gap, when Cl^- will be raised, i.e. hyperchloraemic
- May be an increased anion gap, when Cl^- will be normal, i.e. normochloraemic

Examples:

- Normal anion gap, hyperchloraemia, acidosis — RTA
  - Na^+ 140, Cl^- 110, HCO_3^- 15, anion gap = 15
- Increased anion gap, normochloraemia, acidosis — DKA
  - Na^+ 140, Cl^- 100, HCO_3^- 15, anion gap = 25

6.2 Metabolic alkalosis

A primary increase in plasma bicarbonate and an increase in plasma pH as a result of:

- Chloride depletion, the commonest cause in childhood, leading to low urinary Cl^- and Cl-responsive alkalosis, i.e. as soon as Cl^- is made available (e.g. as intravenous saline) it is retained by the kidney at the expense of HCO_3^-, correcting the alkalosis (see also Pseudo-Bartter syndrome, Section 7.2)
  - Gastrointestinal loss, e.g. pyloric stenosis, congenital chloride diarrhoea
  - Frusemide therapy
  - Cystic fibrosis
- Stimulation of H^+ secretion by the kidney, with normal urinary Cl^- and Cl-unresponsive alkalosis, e.g.
  - Bartter syndrome (see Section 7.2)
  - Cushing syndrome
  - Hyperaldosteronism (see Section 4.3)
- Excess intake of base, e.g. excess ingestion of antacid medicine (rare in childhood)

6.3 Body fluid compartments and regulation

Total body water

Total body water (TBW) represents 85% of the body weight of premature infants 80% in term infants and 65% in children. In children it is distributed between the intracellular (ICF) and extracellular (ECF) fluid compartments as follows:

TBW (%bwt)	ICF (%bwt)	ECF (%bwt)	
		Interstitial	Intravascular
65	40	20	5

Osmotic equlibrium, cell volume regulation

- The major fluid compartments are separated by semi-permeable membranes, which are freely permeable to H_2O. Osmotic equilibrium is maintained between the ICF and ECF compartments by the shift of H_2O from lower to higher osmolality compartments
- ECF osmolality can be calculated as: $[(Na^+ + K^+) \times 2]$ + glucose + urea
- A rise in ECF osmolality, e.g. in DKA, will lead to a shift of H_2O out of the ICF compartment, and thus a reduction in ICF volume, i.e. cell shrinkage. Cell shrinkage stimulates the intracellular accumulation of organic osmolytes which increases ICF osmolality and leads to a shift of H_2O back into the cell, restoring cell volume
- Treatment of DKA may then lead to the **rapid** reduction of ECF osmolality, but the ICF organic osmolytes are degraded **slowly** and thus an **osmotic gradient** may be created during DKA treatment, favouring movement of H_2O into the cells, causing **cerebral oedema**

Osmoregulation

A small (3–4%) increase in ECF osmolality stimulates hypothalamic osmoreceptors to cause posterior pituitary ADH release, leading to water retention and return of osmolality to normal. Increases in ECF osmolality also stimulate thirst and water drinking. Significant (> 10%) ECF depletion, **even if iso-osmolar**, will cause carotid and atrial baroreceptors to stimulate ADH release.

6.4 Electrolyte disturbances

Hyponatraemia

Normal plasma Na^+ is 135–145 mmol/L. Hyponatraemia is usually defined as plasma $Na^+ < 130$ mmol/L. The causes are twofold.

Gain of H_2O in excess of Na^+

- **Excess water intake** — increased volume of appropriately hypotonic urine
  - Iatrogenic — excess hypotonic oral or intravenous fluid
  - Psychogenic polydipsia
- **Acute renal failure** — oedema and hypervolaemia, oliguria with urine $Na^+ > 20$ mmol/L
- **Syndrome of inappropriate ADH secretion** (SIADH) — inappropriately raised urine osmolality, i.e. not maximally dilute; increased body weight; decreased plasma urea and creatinine; absence of overt renal, liver, or cardiac disease
  - Meningitis or central nervous system tumour
  - Pneumonia
  - Intermittent positive pressure ventilation
  - Drugs, e.g. carbamazepine, barbiturates
- **Treatment** is principally water restriction; for severe hyponatraemia (< 120 mmol/L) with neurological symptoms, correction of plasma Na^+ to 125–130 mmol/L over 4 h is usually safe and effective in correcting symptoms

Loss of Na^+ in excess of H_2O

- **Renal losses** — dehydration, but inappropriately high urine volume and urine Na^+ content (> 20 mmol/L); urine isotonic with plasma
  - Loop diuretics
  - Recovery phase of acute tubular necrosis
  - Tubulopathies (see Section 7.1)
  - Salt-wasting congenital adrenal hyperplasia; adrenal insufficiency —hyperkalaemia
- **Extrarenal losses** — dehydration, appropriate oliguria and Na^+ conservation with low urine Na^+ (usually < 10 mmol/L); urine hypertonic
  - Gastrointestinal tract losses — gastroenteritis
  - Skin losses — severe sweating, cystic fibrosis
- Treatment involves
  - Rehydration, and calculation of Na^+ deficit as (140 – plasma Na^+) × 0.65 × body weight (kg)
  - Avoid over-rapid correction of hyponatraemia (risk of cerebello-pontine myelinolysis)

Hypernatraemia

Usually defined as plasma $Na^+ > 150$ mmol/L. There is a shift of H_2O from the ICF to the ECF compartments, so that in hypernatraemic dehydration, ECF volume is not markedly reduced and thus typical signs of dehydration are less obvious. The causes again are twofold.

Loss of H_2O in excess of Na^+

- **Renal losses** — inappropriately high urine output, inappropriately low urine osmolality
  - Reduced renal concentrating ability — premature neonates
  - Diabetes insipidus — pituitary and nephrogenic (see Section 7.4)
  - Osmotic diuresis — DKA
- **Extrarenal losses** — appropriate oliguria and high urine osmolality
  - Gastrointestinal losses
  - Increased insensible H_2O loss, e.g. pyrexia and hyperventilation
- **Inadequate free water intake**
  - Breast-fed neonate with inadequate maternal milk flow
- **Treatment**
  - Safest and best given with standard oral rehydration solution
  - If intravenous treatment is essential, **slow** (48–72 h or 10–15 mmol/L/24 h) correction of hypernatraemia with frequent measurement of plasma electrolytes is safest; a suggested fluid is 1 L dextrose 5% + NaCl 25 mmol + KCl 20 mmol

Gain of Na in excess of H_2O

- Increased volume of urine with high Na^+ content
  - Iatrogenic — excess hypertonic intravenous fluid, e.g. $NaHCO_3$, hypertonic saline
  - Incorrect reconstitution of infant formula
  - Accidental or deliberate (e.g. Munchausen syndrome by proxy) salt poisoning
- **Treatment** — recognition and removal of underlying cause; access to water while kidneys excrete excess salt load

Hypokalaemia

Normal plasma K^+ is 3.4–4.8 mmol/L. The main causes of hypokalaemia are:

- **Inadequate provision of K^+** with prolonged intravenous fluid administration
- **Extrarenal losses**
  - Gastrointestinal losses
- **Renal losses**
  - High plasma renin levels
    - diuretic use — loop and thiazide diuretics
    - osmotic diuresis — DKA (hypokalaemia becomes evident when metabolic acidosis and insulin deficiency are corrected)
    - Fanconi syndrome — see Section 7.1
    - Bartter syndrome — see Section 7.2
    - Gitelman syndrome — see Section 7.3
    - Distal (type 1) RTA

- Low plasma renin levels
  - Conn syndrome – see Section 4.3
  - Liddle syndrome – see Section 4.3
  - Cushing syndrome
- **Shift from ECF to ICF compartment**
  - Correction of metabolic acidosis
  - Insulin treatment
  - High-dose or prolonged salbutamol treatment for asthma

Hyperkalaemia

The main causes are:

- **Excess administration** in intravenous fluid
- **Renal failure** — acute and chronic
- **Shift from ICF to ECF**
  - Metabolic acidosis
  - Rhabdomyolysis — acute tumour lysis (both often associated with acute impairment in renal function which compounds the hyperkalaemia)
- **Hypoadrenal states**
  - Salt-wasting congenital adrenal hyperplasia
  - Adrenal insufficiency
  - Pseudohypoaldosteronism – see Section 4.3
- **Potassium-sparing diuretics** — spironolactone
- **Treatment** includes:
  - Exclusion of K^+ from diet and intravenous fluids
  - Cardiac monitor — peaked T waves → prolonged PR interval → widened QRS → ventricular tachycardia → terminal ventricular fibrillation
  - Calcium gluconate to stabilize myocardium
  - Shift K^+ from ECF to ICF:
    - correct metabolic acidosis if present — in acute renal failure
    - salbutamol: nebulized or short intravenous infusion
    - insulin and dextrose — but extreme caution in young children as there is a risk of hypoglycaemia
  - Remove K^+ from body
    - calcium resonium
    - dialysis

Calcium and hypocalcaemia

Calcium in the body is 40% protein-bound (of which 98% is bound to albumin); 48% ionized and 12% complexed to anions like phosphate or citrate

- Normal values are 2.1–2.6 mmol/L for **total Ca^{2+}**, and 1.14–1.30 for **ionized (Io) Ca^{2+}**
  - Albumin-corrected Ca^{2+} equals measured total plasma Ca^{2+} + [(40 – albumin) × 0.02] — for example, if total Ca^{2+} is 1.98 and albumin is 26; corrected $Ca^{2+} = 1.98 + [(40–26) \times 0.02] = 2.26$
- Degree of protein binding of plasma Ca^{2+} is proportional to plasma pH

Beware in correcting acidosis in renal failure, where total and ionized Ca^{2+} often already low:

- Acute rise in pH with $NaHCO_3$ treatment leads to ↑ protein-bound Ca^{2+} which lead to ↓ ionized Ca^{2+}, which may cause tetany
- Monitoring of ionized Ca^{2+} is useful in intensive-care patients, where changes in acid–base and albumin levels make interpretation of total plasma Ca^{2+} difficult

Hypocalcaemia

The main symptoms are tetany, paraesthesiae, muscle cramps, stridor, seizures. The main causes are:

- **Calcitriol (1,25(OH)$_2$-D$_3$) deficiency**
  - Dietary deficiency of vitamin D
  - Malabsoprtion of vitamin D — fat malabsorption syndromes
  - Renal failure (acute and chronic) — 1α-hydroxylase deficiency
  - Liver disease — 25-hydroxylase deficiency
- **Hypoparathyroidism**
  - Transient neonatal
  - Di George syndrome — 22q11.2 deletion
  - Post-parathyroidectomy
- **Pseudohypoparathyroidism**
  - Autosomal dominant; end-organ resistance to raised levels of PTH
  - Abnormal phenotype with short stature, obesity, intellectual delay, round face, short neck, shortened 4th and 5th metacarpals
- **Acute alkalosis** (respiratory or metabolic); or acute correction of acidosis in setting of already reduced Ca^{2+}
- **Hyperphosphataemia**
  - Renal failure (acute or chronic)
  - Rhabdomyolysis; tumour lysis syndrome
- **Deposition of Ca^{2+}**
  - Acute pancreatitis
- **Treatment** includes:
  - Intravenous 10% calcium gluconate, 0.2 ml (0.045 mmol)/kg, diluted 1 : 5 with dextrose 5%, over 10–15 min with ECG monitoring; followed by intravenous infusion of 10% calcium gluconate at 0.3 ml (0.07 mmol)/kg/day
  - Oral Ca^{2+} supplements
  - Vitamin D, or the analogue alfacalcidol (1α-OH-cholecalciferol) for nutritional deficiency, hypoparathyroidism, and renal failure

Hypercalcaemia

The main symptoms are constipation, nausea, lethargy and confusion, headache, muscle weakness and polyuria and dehydration. The main causes are:

- **Vitamin D therapy**
  - Renal failure
  - Dietary vitamin D deficiency

- **Primary hyperparathyroidism**
  - Neonatal
  - Part of multiple endocrine neoplasia syndromes I and II
- **William syndrome**
  - Heterozygous deletions of chromosomal sub-band 7q11.23 leading to an elastin gene defect in > 90% (detected by fluorescent in situ hybridization)
  - Hypercalcaemia rarely persists beyond 1 year of age
- **Familial hypocalciuric hypercalcaemia**
  - Inactivation of Ca^{2+}-sensing receptor gene in parathyroid cells and renal tubules leads to an inappropriately high plasma PTH level and inappropriately low urine Ca^{2+}
- **↑ Macrophage production of 1,25(OH)2-D3**
  - Sarcoidosis
  - Subcutaneous fat necrosis —prolonged or obstructed labour
- **Malignant disease**
- **Treatment** includes:
  - Intravenous hydration plus a loop diuretic
  - Correction/removal or specific treatment of underlying cause, e.g. steroids for sarcoidosis
  - Rarely, bisphosphonates

Phosphate and hypophosphataemia

Phosphate is excreted from the kidney under the influence of parathyroid hormone (increases excretion), and calcitriol (decreases excretion). In hypophosphataemia, calculation of the **tubular reabsorption of phosphate** (TRP) is useful.

$$TRP = 1 - \text{Fractional excretion of PO}_4$$

i.e.

$$TRP = \frac{1 - \text{urine PO}_4 \text{ (mmol/L)}}{\text{urine creatinine (μmol/L)}} \times \frac{\text{plasma creatinine (μmol/L)}}{\text{plasma PO}_4 \text{ (mmol/L)}} \times 100\%$$

Normally, TRP > 85%. If the TRP is < 85%, in the presence of low plasma PO_4 and a normal PTH level, this implies abnormal tubular leakage of PO_4.

Hypophosphataemia

- With appropriately high TRP ie low urinary PO_4
  - Dietary PO_4 restriction
  - Increased uptake into bone — the 'hungry bone syndrome' seen after parathyroidectomy for prolonged hyperparathyroidism, or after renal transplantation with preceding hyperparathyroidism of CRF; see also Hypocalcaemia
- With inappropriately low TRP, i.e. high urinary PO_4
  - Hypophosphataemic rickets — see Section 7.1
  - Fanconi syndrome – see Section 7.1

Hyperphosphataemia

- With high urinary PO$_4$
  - Tumour lysis syndrome, rhabdomyolysis —see also oliguria, hyperkalaemia
- With low urinary PO$_4$
  - Chronic renal failure — see Section 11.3
  - Hypoparathyroidism; pseudohypoparathyroidism

Magnesium and hypomagnasemia

Most filtered Mg^{2+} is reabsorbed in the distal proximal tubule and the loop of Henle. As with Ca^{2+}, Mg^{2+} transport and NaCl transport are associated. Factors enhancing Mg^{2+} reabsorption include hypocalcaemia and raised PTH levels. Hypomagnesaemia is often found in patients with hypocalcaemia and hypokalaemia, and to correct these the magnesium deficiency must also first be corrected. The main causes of hypomagnesaemia are:

- Poor dietary intake
- Reduced gut absorption
- Increased urinary losses
  - Recovery from acute tubular necrosis
  - Post-transplant diuresis
  - Drug-induced — loop and thiazide diuretics; amphotericin B; cisplatinum
  - Gitelman syndrome — see Section 7.3

7. RENAL TUBULOPATHIES

7.1 Proximal tubulopathies

Cystinuria

- Defect in reabsorption of, and hence excessive excretion of, the dibasic amino acids cystine, ornithine, arginine and lysine
- Not to be confused with **cystinosis** — see below
- Autosomal recessive; two separate cystinuria genes on 2p and 19q
- Cystine is poorly soluble in normal urine pH; has increased solubility in alkaline urine
- Clinical manifestation is recurrent urinary stone formation
- Stones are extremely hard and densely radio-opaque
- Diagnosis based on stone analysis, or high cystine level in timed urine collection
- Treatment based on high fluid intake ($\geq$ 1.5 L/m^2/day) and alkalinization of urine with oral potassium citrate
- If stones still form, oral D-penicillamine leads to formation of highly soluble mixed disulphides with cystine moieties

X-linked hypophosphataemic rickets

- Also known as vitamin-D-resistant rickets
- Mutation in *PEX* gene on X chromosome
- Isolated defect in PO_4 reabsorption leading to:
  - Inappropropriately low tubular reabsorption of PO_4 (TRP) — typically < 85% — with a normal PTH and calcitriol level
  - Hypophosphataemia
- Earliest sign is ↑ alkaline phosphatase (by 3–4 months)
- Plasma PO_4 may be normal until 6–9 months of age

by 12 months, have delayed growth, hypophosphataemia, ↑ alkaline phosphatase, and radiological signs of rickets

- Other features include delayed dentition and recurrent dental abscesses
- Treatment is based on calcitriol or alfacalcidol, and phosphate supplements
- Complications of this treatment include hypercalcaemia and nephrocalcinosis
- Recent evidence suggests that addition of growth hormone treatment may improve growth and biochemical disturbance

Proximal (type 2) RTA

- Failure to reabsorb filtered HCO_3^-
- Renal bicarbonate threshold is low, i.e. HCO_3^- is present in the urine at levels of plasma HCO_3^- lower than normal
- Distal tubular H^+ excretion is intact so acid urine can be produced
- Normal acidification of urine in response to ammonium chloride load
- Normal increase in urine $p(CO_2)$ in response to 3 mmol/kg oral bicarbonate load
- Ability to excrete acid from distal tubule, and the fact that calcium salts are more soluble in acid urine, is the likely reason that nephrocalcinosis is not a feature of proximal RTA
- May occur as an isolated defect or as part of Fanconi syndrome — see below
- Symptoms include faltering growth, vomiting, short stature
- Treatment requires large doses of alkali (5–15 mmol/kg/day)

Fanconi syndrome

- Diffuse proximal tubular dysfunction, leading to excess urinary loss of:
  - Glucose — glycosuria with normal blood glucose
  - Phosphate — hypophosphataemia, low TRP, rickets
  - Amino acids — no obvious clinical consequence
  - HCO_3^- — leading to proximal RTA
  - K^+ — causing hypokalaemia
  - Na^+, Cl^- and water — leading to polyuria and polydipsia, chronic ECF volume depletion, faltering growth
  - Tubular proteinuria — loss of low molecular weight proteins including retinol binding protein, and *N*-acetyl glucosaminidase

- Usual clinical features include polyuria and polydipsia, chronic ECF volume depletion, faltering growth, constipation and rickets; with features of any underlying condition in addition

Main causes of Fanconi syndrome

- Metabolic disorders
  - Cystinosis
  - Tyrosinaemia
  - Lowe syndrome (oculo-cerebro-renal syndrome)
  - Galactosaemia
  - Wilson's disease
- Heavy metal toxicity
  - Lead, mercury, cadmium
- Idiopathic

Cystinosis

Autosomal recessive defect in the transport of cystine out of lysosomes. Gene is localized to chromosome 17p and encodes an integral membrane protein, cystinosin.

- Predominant early clinical features are of:
  - Fanconi's syndrome — see above
  - Photophobia as the result of eye involvement with corneal cystine crystals
  - Hypothyroidism
- Late features include:
  - Renal failure around 8–10 years of age, if untreated
  - Pancreatic involvement with diabetes mellitus
  - Liver involvement with hepatomegaly
  - Gonadal involvement with reduced fertility
  - Neurological deterioration and cerebral atrophy
- Diagnosis is based on:
  - Cystine crystals in cornea seen by slit lamp
  - Peripheral blood white cell cystine level
  - Antenatal diagnosis available for families with positive history

Treatment is:

- **Supportive** — PO_4, NaCl, K^+, and $NaHCO_3$ supplements, and high fluid intake; alfacalcidol; thyroxine
- **Specific** — cysteamine, which increases cystine transport out of the lysosome; commencing treatment in early infancy appears to delay onset of renal failure
- **Other** — indomethacin reduces the GFR, and hence the severe polyuria and secondary polydipsia, and electrolyte wasting

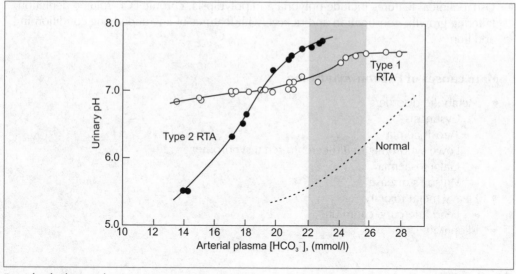

Renal tubular acidosis

In normal subjects, urine pH falls as plasma HCO_3^- decreases through the normal range from 26 to 22 mmol/L. In proximal RTA, the curve has a similar shape but is shifted to the left, such that acid urine is not produced until plasma HCO_3^- has fallen abnormally low, e.g. 16 mmol/L. In distal RTA, acid urine cannot be produced regardless of how low the plasma HCO_3^- falls.

Renal tubular acidosis – classification

	Type 1 (distal)	Type 2 (proximal)
Defect	Impaired excretion of H^+	Failure to reabsorb filtered HCO_3^-; bicarbonate threshold is low
Urine pH	> 5.8 i.e. never 'acid'	Variable; may be < 5.3
Plasma K	Usually ↓	Normal or ↓
Causes	Primary isolated RTA	Primary isolated RTA
	Nephrocalcinosis	Transient infantile
	Obstructive uropathy	Fanconi syndrome
	Amphotericin; cyclosporin	
Clinical features	Nephrocalcinosis; faltering growth; episodes of severe hypokalaemia	Vomiting; faltering growth; short stature
Response to NH_4Cl load	Failure to acidify urine	Production of acid urine
Response to $NaHCO_3^-$ load	No ↑ in urine–blood $p(CO_2)$ gradient	Normal ↑ in urine–blood $p(CO_2)$ gradient
Treatment	1–2 mmol/kg/day of $NaHCO_3$	5–15 mmol/kg/day of $NaHCO_3$; large doses needed to overcome low renal threshold

7.2 Loop of Henle

Bartter syndrome

- This is caused by an inborn autosomal recessive defect, in the $Na^+-K^+-2Cl^-$ co-transporter in the thick ascending limb of the loop of Henle, leading to NaCl and water wasting
- Symptoms are polyuria, polydipsia, episodes of dehydration, faltering growth and constipation; there may be maternal polyhydramnios with an affected fetus
- The resultant ECF volume contraction causes secondary renin secretion and raised aldosterone levels, with avid Na^+ and water reabsorption in the distal tubule, and reciprocal K^+ and H^+ secretion into the urine. (Note that the blood pressure is normal; the hyperreninaemia is a compensatory response to maintain normal blood pressure in the presence of chronic ECF volume depletion). There is also increased renal prostaglandin E_2 production
- The above changes produce the characteristic biochemical disturbance of hypochloraemic hypokalaemic alkalosis
- Crucial to the diagnosis is the finding of inappropriately high levels of urinary Cl^- and Na^+ — usually > 20 mmol/l; urine Ca^{2+} is normal or high (cf Gitelman syndrome — see below)
- Therapy involves K^+ supplementation combined with prostaglandin synthetase inhibitors, usually indomethacin

Pseudo-Bartter syndrome

- The same plasma biochemistry — hypochloraemic hypokalaemic alkalosis — but appropriately low levels of urine Cl^- and Na^+ — < 10 mmol/l
- Main causes are:
  - Cystic fibrosis – sweat loss of NaCl and water
  - Congenital chloride diarrhoea — gastrointestinal loss
  - Laxative abuse — gastrointestinal loss
  - Cyclical vomiting

NB: All the changes of Bartter syndrome, including the high urine electrolyte levels, may be produced by loop diuretics, which block the same site in the thick ascending limb of the loop of Henle.

7.3 Distal tubule

Gitelman syndrome

- This condition is considered a variant of Bartter syndrome
- There is an inborn autosomal recessive defect in the distal tubule Na^+-Cl^- co-transporter
- Often asymptomatic, with transient episodes of weakness and tetany with abdominal pain and vomiting

- Patients have hypokalaemic metabolic alkalosis, raised renin and aldosterone, and **hypomagnesaemia** with increased urinary magnesium wasting, and **hypocalciuria**, a feature which helps distinguish it from classical Bartter syndrome (in which urinary Ca^{2+} is normal or high — see above)
- Biochemical changes resemble those produced by thiazide diuretics, which inhibit this distal tubule co-transporter

7.4 Collecting duct

Nephrogenic diabetes insipidus

- Resistance to action of high circulating levels of ADH
- Associated with ADH-receptor gene mutations (X-linked nephrogenic diabetes insipidus), and aquaporin (water-channel) gene mutations (autosomal recessive nephrogenic diabetes insipidus)
- High volumes of inappropriately dilute urine with tendency to hypernatraemic dehydration

Liddle syndrome — see Section 4.3

Pseudohypoaldosternism — see Section 4.3

8. NEPHROTIC SYNDROME

A triad of oedema, proteinuria and hypoalbuminaemia. It is almost always idiopathic in childhood. It is best classified by response to steroid treatment — steroid-sensitive nephrotic syndrome (SSNS; 85–90% cases) or steroid-resistant nephrotic syndrome (SRNS; 10–15% cases), because this is the best predictor of outcome.

8.1 Definitions

- **Remission** — negative urinalysis on first morning urine for three consecutive mornings
- **Relapse** — 3^+ proteinuria on three or more consecutive first morning urines
- **Frequently relapsing** — two or more relapses within 6 months of diagnosis; or four or more relapses per year
- **Steroid resistant** — no remission after 4 weeks of prednisolone 60 mg/m^2/day

8.2   Clinical features

	SSNS	SRNS
Age at onset	toddler, pre-school	< 1 year; > 8 years
Sustained hypertension	no	often
Microscopic haematuria	mild, intermittent	persistent
Renal function	normal	often reduced
Long term prognosis	excellent, even if frequently relapsing	poor – significant risk of long-term hypertension and renal failure
Usual histology	usually not biopsied; from historical data known to be minimal changes	focal segmental glomerulosclerosis (FSGS)

8.3   Complications

Infection

- Typically with *Streptococcus pneumoniae*
  - Pneumonia
  - Primary pneumococcal peritonitis
- Increased risk as a result of:
  - Tissue oedema and pleural and peritoneal fluid
  - Loss of immunoglobulin in urine
  - Immunosuppression with steroid treatment

Thrombosis

- Increased risk as a result of:
  - Loss of antithrombin III and proteins S and C in urine
  - Increased production of procoagulant factors by liver
  - Increased haematocrit secondary to reduced oncotic pressure
  - Swelling of legs, ascites and relative immobility
  - Steroid therapy

Hypovolaemia

- Reduced plasma oncotic pressure leads to shift of plasma water from intravascular space to interstitial space
- Symptoms include oliguria, abdominal pain, anorexia and postural hypotension

- Signs include cool peripheries, poor capillary refill and tachycardia
- Poor renal perfusion activates the renin–angiotensin–aldosterone system, and urine Na$^+$ will therefore be very low – usually < 10 mmol/L
- Occasionally acute tubular necrosis develops secondary to hypovolaemia

Drug toxicity

- Most morbidity arises from side-effects of steroid treatment
- Nephrotoxicity from cyclosporin A or tacrolimus (see below)

8.4   Treatment

Initial presentation

The most commonly used prednisolone regimen in the UK is:

- Prednisolone 60 mg/m^2/day for 4 weeks; then reduce to 40 mg/m^2 on alternate days for 4 weeks; then stop

However, there is good evidence from controlled trials that longer duration of initial prednisolone treatment is associated with fewer relapses and lower total prednisolone dose over the first 2 years. An example of a 6-month initial course is:

- 60 mg/m^2/day for 4 weeks; then 40 mg/m^2 on alternate days for 4 weeks; 30 mg/m^2 on alternate days for 4 weeks; 20 mg/m^2 on alternate days for 4 weeks; 10 mg/m^2 on alternate days for 4 weeks; 5 mg/m^2 on alternate days for 4 weeks; then stop

Relapse

In cases of relapse the most commonly used prednisolone regimen is:

- Prednisolone 60 mg/m^2/day until in remission; then 40 mg/m^2 on alternate days for three doses; and reduce alternate day dose by 10 mg/m^2 every three doses until 10 mg/m^2 on alternate days is reached; then 5 mg/m^2 on alternate days for three doses; then stop

Frequently relapsing or steroid-dependent nephrotic syndrome

Other drugs that have been successfully used to enable control without steroids, or with much lower doses of steroids, include:

- Cyclosporin A
  - Taken twice daily long-term, e.g. 12–18 months initial trial
  - High relapse rate when weaned/stopped
  - Can cause hirsutism, gum hyperplasia, nephrotoxicity — need to monitor plasma cytochrome A levels and GFR
- Tacrolimus (FK506) — nephrotoxicity
- Cyclophosphamide
  - 2 mg/kg for 12 weeks, or 3 mg/kg for 8 weeks
  - Hair thinning, bone marrow suppression

- Mustine
  - Given as two courses each of four consecutive daily doses intravenously
- Levamisole
  - Need to monitor full blood count for bone marrow suppression
- Mycophenolate mofetil
  - Most recent immunosuppressive drug tried in nephrotic syndrome
  - Gastrointestinal intolerance is commonest side-effect; not nephrotoxic
  - Encouraging early reports

Steroid-resistant nephrotic syndrome

- Patient should be referred to specialist renal unit for assessment including renal biopsy
- Usually resistant to other drug treatments also, so full remission not achieved
- Aim is to reduce proteinuria so that patient is no longer nephrotic
- Commonest treatment is alternate day prednisolone combined with cyclosporin long-term; ACE inhibitor (e.g. enalapril) and/or angiotensin II receptor blocker (e.g. losartan) often used to treat hypertension, with the added benefit of antiproteinuric effect
- Significant chance of hypertension and progression to renal failure
- If histology is focal segmental glomerulosclerosis (FSGS), associated with 20–40% chance of recurrence after transplant

8.5 Congenital nephrotic syndrome

- Onset in first 3 months of life; large placenta — usually 40% of birth weight
- Almost always resistant to drug treatment; clinically severe with high morbidity from protein malnutrition, sepsis
- Main causes are, in decreasing order of frequency:
  - Finnish-type congenital nephrotic syndrome — most severe; autosomal recessive; gene (*NPHS1*) on chromosome 19 normally codes for nephrin, a cell adhesion protein located at the glomerular slit diaphragm
  - Diffuse mesangial sclerosis — less severe; also autosomal recessive
  - Denys–Drash syndrome — includes pseudohermaphroditism and Wilms tumour
  - FSGS
  - Secondary congenital nephrotic syndrome —congenital syphilis
- Treatment is intense supportive care with 20% albumin infusion, nutritional support, and early unilateral nephrectomy (to reduce urinary protein loss) combined with ACE inhibitors and indomethacin (to reduce GFR, and thus protein loss, of remaining kidney)
- Eventual progression to renal failure occurs, when remaining kidney is removed, and the child undergoes dialysis and transplantation

9. GLOMERULONEPHRITIS

9.1 General clinical features

- Inflammation of the glomeruli leading to various clinical features, or renal syndromes, which may include
  - Haematuria and/or proteinuria
  - Nephrotic syndrome
  - Acute nephritic syndrome with reduced renal function, oliguria and hypertension
  - Rapidly progressive crescentic glomerulonephritis — rapid onset severe renal failure and hypertension, usually associated with the histological lesion called a crescent
- These renal syndromes are not specific to particular conditions and the same condition may present with different renal syndromes in different patients
- Chronic glomerulonephritis may lead to scarring of the tubulo-interstitial areas of the kidney, with progressive renal impairment
- The main causes of glomerulonephritis, and the associated changes in serum complement, include the following.

The main causes of glomerulonephritis

Normal complement	Reduced complement
Primary renal disease 　FSGS 　IgA nephropathy	Primary renal disease 　Acute post-streptococcal GN 　↓ C_3, normal C_4 　Mesangiocapillary GN (MCGN) 　↓ C_3 and C_4
Systemic disease 　Henoch–Schönlein nephritis	Systemic disease 　Systemic lupus erythematosus 　↓ C_3 and C_4 　'Shunt nephritis' 　↓C_3 and C_4

GN, glomerulonephritis

9.2   Acute post-streptococcal glomerulonephritis

- Onset of reddish-brown ('Coca-Cola-coloured') urine 10–14 days after streptococcal throat or skin infection
- May have any of the renal syndromes described above
- Deposition of immune complexes and complement in glomeruli
- Investigations include:
  - Throat swab
  - Antistreptolysin O (ASO) titre; anti-DNAase B
  - Typically, ↓ C_3, normal C_4
  - Biopsy if there is significant renal involvement — diffuse proliferative glomerulonephritis is seen, with crescents, in severe cases
- Treatment is mainly supportive, with an excellent prognosis for recovery; in very severe cases involving renal failure, steroids have been used

NB: Always check C_3 and C_4 3 months after acute illness — should normalize; if still lowered there may be another diagnosis, e.g. systemic lupus erythematosis or MCGN, which have much worse prognoses.

9.3   Henoch–Schönlein nephritis

- 70% of children with Henoch–Schönlein purpura will have some degree of renal involvement, usually just microscopic haematuria with/without proteinuria
- They may have any of the renal syndromes described above.
- They may have a relapsing course
- Refer to specialist renal unit if nephrotic, or nephritic, or sustained hypertension as these patients may require biopsy
- Prognosis is difficult to be certain about, but initial clinical severity and histological score on biopsy guide the prognosis
- Treatment of severe cases includes steroids, azathioprine; and for very severe crescentic nephritis with renal failure, methylprednisolone combined with cyclophosphamide and plasma exchange has been used
- Histologically identical to IgA nephropathy — see Section 9.4
- Follow-up should continue for as long as there continues to be any abnormality on urinalysis
- Accounts for 5–8% of children in end-stage renal failure

9.4   IgA nephropathy

- Presents with incidental finding of persistent **microscopic haematuria** or with an episode of **macroscopic haematuria** which is typically associated with concurrent upper respiratory infection — these episodes may be recurrent
- Again, may have any of the renal syndromes described above
- Prognosis for childhood presentation is quite good, though 10–15% will develop proteinuria, hypertension with/without renal failure during long-term follow-up

- Treatment as for Henoch–Schönlein purpura nephritis; ACE inhibitors used for long-term control of hypertension and to minimize proteinuria

9.5   Systemic lupus erythematosus nephritis

- Again, may present with various renal syndromes
- Histologically variable and the condition may change its clinical and histological features and severity over time
- Patients may also manifest the antiphospholipid/anticardiolipin antibody syndrome, with thrombotic complications affecting the renal vasculature

9.6   'Shunt' nephritis

- Classically associated with infected ventriculo-atrial shunts — these are now rarely used so the condition is rare
- Histologically similar to nephritis of subacute bacterial endocarditis

10.   ACUTE RENAL FAILURE

An acute disturbance in fluid and electrolyte homeostasis, typically associated with oliguria (< 300 ml/m^2/day) and retention of urea, potassium, phosphate, H$^+$ and creatinine. It is rare in childhood compared with the incidence in the elderly. The main cause of severe acute renal failure in otherwise normal children is haemolytic–uraemic syndrome.

10.1   Classification of acute renal failure

Pre-renal failure with reduced renal perfusion

- In early stages, kidney reacts appropriately producing small volumes of urine with very low Na$^+$ and high concentration of urea; may be reversible at this stage with fluid therapy (with/without inotropic support)
- If uncorrected, progresses to established **acute tubular necrosis**
- Main causes are:
  - ECF volume deficiency — haemorrhage, diarrhoea, burns, DKA, septic shock with 'third space' fluid loss
  - Cardiac ('pump') failure — congenital heart disease, e.g. severe coarctation, hypoplastic left heart, aortic cross-clamping and bypass for correction of congenital heart disease, myocarditis

Intrinsic renal failure

- Acute tubular necrosis as a result of:
  - Uncorrected pre-renal failure as above
  - Toxins — gentamicin; X-ray contrast; myoglobinuria; and gentamicin toxicity most common in neonates, and may cause non-oliguric renal failure
    - Acute glomerulonephritis — see Section 9
- Vascular
  - Small vessel occlusion — haemolytic–uraemic syndrome
  - Bilateral renal vein thrombosis — neonates
  - Acute renal cortical necrosis — neonatal birth asphyxia
- Tubulo-interstitial nephritis
  - Drugs — non-steroidal anti-inflammatories; frusemide; penicillin; cephalosporins

Post-renal (obstructive) renal failure

- Posterior urethral valves is main lesion, but not **acute** renal failure
- Neuropathic bladder — may be **acute** in:
  - Transverse myelitis
  - Spinal trauma or tumour
- Stones
  - Bilateral pelviureteric junction or ureteral stone or bladder stone
  - Urethral prolapse of bladder ureterocoele

10.2 Differentiating pre-renal oliguria and intrinsic renal failure/acute tubular necrosis

- Clinical assessment of circulation in oliguric child is crucial:
  - Low blood pressure, poor capillary refill and cool peripheries suggest pre-renal cause: may respond to fluid challenge
  - Normal/raised blood pressure, raised JVP, good peripheral perfusion, gallop rhythm suggest intravascular volume overload and thus not pre-renal, and fluid challenge is contraindicated (though challenge with loop diuretic may improve urine output)
- Urine biochemical indices may help

Urine indices in pre–renal and intrinsic renal failure

Urine indices	Pre-renal failure	Intrinsic renal failure
Osmolality	> 500	< 300
Urine Na	< 10	> 40
Urine : plasma urea ratio	> 10 : 1	< 7 : 1
Fractional excretion of Na	< 1%	> 1%

10.3   Initial assessment of acute renal failure

- History may give clues to diagnosis
  - Sore throat and fever 10 days earlier suggests post-streptococcal glomerulonephritis
  - Bloody diarrhoea and progressive pallor suggest haemolytic–uraemic syndrome
  - Drug history may reveal use of non-steroidal anti-inflammatories (increasingly used for childhood fever, earache etc.)
- Examination aims to:
  - Assess circulation — see Section 10.2
  - Look for clues to diagnosis — drug rash suggests interstitial nephritis; large palpable bladder suggests acute obstructive nephropathy
- Initial investigations
  Blood
  - electrolytes, chloride, urea, creatinine, phosphate, calcium, magnesium, urate, liver function tests, venous or capillary blood gas
  - full blood count, blood film (red blood cell fragments in haemolytic–uraemic syndrome)

  Urine
  - urinalysis for blood, protein; glucose (a clue to interstitial nephritis)
  - urine microscopy for casts
  - urine Na^+, urea, creatinine, osmolality — see table above

  Ultrasound of urinary tract
  - with most causes of acute renal failure, kidneys appear normal or increased in size and echogenicity (if kidneys appear small with poor corticomedullary differentiation, renal failure is **chronic**)
  - rules out or confirms obstruction of urinary tract; stones
  - can detect clot in renal vein thrombosis

Renal biopsy if diagnosis not clear from above assessment

10.4   Initial management of child with acute renal failure

- Early liaison with paediatric renal unit
- Fluid therapy determined by clinical assessment and urine indices, as above
  - Pre-renal failure: fluid challenge with normal saline
  - Intrinsic renal failure
    - if clinically euvolaemic, give fluid as insensible loss (300 ml/m²/day) + urine output
    - if clinically overloaded, challenge with loop diuretic and restrict to insensible losses
- If hypertensive because of ECF volume overload
  - Challenge with loop diuretic
  - Nifedipine or hydrallazine as simple vasodilating hypotensives
- If hyperkalaemic, treat as in Section 6.4

NB: If anaemic, e.g. in hameolytic–uraemic syndrome, transfusion usually delayed until dialysis access is established (i.e. until transferred to renal unit), as hyperkalaemia and fluid overload may be worsened

10.5   Indications for acute dialysis

- Severe ECF volume overload — severe hypertension; pulmonary oedema; no response to diuretics
- Severe hyperkalaemia, not responding to conservative treatment
- Severe symptomatic uraemia — usually urea > 40 mmol/L
- Severe metabolic acidosis not controllable with intravenous bicarbonate
- To remove fluid to 'make space' for nutrition (intravenous or enteral), intravenous drugs — a common reason in intensive care patients
- Removal of toxins — haemodialysis will be most effective for small molecular weight substances that are not highly protein bound. These include:
  - Drugs — gentamicin, salicylates, lithium
  - Poisons — ethanol, ethylene glycol
  - Metabolites from inborn errors of metabolism — leucine in maple syrup urine disease, ammonia

10.6   Haemolytic–uraemic syndrome

- Commonest cause of acute renal failure in children
- Diarrhoea-associated (D$^+$-HUS) is the major type, usually as the result of *Escherichia coli* 0157, which produces verocytotoxin (also called shiga toxin)
- Toxin is released in gut and absorbed, causing endothelial damage especially in renal microvasculature, leading to microangiopathic haemolytic anaemia with thrombocytopenia and red blood cell fragmentation (seen on blood film)
- The microangiopathy leads to patchy focal thrombosis and infarction, and renal failure which is often severe and requires dialysis
- Brain (fits, focal neurology), myocardium, pancreas and liver are sometimes affected
- Treatment is supportive; antibiotic treatment of the *E. coli* gastroenteritis increases the incidence and severity of haemolytic–uraemic syndrome, and is thus contraindicated
- Long-term follow-up shows the 10–15% will develop hypertension, proteinuria, or impaired renal function
- Prevention with a synthetic Shiga toxin-binding trisaccharide linked to silica beads, taken orally, is undergoing clinical trials in Canada and USA, but early results are disappointing
- Atypical D$^-$-HUS is rare but more serious, with recurrent episodes, progressive renal impairment, and higher incidence of neurological involvement
  - Autosomal recessive forms associated with disturbances of complement regulation
  - Rare complication of bone marrow transplant

11. CHRONIC RENAL FAILURE, DIALYSIS, AND TRANSPLANTATION

A persistent impairment of renal function, classified according to the GFR as mild (60–80 ml/min/1.73 m^2), moderate (40–59 ml/min/1.73 m^2), and severe (< 40 ml/min/1.73 m^2). End-stage renal failure, where dialysis or transplantation are needed, is reached once GFR < 10 ml/min/1.73 m^2.

11.1 Main causes

The main causes are:

- Congenital dysplasia +/– obstruction
- Reflux nephropathy
- Chronic glomerulonephritis – FSGS; MCGN
- Genetically inherited disease
  - hereditary nephritis — Alport syndrome, nephronophthisis
  - polycystic kidney disease
- Systemic disease — Henoch–Schönlein purpura; systemic lupus erythematosus

11.2 Clinical presentations

- Antenatal diagnosis
- Faltering growth, poor growth; pubertal delay
- Malaise, anorexia
- Anaemia
- Incidental — blood test; urinalysis
- Hypertension

11.3 Main clinical features

Poor growth

- Anorexia, vomiting (uraemia)
- Anaemia, acidosis, and renal osteodystrophy — see below
- Reduced effectiveness of growth hormone, probably as the result of raised levels of insulin-like growth factor (IGF) binding protein, and hence less free IGF; levels of growth hormone are normal
- Recombinant human growth hormone is effective in improving growth in children with chronic renal failure, and is licensed for this use

Dietary considerations

- Inadequate calorie intake and catabolism worsens acidosis, uraemia and hyperkalaemia in chronic renal failure; aggressive nutritional management is crucial to control these, and to achieve growth

- Children with chronic renal failure often have poor appetite, and infants in particular benefit from nasogastric or gastrostomy tube feeding
- Congenital dysplasia +/– obstruction typically causes polyuria, with NaCl and HCO_3^- wasting, and these need supplementing along with generous water intake; note that salt and water restriction is **inappropriate** in many children with chronic renal failure, until they reach end-stage renal failure
- Protein intake should usually be the recommended daily intake for age; note that protein restriction is **inappropriate** for children with chronic renal failure
- Dietary restriction of PO_4 (dairy produce) combined with use of PO_4 binders (e.g. calcium carbonate) is essential in controlling secondary hyperparathyroidism
- Dietary restriction of K^+ (fresh fruits, potatoes) is also commonly needed

Anaemia

- Dietary iron deficiency
- Reduced red blood cell survival in uraemia
- Erythropoietin deficiency; recombinant human erythropoietin is available for treatment

Renal osteodystrophy

There are two main contributing processes:

- Phosphate retention leads to hypocalcaemia, and both increased PO_4 and decreased Ca^{2+} stimulate secondary hyperparathyroidism
  - Subperiosteal bone resorption
- Deficient renal 1α-hydroxylase activity and deficient $1,25(OH)_2$-D_3 also contributes to hypocalcaemia, and leads to **rickets**
- Treatment includes control of hyperphosphataemia (see above); and alfacalcidol (1α-OH-cholecalciferol) or calcitriol

Metabolic acidosis

- Contributes to bone disease, because chronic acidosis is significantly buffered by the uptake of H^+ into bone in exchange for Ca^{2+} loss from bone

Hypertension

- Depends on the underlying cause of the chronic renal failure
  - Congenital dysplasia +/– obstruction — patients tend to be polyuric, salt wasting and normotensive
  - Chronic glomerulonephritis, polycystic kidney disease, systemic disease — hypertension is common; usually secondary to increased renin, so ACE inhibitors are often effective

11.4 Dialysis

Once the GFR falls to 10 ml/min/1.73 m^2, the child will usually need dialysis, or transplantation, to be maintained safely. The two main types of dialysis, peritoneal dialysis and haemodialysis, both use a semi-permeable membrane to achieve solute removal (K^+, urea, PO_4, creatinine, etc), and fluid removal.

Infants and small children are better suited to peritoneal dialysis, which is more 'physiological' and avoids abrupt haemodynamic changes

	Peritoneal dialysis	**Haemodialysis**
Semipermeable	peritoneum membrane	synthetic membrane
Access	peritoneal catheter	central venous catheter or arteriovenous fistula in arm
Frequency and duration	daily (usually overnight) via automated PD machine	thrice weekly, 4-h/session
Where	home	hospital
Complications	peritonitis; catheter blockage or leakage	catheter sepsis; haemodynamic instability in infants
Advantages	independence from hospital; schooling uninterrupted; PD machine portable so can travel on holidays	no burden of care for dialysis procedure on family
Disadvantages	burden of care on family	missed school; travel to and from hospital; limited holiday options

PD, peritoneal dialysis

11.5 Transplantation

- The proportion of living related donor transplants in paediatric units (~50% of transplants) is higher than the national figure overall — a parent is usually the donor
- Transplantation before the need for dialysis is usually the aim
- There are advantages to living related donor transplantation
  - Better long-term survival of the graft kidney: approximate figures are 90% at 1 year; 75–80% at 5 years; 60% at 10 years
  - Surgery is planned, so family life can be organized to deal with it
  - Increases the chance of achieving transplantation without dialysis
- Human leukocyte antigen (HLA) matching is based around HLA-A, -B and -DR; on average a parent and child will be matched for one allele, and mismatched for one allele, at each site
- The main immunosuppressive drugs are prednisolone, tacrolimus and azathioprine

- Children should be immune to tuberculosis, measles and chicken pox before transplantation — immunization is available for all these infections
- Children must weigh ⩾ 10 kg for transplantation to be performed
- The main complications of transplantation include
  - Early surgical complications — bleeding; transplant artery thrombosis; wound infection
  - Rejection — diagnosed on biopsy; usually treatable with extra immune suppression
  - Opportunistic infection — fungal infections; cytomegalovirus; *Pneumocystis pneumoniae*
  - Drug toxicity — hypertension; Cushingoid changes; hirsutism and nephrotoxicity from cyclosporin
  - Post-transplantation lymphoproliferative disorder — lymphoma-like condition, especially associated with primary Epstein–Barr virus infection when immunosuppressed

12. URINARY TRACT INFECTION, NEUROPATHIC BLADDER

12.1 Urinary tract infection

- Commonest presenting urinary tract problem — 1% boys and 3% girls
- Boys outnumber girls until 6 months (posterior urethral valves); thereafter girls outnumber boys
- Significance of UTI
  - Renal scar gives 15–20% risk hypertension
  - Reflux nephropathy causes 15–20% end-stage renal failure
- Age at greatest risk for renal damage, age in which symptoms of UTI are least specific, age group most often seen with fever by general practitioners, and age at which proper urine sample are hardest to obtain — infancy
- Collection of an uncontaminated urine sample is crucial to accurate diagnosis of UTI — methods include
  - Adhesive bag — problems with leakage and faecal contamination
  - Absorbent pad —also prone to contamination
  - Clean catch
  - Catheter specimen, or suprapubic aspirate — suitable if urine sample is needed urgently, e.g. septic screen in ill infant

Predisposing factors for UTI

- Vesicoureteric reflux (VUR)
  - Familial, behaves as autosomal dominant condition
  - May be graded according to severity on MCUG
  - Management based on long-term, low-dose antibiotic prophylaxis (although no convincing randomized prospective controlled trials have been reported, this remains the standard of care currently)
  - Significant spontaneous resolution rate; less likely in grades IV and V

- Controlled studies show no benefit for surgery over conservative management for grades I–III
- Surgery may be indicated where prophylaxis fails to control infection and where there is progressive reflux nephropathy; options are reimplantation of ureters or endoscopic injection of synthetic material at ureteric orifice
- Screening of newborn siblings or offspring of index children or parents should be considered
- In children who have normal bladder control and no symptoms of detrusor dysfunction, and who have been free of infection on prophylaxis, evidence suggests that there is little benefit from continuing prophylaxis beyond 5 years old
- Incomplete bladder emptying
  - Posterior urethral valves
  - Neuropathic bladder
- Catheterization or instrumentation of urinary tract
- Stones

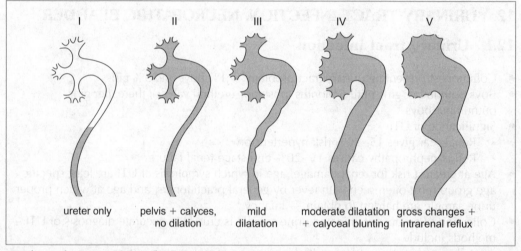

I	II	III	IV	V
ureter only	pelvis + calyces, no dilation	mild dilatation	moderate dilatation + calyceal blunting	gross changes + intrarenal reflux

Grading of vesicoureteric flux

Investigation of UTI

- Aims
  - To identify scarring
  - To identify underlying abnormalities likely to cause recurrent infection — VUR; incomplete emptying
- Suggested protocol
  - under 1 year — ultrasound + DMSA + MCUG
  - over 1 year — ultrasound + DMSA; MCUG only if
    - ultrasound or DMSA is abnormal
    - pyelonephritis clinically
    - recurrent UTI
    - family history

- There is much debate about the investigation of UTI but the above scheme is cautious and commonly used
- Indirect radioisotope reflux study (e.g. DTPA) — see Section 5.5
  - May be adequate for initial investigation for VUR in girls, but initial contrast MCUG should always be performed in boys to exclude posterior urethral valves

Prevention of UTI

- Non-pharmacological methods
  - Avoidance of constipation; correct bottom wiping
  - Frequent voiding and high fluid intake; double voiding
  - Lactobacilli in live yoghurt; cranberry juice
  - Clean intermittent catheterization
- Prophylactic antibiotics

Treatment of UTI

- Empirical antibiotic treatment until culture and sensitivity results are known; > 90% childhood UTIs are *E. coli*
- Intravenous antibiotics for unwell infants and children with clinical pyelonephritis — high fever and rigors, loin pain, vomiting, neutrophilia, raised C-reactive protein
- Obstructed kidneys may need drainage
- Stones may need removing
- Augmented bladders may improve with mucolytic and bacteriostatic washouts
  - Parvolex washouts; chlorhexidene washouts

12.2   Neuropathic bladder

Important cause of renal damage

- UTI caused by incomplete emptying
- High-pressure vesicoureteric reflux
- Progressive renal scarring

Causes

- Spina bifida; sacral agenesis (maternal diabetes)
- Tumour; trauma
- Transverse myelitis

Types

- Hyper-reflexic — high pressure; detrusor-sphincter dyssynergia
- Atonic — large, chronically distended, poorly emptying

Principles of management

- Videourodynamic assessment of type of bladder dysfunction
- Careful assessment of kidney structure, scarring, function, blood pressure
- Improve emptying with clean intermittent catheterization
- Anticholinergics (oxybutinin) may help reduce unstable contractions
- Augmentation cystoplasty — larger capacity, lower pressure

13. NOCTURNAL ENURESIS

This is a common condition which is benign but which may cause distress and psychological upset to the child and family. Most children become dry at night 6–9 months after becoming dry by day, which is usually by 3 years. As a simple guide, 10% of 5-year-olds and 5% of 10-year-olds wet the bed at least 1 night per week. It is commoner in boys.

13.1 Definitions

- Primary nocturnal enuresis (~80%) — never achieved night-time dryness
- Secondary nocturnal enuresis — recurrence of bedwetting having been dry for $\geqslant 1$ year
- Initial successful response — 14 consecutive dry nights within 16 weeks of starting treatment
- Relapse — more than two wet nights in 2 weeks
- Complete success — no relapse within 2 years of initial success

13.2 Aetiology

- Rarely an organic cause; should be distinguished from true **incontinence**, e.g. as a result of neuropathic bladder or ectopic ureter, when child is never dry
- Genetic component
  - More common where there is a first-degree relative with history of enuresis
  - Concordance in monozygotic twins twice that in dizygotic twins
- No significant excess of major psychological or behavioural disturbance, though family stress, bullying at school etc. may trigger secondary enuresis and such factors should be sought in the history
- Evidence from studies that
  - In younger children, bladder capacity is reduced compared with non-enuretic children
  - In older children and adolescents, there is reduction in the normally observed rise in nocturnal ADH levels and in the decrease in nocturnal urine volume (hence rationale for DDAVP treatment — see Section 13.4)

13.3 Assessment

- Careful history is crucial
- Examination should exclude abnormalities of abdomen, spine, lower limb neurology, hypertension
- Investigations should be limited to urinalysis

13.4 Treatment

Sustained and frequent support and encouragement for child and parents from an enthusiastic carer (doctor, nurse) is the most essential factor in seeing improvement. Any treatment must involve the child, and depends for success on their motivation.

- Star charts; colouring-in charts — simple behavioural therapy that is successful in many children; and should be part of the monitoring of all interventions
- Enuresis alarms
  - Mat on bed attached to bed-side buzzer, *or*
  - Small moisture sensor worn between two layers of underwear with vibrator alarm attached to pyjamas (has the advantage of detecting wet underwear rather than waiting to detect a wet bed)
  - May see 85% dry within 4 months, with a low 10% relapse rate
  - More effective than drug therapies in direct comparative trials
  - Should be mainstay of treatment, but enthusiastic and supportive care, and involvement of child (e.g. they should get up and change bedding) is crucial to success
- Drug therapy
  - Imipramine — low long-term success rate; high relapse rate; potentially serious side-effects; rarely used
  - Desmopressin (oral or intranasal) — meta-analysis of all published trials showed relatively poor short-term complete response rate, high relapse rate, and poor long-term cure rate; more effective in older children; useful for short-term control for special situations, e.g. school trip
  - Oxybutinin — should be restricted to those children with a clear history of **detrusor instability** — daytime urgency, frequency, urge incontinence —many of whom also wet the bed

14. HYPERTENSION

Most significant hypertension in childhood is secondary to an underlying cause. **Essential hypertension** is a diagnosis of exclusion; the typical patient is an obese adolescent with mild hypertension and a family history of hypertension.

What is normal?

- Blood pressure rises throughout childhood, related to age and height
- Depends on method and frequency of measurement
- US Task Force on Blood Pressure Control produce centile charts based on 60,000 normal children and teenagers

What is abnormal?

- **Consistently** above the 95th centile for age
- Loss of normal diurnal pattern
- Infants and toddlers may require admission to hospital for blood pressure monitoring to make diagnosis

14.1 Ambulatory blood pressure monitoring

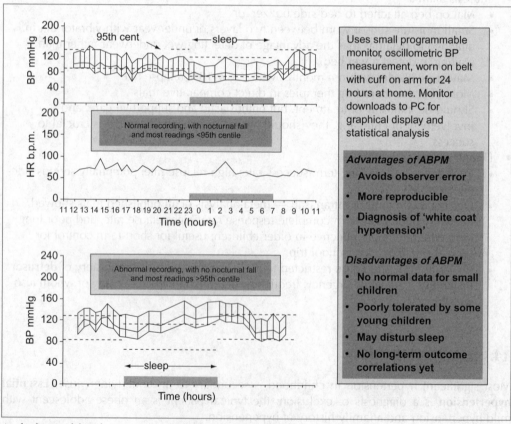

Uses small programmable monitor, oscillometric BP measurement, worn on belt with cuff on arm for 24 hours at home. Monitor downloads to PC for graphical display and statistical analysis

Advantages of ABPM
- **Avoids observer error**
- **More reproducible**
- **Diagnosis of 'white coat hypertension'**

Disadvantages of ABPM
- **No normal data for small children**
- **Poorly tolerated by some young children**
- **May disturb sleep**
- **No long-term outcome correlations yet**

Ambulatory blood pressure monitoring (ABPM)

14.2 Causes of secondary hypertension

Cause	Potentially curable by surgery/intervention
Renal	
Reflux nephropathy	if unilateral only
Polycystic kidney disease	✗
Glomerulonephritis, e.g. FSGS	✗
Renal artery stenosis	✔
Middle aortic syndrome e.g. NF1; William syndrome	✔
Coarctation	✔
Endocrine	
Phaeochromocytoma	✔
Cushing syndrome	✔
Other	depends on cause

14.3 Evaluation of hypertension by increasing level of invasiveness

Level 1	Level 2	Level 3
Assessment of risk factors	*Further renal imaging*	*Arteriography*
Family history; obesity	DMSA scan	Renal artery stenosis
Consequences of HT	*Urine catecholamines*	*Renal vein renin sampling*
Symptom history	24-h total Catecholamine :	*IVC catecholamine*
Fundoscopy	creatinine ratio on spot	sampling
Echocardiography	sample	
Secondary renal causes of HT	*Further blood samples*	*Renal biopsy*
Urinalysis	Renin, aldosterone	
U&E, creatinine, pH	Plasma catecholamines	
Renal ultrasound scan		
	Other imaging	
	MIBG scan for	
	phaeo-chromocytoma	

HT, hypertension

14.4 Treatment of hypertension

Short term treatment of acute hypertension

- Commonest clinical indication is **acute nephritis** with salt and water retention; simple and well tolerated combination would be a loop diuretic, e.g. frusemide, plus a vasodilating Ca^{2+}-channel blocker, e.g. nifedipine
- **Phaeochromocytoma** — α- and β-blockers, e.g. phenoxybenzamine + labetolol

Urgent treatment of hypertensive encephalopathy

- Severe hypertension with headache, vomiting, hyperreflexia, seizures
- Principle of treatment is
  - **Controllable** reduction with intravenous infusions — labetolol; sodium nitroprusside
  - **Gradual** reduction — end-organ damage, e.g. seizures often controlled before normal blood pressure is seen
  - Risk of treatment is too rapid reduction causing stroke; cortical blindness

Long term treatment of chronic hypertension

- Aim to use single agent if possible; and select long-acting once-daily agent to aid compliance, e.g.
  - β-blocker — atenolol
  - Ca^{2+}-channel blocker — amlodipine
  - ACE inhibitor — enalapril; logical choice for hypertension secondary to chronic renal disease (e.g. reflux nephropathy; FSGS); also has an antiproteinuric effect; relatively contraindicated in renal artery stenosis

15. INHERITED DISEASES

15.1 Polycystic kidney disease

Autosomal recessive polycystic kidney disease (ARPKD)

- Gene is on Chromosome 6
- Tubular dilatation of distal collecting ducts, i.e. not true cysts
- Clinical presentation
  - Antenatal ultrasound — large echobright kidneys; oligohydramnios
  - At birth or early infancy — large palpable renal masses; respiratory distress secondary to pulmonary hypoplasia
  - At any time — signs and symptoms of chronic renal failure; hypertension — often very severe
- Median age for onset of end-stage renal failure around 12 years, though may cause severe renal failure in infancy; very variable disease severity even within same family
- Always associated with **congenital hepatic fibrosis** which may vary from subclinical to causing liver disease which is the dominant clinical feature; complications include ascending cholangitis

Autosomal dominant polycystic kidney disease (ADPKD)

- At least two gene loci; commonest on chromosome 16 (adjacent to tuberous sclerosis gene); normal gene product is polycystin
- True cysts arising from tubules — get larger and more numerous with time and hence cause progressive decline in renal function
- An important cause of hypertension and renal failure in adults though may present in childhood
- Clinical presentation —again, very variable in age and severity
  - Antenatal ultrasound — discrete cysts in fetal kidneys (**NB:** always scan parent's kidneys)
  - Microscopic haematuria
  - Hypertension; renal failure
  - Incidental finding of renal cysts during abdominal ultrasound — first cysts may not appear until patient is in 20s; may be unilateral
- Associated with cerebral aneurysms and subarachnoid haemorrhage

15.2   Alport syndrome

- Hereditary nephritis with sensorineural deafness and anterior lenticonus (conical deformity of lens of eye seen with slit lamp)
- X-linked (commonest) and autosomal recessive forms
  - X-linked — males affected; female carriers all have microscopic haematuria; with Lyonization some females may develop hypertension and renal disease, but with milder and later onset
  - Autosomal recessive (chromosome 2) — both sexes equally severe
- Basic defect is in production of subunits for type IV collagen (two subunits coded for on X chromosome, two on chromosome 2); type IV collagen is located in kidney, eye and inner ear — hence the main clinical features
- Presents with incidental finding of microscopic haematuria, or episode of macroscopic haematuria
- Deafness around 10 years
- Hypertension mid-teens
- Eye signs mid-late teens (not before 12 years)
- Average age for end-stage renal failure 21 years

15.3   Nephronophthisis

- Autosomal recessive condition; gene (called *NPHP1*) on chromosome 2
- Produces polyuria (concentrating defect), growth delay, and often severe anaemia
- Urinalysis typically 'bland' — sometimes a trace of glucose
- Progresses to end-stage renal failure towards the end of the first decade
- Sometimes associated with tapeto-retinal degeneration: Senior–Löken syndrome

16. NEPHROCALCINOSIS AND NEPHROLITHIASIS

16.1 Nephrocalcinosis

Diffuse speckling calcification is seen on ultrasound scans or plain X-ray.

Main causes are:

- Distal RTA
- Ex-premature neonates
  - Frusemide — hypercalciuria
  - Steroids — hypercalciuria
- Vitamin D treatment for hypophosphataemic rickets
  - Enhances tubular reabsorption Ca^{2+}
- Oxalosis
  - Autosomal recessive disorder
  - Primary hyperoxaluria associated with defect in alanine : glyoxylate aminotransferase (AGT) enzyme, which leads to excess oxalate production and urinary oxalate excretion
  - Calcium oxalate precipitates, nephrocalcinosis and obstructing stones form, renal failure ensues
  - Systemic oxalosis — joints, heart, blood vessels
  - Treatment — liver and kidney transplantation

16.2 Nephrolithiasis — stones

- Uncommon in paediatrics
- Clinical presentation
  - Painful haematuria
  - Revealed during investigation into UTI
- Important to undertake metabolic analysis of timed urine collection, or of stone itself if possible, because several metabolic diseases cause stones which may be recurrent

Type	Cause	Radio–opaque
Mg-ammonium-phosphate	*Proteus* UTI; urinary stasis	+/–
Calcium phosphate	RTA; hypercalciuria	+
Calcium oxalate	oxalosis	+
Cystine	cystinuria	+
Uric acid	Lesch–Nyhan; tumour lysis	–
Xanthine	xanthinuria	–

17. FURTHER READING

Webb, NJ, Postlethwait RJ (eds). 2002. *Clinical Paediatric Nephrology*, 3rd edition. Oxford: Oxford University Press.

Avner E, Harmon W, Niaudet P (eds). 2000. *Pediatric Nephrology*, 5th edition. Baltimore, US: Lippincott, Williams and Wilkins.

Rose BD, Post TW (eds). 2001. Clinical Physiology of Acid-Base and Electrolyte Disorders, 5th edition. New York: McGraw Hill.

Chapter 18

Neurology
Neil H Thomas

CONTENTS

Neurology

1. DEVELOPMENTAL ABNORMALITIES OF THE NERVOUS SYSTEM

1.1 Normal development of the nervous system

The exact details of the normal development of the nervous system are complex, but the important stages can be summarized in the table below:

Stage	Time	Event	Potential Disorder
Organ induction: (a) Dorsal	3–7 weeks	Neural tube closure	Anencephaly, spina bifida
(b) Ventral	5–6 weeks	Forebrain, facial development	Holoprosencephaly
Neuronal and glial proliferation	8–16 weeks	Neural proliferation and early cellular differentiation	Microcephaly
Neuronal migration	12–19 weeks	Neuronal migration and formation of corpus callosum	Lissencephaly, pachygyria, agenesis of corpus callosum
Neuronal organization	22 weeks to postnatal	Orientation of cortical structures	Cortical dysplasia
Myelination	24 weeks through early childhood years		Dysmyelination

1.2 Neural tube defects

Spina bifida occulta

Asymptomatic condition characterized by failure of closure of vertebral arch. Occurs in up to 5% of population.

Anencephaly

Failure of closure of the rostral aspect of the neural tube; 75% of affected infants are stillborn.

Encephalocele

Protrusion of cerebral tissue through midline cranial defect located in frontal or occipital regions.

Meningocele

Cyst formed by herniation of meninges, usually over dorsum of spine. Neurological disability minimal, risk of bacterial meningitis.

Meningomyelocele

Herniation of meninges, nerve roots and spinal cord through dorsal vertebral defect. Leads to motor and sensory deficits below lesion, including sphincter disturbance. May be associated with other malformations of spinal cord including Arnold–Chiari malformation (downward displacement of cerebellar tonsils through foramen magnum). Hydrocephalus may coexist, secondary to Arnold–Chiari malformation or aqueduct stenosis.

Prevention of neural tube defects

There is clear evidence that preconceptual folate supplementation prevents production of neural tube defects.

Treatment of neural tube defects

- Operative repair of encephalocele, meningocele, myelomeningocele
- Close observation for development of hydrocephalus and operative treatment
- Management of bladder and bowels. Possible intermittent bladder drainage
- Orthopaedic management of limb deformities
- Assessment of cognitive abilities
- Treatment of seizures

1.3 Hydrocephalus

Defined as excess fluid within the cranium. Usually refers to increased volume of cerebrospinal fluid (CSF).

Production of CSF

- Secreted by choroid plexus (as plasma ultrafiltrate which is then modified)
- Flows through lateral ventricles, through third and fourth ventricles into posterior fossa and basal cisterns
- Reabsorbed through arachnoid granulations

Terms such as 'communicating' and 'non-communicating' or 'obstructive' hydrocephalus are now obsolete.

Main aetiological mechanisms of hydrocephalus:	
Over secretion	Choroid plexus papilloma
Obstruction	
Intraventricular	Tumours, malformations, inflammation (post-haemorrhagic)
Extraventricular	Inflammation, tumours, mucopolysaccharidoses
Impaired resorption	Venous sinus compression

Diagnosis (clinical)

- May be asymptomatic
- Irritability
- Headache
- Vomiting
- Drowsiness
- Increased head circumference
- Tense anterior fontanelle
- Splayed sutures
- Scalp vein distension
- Loss of upward gaze (sunsetting)
- Neck rigidity
- Decreased conscious level
- Cranial nerve palsies

Investigations

- Ultrasonography (when fontanelle open)
- Computerized tomography (CT)
- Magnetic resonance imaging (MRI)
- Measurement of CSF pressure by neurosurgical intervention may be indicated

Management

- Decide need for operation by considering symptoms and rate of head growth
- Surgical:
  - Ventriculostomy
  - Shunting (ventriculoperitoneal, ventriculoatrial)

1.4 Disorders of cortical development

Lissencephaly

Brain has very few or no gyri, leaving the surface of the brain smooth. Leads to severe motor and learning disability. Lissencephaly may be associated with facial abnormalities and a deletion on chromosome 17p13.3 in the Miller–Dieker syndrome. X-linked lissencephaly and subcortical band heterotopia ('double cortex') linked to mutations in either the doublecortin (*DCX*) or *LIS1* genes.

Polymicrogyria

Increased numbers of small gyri, especially in temporoparietal regions.

Periventricular heterotopia

Aggregation of neurones arrested in their primitive positions. May be part of complex brain malformation syndromes. X-linked periventricular nodular heterotopia is seen in females, characterized often by focal epilepsy and is associated in a proportion of cases with mutations in the *FLN1* gene.

Pachygyria

Thickened abnormal cortex. Depending on extent, it may lead to cerebral palsy or to epilepsy.

Agenesis of corpus callosum

Corpus callosum develops between the 10th and 12th weeks of embryonic life. Agenesis may be isolated or associated with other malformations. Extent of other malformations determines disability.

1.5 Other nervous system maldevelopments

Dandy–Walker malformation

Classical Dandy–Walker malformation includes:

- Complete or partial agenesis of cerebellar vermis
- Large cystic formation in posterior fossa as a result of dilatation of fourth ventricle
- Hydrocephalus, which may not develop until adulthood.

May be associated with other cerebral malformations. Considered part of a continuum including Dandy–Walker variant (part of vermis present, posterior fossa not enlarged) and megacisterna magna (complete vermis, large retrocerebellar cyst).

Aqueduct stenosis

Cause of hydrocephalus in 11% of cases. Aqueduct may be reduced in size or may be represented by numerous channels within aqueduct location. Can occur in X-linked syndrome.

2. NEONATAL NEUROLOGY

2.1 Neonatal seizures

Seizures are a major neurological problem in the first 28 days of life.

Classification

Tonic seizures	— stiffening of trunk and extremities
Mulitfocal clonic seizures	— rhythmic clonic movements of different parts of the body and various seizures
Focal clonic seizures	— repetitive clonic movements of the same part of the body
Subtle seizures	— episodes of stereotyped bicycling, sucking and swallowing movements
Myoclonic seizures	— isolated repetitive brief jerks of the body

Causes

- Hypoxic–ischaemic encephalopathy
- Intracranial haemorrhage
- Intracranial infection
- Cerebral malformations
- Metabolic disturbances
- Withdrawal seizures
- Familial neonatal convulsions

2.2 Hypoxic–ischaemic encephalopathy

The neonatal brain is highly resistant to hypoxia–ischaemia compared with that of an adult. The degree of hypoxia–ischaemia necessary to damage the neonatal brain usually leads to impairment of other organs.

Hypoxia–ischaemia leads to depletion of brain phosphocreatine and ATP. Lactate increases.

Clinical features

Five-minute Apgar score of less than 6, a metabolic acidosis and hypotension are all suggestive of asphyxia in term infants.

Hypoxic–ischaemic encephalopathy in term infants
Stage 1 — Hyper-alert, tremulousness, poor feeding; seizures infrequent
Stage 2 — Lethargic, obtunded, hypotonic; seizures may occur
Stage 3 — Comatose; seizures within 12–24 h

Outcome according to severity of hypoxic–ischaemic encephalopathy
Stage 1 — Largely normal
Stage 2 — 5% die, 25% suffer neurological injury
Stage 3 — 80% die, 20% suffer neurological injury

2.3 Periventricular–intraventricular haemorrhage

Usually a disease of preterm infants. Majority of haemorrhages originate in subependymal germinal matrix.

Potential consequences

- Asymptomatic
- Catastrophic collapse
- Cerebral infarction
- Post-haemorrhagic hydrocephalus

2.4 Periventricular leukomalacia

A pathological term to describe bilateral necrosis of periventricular white matter. Gliosis ensues. Leads to interruption of the fibres that are responsible for lower limb and optic function, so that periventricular leukomalacia is often the underlying pathology to the spastic diplegia and visual impairment seen in survivors of preterm birth.

2.5 Brachial plexus injuries

Traction injury to the brachial plexus can follow difficulty in delivery of the shoulders and head during birth. A large baby, narrow birth canal and malpresentation may all contribute. Usually, the nerve roots are stretched but not completely avulsed. Clavicular or humeral fractures may also occur.

Erb's palsy

- C5–C6 lesion
- Affects deltoid, serratus anterior, supraspinatus, infraspinatus, biceps, brachioradialis muscles
- Arm is flaccid, adducted and internally rotated
- Elbow is extended, wrist is flexed ('waiter's tip')

Klumpke's paralysis

- C8–T1 lesion
- Affects intrinsic hand muscles so that flexion of wrist and fingers is affected
- Cervical sympathetic involvement may lead to an ipsilateral Horner syndrome

Management

- Physiotherapy
- Consideration of nerve root surgery

3.   DISORDERS OF MOVEMENT

3.1   Cerebral palsy

Cerebral palsy may be defined as a disorder of tone, posture or movement, which is the result of a static lesion affecting the developing nervous system. Despite the unchanging nature of the causative lesion, its existence in a developing nervous system means that its manifestations may change over time.

Causes of cerebral palsy
Prenatal insults

- Intrauterine hypoxic-ischaemic injury
- Intrauterine infection
- Toxins
- Chromosomal disorders

Perinatal insults

- Hypoxic–ischaemic injury
- Intracranial haemorrhage
- Bilirubin encephalopathy

Postnatal insults

- Trauma
- Bacterial meningitis
- Viral encephalitis

Epidemiological studies suggest that at least 80% of cases of cerebral palsy are the result of prenatally acquired causes. A minority are the result of intrapartum asphyxia.

Classification

Based on the distribution of motor impairment and tone variations.

- **Spastic** (characterized by fixed increase in muscular tone)
  - Hemiplegia
  - Diplegia
  - Quadriplegia

- **Athetoid** (dyskinetic, dystonic)
  - Athetoid — writhing, involuntary pronation and flexion of distal extremity
  - Choreiform ('dancing') — involuntary rapid semi-purposeful movements of proximal segments of body
- **Ataxic**
  - Mixed

Spastic diplegia is most frequently seen as the result of periventricular leukomalacia in preterm infants.

Athetoid cerebral palsy may result from bilirubin encephalopathy or from brief profound anoxic–ischaemic episodes.

Associated clinical features

- Developmental delay
- Tendency to joint contractures
- Epilepsy
- Perceptual difficulties
- Visual and hearing impairment
- Poor growth
- Feeding difficulties

Children with cerebral palsy need the care of a multidisciplinary team.

3.2   Ataxia

Acute cerebellar ataxia may occur following viral infection. It appears to be the result of both infectious and post-infectious processes; most commonly following varicella virus infection. Also measles, mumps, herpes simplex and Epstein–Barr viruses, coxsackievirus and echovirus.

Occult neuroblastoma may also lead to acute ataxia.

A common cause is overdosage of drugs such as carbamazepine, phenytoin, benzo-diazepines. Also piperazine, antihistamines.

Other causes

- Posterior fossa tumour
- Migraine

Ataxia-telangiectasia

See section 13.3 in this chapter.

Friedreich's ataxia

- Classified as a spinocerebellar degeneration
- Autosomal recessive condition (9q13)
- Gene product frataxin
- Involved in modulation of mitochondrial function
- Clinical characteristics:
  - Onset of symptoms in first or second decade
  - Loss of proprioception
  - Increasing impairment of cerebellar function
  - Development of pes cavus
  - Cardiomyopathy develops
  - Deterioration so that patients are usually not ambulant in their 20s or 30s
- Treatment:
  - Currently symptomatic
  - Physiotherapy
  - Suitable aids and appliances

3.3 Dystonia

Dystonia is a condition in which muscle tone is abnormal without pyramidal involvement. In many dystonias, muscular tone varies with the position of the limbs. There may be a dystonic component to cerebral palsy of hypoxic–ischaemic origin, but there are a number of clearly defined syndromes in which dystonia is the main feature.

Torsion dystonia (dystonia musculorum deformans)

- Genetically determined
- Autosomal dominant with incomplete penetrance
- Gene maps to 9q34 in Jewish families
- Other unidentified gene responsible in some non-Jewish families
- Clinical characteristics:
  - Onset usually after 5 years
  - May be focal or generalized
  - Dystonia may be task-specific, for example, affected children may not be able to walk forwards but can walk backwards normally
  - Often has gradual spread to other parts of the body
  - Wilson disease should always be excluded
- Treatment:
  - High-dose anticholinergic drugs
  - Occasionally L-dopa

Dopa-responsive dystonia

- Described by Segawa
- Idiopathic dystonia
- Symptoms vary throughout the day

- Onset may be in the first 5 years
- Gene maps to 14q22.1-q22.2
- Symptoms respond dramatically to low-dose L-dopa, which should be continued for life

Other important causes of dystonia

- Wilson disease
- Juvenile Huntington disease

3.4 Tics, Tourette syndrome

Tics are involuntary movements affecting specific groups of muscles so that that the affected individual appears to have brief purposeless movements or actions. Tics may be motor or vocal.

Simple tics

- Commonly affect children for a few months in mid-childhood
- Up to 25% of children
- Spontaneous resolution

Multiple tics

- Some children are prone to tics of different types
- Different motor tics, vocal tics
- May not remit entirely

Tourette syndrome

This is defined by:

- Multiple motor tics
- One or more vocal tics
- Onset before 21 years of age
- Duration of > 1 year

There is probably a continuum between multiple tics and Tourette syndrome.

Other characteristic features of Tourette syndrome

- Echolalia (compulsive repetition of words or phrases just heard)
- Coprolalia (compulsive swearing)
- Attention-deficit disorder and obsessive compulsive features are present in 50%

Treatment

Tics may respond to haloperidol.

4. DEVELOPMENTAL DISABILITIES

4.1 Learning disability

The term 'learning disability' is now generally used in preference to the term mental retardation. It covers a wide variety of conditions in which cognitive functioning is depressed below average levels. In the United States, the term mental retardation is retained, with learning disability being used to refer to failure to achieve cognitive potential.

Learning disability tends to be grouped according to severity: moderate learning disability usually refers to IQ 50–70, with severe learning disability being defined as IQ <50. The term profound learning disability is sometimes used to refer to IQ <20.

The prevalence of learning disability is difficult to estimate. The prevalence of severe learning disability has been estimated at 3 to 4 per 1000 but although moderate learning disability is clearly more common, its exact prevalence remains obscure.

Aetiology

This is easier to determine in severe learning disability.

In **severe learning disability**, the following potential causes are recognized:

- Chromosomal
- Genetic
- Congenital anomalies
- Intrauterine insults
- Central nervous system infection
- Familial
- Unknown (20%)

In **moderate learning disability**, the following potential causes are recognized:

- Same range of problems as severe learning disability
- Unknown (55%)

Associated problems with learning disability

- Cerebral palsy
- Visual impairment
- Hearing impairment
- Behavioural difficulties

Baseline medical investigations for all children

- Full history and examination
- Karyotype, including a test for fragile X
- Thyroid function tests
- Plasma amino acids

- Urine mucopolysaccharide screen
- Plasma creatine kinase (in boys < 5 years)

Other tests may be indicated, depending on the clinical features.

4.2 Autism

Autism is a disorder characterized by:

- Disturbance of reciprocal social interaction
- Disturbance of communication (including language, comprehension and expression)
- Disturbance of behaviour, leading to restriction of behavioural range

All the above findings may be seen in learning disabled individuals.

See also Chapter 2 — Child Development, Child Psychiatry and Community Paediatrics, section 5.

Associated features in autism

- Learning disability
- Epilepsy
- Visual impairment
- Hearing impairment

Asperger syndrome

Often considered to be on the autistic spectrum. It is characterized by autistic features in individuals of otherwise normal intelligence. Specifically characterized by:

- Impairment in social interaction
- Stereotypic behaviour
- No specific impairment of language

4.3 Attention-deficit hyperactivity disorder

Some children show impulsive, hyperactive behaviour in conjunction with poor concentration and attention. These children are usually of normal intelligence, although functionally they may achieve less than their peers. Medication such as methylphenidate or dexamphetamine may be effective.

See also Chapter 2 — Child Development, Child Psychiatry and Community Paediatrics, section 8.

4.4 Deficits in attention, motor control and perception (DAMP)

- Often described as 'minimal brain damage' in the older literature
- Deficit in motor control and perception is often referred to as 'dyspraxia'
- Children have difficulties as described in varying degrees

- Treatment needs to include not only assessment but also educational help and a physical programme (occupational therapy)

5. EPILEPSY

5.1 Diagnosis

Diagnosis of 'fits, faints and funny turns' is based primarily on clinical assessment of such events with recognition of characteristic patterns, supported by the results of special investigations.

5.2 Definition and classification

Epileptic seizures are clinical events which result from abnormal, excessive electrical discharge from cerebral neurones.

Epilepsy is the tendency to have recurrent, usually unprovoked, epileptic seizures.

The classification of epilepsy can be approached from the viewpoint of the characteristics of individual seizures or by identification of epileptic syndromes.

International Classification of Epileptic Seizures (modified from the International League against Epilepsy Classification)

Partial seizures	Simple partial seizures (no disturbance of consciousness)	with motor signs with somatosensory symptoms with autonomic symptoms with psychic symptoms
	Complex partial seizures (disturbance of consciousness) Partial seizures with secondary generalization	
Generalized seizures	Absence seizures (typical and atypical) — myoclonic seizures — clonic seizures — tonic seizures — tonic–clonic seizures — atonic seizures	

Classification of epileptic syndromes

Localization related epilepsies	Idiopathic	Benign childhood epilepsy with centrotemporal spikes ('benign rolandic epilepsy') Childhood epilepsy with occipital paroxysms
	Symptomatic	Temporal lobe epilepsy Frontal lobe epilepsy Parietal lobe epilepsy Occipital lobe epilepsy Epilepsia partialis continua
Generalized epileptic syndromes	Idiopathic	Benign neonatal familial convulsions Benign neonatal convulsions Benign myoclonic epilepsy of infancy Childhood absence epilepsy Juvenile absence epilepsy Juvenile myoclonic epilepsy Epilepsy with grand mal seizures on wakening
	Symptomatic/cryptogenic	West syndrome (infantile spasms) Lennox–Gastaut syndrome Myoclonic–astatic epilepsy
	Symptomatic	Early myoclonic encephalopathy Ohtahara syndrome
Epileptic syndromes unclassified as focal or generalized		Neonatal seizures Severe myoclonic epilepsy in infancy Epilepsy with continuous spike-waves in slow-wave sleep Landau–Kleffner syndrome

5.3   Generalized epilepsies

Absence seizures

Typical absence seizures — previously termed petit mal epilepsy, are characterized by brief (5–20 seconds) episodes of staring during which the child is unaware of his surroundings. Associated with 3-Hz spike and wave discharge on electroencephalogram (EEG). Can be precipitated by hyperventilation. Drugs of choice are sodium valproate, ethosuximide, lamotrigine.

Atypical absences — EEG shows pattern of different frequency.

Myoclonic seizures

Brief sudden generalized muscular jerks. Drugs of choice are sodium valproate, benzodiazepines, lamotrigine. May be exacerbated by carbamazepine.

Infantile spasms

Onset in first 12 months. Brief sudden muscular contractions resulting in extension or flexion of the body. Attacks occur in runs. Associated with disorganized EEG described as hypsarrhythmia, as well as developmental arrest or regression. May be idiopathic or symptomatic (causes include tuberous sclerosis, perinatal hypoxic–ischaemic injury, inborn errors of metabolism). Treatment of choice is corticosteroids (or adrenocorticotropic hormone) or vigabatrin.

Juvenile myoclonic epilepsy

Onset in adolescence — myoclonic seizures on wakening from sleep. Treatment of choice is sodium valproate; carbamazepine may exacerbate seizures.

5.4 Partial epilepsies

Benign childhood epilepsy with centrotemporal spikes ('benign rolandic epilepsy')	Characterized by predominantly nocturnal partial seizures with a slight male preponderance. Seizures may affect face or upper limbs; speech arrest may occur. Excellent prognosis for remission.
Complex partial seizures	Characterized by stereotypic behaviour, loss of consciousness and focal EEG abnormalities. Often arise from temporal lobe foci. May respond to carbamazepine or sodium valproate.

5.5 Assessment and treatment of epilepsy

- Clinical assessment of seizure type and frequency
- EEG allows more specific classification of seizure type; if standard EEG is normal and further EEG confirmation is necessary in the face of clear clinical history of epileptic seizures, then sleep or sleep-deprived EEG may document abnormalities
- Imaging (MRI) is indicated in partial seizures and generalized seizures that are resistant to treatment

Management

- Explanation of potential risks and benefits of different therapies
- Medication — start, depending on frequency and number of seizures
- Maintenance of seizure freedom with medication for perhaps 2 years
- Subsequent withdrawal of medication

- Some forms of partial epilepsy may be amenable to epilepsy surgery — when seizure disorder is intractable — site of seizure onset can be localized — site is non-eloquent brain
- Other forms of treatment — steroids, ketogenic diet, vagal nerve stimulation

5.6 Anticonvulsant drugs

Drug	Used for seizure types	Dose range	Side-effects	Notes
Carbamazepine	Partial seizures Generalized tonic–clonic seizures	15–25 mg/kg per day	Ataxia, sedation, leukopenia, thrombocytopenia, rash	
Sodium valproate	All seizure types	20–40 mg/kg per day	Nausea, vomiting, abdominal pain, tremor, hair loss, thrombocytopenia, liver function abnormalities	
Lamotrigine	All seizure types	With valproate: 5 mg/kg per day Without valproate: 15 mg/kg per day	Rash	Not licensed as monotherapy for under 12 years
Vigabatrin	Partial seizures West's syndrome	50–150 mg/kg per day	Sedation, visual field constriction	
Ethosuximide	Absences	20–50 mg/kg per day	Gastrointestinal disturbance, rash	
Gabapentin	Partial seizures	Up to 45 mg/kg per day	Sedation	
Oxcarbazepine	Partial/generalized seizures	30 mg/kg per day	Sedation, rash	
Topiramate	All seizure types	6–9 mg/kg per day	Sedation, anorexia, paraesthesiae	
Clobazam	All seizure types	2 mg/kg per day	Sedation	
Clonazepam	All seizure types		Sedation	
Phenytoin	All seizure types	5 mg/kg per day	Nausea, vomiting, diarrhoea, rash, peripheral neuropathy	Measure level
Phenobarbital	All seizure types	5–8 mg/kg per day	Sedation	Measure level
Levetiracetam	Partial seizures		Sedation	Not licensed for under 16 years
Tiagabine	Partial seizures		Sedation	Not licensed for under 12 years

5.7 Management of status epilepticus

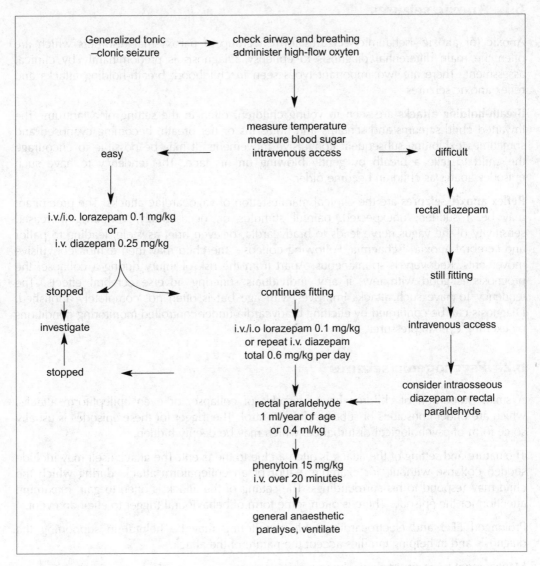

Generalized tonic –clonic seizure → check airway and breathing administer high-flow oxyten

measure temperature measure blood sugar intravenous access

easy ← → difficult

i.v./i.o. lorazepam 0.1 mg/kg or i.v. diazepam 0.25 mg/kg

rectal diazepam

still fitting

stopped — continues fitting — intravenous access

investigate

i.v./i.o lorazepam 0.1 mg/kg or repeat i.v. diazepam total 0.6 mg/kg per day

stopped ←

consider intraosseous diazepam or rectal paraldehyde

rectal paraldehyde 1 ml/year of age or 0.4 ml/kg ←

phenytoin 15 mg/kg i.v. over 20 minutes

general anaesthetic paralyse, ventilate

Prognosis

70% of children with epilepsy are seizure-free by their 16th birthday. Remission is less likely in: partial epilepsy, symptomatic epilepsy, some epilepsy syndromes such as juvenile myoclonic epilepsy or epileptic encephalopathies such as Lennox–Gastaut syndrome.

6. NON-EPILEPTIC SEIZURES

6.1 Anoxic seizures

Anoxic (or anoxic–ischaemic) seizures form a group of paroxysmal disorders which are often the main differential diagnosis to epilepsy. Diagnosis is predominantly by clinical assessment. There are two important types seen in childhood: breath-holding attacks and reflex anoxic seizures.

Breath-holding attacks are seen in young children, often in the setting of a tantrum. The thwarted child screams and screams and holds his or her breath, becoming cyanosed and sometimes exhibiting subsequent convulsive movements. It may be possible to encourage the child to take a breath by gently blowing on his face. The tendency to have such episodes abates as children become older.

Reflex anoxic seizures are the clinical manifestation of vagocardiac attacks. The precipitant may be a sudden, unexpected, painful stimulus or, occasionally, vomiting. Increased sensitivity of the vagus nerve leads to bradycardia, or even brief asystole, leading to pallor and cerebral anoxia–ischaemia. Following collapse, the child may then exhibit convulsive movements. Recovery is spontaneous. Apart from the risk of injury during a collapse, the prognosis is good with few, if any, individuals suffering adverse cerebral effects. The tendency to have such attacks improves with age but is often not completely abolished. Diagnosis can be confirmed by eliciting bradycardia under controlled monitoring conditions by exerting eyeball pressure.

6.2 Psychogenic seizures

A small proportion of children have episodes of collapse, or even epileptiform attacks, which are under conscious or subconscious control. The trigger for these episodes is usually some form of psychological disturbance, which may be deeply hidden.

The nature and setting of the attack is often a clue to the event. The attack itself may include sudden collapse without, for example, pallor or an epileptiform attack, during which the child may respond to his surroundings. The setting of the attack is often to gain maximum attention for the episode. There is often some form of behavioural trigger to elicit an event.

Prolonged EEG and electrocardiographic monitoring may be helpful in supporting the diagnosis and in helping families accept the nature of the attack.

Management is via psychological or psychiatric treatment.

7. HEADACHES

Headache is a common complaint in childhood. Population studies estimate that up to 35% of children have complained of headache at some time. The commonest cause of headache in Western populations is tension or psychogenic headache.

Classification of headache

Tension or psychogenic headache

Migraine

Vascular disorders	• Subarachnoid haemorrhage • Hypertension • Arteriovenous malformation
Headaches related to raised intra-cranial pressure	• Tumours • Hydrocephalus • Benign intracranial hypertension • Subdural haematomata
Inflammatory disorders	• Meningitis • Vasculitis
Referred pain	• Sinusitis • Optic neuritis • Otitis media
Miscellaneous	• Refractive errors • Carbon monoxide poisoning • Substance abuse

7.1   Tension headaches

- Often occur daily
- Generalized, dull — may involve band-like compression around head
- Worsens over the day
- Worse with stress
- Normal examination
- Anxious or depressed affect
- Depressive features in history

Management

- Reassurance
- Supportive psychotherapy

7.2 Migraine

Defined as 'familial disorder characterized by recurrent attacks of headache widely variable in intensity, frequency and duration. Attacks are commonly unilateral and are usually associated with neurological and mood disturbance. All of the above characteristics are not necessarily present in each attack or in each patient'.

Classification of migraine

- Common migraine (no aura)
- Classical migraine (aura preceding onset of headache)
- Complicated migraine (persisting neurological deficit after migraine attack)
- Basilar migraine
- Migraine variance
- Cluster headaches

Treatment

- **Acute** — analgesics, relaxation, occasionally antiemetics
- **Prophylaxis** — avoidance of triggers such as cheese, pizotifen, propranolol

7.3 Other headaches

Post-traumatic headache

Following concussive head injury. May last several months then resolve. May persist in the setting of depression or ongoing litigation.

Headache as a result of raised intracranial pressure

Worse in early morning. Worse with coughing and bending.

8. ABNORMALITIES OF HEAD SIZE AND SHAPE

Brain growth is usually the most important determinant of head growth. In full-term infants, the rate of head growth is 2 cm per month in the first 3 months, in the second 3 months it is 1 cm per month and in the subsequent 6 months it is 0.5 cm per month.

8.1 Macrocephaly

Consider

- Familial macrocephaly
- Hydrocephalus
- Chronic subdural haematomata
- Associated disorders such as tuberous sclerosis or neurofibromatosis
- Metabolic conditions

Investigations depend on rate of growth, deviation from normal and presence or absence of abnormal neurological signs.

Treatment

If necessary, this is based on the underlying pathology.

8.2   Microcephaly

Defined as occipitofrontal head circumference, below two standard deviations for age, sex and gestational age.

Consider

- Insults during pregnancy
- Perinatal insults
- Encephalopathies in infancy
- Autosomal recessive microcephaly

Investigations

- Chromosomes
- Antibodies to congenital infections
- Metabolic screen
- MRI scan
- Consider measurement of maternal plasma amino acids to exclude maternal phenylketonuria

8.3   Abnormal head shape

May be associated with a specific syndrome, e.g achondroplasia or Down syndrome. May be the result of craniosynostosis.

Craniosynostosis

Premature closure of one or more cranial sutures. Ultimate skull deformity will depend upon which sutures are involved and the timing of their fusion.

Head shape	Description	Sutures involved	Problems
Scaphocephaly	Elongated narrow skull	Sagittal	Cosmetic
Brachycephaly	Short, broad skull	Both coronal	Associated anomalies such as learning disability
Plagiocephaly	Unilateral flattening of skull	Single coronal (occasionally lambdoid)	Cosmetic
Trigonocephaly	Narrow, pointed forehead	Metopic	Possible associated forebrain abnormalities
Oxycephaly (acrocephaly)	High pointed head	Coronal, sagittal, lambdoid	Apert and Crouzon syndromes (see below)

Apert syndrome

Acrocephaly, facial underdevelopment, syndactyly, learning disability.

Crouzon syndrome

Acrocephaly, scaphocephaly or brachycephaly, hypertelorism, exophthalmos, increased intracranial pressure, learning disability.

9.   NEUROMUSCULAR DISORDERS

9.1   The floppy infant

It is important to realize that much of the process leading to a diagnosis in the floppy infant is the clinical assessment of the infant by history and examination. It is this assessment which should direct diagnostic investigations. In an era when specific genetic tests for conditions are increasingly available, a clearer idea of possible diagnoses is even more important.

Causes of hypotonia in infants

General health

- Prematurity
- Intercurrent illness
- Ligamentous laxity

General: neurological

- Chromosomal abnormalities
  e.g Down syndrome
- Prader–Willi syndrome
- Hypoxic–ischaemic brain injury
  (especially early basal ganglia injury)

- Metabolic conditions
  - aminoacidurias
  - organic acidurias
  - peroxisomal disorders

Muscle

- Congenital muscular dystrophy
- Congenital myopathies
- Congenital myotonic dystrophy

Spinal

- Cervical cord injury

Anterior horn cell

- Poliomyelitis
- Spinal muscular atrophy

Peripheral nerve

- Peripheral neuropathies

Neuromuscular junction

- Transient myasthenia
- Congenital myasthenic syndrome

9.2 Duchenne muscular dystrophy

Duchenne muscular dystrophy is easily the commonest neuromuscular condition seen in western European practice.

- Inherited as an X-linked recessive condition
- One-third are new mutations
- Incidence is 1 in 3500 male births
- Female carriers are usually asymptomatic, occasionally manifesting carriers

Molecular genetics

- Caused by mutations in the dystrophin gene
- Gene comprises approximately 2 million base pairs
- Duchenne muscular dystrophy patients produce no dystrophin
- Becker muscular dystrophy (allelic, milder form) patients produce abnormal but functional protein
- Dystrophin is localized to muscle cell membranes

Clinical features

- Onset in early years
- Some cases are identified presymptomatically by abnormal transaminases measured during intercurrent illness
- Sometimes leads to faltering growth
- Early delay in motor milestones
- Difficulties in climbing stairs
- Lordosis with waddling gait
- Pseudohypertrophy of calves
- Progressive muscular weakness
- Tendency to joint contractures
- Typically, boys lose ability to walk between 8 and 12 years
- When dependent on wheelchair, boys are prone to develop scoliosis
- Respiratory failure supervenes

Also

- Increased incidence of learning disability
- Cardiomyopathy occurs
- Survival to late teens, early twenties

Diagnosis

- High plasma creatine kinase (greater than 5000 IU/l)
- Mutations in dystrophin gene
- Muscle biopsy – dystrophic picture with absent dystrophin

Treatment

- There is no curative treatment
- Physiotherapy
- Appropriate seating
- Management of scoliosis
- Non-invasive respiratory support
- Corticosteroids improve muscular power, but it is unclear as to when, how and for how long they should be administered

9.3 Becker muscular dystrophy

- Allelic disease to Duchenne muscular dystrophy
- Milder than Duchenne muscular dystrophy
- Patients walk beyond 16 years of age
- Similar clinical pattern to Duchenne muscular dystrophy
- Cramps can be problematical ✗
- Prone to cardiomyopathy

Diagnosis

Duchenne and Becker muscular dystrophies are distinguished clinically and on muscle biopsy findings. Nature of genetic mutation can provide a pointer as to the severity of the condition but current routine genetic testing does not distinguish reliably between Duchenne muscular dystrophy and Becker muscular dystrophy; it just identifies a dystrophinopathy.

9.4   Other muscular dystrophies and congenital myopathies

Muscular dystrophies are characterized by dystrophic muscle histopathology: muscle fibre necrosis and regeneration with increased fat and connective tissue. May be progressive or static.

Emery–Dreifuss muscular dystrophy

- Uncommon X-linked muscular dystrophy (Xq28)
- Mild proximal muscular weakness
- Joint contractures
- Cardiac involvement — affected individuals may be prone to sudden cardiac death

Fascio-scapulohumeral muscular dystrophy

- Autosomal dominant muscular dystrophy (4q35)
- Facial, scapular and humeral wasting and weakness
- Slowly progressive
- Other muscles may be involved
- Variable expression within families

Limb-girdle muscular dystrophies

- Common on a world-wide basis
- May be inherited as autosomal dominant or autosomal recessive traits (at least three separate autosomal dominant and nine autosomal recessive limb-girdle muscular dystrophies have been identified so far)
- Variations in clinical phenotype
- Many are similar to Duchenne muscular dystrophy or Becker muscular dystrophy

Congenital muscular dystrophies

This is a group of disorders in infants characterized by muscular weakness, hypotonia and joint contractures from birth.

- Muscle biopsy shows typical dystrophic changes
- Different subtypes now being described

Merosin-negative congenital muscular dystrophy

- Characterized by absence of merosin on muscle biopsy
- Clinically hypotonia, weakness, contractures
- Often associated with learning disability
- Functionally, affected children do not achieve independent walking
- Autosomal recessive (6p2)

Merosin-positive congenital muscular dystrophy

- Clinically less severe than merosin-negative congenital muscular dystrophy

Fukuyama congenital muscular dystrophy

- Autosomal recessive (9q31–q33)
- As well as severe weakness, affected individuals have brain malformations

Congenital myopathies

A group of disorders characterized by hypotonia and weakness from birth. Differentiated on clinical and histological features.

- Central cord disease
- Nemaline myopathy
- Myotubular myopathy

Myotonic dystrophy

- Common (incidence 13.5 per 100,000 live births) neuromuscular condition
- Autosomal dominant inheritance (19q13)
- Severity appears to be related to size of triplet repeat (CTG) in gene mutation

Congenital myotonic dystrophy

- Condition often unrecognized in mothers
- Preceding polyhydramnios
- Baby often born unexpectedly 'flat'
- Facial weakness, hypotonia
- Often requires respiratory support
- Joint contractures, especially talipes

Myotonic dystrophy in older children and adults

- Facial weakness initially
- Then weakness affecting temporalis, sternomastoid, distal leg muscles
- Progressive weakness
- Difficulties in relaxing muscular contraction, e.g. difficulties in relaxing grip
- Cardiac involvement

Diagnosis

- Gene mutation analysis
- Electromyogram in older children upwards (>3 to 4 years of age) shows characteristic 'dive bomber' discharges

Myotonia congenita (Thomsen disease)

- Rare
- Autosomal dominant inheritance
- Characterized by myotonia, cramps
- Muscular hypertrophy is typical

9.5 Anterior horn cell disease

Spinal muscular atrophy

The spinal muscular atrophies are a group of heterogeneous conditions which are characterized by the clinical effects of anterior horn cell degeneration. The commonest in childhood are the autosomal recessive proximal spinal muscular atrophies.

Clinical

- Symmetrical muscle weakness of trunk and limbs, more marked proximally than distally and in legs more than arms
- Tongue fasciculation
- Investigations confirming neurogenic abnormalities

Genetics

- Autosomal recessive
- Gene at chromosome 5q11-13
- Disease caused by mutations of the *SMN* gene
- Severity-determining mechanism remains unclear

Childhood onset proximal spinal muscular atrophies

Severity	Synonyms	Functional abilities
Severe	Type I, acute, Werdnig–Hoffmann disease	Unable to sit or walk
Intermediate	Type II	Able to sit but not walk
Mild	Type III, Kugelberg–Welander disease	Able to walk

Severe spinal muscular atrophy

- Incidence 1 in 20,000 live births
- In approximately 30% onset is prenatal
- Symmetrical weakness
- Paralysis of intercostal muscles
- Absent deep tendon reflexes
- Tongue fasciculation
- Death occurs within first 18 months from respiratory failure/infection

Diagnosis

- Electromyography
- Muscle biopsy
- Genetic analysis

Intermediate spinal muscular atrophy

- Autosomal recessive
- Usual onset after 3 months
- Infant learns to sit
- Prone to early scoliosis
- Prognosis depends on degree of respiratory muscle involvement

Mild spinal muscular atrophy

- Autosomal recessive
- Able to walk, but proximal weakness is evident
- Tendon jerks may not be absent

9.6   Neuropathies

Hereditary motor and sensory neuropathies are the most common degenerative disorders of the peripheral nervous system. Often known by their eponymous title Charcot–Marie–Tooth disease or peroneal muscular atrophy.

Previously X-linked, autosomal recessive and autosomal dominant forms were recognized, but the advent of molecular genetics has identified numerous genetically distinct forms (see table below).

Clinically, affected individuals develop slowly progressive distal weakness with areflexia. In the early phases, foot drop is often the main clinical problem. In later stages, which in the common forms may be several decades after onset, hand weakness, joint deformity and distal sensory loss may be problematic.

Hereditary motor and sensory neuropathies (Charcot–Marie–Tooth disease)

Type	Inheritance	Genetic defect	Gene	Neurophysiology	Onset
Type I (Demyelinating)					
CMT 1A	AD	Duplication 17p11.2	PMp22	Low motor nerve conduction velocity	First decade
CMT 1B	AD	1q21-q23	PO		
CMT 1C	AD	?	?		
CMT 4	AR	8q (one type)	?		
Type II (Axonal)					
CMT 2A	AD	1p36	?	Normal motor nerve conduction velocity	Second to third decade
CMT 2B	AR	3q13-q22	?		
Type III (Hypertrophic)					
Déjerine–Sottas AD		17p11.2	PMP22	Low motor conduction velocity	First year
		1q21-q23	PO		
X-linked forms					
CMTX	XL	Xq13	connexin 32		

Hereditary motor and sensory neuropathies and Friedreich's ataxia are sometimes confused. In the hereditary motor and sensory neuropathies, there is areflexia and evidence of distal weakness. In Friedreich's ataxia is there much clearer ataxia with evidence of loss of joint position sense. On neurophysiological testing, the patients with hereditary motor and sensory neuropathy have abnormal motor conduction, whereas Friedreaich's ataxia patients have evidence of a sensory neuropathy.

9.7 Acute neuromuscular disorders

Guillain–Barré syndrome

An acute demyelinating disease of peripheral nerves characterized by progressive weakness.

- Usually follows viral infection or immunization
- Numerous other infections, including *Campylobacter jejuni* gastroenteritis, have been implicated

Clinical features

- Sudden onset of weakness, usually affecting lower limbs
- Ascending paralysis
- Usually symmetrical weakness
- Pain often a prominent feature
- Sensory involvement in about 50%
- Respiratory muscle weakness may occur

Diagnosis

- High CSF protein
- A marked slowing of motor neurone conduction velocity
- Conduction block

Course

- Deterioration over the first 10–20 days
- Plateau
- Recovery
- Mortality is 2–3% in children

Treatment

- Symptomatic
- Respiratory support
- Plasma exchange
- High-dose immunoglobulin

Juvenile dermatomyositis

A systemic illness affecting primarily the skin, muscles and gastrointestinal tract.

Unlike adult dermatomyositis, juvenile dermatomyositis is not associated with malignancy.

Clinical

- Age of onset between 5 and 10 years
- May present with fever, muscle pain
- Onset can be insidious
- Increasing muscular weakness, mainly proximal
- Rash involving upper eyelids (heliotrope rash) and periorbital region develops
- Rash on extensor surfaces. Calcinosis is a feature
- May have difficulty swallowing
- Children are often miserable in advance of other symptoms

Diagnosis

- Creatine kinase may or may not be raised
- Muscle biopsy may show perifascicular atrophy, but changes can be patchy

Treatment

- Corticosteroids
- Other immunosuppressive treatment such as methotrexate or cyclosporin

9.8 Disorders of neuromuscular junction

Myasthenia gravis

- Commonest disease of neuromuscular junction
- Caused by antibodies directed against postsynaptic acetylcholine receptors

Clinical features

- Onset after 1 year
- Adolescent girls most commonly affected
- Generalized form affects extraocular muscles first
- Then goes on to affect proximal limbs and bulbar muscles
- Variable natural course

Diagnosis

- Edrophonium test
- Electromyography confirming neuromuscular block
- Demonstration of anti-acetylcholine receptor antibodies

Treatment

- Anticholinesterase drugs
- Immunosuppressants
- Thymectomy
- Plasma exchange or immunoglobulin infusion acutely

Other myasthenic syndromes

There are rare congenital myasthenic syndromes which result from specific defects in the process of neuromuscular transmission. Some affect presynaptic mechanisms, other affect postsynaptic components. Some of these infants may have joint contractures.

10. CENTRAL NERVOUS SYSTEM INFECTIONS AND PARAINFECTIOUS DISORDERS

10.1 Meningitis

Acute bacterial meningitis remains an important cause of neurological morbidity in childhood. Causative organisms vary depending on the age of the child. The pattern of infection has been altered by changing immunization patterns.

Age	Organism
Neonatal	Group B streptococcus
	Escherichia coli
	Listeria monocytogenes
	Staphylococcus aureus
First 2 months	Group B streptococcus
	Escherichia coli
	Haemophilus influenzae
	Streptococcus pneumoniae
Older infants and	*Haemophilus influenzae*
young children	*Neisseria meningitidis*
	Streptococcus pneumoniae

Clinical features

- In neonates meningitis is usually part of a septicaemic illness. Symptoms and signs may be non-specific, e.g. lethargy, poor feeding, respiratory distress. Neck stiffness is rarely seen
- In young infants also, signs may be non-specific and meningeal irritation may be absent
- In older children, signs are more typical — lethargy, headache, photophobia, neck stiffness. Meningococcaemia is associated with a haemorrhagic rash

Outcome

- Neurological sequelae may occur in up to 30% of children — focal neurological deficits, learning disability, hydrocephalus and deafness may all occur
- Mortality is improving with earlier diagnosis and treatment

Diagnosis

- Lumbar puncture and CSF analysis are definitive
- White cell count is raised with a predominance of neutrophils, CSF glucose is reduced and protein is raised
- Gram staining of CSF and immunoassays may allow identification of the organism
- Lumbar puncture is contraindicated if there are signs of raised intracranial pressure or if consciousness is impaired. Treatment then needs to be aimed at the most likely organisms. Blood cultures can be taken before starting treatment

Management

- Antibiotic treatment — agent will depend on age of patient and probable infecting organism
- Watch for subdural effusions and hydrocephalus — measure head circumference
- Evidence concerning steroid use to prevent neurological sequelae is unclear — some evidence to support the prevention of deafness in *Haemophilus influenzae* meningitis

Viral meningitis may result from a wide variety of viruses: coxsackievirus, echoviruses, and mumps, measles, herpes simplex, poliomyelitis and varicella zoster viruses.

- Symptoms similar to bacterial meningitis, but less pronounced
- Specific diagnosis may be suggested by other disease stigmata
- CSF clear with lymphocytosis
- Prognosis of uncomplicated viral meningitis is good

Tuberculous meningitis

Generally occurs within 6–8 weeks of primary pulmonary infection or during miliary tuberculosis (TB). Commonest in age range 6 months to 3 years.

Leads to basal arteritis, which may cause hydrocephalus and cranial neuropathies. Symptoms otherwise are often non-specific, lethargy, fever, headache.

CSF — high white cell count, predominantly lymphocytes, raised protein often > 2 g/l, low glucose, tuberculous cultures may be positive.

Treatment

- Antituberculous chemotherapy
- Optimal treatment not determined
- Usually triple therapy (rifampicin, isoniazid, pyrazinamide) for at least 6 months but many authorities suggest a fourth drug for the first 2 months
- The place of corticosteriods in treatment is unclear but these are often used in the first few months to reduce inflammation

Mortality and morbidity remain high despite treatment.

10.2   Encephalitis

Numerous viruses may lead to inflammation of the brain: herpes viruses, adenoviruses, arboviruses and enteroviruses for example. The underlying causative agent in undiagnosed encephalitis may remain obscure. It is therefore usual practice to treat with cefotaxime/ceftriaxone, aciclovir and erythromycin/azithromycin until results are available.

- Clinical features — confusion, coma, seizures, motor abnormalities
- Infection usually starts to resolve 7–14 days after the onset. However, recovery may be delayed for several months

Herpes simplex encephalitis

- Common
- Often focal brain inflammation, located in temporal lobes
- High mortality, high morbidity (50%)
- Specific treatment: aciclovir

Investigations for encephalitis

- CSF examination/cultures
- Electroencephalogram
- Brain imaging
- Occasionally, brain biopsy

Treatment

- Supportive (fluid management/ventilation if necessary)
- Aciclovir

10.3   Immune-mediated and other infectious disorders

Sydenham's chorea

- Main neurological feature of rheumatic fever
- Chorea results from immune reaction triggered by Group A streptococcal infection
- May be associated with emotional lability
- Probably overlaps with PANDAS (psychiatric and neurological diseases associated with streptococcal infection)
- In about 75% of cases the chorea resolves within 6 months

Subacute sclerosing panencephalitis

A slow viral infection, caused by an atypical response to measles infection. Exposure to measles virus is usually in the first 2 years. Risk is higher after contracting natural measles, compared with that after measles immunization. Median interval between measles and subacute sclerosing panencephalitis is 8 years.

- Subtle deficits initially
- Increasing memory difficulties
- Worsening disabilities — seizures, motor difficulties, learning disability

Mycoplasma encephalitis

Mycoplasma pneumoniae is the commonest cause of community-acquired pneumonia in adults and commonly leads to infection in the paediatric age range. It may cause encephalitis, predominantly through immune-mediated mechanisms which may respond to steroid administration. The evidence base is small.

Acquired immune deficiency syndrome

Caused by human immunodeficiency virus, an RNA retrovirus which eventually leads to the death of its host cell CD4-positive T lymphocyte.

Neurological features include:

- Neurological features of opportunistic infection such as meningitis or encephalitis
- Dementia

11. CEREBROVASCULAR DISEASE

11.1 Arterial occlusion

May result from embolism or thrombosis.

Effects of arterial occlusion

Internal carotid artery	Hemiplegia, hemianopia, aphasia if dominant hemisphere
Middle cerebral artery	Hemiplegia with upper limb predominance, hemianopia, aphasia if dominant hemisphere
Anterior cerebral artery	Hemiplegia affecting predominantly lower limbs
Posterior cerebral artery	Homonymous hemianopia, ataxia, hemiparesis, vertigo

Investigations
MRI
MR angiography
Possible formal angiography
Carotid Doppler studies
Echocardiography
Full blood count, plasma homocysteine
Clotting studies, especially factor V Leiden, prothrombin 20210A, lipoprotein(a)

The place of measurement of antithrombin III protein C and protein S in the genesis of childhood stroke remains controversial.

11.2 Venous thrombosis

- Less common than arterial occlusion
- Produces a variable clinical picture
  - Intracranial hypertension
  - Seizures
  - Focal neurological signs

Causes

- Sepsis
  - Otitis media
  - Sinusitis
  - Cutaneous infection
- Dehydration
- Coagulopathy

Treatment

- Disputed
- Heparin may be given in the acute phase

12. NEURO-ONCOLOGY

Brain tumours are the second commonest malignancy in children after leukaemia. In infants, supratentorial tumours predominate, whereas in older children, infratentorial tumours are much more common. The trend reverses in children over 8 years of age with a slight preponderance of supratentorial tumours.

Central nervous system tumours are of varying degrees of malignancy. Those which do metastasize tend to do so within the central nervous system. It is also important to note that a 'benign' tumour situated so that it cannot be removed may have a more serious effect than a 'malignant' tumour that is differently situated.

General symptoms and signs associated with brain tumours in children may include headache, vomiting, papilloedema, cranial nerve palsies, and other focal symptoms such as ataxia.

12.1 Posterior fossa tumours

Cerebellar astrocytoma

The commonest tumour in children; may involve vermis, cerebellar hemispheres or both. Majority are cystic, slow growing.

- Treatment — surgical. Occasionally more malignant tumours require radiotherapy also.

Medulloblastoma

A common tumour. Highly malignant, rapidly growing. Arises from the cerebellar vermis. Often leads to hydrocephalus. May metastasize along CSF pathways. Often solid tumours.

- Treatment — surgery and radiotherapy. Trials have sought to clarify the position of chemotherapy
- Outlook has improved — 75% 5-year survival, 50% 10-year survival. Prognosis is poorer in young children. Evidence is emerging that the specific genetic constitution of tumour is most important in determining outcome

Ependymoma

6–10% of childhood tumours. Arises from fourth ventricle. May lead to hydrocephalus and may metastasize.

- Treatment — surgical resection and radiotherapy
- Poor five-year survival often related to localization of tumour

	Percentage total tumours in childhood	Spread	Location	Structure	Treatment	Five-year survival
Astrocytoma	14–20	Local	Vermis cerebellar hemispheres	Cystic	Surgery	c 100%
Medulloblastoma	14–20	CSF pathways	Vermis	Usually solid	Surgery radiotherapy/ chemotherapy	75%
Ependymoma	6–10	CSF pathways	Floor fourth ventricle	May be cystic	Surgery/ radiotherapy	40%

12.2 Brainstem tumours

Brainstem gliomas, which may vary in their degree of malignancy, form approximately 15% of brain tumours in childhood. Peak incidence is 5–9 years of age. Present with multiple cranial nerve palsies plus long tract signs. Vomiting may be a feature.

- Treatment — radiotherapy
- Survival — poor

12.3 Supratentorial tumours

Cerebral astrocytomas

- Presentation depends on location
- Often leads to seizures
- Low-grade astrocytomas (benign) — more common in children
- High-grade astrocytomas — fortunately, more rare

Ependymoma

- 30–40% of ependymomas are supratentorial
- These are more malignant than their infratentorial counterparts
- They have a tendency to metastasize and so prognosis is poor

Optic gliomas

- One-third are prechiasmatic, two-thirds are chiasmatic or postchiasmatic
- Generally, these tumours are pilocytic astrocytomas. One-quarter occur in the setting of neurofibromatosis type 1

- Clinical presentation — prechiasmatic lesions may present late with proptosis with associated visual loss. Postchiasmatic lesions lead to visual loss
- Treatment — controversial. Often conservative, but surgery and radiotherapy may be indicated

Craniopharyngioma

Tumour arises from small aggregates of cells which are remnants of Rathke's pouch. Tumour is either suprasellar or suprasellar and intrasellar. Often cystic.

Clinical features related to:

- Endocrine disturbance:
  - Delayed growth
  - Hypothyroidism
  - Diabetes insipidus
- Raised intracranial pressure:
  - Headache
  - Ataxia
- Local features:
  - Visual disturbance (bitemporal hemianopia)
  - Depressed consciousness
  - Vomiting
  - Nystagmus

Investigations

- Skull X-ray may show erosion of dorsum sellae, also calcification
- MRI scan will delineate lesion better
- Also, endocrine investigations and visual field mapping

Treatment

- Controversial
- Surgery
- Radiotherapy

13. NEUROCUTANEOUS SYNDROMES

Neurocutaneous syndromes form a group of unrelated disorders in which skin and neurological features coexist. Most are genetically determined.

13.1 Neurofibromatosis

Neurofibromatoses are predominantly inherited disorders.

Neurofibromatosis type 1

Gene is localized to chromosome 17q11.2.

Diagnostic criteria (two or more are necessary for diagnosis):

- Six or more café-au-lait spots > 5 mm in diameter in prepubertal patients and > 15 mm in postpubertal patients
- Two or more neurofibromas or one plexiform neurofibroma
- Axillary or inguinal freckling
- Optic glioma
- Two or more iris hamartomas (Lisch nodules)
- Typical osseous lesions such as sphenoid dysplasia
- First-degree relative affected

Neurological manifestations

- Macrocephaly
- Learning disability
- Epilepsy
- Optic gliomas

Neurofibromatosis type 2

Gene is localized to chromosome 22q11.2.

Diagnostic criteria

- Bilateral VIIIth nerve neurofibromas
- Unilateral VIIIth nerve mass in association with any two of the following:
  - meningioma, neurofibroma, schwannoma, juvenile posterior capsular cataracts
- Unilateral VIIIth nerve tumour or other spinal or brain tumour as above in first-degree relative

13.2 Tuberous sclerosis

Dominantly inherited disorder with variable expression. Characterized by skin and central nervous system abnormalities, although there may be cardiac, renal and bony abnormalities as well. At least two mutant genes on chromosomes 9p34 (*TSC1*) and 16p13 (*TSC2*).

Clinical features

- Seizures
- Neurodevelopmental impairment
- Cutaneous manifestations
  - Adenoma sebaceum
  - Periungual fibromata
  - Hypopigmented patches
  - Shagreen patch

- Retinal hamartomas
- Renal angiolipomatas
- Cardiac rhabdomyomata

Brain imaging may reveal cortical tubers, subependymal nodules with calcification.

13.3   Other neurocutaneous disorders

Ataxia-telangiectasia

Characterized by conjunctival telangiectasia, progressive cerebellar degeneration and immunological impairment. Multisystem disease with autosomal recessive inheritance. Responsible gene, at least in some families, is mapped to chromosome 11q22-23.

Clinical features

- Progressive ataxia
- Scleral telangiectasia
- Abnormalities of cell-mediated and humoral immunity leading to increased sinopulmonary infections and high incidence of reticuloendothelial malignancies in later life

Diagnosis

- Elevated α-fetoprotein level
- Reduced IgA
- Reduced IgD
- Inversions and translocations involving chromosomes 7 and 14
- Gene mutation analysis

Sturge–Weber syndrome

Characterized by port wine stain, facial naevus and ipsilateral leptomeningeal angioma which leads to ischaemic injury to the underlying cerebral cortex leading to focal seizures, hemiparesis and variable degrees of intellectual deficit.

Incontinentia pigmenti

- Rare
- Probably inherited as X-linked dominant
- Characterized by skin lesions — initially erythematous, papular, vesicular or bullous lesions on trunk and limbs, then pustular lesions, then pigmented lesions
- 30–50% of neurological features:
  - seizures
  - encephalopathy
- Eye lesions in 30%

Hypomelanosis of Ito

- Also rare
- Sporadic inheritance
- Hypopigmented areas
- Central nervous system involement common including seizures, hemimegalencephaly

14. NEUROMETABOLIC DISEASES

Disorders of the intermediary metabolism form a huge group of heterogeneous conditions which have effects on the nervous sytem of different natures and severities.

14.1 Amino and organic acid disorders

Phenylketonuria (PKU)

See Chapter 15 — Metabolic Medicine, Section 3.1.

Branched chain amino acid disorders

See Chapter 15 — Metabolic Medicine, Section 3.3.

Glutaric aciduria type I

- Inborn error of lysine and tryptophan catabolism
- Leads to extrapyramidal syndrome
- Initially, children may develop normally
- May be hypotonic or irritable
- Chronic subdural haematomata may be present
- Acute neurological deterioration occurs
- Brain imaging shows striatal changes

Canavan disease

- *n*-Acetylaspartic aciduria
- Autosomal recessive (17p13-ter)
- Leads to spongy degeneration of the subcortical white matter
- Progressive neurological impairment occurs
- Death in first decade

14.2 Neurotransmitter disorders

Non-ketotic hyperglycinaemia

- Autosomal recessive
- Glycine accumulates in body fluids
- Neuropathology — identifies poor myelination

- Clinical
  - Poor respiratory effort at birth
  - Hypotonia
  - Gradual improvement over first week
  - Evolution of myoclonic encephalopathy
- Severe seizure disorder and major developmental delay ensues

14.3   Mitochondrial disease

Respiratory chain disorders

Abnormalities of mitochondrial energy production produce a variety of clinical syndromes, many of which have significant neurological features.

Potential clinical features of respiratory chain disorders

- Lactic acidosis
- Faltering growth
- Progressive external ophthalmoplegia
- Myopathy
- Seizures
- Dementia
- Movement disorders
- Cardiomyopathy
- Retinopathy
- Deafness

Specific syndromes	
Kearns–Sayre syndrome	Progressive external ophthalmoplegia, heart block, cerebellar dysfunction
MERRF	Myoclonic epilepsy with ragged red fibres (on muscle biopsy)
MELAS	Mitochondrial myopathy, encephalopathy, lactic acidosis and stroke-like episodes
Leigh disease	Subacute necrotizing encephalopathy — hypotonia, progressive deterioration in neurological abilities
Alpers disease	Grey matter disease — seizures are a prominent feature; liver abnormalities are seen, often late in the course of disease

14.4 Abnormalities of copper metabolism

Wilson disease

- Autosomal recessive
- Excessive accumulation of copper in nervous system and liver as a result of a lack of binding globulin (caeruloplasmin)
- Approximately 30% present with neurological symptoms alone, one-third with central nervous sytem and liver changes
- Leads to movement disorder which may include dystonia, rigidity, chorea and which may also be characterized by intellectual deterioration and behavioural lability
- Diagnosis by biochemical means
- Treatment — copper chelation therapy with penicillamine

Menkes disease (Kinky hair disease)

- Uncommon X-linked disorder
- Low serum copper and caeruloplasmin
- Gene maps to Xq13.3

Clinical

- Onset in the neonatal period or early infancy
- Hypothermia, poor weight gain
- Hair is sparse, brittle
- Progressive cerebral infarction occurs leading to seizures and neurological impairment
- Diagnosis is confirmed by biochemical or genetic means or by hair examination
- Death in first 2 years

14.5 Storage disorders

In these conditions, an enzymatic block leads to accumulation of products of cellular metabolism in the nervous system.

Sphingolipidoses

These are lysosomal diseases involving disorders of the sphingolipid metabolism. Sphingolipids are important components of central nervous system membranes. See Chapter 15 — Metabolic Medicine, Section 12.

- **GM$_2$ gangliosidosis (Tay–Sachs disease)** — neurodegenerative, onset 3–9 months, startles, seizures, blindness
- **Gaucher disease** — types 2 and 3 have neurological involvement: hypotonia, progressive deterioration, hepatosplenomegaly
- **Niemann–Pick disease** — types A and C have neurological involvement leading to progressive deterioration
- **Fabry disease** — presents with painful hands and feet. May run a slow progressive course with renal involvement

Mucopolysaccharidoses

These are disorders characterized by accumulation of mucopolysaccharides or glycosaminoglycans in lysosomes. There are numerous different types. See Chapter 15 — Metabolic Medicine, Section 11.

- **Hurler disease** (MPS 1H) — characteristic facies, marked dwarfism, corneal clouding, neurological involvement progressive. Hydrocephalus may ensue
- **Sanfilippo disease** (MPS III) — typical mucopolysaccharidosis features may be mild. However, severe neurological involvement with intellectual deterioration and seizures

Peroxisomal disorders

See Chapter 15 — Metabolic Medicine, Section 10.

Zellweger syndrome

- Presents in the neonatal period
- High forehead, patent fontanelles. Severe hypotonia and poor sucking or swallowing
- Very poor subsequent neurological development
- Often associated with cerebral gyral abnormalities

X-linked adrenoleukodystrophy

- Relatively common disease which involves the central nervous system and adrenal glands
- Over half present with central nervous system features. This group present at 4–8 years with cognitive decline and progressive gait disturbance
- Brain imaging shows leukodystrophy
- Levels of very-long-chain fatty acids (VLCFAs) are elevated

14.6 Leukodystrophies and other neurodegenerative disorders

Leukodystrophies are degenerative disorders which affect the white matter of the brain through abnormalities of myelin. In some, the metabolic features are known, in others the diagnosis is based on clinical features.

Leukodystrophies

- With known metabolic defect
  - Metachromatic leukodystrophy
  - Krabbe leukodystrophy
  - Adrenal leukodystrophy
  - Canavan disease (see Section 14.1 above)
- Without recognized metabolic defect
  - Pelizaeus–Merzbacher disease
  - Cockayne disease
  - Alexander disease
  - Leukodystrophy with subcortical cysts
  - Leukodystrophy with vanishing white matter

Grey matter disorders

Neuronal ceroid-lipofuscinoses (Batten disease)
These disorders are characterized by storage of pigments which are similar to ceroid and lipofuscin. Although originally thought to be related, genetic analysis has shown them to be separate disorders.

The neuronal ceroid-lipofuscinoses

Disease	Onset	Clinical features	Course
Infantile NCL	8–18 months	Myoclonus, ataxia, extrapyramidal features, visual impairment slight	Death in first 5 years
Late infantile NCL	18 months to 4 years	Epilepsy, marked ataxia, late visual deficit	Death 5–15 years
Juvenile NCL	4–7 years	Visual failure, later dementia	Death 15–30 years
Adult NCL	Adulthood	Slow cognitive decline, normal vision	Slow

Rett syndrome
A syndrome of dementia, autistic behaviour and motor stereotypes seen in girls.

Classical clinical features include:

- Normal perinatal period and normal first year
- Deceleration of head growth from around 9 months
- Loss of neurological skills
- Hand wringing
- Hyperventilation
- Gait apraxia
- May develop scoliosis

Diagnosis was clinical but is now by mutation analysis of *MeCP2* gene (Xq28).

Mutation analysis has shown that mutations in this gene lead to severe neonatal encephalopathy in boys.

Angelman's syndrome
Previously known as 'happy puppet' syndrome, this syndrome is caused by the deletion of chromosome 15q11.2-12, which is maternally inherited. Deletion includes the gene for β3 subunit of GABA receptor.

Clinical features include:

- Severe learning disability
- Ataxia
- Jerky movements
- Seizures
- Often cheerful demeanour

15. HEAD INJURY

It has been estimated that one in ten children suffer a head injury severe enough to impair consciousness. Boys outnumber girls by 2–3 to 1. The overall incidence of head injury is 2–3 per 1000 population. Around 5% are severe (Glasgow Coma Scale ≤ 8), 5–10% are moderate (Glasgow Coma Scale 9–12) and 85–90% are minor.

15.1   Mild closed head injury

Clinical features

- Impaired consciousness
- Lethargy
- Crying
- Vomiting
- Ataxia

Develops immediately or within 6–8 h of injury. There is usually complete resolution of symptoms within 24 h of the injury.

15.2   Severe closed head injury

Characterized by major loss of consciousness which is deeper and persists longer than in milder head injury. The greatest neurological deficit usually occurs immediately after the injury. Injuries may be the result of:

- Primary trauma to brain
- Secondary changes as a result of inflammation and ischaemia

Paediatric Glasgow Coma Scale

Eye opening (E)	Spontaneous	4
	To speech	3
	To pain	2
	None	1
Best verbal response (V)	Oriented	5
	Words	4
	Inappropriate sounds	3
	Vocalization	3
	Cries	2
	None	1
Best motor response (M)	Obeys command	6
	Localizes pain	5
	Withdraws to pain	4
	Abnormal flexion to pain	3
	Abnormal extension to pain	2
	None	1

Clinical assessment

- Level of consciousness
- Respiratory pattern
- Pupil size and reaction
- Brainstem signs
- Leakage of cerebrospinal fluid
- Focal signs
- Consider potential of cervical spine fracture

Management

- Airway, breathing, circulation
- X-ray cervical spine
- Assess intracranial pressure
- CT scan
- Fluid restriction
- After first 4–5 days — supportive care

Late complications

- Learning disability (global and specific)
- Behavioural disturbance
- Motor deficits
- Post-traumatic epilepsy
- Headaches

15.3   Non-accidental head injury

The incidence of non-accidental head injury is unknown but most estimates almost certainly under-diagnose the problem. Non-accidental head injury may include blunt trauma, sometimes leading to skull fracture, and the so-called shaken (or shaken-impact) baby syndrome.

Clinical features of 'shaken baby syndrome'

- Peak incidence is 5 months of age
- History inconsistent with severity of injury
- Baby presents shocked, possibly apnoeic, following apparent sudden spontaneous collapse at home
- Impaired consciousness
- Shocked
- Irregular breathing
- Retinal haemorrhages
- Possible bruising on arms or trunk
- Brain imaging identifies acute and/or chronic intracranial bleeding with brain swelling
- There may be signs of other non-accidental injury

Mechanism

- Unclear
- Cerebral parenchyma may be damaged by blunt trauma
- Recent evidence suggests brainstem injury leading to apnoea and ischaemic injury

Prognosis

- Non-accidental head injury may lead to death
- Prognosis for neurological recovery is guarded

16.   SPECIFIC NEUROLOGICAL LESIONS

16.1   Cranial nerve lesions

Facial nerve paralysis

Symptoms and signs will depend on the location of the lesion in the course of the nerve with potential abnormalities of taste, lachrymation and salivation as well as hyperacusis.

Congenital facial paralysis

- May be the result of birth trauma or prenatal compression
- May also be non-traumatic as the result of anomalies of nerve and nerve cell body

Moebius syndrome

- Bilateral facial paralysis with bilateral abducens paralysis
- Other lower cranial nerves may be affected
- Up to one-quarter have learning disability

Acquired facial palsy (Bell's palsy)

- Acute, usually idiopathic, paralysis which is unilateral
- Weakness maximal for 2–4 weeks
- Complete recovery is usual
- Steroids often given, but no evidence to support their use

Other facial paralyses

- Lyme disease
- Otitis media/mastoiditis
- Hypertension

Lower cranial nerve palsies (VII–XII)

- Congenital — often present in Chiari I and II malformations

16.2   Disorders of eye movement

Acquired ophthalmoplegia

IIIrd nerve palsy

- Common
- Most frequently the result of closed head trauma, infections and tumours

IVth nerve palsy

- Traumatic

VIth nerve palsy

- The result of raised intracranial pressure:
  - Tumours
  - Benign intracranial hypertension

Congenital ophthalmoplegia

- Can affect all the above nerves

Nystagmus

- Involuntary, rhythmical, conjugate, oscillatory movements of the eyes which may occur in any plane
- Results from dysfunction of complex mechanisms that maintain ocular fixation

Type	Cause
Pendular	Congenital
	Acquired – disease of brainstem/cerebellum
Horizontal jerk:	
Vestibular	End organ
Gaze evoked	Posterior fossa
Rotary	Vestibular or medullary lesions

Differential diagnosis

- Roving eye movements of blind children
- Opsoclonus

16.3   Unequal pupils

- May be the result of physiological anisocoria
- Establish which pupil is abnormal
- Ptosis and large pupil — IIIrd nerve palsy
- Ptosis and constricted pupil — Horner syndrome
- Extremely important in unconscious patient (much more so than establishment of papilloedema, for example)

17.   NEUROLOGICAL INVESTIGATIONS

17.1   Electroencephalography (EEG)

The EEG allows an assessment of changes in cortical function. Electrodes applied to the scalp allow the cortical action potential between two electrodes to be amplified and displayed. The quality of the normal EEG will depend upon:

- Age of the patient
- Whether the patient is awake or asleep

Uses

- Investigation of patients with seizures
- Detection of cerebral dysfunction
- Evaluation of depressed consciousness
- Investigation of neurodegenerative disorders

Typical EEG appearances

Epilepsies

- Three cycles per seond (c/s) spike and wave in typical absences ('petit mal')
- Four c/s spike and wave and poly-spike and wave bursts in juvenile myoclonic epilepsy
- Clusters of high-amplitude spike and wave complexes in one or both Rolandic areas in benign focal epilepsy with Rolandic spikes

Epileptic encephalopathies

- High-voltage chaotic slow waves and spike and sharp waves in hypsarrythmia
- Spike and waves in absence of seizures and loss of language skills in Landau–Kleffner syndrome
- Slow spike wave discharges at 1.5–2.5 c/s in Lennox–Gastaut syndrome

Undiagnosed neurological illness

- Burst suppression in asphyxia, early myoclonic epilepsy, glycine encephalopathy
- Slowing of background in encephalopathies generally
- Focal slowing may indicate structural lesions such as cerebral abscess
- Focal flattening may indicate subdural haemorrhage or effusion
- Diffuse moderate amplitude fast beater activity is the result of some drug intoxications

Suspect cerebral malformation or mental handicap

- High-voltage activity in the α-frequency or lower part of β-characteristic of lissencephaly or pachygyria
- High-voltage posterior spike and wave accentuated by passive eye closure is a feature of Angelman syndrome
- Trains of spikes or sharp waves, at first in sleep, with poorly organized background activity develop in Rett syndrome

Suspect neurodegenerative disorder

- Stereotyped high-voltage polyphasic complexes repeated every few seconds and often associated with transient reduction in tone — subacute sclerosing panencephalitis
- Progressive reduction in EEG amplitude after infancy is typical of infantile neuronal ceroid lipofuschinosis
- High-voltage posterior complexes induced by slow stroboscopic activation at less than 0.5 c/s is typical of late infantile neuronal ceroid lipofuschinosis
- β-activity of moderate amplitude develops after 2 years in infantile neuraxonal dystrophy
- Multiple spikes superimposed on lateralized large slow waves suggest progressive neuronal degeneration of childhood, and predict later hepatic involvement

17.2 Evoked potentials

Used to assess the function of auditory, visual and somatosensory pathways.

Auditory brainstem evoked potentials

• Assessment of peripheral hearing in infants and young children

Visual evoked potentials

• Detection of disease in anterior visual pathway

Electroretinogram (ERG)

• Measures response of retina to repeated light flashes
• Used in investigation of low vision and in neurological regression

Somatosensory evoked potentials

• Diagnosis of spinal cord disease
• Intraoperative monitoring

17.3 Peripheral neurophysiology

Measurement of peripheral nerve conduction allows the assessment of the function of the motor unit — the anterior horn cell, the peripheral axon and the innervated muscle.

Nerve conduction studies allow the measurement of:

• Motor nerve conduction velocity — reduced in demyelination
• Amplitude of action potential — reduced in axonal neuropathies
• Sensory nerve conduction velocity — reduced in Friedreich's ataxia, for example

Electromyography

• Denervation — shorter and lower voltage action potentials; later giant potentials
• Myopathic change — reduced action potentials

17.4 Brain imaging

Computerized axial tomography (CT) scanning

Useful in:

• Initial evaluation of coma
• Trauma
• Calcification

Magnetic resonance imaging (MRI) scanning

Useful in:

- Detection of parenchymal lesions, especially white matter lesions
- Posterior fossa lesions

17.5 Lumbar puncture

Useful in the diagnosis of:

- Infection
- Demyelinating diseases
- Subarachnoid haemorrhage
- Benign intracranial hypertension (measure pressure)

18. FURTHER READING

Aicardi J. 1998. *Diseases of the Nervous System in Childhood. Clinics in Developmental Medicine*, 2nd edn. London: MacKeith Press.

Patten J. 1995. *Neurological Differential Diagnosis*, 2nd edn. New York: Springer Verlag.

Stephenson JBP, King MD. 1989. *Handbook of Neurological Investigations in Childhood*. London: Wright.

Volpe J. 2001. *Neurology of the Newborn*, 4th edn. Philadelphia, USA: W B Saunders.

Chapter 19

Ophthalmology

William H Moore and Ken K Nischal

CONTENTS

771

Ophthalmology

1. BASIC ANATOMY OF THE EYE

1.1 Orbits

The orbits are related to the frontal sinus above, the maxillary sinus below and the ethmoid and sphenoid sinuses medially. The orbit houses the eyeball (which occupies only one-fifth of the space), the lacrimal glands, fat and muscle account for the bulk of the remainder.

1.2 Extraocular muscles

Six extraocular muscles (four rectus and two oblique) control the movement of each eye.

Muscle	Nerve supply	Primary action	Secondary action
Lateral rectus	VI (abducens)		AbductionNone
Medial rectus	III (oculomotor)		AdductionNone
Superior rectus	III	Elevation	Adduction/Intorsion
Inferior rectus	III	Depression	Adduction/Extorsion
Superior oblique	IV (trochlear)	Depression	Intorsion/Abduction
Inferior oblique	III	Elevation	Extorsion/Abduction

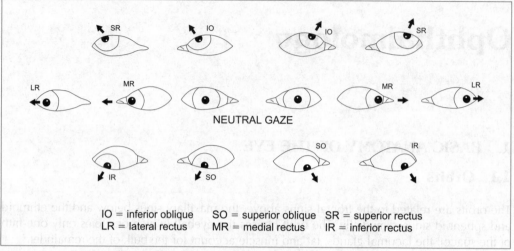

IO = inferior oblique   SO = superior oblique   SR = superior rectus
LR = lateral rectus   MR = medial rectus   IR = inferior rectus

The action of the external ocular muscles with the patient confronting the examiner.

1.3   The globe

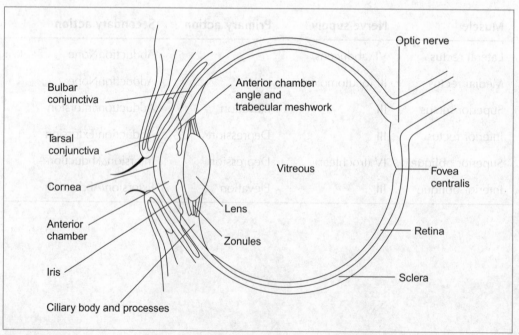

The eyeball.

Cornea

A transparent avascular tissue joined to the sclera at the limbus that refracts light en route to the retina. Sensory innervation is supplied by the first division of the trigeminal nerve. The transparency of the cornea is the result of its uniform structure, avascularity and the active transport functions of the corneal endothelium, which keep it relatively dehydrated.

Conjunctiva

Thin, transparent membrane that covers the posterior surface of the eyelids and the anterior surface of the sclera (bulbar conjunctiva).

Sclera

The fibrous outer protective coating of the eye.

Uveal tract

Consists of iris, ciliary body and choroid, each of which has a rich vascular supply and pigment. The choroid's vasculature provides nutrition for the outer sensory retina (photo-receptors and outer nuclear layer).

Anterior chamber

Fluid-filled space between the cornea and iris diaphragm. The aqueous fluid is secreted by the ciliary body and provides nutrition for the corneal endothelium. It reaches the anterior chamber through the pupillary space and drains via the trabecular meshwork and canal of Schlemm (in the periphery of the anterior chamber) into the venous circulation.

Lens

Lies posterior to the iris and anterior to the vitreous humour, suspended by zonules from the ciliary body. Anterior to the lens is the aqueous humour. The lens of the newborn infant is more spherical than that of the adult and as such has a greater refractive power which can compensate for the relative shortness of the young eye.

Vitreous

A transparent gelatinous structure which fills the posterior four-fifths of the globe. It is firmly attached to the pars plana anteriorly and has a loose attachment to the retina and optic nerve posteriorly. The vitreous is ~99% water.

Retina

The retina contains the sensory receptors (rods and cones) and their complex network of connections leading to the optic nerve. The fovea centralis is the centre of the macula; it has the greatest concentration of cones and subsequently the best potential for visual acuity. Light falling onto the retina is converted into nerve impulses by the rods and cones. Nerve fibres from the ganglion cell layer of the retina coalesce to form the optic nerve and synapse in the lateral geniculate body. Fibres from the temporal retina travel without crossing at the chiasm to the ipsilateral visual cortex. Nerve fibres from the nasal retina will decussate at the chiasm and are directed toward the contralateral visual cortex. The decussation of nerve fibres causes portions of each retina to be represented in each visual cortex (see visual fields box on page 776)

2. AMBLYOPIA

This is the commonest cause of decreased vision in childhood between birth and 8 years of age. It is the reversible decrease in vision as a result of abnormal visual experience during the first few years of life. It is reversed in unilateral cases by occluding the good or better seeing eye. Causes include strabismic, ammetropic (bilateral large refractive errors), anisometropic (difference in refraction of the two eyes) and meridional (due to astigmatism) amblyopia. In bilateral cases alternate eye occlusion may be attempted.

3. OPHTHALMIC EXAMINATION

Examination begins with observation of the child in the waiting area or in bed, in their parents' arms and as they enter the examination room. Note eye movements, eye contact, sensitivity to lighting changes and gross and subtle dysmorphic features. Observation of the family may give clues to inherited conditions.

History, as in all medicine, is paramount to a correct diagnosis. This time is also useful for examining the behaviour of the child and building the rapport and trust needed to produce a fruitful examination.

Visual acuity measurement is the most important test of visual function. The age of the child and their level of development dictate which type of test is used. The table of observable visual behaviour indicates expected levels of vision up to the age of 1 year.

Behaviours	Neo.	6 wk	3 m	4 m	5 m	6 m	9 m	12 m
Blink to flash	+	+	+	+	+	+	+	+
Turn to diffuse light	+	+	+	+	+	+	+	+
Fix & Follow near face	+/−	**+/−**	+	+	+	+	+	+
Watches adult 0.75 m	+/−	**+**	+	+	+	+	+	+
Fix & Follow 6.5 cm ball	−	+/−	**+**	+	+	+	+	+
Watches adult 1.5 m	−	+/−	+/−	**+**	+	+	+	+
Converges to 6.5 cm	−	−	+/−	**+**	+	+	+	+
Fixates 2.5 cm brick 0.3 m	−	−	−	+/−	**+**	+	+	+
Blinks to Threat	−	−	−	+/−	**+**	+	+	+
Watches adult 3 m	−	−	−	−	+/−	**+**	+	+
Fixates 1.25 cm (Smarties)	−	−	−	−	+/−	**+**	+	+
Fixates 1.25 mm (100s & 1000s)	−	−	−	−	−	+/−	**+**	**+**

Bold text indicates upper limit of normal; Neo. neonate; wk, weeks; m, months.

Observable visual behaviour (after Blanche Stiff and Patricia Sonksen)

- Quality of visual behaviour and stereoacuity tests are useful in the pre-verbal child.
- From $2\frac{1}{2}$–3 years objective measurements of visual acuity are possible. Picture matching tests are available, e.g. Kay's picture tests, illiterate E. Letter matching tests are available.
- Snellen or Logmar acuity tests are the tests of choice for the older child.

3.1 Refractive errors

Errors in the refractive state of the eye may arise from variation in the corneal curvature, variation in the size and shape of the crystalline lens in the eye or variation in the axial length of the eye. A significant refractive error or a difference between the two eyes can lead to amblyopia, if not suitably corrected, because one or both eyes will have a blurry image falling on the retina.

In children, measuring the refraction is an objective test requiring cycloplegic drops to prevent accommodation and facilitate viewing the light reflection from the retina. Co-operative older children and adults can be refracted subjectively with trial-frame glasses.

- **Myopia (short-sightedness)** — objects further away are blurred. Inheritance is multifactorial but may be associated with systemic conditions such as Stickler syndrome. Concave lenses are used to correct myopia
- **Hypermetropia (long-sightedness)** — images further away are generally clearer than nearer ones. Convex lenses are used
- **Astigmatism** — this occurs when the curvature of the cornea, lens or retina is more curved in one axis with respect to another [rugby ball (toric shape) versus football (spherical shape)]. This produces a blurred retinal image of an object at any distance. Toric lenses are used to correct this. A degree of astigmatism is normal (< 1 dioptre)

- **Anisometropia** — this is where the two eyes have differing refractive errors. A small degree may be acceptable for visual development but amblyopia will almost certainly develop if hypermetropic and > 1 dioptre

3.2   Slit-lamp biomicroscopy

This illuminating microscope allows visualization of many of the structures of the eye.

3.3   Fundoscopy

By direct/indirect ophthalmoscope, facilitated by dilatation of the pupil.

3.4   Visual fields

Assessment of visual fields depends on the age and ability of the child. Simple confrontational fields, bringing toys/objects silently into the visual field from the periphery, can be performed, with the infant/child on their carer's lap, looking for the movement of eyes or head towards the object at the end-point. Older children can be tested with more formal Goldman visual field testing or some of the automated visual field machines.

Visual fields

Homonymous hemianopia
Optic tract or lateral geniculate body lesion; temporal, parietal or occipital lobe lesion of the brain (tumour, ischaemia; aneurysm, trauma). Migraine may cause transient homonymous hemianopia.

Bitemporal hemianopia
Chiasmal lesion (pituitary tumour, craniopharyngioma, glioma, mid-line developmental abnormalities)

- Tilted optic discs
- Nasal retinal disease (retinitis pigmentosa)

Binasal hemianopia
Glaucoma, temporal retinal disease (retinitis pigmentosa)
Bilateral occipital disease, tumour/aneurysm compressing both optic nerves/chiasm

Central scotoma
Macular disease, optic neuritis, optic atrophy (compressive/degenerative)

Arcuate scotoma
Glaucoma, ischaemic optic neuropathy (craniosynostoses), optic disc drusen, high myopia

Altitudinal field defect
Glaucoma, optic nerve/chiasmal lesion, optic nerve coloboma
Ischaemic optic neuropathy, hemibranch artery/vein occlusion

Acquired visual loss

Acquired visual loss is rare in children. A thorough ovular examination including visual field analysis is very important.

History is vital to ascertaining whether this is acquired rather than present from birth.

- Cortical blindness
- Post-traumatic anoxia
- Hypotension
- Hypoglycaemia
- Migraine
- Occipital epilepsy
- Vitreous haemorrhage
- Retinal disease
- Optic nerve disease/optic neuritis
- Ischaemia
- Trauma — cerebral contusion, haemorrhage
- Drugs — lead, quinine, methyl alcohol
- Benign intracranial hypertension/pituitary tumour
- Functional visual loss/hysteria

Electrophysiology is particularly helpful in differentiating many of these causes.

Infant with decreased vision

Most common causes are:

- Anterior segment anomalies
- Glaucoma
- Cataract
- Optic nerve hypoplasia
- Optic atrophy
- Coloboma
- Leber congenital amaurosis
- TORCH/congenital infection
- Albinism
- X-linked retinoschisis
- Retinopathy of prematurity
- Achromatopsia (rod monochromatism)
- Congenital motor nystagmus
- Delayed visual maturation
- Cortical blindness

Blind spot enlargement

Papilloedema, glaucoma, optic nerve drusen, optic nerve coloboma, myelinated nerve fibres from the disc, myopic disc/crescent, drugs

Constriction of peripheral fields leaving a residual central visual field

Glaucoma, retinitis pigmentosa/peripheral retinal disorder, chronic papilloedema, central retinal artery occlusion with cilioretinal artery sparing, bilateral occipital lobe infarction with macular sparing, non-physiological visual loss (reducing spiral visual fields), carcinoma-associated retinopathy, drugs

3.5 Colour vision

Usually this is tested using standard Ishihara colour plates, which test only red/green colour deficiency; other plates may be used for blue/yellow testing.

Red/green colour vision defects are inherited as X-linked disorders but can also be acquired, usually secondary to optic nerve disease.

More detailed colour vision tests exist (Farnswell–Munsell 100 Hue tests) but are rather too complicated for paediatric use.

3.6 Electrophysiology

- Visual evoked potentials — can be used to define visual development in infants. This measures the time taken for light stimuli to induce excitation of the visual pathways from the retina to the occipital cortex and gives an indication of the latency and amplitude of the response. A measure of visual acuity can be extrapolated from this with varying size of stimuli
- Electroretinogram — this is an electrical recording of the response of the retina to a visible stimulus, e.g. flash of light. Useful in retinal disease.

4. EYELID ABNORMALITIES

4.1 Congenital eyelid abnormalities

Cryptophthalmos

A rare condition. The eyebrow is usually absent and the globe is microphthalmic (complete cryptophthalmos), may be part of Fraser syndrome; evaluation by electrodiagnostics and ultrasound is required before surgery can be considered.

Coloboma

Incomplete formation of upper or lower lids. May be associated with Goldenhar syndrome (upper lid), First Arch syndrome, amniotic band syndrome and other clefting syndromes (usually lower lid). In the first instance management is with lubricants to prevent exposure keratopathy, followed by reconstruction of the lids.

Ablepharon

Congenital absence of the lids. Copious lubricants are required until reconstruction is performed.

Ankyloblepharon

Partial or complete fusion of the eyelid margins. Surgical division may be required.

Euryblepharon

Sagging of lateral part of lower eyelid reducing apposition to globe, e.g. in Kabuki syndrome.

Ectropion

Congenital ectropion is an outward rotation of the upper or lower eyelid margin. It may be idiopathic or associated with conditions such as ichthyosis (collodion baby) or Down syndrome. Management may consist of lubrication alone or surgery +/− skin graft to prevent exposure keratopathy.

Entropion

Inward rotation of the lid margin with eyelashes rubbing against the cornea and conjuncti-va. Usually seen in conjunction with epiblepharon or microphthalmos. Simple lubrication alone may be required or surgery may be indicated to prevent keratopathy.

Epiblepharon

The presence of a fold in the skin and orbicularis muscle of the lower eyelids which may cause lashes to rub against the cornea. Most commonly seen in oriental patients and usually self-resolving. It is more common than congenital entropion, which more frequently affects the upper lid.

Symblepharon

An abnormal connection between the lid and the conjunctiva usually acquired (e.g. Stevens–Johnson syndrome) but may be congenital. Management is best with lubrication to prevent occurrence.

Epicanthus

Epicanthal folds are folds of skin that extend from the upper lid towards the medial canthus. This may give rise to the false appearance of strabismus (pseudosquint). Epicanthus inversus extends from the lower lid to the medial canthus.

Telecanthus

There is an increased width between the medial canthi with normal interpupillary distance.

Hypertelorism

Increased interorbital distance. May be idiopathic (e.g. Greig syndrome), congenital (e.g. craniosynostoses, clefting syndromes), or acquired (e.g. trauma, fibrous dysplasia).

Hypotelorism

Reduced interorbital distance. May be idiopathic or congenital, e.g. craniosynostoses (metopic suture).

Blepharophimosis

Small eyelids. Horizontal and vertical narrowing of the palpebral fissure, usually seen in blepharophimosis syndrome (ptosis, telecanthus and epicanthus inversus).

4.2 Infections and inflammations of the lids

Hordeolum (stye)

Staphylococcal infection of the lid hair follicle. Lash removal +/− topical antibiotic as necessary.

Chalazion

A chronic, painless, granulomatous inflammation of the Meibomian gland which results from obstruction of the gland duct. Treatment includes warm compresses, hygiene and massage to try to encourage drainage of the lipid material. Most small chalazia resolve spontaneously but incision and drainage may be required for persistent ones.

Molluscum contagiosum

Common eyelid lesion caused by a poxvirus. Often situated on the lid margin and associated with chronic conjunctivitis. Usually self-limiting but curettage of the lid lesion may hasten resolution.

Preseptal cellulitis

Occurs when the infection is anterior to the orbital septum. More common than orbital cellulitis. Causes include eyelid trauma, extraocular infection and upper respiratory tract infection. Usually unilateral with no proptosis. Causative organisms vary with age: streptococcal pneumonia and staphylococcal abscess in the neonatal period and *Haemophilus influenzae* in later infancy. Treatment is with antibiotics.

4.3 Haemangiomas

Capillary haemangioma

The commonest tumour of the eyelids or orbits in childhood. May be associated with dermal Kasabach–Merritt syndrome.

Capillary haemangiomas appear 2 or 3 weeks after birth, grow rapidly until 4 months of age and then stop growing by 6 months, regressing thereafter. They may cause ptosis, amblyopia from astigmatism or rarely compress the optic nerve. Treatment may involve intralesional and/or systemic steroids, and/or surgical excision; it almost always involves amblyopia therapy.

Port wine stain

A dermal capillary vascular anomaly which may occur in the periocular region. Ocular associations include episcleral haemangioma, iris heterochromia (affected iris is darker than unaffected one), choroidal haemangioma and glaucoma. Systemic associations include Sturge–Weber syndrome and congenital cutis marmorata telangiectasia.

4.4 Ptosis

Drooping of the upper lid, which may be uni- or bilateral, congenital or acquired.

Ptosis may be measured in terms of palpebral aperture or margin reflex distance. The latter is the distance between the upper lid margin and the central corneal light reflection when using a torch as a target for the patient to look at. This should be 3.5–4.5 mm.

Causes of ptosis

- **Congenital ptosis**
  - Idiopathic — simple congenital dystrophy
  - Syndromic — blepharophimosis syndrome, Noonan syndrome, Turner syndrome
- **Acquired ptosis**
  - Aponeurotic (trauma or oedema)
  - Lid inflammation (trauma or oedema)
  - Neurogenic (third-nerve palsy, Horner syndrome, Marcus Gunn jaw winking)
  - Myogenic (progressive external ophthalmoplegia, includes Kearns–Sayre syndrome, ocular myopathies, myasthenia gravis and myotonic dystrophy
  - Mechanical (lid tumours and lacerations)
  - Infections (encephalitis and botulism)
  - Syndromes (neurofibromatosis)
  - Drugs (vincristine)

Horner syndrome

This is caused by sympathetic denervation. It may be congenital (caused by obstetric trauma, with cervical vertebral abnormalities; rarely it may also be seen as a result of neuroblastoma) or acquired (caused by trauma, surgery or tumours). Features include, ptosis (partial), miosis (pupil constriction), enophthalmos, anhidrosis (ipsilateral), heterochromia iridis (congenital type) and normal direct and consensual reflex to light.

Marcus Gunn jaw-winking syndrome

This is the result of an abnormal synkinesis between the levator and the lateral pterygoid muscle. The affected lid is usually ptotic but elevates when the jaw opens and deviates to the contralateral side.

Treatment of ptosis

Ptosis of sufficient degree to interfere with vision requires early correction to prevent permanent loss of vision (amblyopia). Surgical treatment includes levator resection or brow suspension.

4.5 Lid retraction

Usually retraction of the upper lids. Associations include thyroid eye disease (lid lag/retraction seen in 25–60% of paediatric cases), Parinaud syndrome (see later in Sections 17.2 and 19.4), Marcus Gunn jaw winking and primary congenital idiopathic lid retraction.

Lower lid retraction is seen in cherubism (a rare inherited condition with fibro-osseous lesions of the maxilla and mandible linked to chromosome 4p16.3). No treatment is required except lubrication if lid lag/incomplete lid closure is noticed while asleep.

4.6 Lid lag

Delay or absence of normal downward excursion of upper lid on down-gaze. Most commonly seen in congenital ptosis (usually unilateral) but also seen in thyroid eye disease and, rarely, polyneuritis. May require lubrication if there is incomplete lid closure at night.

5. LACRIMAL SYSTEM DISORDERS

The function of the lacrimal system is to produce and remove the tears.

5.1 Congenital nasolacrimal sac dilatation (mucocele or dacryosystocele)

This presents shortly after birth as a bluish mass site because of fluid trapped in the nasolacrimal sac. Treatment varies from massage to probing within a few days.

5.2   Dacryocystitis

This may be caused by bacterial infection of the nasolacrimal sac associated with nasolacrimal duct obstruction. It presents with swelling of the nasolacrimal sac region with cellulitis of the surrounding tissues. Systemic and topical antibiotics are required. Persistence may require surgical incision and washout.

5.3   Stenosis or obstruction of the nasolacrimal duct

This may occur in 30% of newborn infants. Signs include tearing or mucopurulent discharge which may start 3–5 weeks later. Gentle pressure over the nasolacrimal sac expresses tears and mucopurulent material from the sac. Spontaneous resolution is common but probing of the nasolacrimal duct may be required.

5.4   The watering eye (lacrimation and epiphora)

Lacrimation is excessive production of tears, e.g. crying, whereas epiphora means watering of the eyes, i.e. overflow of tears because of inadequate drainage. The newborn baby does not usually shed tears during crying for the first 4–6 weeks of life.

Causes of a watering eye

- Blocked nasolacrimal system (usually painless)
- Congenital glaucoma (+ photophobia)
- Facial palsy (usually painless)
- Acquired foreign body (photophobia + pain)
- Keratitis (+ photophobia)
- Chronic blepharitis
- Migraine (cluster headache)
- Contact lens related
- Drugs (e.g. maternal heroin addiction)

5.5   The dry eye

The child with a dry eye rarely complains that it is dry but may complain of sore, red, itchy eyes and may rub them. It is a relatively uncommon problem but should be looked for in certain systemic diseases, (see below).

Causes of dry eye

- **Tear mucin deficiency** — vitamin A deficiency (xerophthalmia), trachoma, burns and Stevens–Johnson syndrome
- **Tear lipid-layer deficiency** — blepharitis
- **Tear aqueous deficiency** — keratoconjunctivitis sicca
- **Congenital alacrima** — rule out AAA syndrome (**a**lacrima, **a**chalazia, hypoadrenalism)
- **Ectodermal dysplasia** — dry skin, the anhidrotic type – absence of sweat and sebaceous glands, poor hair formation and abnormalities of nails and teeth
- **Familial dysautonomia** — (Reilly–Day syndrome – autosomal recessive) emotional lability, paroxysmal hypertension, sweating, cold hands/feet and blotchy skin
- **Sjögren syndrome** — uncommon in childhood, arthritis, dryness of mouth and mucous membranes, tendency to bronchitis and pneumonia with pulmonary disease
- **Drug-induced**

The mainstay of treatment is artificial tears but punctual occlusion should be considered.

6. THE ORBIT

6.1 Abnormalities of the position of the globe

Enophthalmos

This is when the globe sits further back in the orbit than normal causing a narrowing of the palpebral fissure. It is most commonly seen after a traumatic blow-out fracture of the orbit or in cases of microphthalmos.

Exophthalmos (or Proptosis)

This is when the globe sits further forward than normal. It is best described as proptosis and best observed when viewed from directly above the patient with the patient looking straight ahead.

Pseudo-proptosis is seen when there is an abnormally large globe (e.g. high myopia or buphthalmos (congenital glaucoma)) or if the lids are retracted or if there is contralateral microphthalmos.

True proptosis may be axial or non-axial. Axial proptosis is causes by intraconal lesions while non-axial proptosis (globe is displaced out and either laterally, inferiorly, superiorly or medially) is caused by extraconal lesions. Occasionally intermittent (as a result of lymphangioma, capillary haemangioma), non-pulsatile (as a result of encephalocele, orbital roof fracture), or pulsatile (with-a-bruit proptosis; congenital arteriovenous malformation).

Causes of proptosis

In neonates and infants

- Tumours such as capillary haemangioma, juvenile xanthogranuloma, teratoma, rhabdomyosarcoma, very rarely retinoblastoma and acute leukaemia
- Cystic lesions including microphthalmos with cyst, anterior and posterior orbital encephalocele
- Shallow orbits may be seen in the syndromic craniosynostoses such as Crouzon syndrome

In children

- **Inflammatory causes**
  - Infection — this is more frequent in children over 5 years of age and is usually secondary to ethmoiditis. It may be the result of *Haemophilus influenzae, Staphylococcus aureus* or *Streptococcus pneumoniae*. In severe cases there may be visual compromise and/or cavernous sinus thrombosis. The child usually presents with pyrexia, chemosis, lid oedema and axial proptosis with limitation of eye movements. After admission, the child needs an Ear, Nose & Throat opinion, orbital and brain imaging and intravenous antibiotics to cover anaerobic and aerobic organisms
  - Orbital pseudotumour — idiopathic orbital inflammatory condition in children between 6 and 14 years. If bilateral then Wegener's granulomatosis must be excluded. Orbital imaging is essential to differentiate from orbital cellulitis. Treatment is with steroids though biopsy may be needed first
  - Dacryoadenitis — usually the result of viral infection of the lacrimal gland Present with 's'-shaped upper lid, and extreme pain. Antibiotics and non-steroidal anti-inflammatory treatment is needed with orbital imaging
- **Benign tumours**
  - Lymphangioma — occurs between 1 and 15 years of age. May cause sudden painless proptosis as a result of a bleed ('chocolate cyst') or upper respiratory tract infection
  - Dermoid cysts — rarely cause proptosis but may be seen as a lump on the lateral brow
  - Plexiform neurofibromatosis — seen in patients with neurofibromatosis. The lid often has an 's'-shaped curve
  - Optic nerve glioma — usually seen in neurofibromatosis type 1. The eye is often turned down slightly and proptosed. Neuroimaging is essential
- **Malignant tumours**
  - Rhabdomyosarcoma — presents around 7 years of age with chemosis, proptosis and pain, but usually no pyrexia. Orbital imaging may show bony involvement
  - Metastatic neuroblastoma — similar presentation to rhabdomyosarcoma but in the younger child (under 5 years). Two-fifths are bilateral
  - Langerhans cell histiocytosis — orbital involvement is usually in the upper outer orbit and is painless
  - Acute leukaemia — rare but presents around 7 years of age with ecchymosis (bruising of eyelids) and mild proptosis. Blood film confirms diagnosis

7. THE CONJUNCTIVA

7.1 Conjunctivitis

Neonatal

This is inflammation of the conjunctiva occurring during the first month of life affecting 7–19% of all newborns (ophthalmica neonatorum). It may be chemical (diffuse without discharge), gonococcal (profuse green discharge), herpetic, chlamydial, or bacterial. It is a notifiable condition.

- Gonococcal — may cause corneal perforation. Needs topical and systemic antibiotics and admission to hospital
- *Chlamydia trachomatis* — potentially blinding and treatment is with erythromycin (topical and systemic). Pneumonitis must be excluded
- *Pseudomonas aeruginosa* — usually acquired in the nursery. Lid oedema and discharge are seen at day 5–18. Treatment is with topical and systemic antibiotics (usually fluoroquinolones)

Bacterial

Very common. Bilateral purulent discharge. Broad topical antibiotics are treatment of choice. If these do not work then swab for culture and sensitivities for second-line antibiotic (topical).

Viral

Common contagious usually bilateral condition. Commonest cause is adenoviral and presents with watery discharge, hyperaemia, follicular conjunctivitis, preauricular lymphadenopathy. Rarely may be caused by herpes simplex virus.

Allergic

Presents with hyperaemia, itching, chemosis (conjunctival oedema). May be seasonal or perennial. Topical antihistamines and/or mast cell stabilizers are helpful. Sometimes systemic antihistamines are also helpful.

Vernal

Usually occurs later in the prepubertal period. Atopy may be a factor. It results in a cobblestone appearance of the palpebral conjunctiva. Treatment consists of systemic antihistamines, topical mast cell stabilizers and/or antihistamines. Topical steroids may be needed and occasionally, topical ciclosporine.

Miscellaneous

Kawasaki disease causes marked hyperaemia and Stevens–Johnson syndrome and toxic-epidermal necrosis cause marked conjunctival erosions and discharge. These last two need topical steroids and lubrication.

Red eye

- Infectious conjunctivitis
  - Bacterial
  - Viral
  - Chlamydial
- Blepharoconjunctivitis
- Allergic conjunctivitis
- Trauma
- Foreign body
- Iritis
- Episcleritis/scleritis
- Drug, toxin, chemical
- Secondary infection with nasolacrimal duct obstruction
- Sub-conjunctival haemorrhage
- Orbital disease — cellulitis, tumour (rhabdomyosarcoma)

7.2   Conjunctival pigmentation

Flat pigmentation

- Benign melanosis — congenital brown patches near limbus usually in pigmented races
- Nevus of Ota — slate-grey appearance of the eye which may be isolated to the eye but is usually associated with similar pigmentation of the surrounding skin. This is associated with an increased risk of glaucoma and malignant change (in non-pigmented races)
- Nevus — a mole
- Telangiectasia — dilated and tortuous bulbar vessels. May be associated with ataxia telangiectasia (only seen in interpalpebral fissure), metabolic causes (e.g. Fabry disease)

Non-pigmented lesions

- Phlycten — uncommon, straw yellow, limbal lesion. It is most commonly caused by *S. aureus* hypersensitivity seen in blepharitis. May also be caused by tuberculosis or herpes simplex infection. Treatment is with topical steroid and antibiotics
- Limbal dermoid — white or cream coloured limbal lesion. May have hairs growing on the surface. It may be associated with Goldenhar or Treacher–Collins syndromes. Surgical removal may be needed but usually topical lubrication is adequate
- Bitot spot — foamy plaques temporal to the limbus as a result of vitamin A deficiency
- Plexiform neurofibroma — diffuse, elevated lesion extending from lid to the superior conjunctiva. Associated with neurofibromatosis type 1

8. THE SCLERA

8.1 Pigmentation of the sclera

- Blue sclera — may be seen in high myopes, osteogenesis imperfecta I, Marshall–Smith, Russell–Silver and Ehlers–Danlos syndromes
- Yellow sclera — seen in jaundice
- Black pigmentation — metabolic causes include alkaptonuria and haemochromatosis. Thinning of the sclera will result in the choroid showing through

8.2 Scleral inflammation

Episcleritis

Diffuse, non-tender inflammation which is often self-limiting. However, persistent inflammation or nodular episcleritis may be associated with juvenile idiopathic arthritis, inflammatory bowel disease, and systemic lupus erythematosus. Topical steroids may be needed but usually systemic non-steroidal anti-inflammatory drugs.

Scleritis

This is tender and painful. It may be diffuse, nodular or necrotizing. A systemic association must be excluded, e.g. connective tissue disorders, vasculitides, enteropathies, or granulomatous disorders. Treatment of the underlying condition together with systemic anti-inflammatory drugs are needed.

9. THE CORNEA

9.1 Developmental anomalies

Microcornea

Corneas < 10 mm in diameter, may be associated with various syndromes, e.g. Warburg syndrome and glaucoma.

Cornea plana

A flat cornea most commonly seen with sclerocornea.

Sclerocornea

Congenital, non-inflammatory extension of opaque scleral tissue and fine vascular tissue into the cornea. Usually bilateral and may be associated with cornea plana, glaucoma and microphthalmos.

Megalocornea

A cornea > 13 mm in the absence of glaucoma. Usually X-linked condition. Megalocornea with glaucoma is called buphthalmos and is the result of congenital or infantile glaucoma.

Peters' anomaly

Usually a bilateral opacity of the cornea as a result of a defect in the posterior cornea, with or without iridocorneal or keratolenticular adhesions. May be associated with aniridia, Axenfeld–Rieger anomaly (see Section 12.5) or systemic conditions e.g. Peters' Plus syndrome. Glaucoma should be excluded and corneal transplant considered.

Posterior embryotoxon

This is a prominent, anteriorly displaced white line usually seen on the slit-lamp. It is seen in 20% of normals but in the presence of prolonged jaundice in a neonate, Alagille syndrome should be excluded.

9.2 Corneal clouding

Causes of clouding include:

- Developmental anomalies — see above
- Congenital glaucoma — enlarged corneas (buphthalmos) with increased intraocular pressure and hazy corneas
- Infections — keratitis as a result of neonatal herpes simplex virus infection. Rubella virus or *Neisseria gonorrhoeae* may cause corneal haze
- Metabolic — mucoploysaccharidoses (not Hunter), mucolipidoses, cystinosis, tyrosinaemia type II, or lecithin cholesterol acyltransferase deficiency
- Non-metabolic — corneal blood staining (seen after a traumatic hyphaema where the intraocular pressure has not been adequately controlled), band-shaped keratopathy (calcium deposition most commonly seen in patients with juvenile idiopathic arthritis and iritis), amyloid deposition
- Corneal dystrophies — there are a number of dystrophies that cause corneal haze
- Trauma — tears in Descemet's membrane, usually seen after forceps delivery in neonates, cause unilateral corneal oedema. Perforations of the cornea can be seen in neonates born after amniocentesis

9.3 Keratitis

This is inflammation of the cornea as a result of infections, exposure keratopathy, or neuropathy (usually seen in patients with facial nerve palsy and/or corneal anaesthesia).

Infectious keratitis needs prompt diagnosis and topical/systemic treatment. Exposure and neuropathic keratitis demand frequent ocular lubrication.

9.4 Keratoconus

This condition results in corneal thinning leading to a conical shape of the cornea with high levels of astigmatism. It may be associated with systemic disorders, e.g. Ehlers–Danlos syndrome type IV

10. DEVELOPMENTAL ANOMALIES OF THE GLOBE

10.1 Nanophthalmos

This is a small but structurally normal eye. The child is hypermetropic and predisposed to glaucoma and choroidal effusions.

10.2 Simple microphthalmos

This is a small but structurally normal eye which is usually associated with a systemic abnormality, e.g. fetal alcohol syndrome, but the late complications of choroidal effusions seen in nanophthalmos are not seen here.

10.3 Complex microphthalmos

Usually a bilateral condition associated with colobomas of the eye and sometimes orbital cyst. Usually associated with a systemic condition e.g. CHARGE (**c**oloboma/**h**eart defects/**a**tresia of choanae/**r**etardation of growth and developmental delay/**g**enital anomalies/**e**ar anomalies) syndrome or chromosomal abnormalities.

10.4 Anophthalmia

In this condition there may be an actual absence of the globe or a clinically absent globe. Patients with clinical anophthalmos have a high incidence of developmental anomalies involving both eyes (88%), the brain (71%) and the body (58%). Orbital expanders are needed to provide normal stimulus for normal facial growth.

11. THE IRIS

11.1 Congenital iris defects

Iris coloboma

These are typical if they occur in the infero-nasal quadrant and are the result of non-closure of the embryonic fissure during the 5th week of gestation. Typical iris colobomas may involve the ciliary body, choroid, retina and optic nerve.

Associations

It may be isolated or associated with ocular features such as retinochoroidal/optic nerve coloboma, microcornea, microphthalmos, microphthalmos with cyst, nystagmus and cataracts. Although iris coloboma can be associated with almost any chromosomal abnormality they are frequently seen in:

- Cat-eye (tri-tetrasomy 22), colobomatous microphthalmia, anal atresia and pre-auricular skin tags
- CHARGE association
- Rubinstein–Taybi syndrome
- Triploidy, trisomy 13 (Patau syndrome)

Treatment

Review for correction of refractive error and cataract progression if lens opacity is present.

Aniridia

Autosomal dominant aniridia is a bilateral panocular disorder (as a result of mutation on the *PAX6* gene on the short arm of chromosome 11). The most obvious finding is absence of much/most of the iris tissue.

In addition to iris involvement, foveal and optic nerve hypoplasia may be present, resulting in a congenital sensory nystagmus and leading to a reduced visual acuity of 6/30 or worse. Anterior polar cataracts (50–85%), glaucoma (~50%) and corneal opacification often develop later in childhood and may lead to progressive deterioration of vision.

Associations

Wilms' tumour, genitourinary abnormalities and retarded growth or development (AGR triad) or both (WAGR) or associated with ataxia and neurodevelopmental delay (Gillespie syndrome).

Treatment

All children with sporadic aniridia should have repeated abdominal ultrasonographic and clinical examinations. The child should be seen 3-monthly until 5 years, 6-monthly until 10 years, then yearly to 16 years. However, the examinations are best continued until chromosomal and then intragenic mutational analyses have confirmed a *PAX6* mutation only. If chromosomal deletion is found, 3-monthly scans should be performed.

Iris transillumination

The congenital causes include albinism (both ocular and oculocutaneous). Small iris transillumination defects just visible near the iris root in blue-eyed children may be idiopathic with no clinical significance.

Ocular albinism (usually X-linked)

Males with photophobia, foveal hypoplasia causing nystagmus and reduced visual acuity, iris transillumination defects and scanty retinal pigmentation.

Oculocutaneous albinism (autosomal recessive)

Tyrosine-negative (incapable of synthesizing melanin)

Steely-white hair, very pale skin (sunburn), pink–blue eyes, nystagmus and reduced visual acuity < 6/60, reduced number of nerve fibres crossing at the chiasm.

Tyrosine-positive (can synthesize variable amounts of melanin, appear pale to almost normal)

Foveal hypoplasia-reduced visual acuity, variably hypopigmented fundus, blue to dark brown iris with variable translucency, associated syndromes:

- Chediak–Higashi syndrome — autosomal recessive, albinism, white cell abnormalities, recurrent infections, mild bleeding diathesis, hepatosplenomegaly, peripheral and cranial neuropathy
- Hermansky–Pudlak syndrome — autosomal recessive, albinism, platelet dysfunction, pulmonary fibrosis and inflammatory bowel disease

11.2   Acquired iris defects

Iris transillumination

Causes include:

- Iatrogenic — post-surgical
- Herpes zoster ophthalmicus causes sector iris atrophy
- Trauma — blunt ocular trauma may cause iridodialysis (disinsertion of the iris root) which may result in pseudopolycoria (more than one pupil)

11.3   Changes in iris colour

Benign primary iris tumours

Brushfield spots

These occur in 38–90% of patients with Down syndrome (silvery-grey spots, circumferentially placed in mid-peripheral iris) but are also seen in 24% of normal individuals (Wolfflin nodules)

Secondary tumours

Juvenile xanthogranuloma

Iris involvement occurs almost exclusively in infants. Usually unilateral yellow nodules or diffuse infiltration may be seen. Spontaneous hyphaema (blood in anterior chamber) and/or unilateral glaucoma may occur. All children with juvenile xanthogranuloma should have ocular screening because even asymptomatic ocular lesions may be associated with glaucoma. Most ocular lesions will regress with topical steroids. Some cases may need systemic steroids and others a small dose of radiotherapy treatment.

Lisch nodules

Neural crest hamartomas, usually light brown and usually seen in neurofibromatosis 1 (ocular findings in this condition include optic nerve glioma, glaucoma, plexiform neurofibroma of lid or conjunctiva or both, hamartoma of optic disc and retina, meningioma) but also seen in neurofibromatosis 2 (bilateral acoustic neuromas and other central nervous system tumours, cataract, 66% before 30 years of age, combined hamartomas of retina and retinal pigment epithelium).

Langerhans cell histiocytosis

Includes eosinophilic granuloma, Letterer–Siwe and Hand–Schüller–Christian disease, although similar to juvenile xanthogranuloma; these are systemic malignancies and need appropriate management/chemotherapy.

Usually limited to orbital involvement but iris nodules or choroidal involvement may rarely occur in Letterer–Siwe disease.

Leukaemia/lymphoma

Leukaemia iris infiltrates, although rare, have been reported with most types of childhood leukaemia (most commonly in acute lymphoblastoid leukaemia) and lymphoma and is an ominous finding since the median survival time after discovery of leukaemic iris involvement is 3 months.

Anterior chamber paracentesis or iris biopsy may be required to exclude an infectious aetiology. Chemotherapy may not be effective and low dose radiotherapy has been used successfully.

11.4 Heterochromia irides

The differential diagnosis of paediatric heterochromia irides is extensive but may be classified on the basis of whether the condition is congenital or acquired and whether the affected eye is hypo- or hyper-pigmented.

Hypochromic heterochromia

- Congenital
  - Horner syndrome
  - Waardenburg syndrome (autosomal dominant), telecanthus, prominent root of the nose, white forelock and sensorineural deafness
  - Piebaldism trait
- Acquired
  - Fuch's heterochromic iridocyclitis — rare type of unilateral uveitis
  - Non-pigmented iris tumours

Hyperchromic heterochromia

- Congenital
  - Iris mammilations — unilateral villiform protuberances that cover the iris, usually in association with oculodermal melanosis or neurofibromatosis
  - Congenital iris ectropion
  - Unilateral iris coloboma (affected iris is darker)
  - Port wine stain (haemangioma)
- Acquired
  - Cataract surgery in children (operated eye is darker if operated early in life)
  - Topical medications (latanaprost — a prostaglandin analogue used in treatment of glaucoma — darkens iris)
  - Pigmented iris tumours (naevus, melanoma)
  - Rubeosis iridis (iris neovascularization) — causes include; retinopathy of prematurity, retinoblastoma, Coats disease, iris tumours
  - Siderosis — as a resulst of intraocular metallic foreign body

12. PUPIL ANOMALIES

12.1 Leukocoria

A white pupil reflex, caused by

- Congenital cataract (uni- or bi-lateral)
- Persistent hyperplastic primary vitreous (rare congenital, usually unilateral condition resembling cataract on examination)
- Inflammatory cyclitic membrane
- Retinal dysplasia (very rare, may be associated with Norrie disease, Bloch–Sulzberger syndrome (incontinentia pigmenti), Warburg, Patau (trisomy 13), Edward (trisomy 18) syndromes
- Tumours — retinoblastoma, retinal astrocytoma
- Granuloma — toxocaral granuloma
- Retinal detachment — retinopathy of prematurity, Coats disease, toxocaral granuloma, Stickler syndrome
- Miscellaneous — extensive nerve fibre layer myelination, large chorioretinal coloboma

12.2 Dyscoria

An abnormality of the shape of the pupil.

- Congenital causes— persistent pupillary membrane, iris coloboma, iris hypoplasia and ectopia lentis et pupillae
- Acquired causes — most commonly uveitis, trauma (accidental/surgical)

12.3 Miosis

A small pupil usually < 2 mm, which reacts poorly to dilating drops.

- Congenital miosis (microcoria) may be the result of an absence of the dilator pupillae muscle or fibrous contraction secondary to persistent pupillary membrane. It can be seen in congenital rubella syndrome, Marfan syndrome, in 20% of Lowe (oculocerebrorenal) syndrome and in ectopia lentis et pupillae

12.4 Mydriasis

A large pupil usually > 4 mm. May be true mydriasis or pseudo-mydriasis.

True mydriasis

This may be congenital but blunt trauma causing iris sphincter rupture, ciliary ganglionitis (unilateral most commonly after chickenpox/varicella zoster virus infection — also known as Adie pupil) or acquired neurological disease must be excluded (especially third-nerve palsy)

Pseudo-mydriasis

Many cases of congenital mydriasis are actually part of the aniridia spectrum. Congenital iris ectropion is often mistaken as an enlarged pupil. Iris ectropion is eversion of the posterior pigment epithelium onto the anterior surface of the iris. Iris ectropion can occur as an acquired tractional abnormality, often in association with rubeosis iridis or as a congenital non-progressive abnormality. Congenital iris ectropion may be associated with congenital and/or developmental glaucoma. Associated conditions include neurofibromatosis type 1, Prader–Willi syndrome and facial hemihypertrophy. Review to exclude glaucoma or associations.

12.5 Corectopia

Displacement of the pupil. Normally the pupil is displaced inferonasally, about 0.5 mm, from the centre of the iris.

Sector iris hypoplasia, colobomas, ectopia lentis et pupillae, Axenfeld–Reiger anomaly (an autusomal dominant form of iris hypoplasia with posterior embryotoxon with or without iris adhesions, corectopia, dyscoria, pseudopolycoria and glaucoma in 50% of cases), anterior segment dysgenesis syndromes, and iridocorneal endothelium syndromes.

12.6   Anisocoria

A difference in the size of the two pupils > 1 mm. The three main causes that need differentiation in children are:

- Physiological
- Horner syndrome
- Adie pupil (ciliary ganglionitis)

Examination

The child should be examined in bright light and then in the dark. If the anisocoria is physiological then the difference between the two pupils will remain constant and is usually < 2 mm. If the anisocoria is accentuated in bright surroundings then the larger pupil is at fault because it cannot constrict (parasympathetic). The commonest cause for this is ciliary ganglionitis (Adie pupil). If the anisocoria is accentuated in the dark then the smaller pupil is at fault (sympathetic nervous system). The commonest cause for this is Horner syndrome.

Horner syndrome

Miosis, with ipsilateral ptosis (1–2 mm) and sometimes anhidrosis.

Congenital Horner syndrome is associated with hypopigmentation of the iris on the affected side.

Acquired Horner syndrome may be the result of:

- Central (first-order neurone) lesions (posterior hypothalamus down to spinal cord C8–T2)
- Pre-ganglionic (second-order) lesions (C8–T2 to superior cervical ganglion in the neck)
- Post-ganglionic (third-order) lesions (from cervical ganglion via internal carotid to cavernous sinus then via VI to nasociliary and ciliary nerves to eye)

Even if there is heterochromia irides, metastatic neuroblastoma should be excluded. In an otherwise healthy child, at least a chest X-ray and spot urine vanillylmandelic acid (VMA) should be performed.

Adie syndrome

Commonest association is chickenpox infection but other viral infections may also cause ciliary ganglionitis.

Accommodation is usually affected and the child may need reading spectacles.

13. INFLAMMATION OF THE IRIS

13.1 Irisitis/iridiocyclitis/uveitis

Inflammation of the uveal tract. Cells and flare can be seen in the anterior chamber, with deposition on the corneal endothelium (keratatic precipitates) seen on slit-lamp examination. Symptoms range from asymptomatic white eyes (pauciarticular arthritis) to photophobia, injected/red eyes with pain and reduced visual acuity.

Causes are idiopathic (35–50%), oligoarticular arthritis (juvenile idiopathic arthritis) – 33% are involved, female : male ratio of 3 : 1. Bilateral and asymptomatic and may precede arthritis (follow-up 3- to 6-monthly). Accounts for about 40% of paediatric uveitis.

Other causes are measles, mumps, chickenpox, Lyme disease, Kawasaki disease, Reiter syndrome, Behçet disease and sarcoidosis.

Treatment is with topical steroids and mydriatics (to prevent posterior synechiae between lens and iris) and anti-glaucoma medications as needed. Local steroid injections (triamcinolone/betnesol/dexamethasone) may be indicated as may systemic immunosuppression (steroids and steroid-sparing agents).

Complications of the disease and/or treatment include Band keratopathy, cataract and secondary glaucoma.

Photophobia
Common causes are:

- Glaucoma
- Uveitis
- Corneal abrasion/trauma/foreign body/ulcer
- Achromatopsia
- Cataract (glare from bright lights)
- Albinism
- Conjunctivitis (mild)

With normal ocular examination:

- Migraine
- Meningitis
- Retrobulbar optic neuritis
- Subarachnoid haemorrhage
- Trigeminal neuralgia

14. LENS ANOMALIES

14.1 Aphakia

Absent lens

The commonest cause is after cataract extraction without lens implantation because of congenital cataracts.

Treatment

Refractive correction of aphakia and surveillance to exclude glaucoma, which can develop at any time.

14.2 Abnormal shape

- Anterior lenticonus — rare bilateral condition with a conoid projection of the anterior surface of the lens centrally. Associated with Alport syndrome
- Posterior lenticonus — posterior conoid projection of the lens. Associated with Lowe syndrome but usually isolated

14.3 Dislocated lens

- Subluxed lens — partially displaced, remaining within pupillary space
- Luxated lens — displaced from the pupil

Ocular associations include megalocornea, severe buphthalmos, very high myopia and aniridia. Familial ectopia lentis, ectopia lentis et pupillae and isolated familial microspherophakia (autosomal recessive condition where displacement of the lens and pupil occur in opposite directions).

Systemic associations include Marfan syndrome (fibrillin gene mutation spectrum), Weill–Marchesani (short stature, brachydactyly, microspherophakia with or without lens dislocation), Ehlers–Danlos, Stickler (progressive early myopia, retinal detachment, joint anomalies, cleft palate) and Kniest (short stature, hearing loss, myopia, retinal detachment) syndromes, mandibulofacial, dysostosis and osteogenesis imperfecta. Metabolic disorders include homocystinuria, hyperlysinaemia and molybdenum cofactor deficiency (including sulphite oxidase deficiency).

Treatment comprises exclusion of systemic associations. Careful observation with refractive correction to ensure adequate visual development. May need lensectomy to improve visual function.

14.4 Lens opacity

These may be defined in terms of age of presentation or in terms of characteristic opacities for certain systemic associations.

Congenital or infantile cataract

In the UK two-thirds are bilateral; 31% have systemic associations (6% unilateral, 25% bilateral) and 61% are associated with ocular disease (47% unilateral, 14% bilateral). No underlying cause or risk-factor can be found in 92% of unilateral and 38% of bilateral cases. Hereditary disease may be associated with 56% of bilateral and 6% of unilateral cases.

Therefore if no hereditary risk or ocular disease is detected all bilateral cases should be considered for investigation of:

- Urine — reducing substances (galactosaemia), protein (Alport), amino acids (Lowe)
- Serology — TORCH (**t**oxoplasmosis, **o**ther infections, **r**ubella, **c**ytomegalovirus, and **h**erpes simplex), red blood cell galactokinase deficiency, red blood cell galactose-1-phosphate uridyltransferase activity, serum ferritin, karyotype, calcium, glucose, VDRL, phosphorus and alkaline phosphatase
- Maternal factors — diabetes mellitus, drugs in pregnancy (steroids, chlorpromazine)

Possible associations include:

- Hereditary
- Ocular — persistent hyperplastic primary vitreous, aniridia, iris coloboma, microphthalmos
- Systemic
  - Infection — intrauterine infection (TORCH)
  - Metabolic disease — galactosaemia, neonatal hypoglycaemia, hypocalcaemia
  - Renal disease — Lowe syndrome, congenital haemolytic syndrome
  - Chromosomal disorder — trisomy 13, trisomy 18 and Patau syndrome
  - Neurological disease — Marinesco–Sjögren syndrome (ataxia), Smith–Lemli–Opitz syndrome, Zellweger syndrome and Sjögren–Larsson syndrome
  - Skeletal disorders — Conradi syndrome
  - Skin disorders — Ectodermal dysplasia syndromes, incontinentia pigmenti syndrome, Cockayne syndrome.
  - Miscellaneous — Norrie syndrome (retinal dysplasia, mental retardation, microcephaly), Rubinstein–Taybi, Turner syndromes

Treatment

Lensectomy with sparing of the capsule for possible secondary lens implantation is one option, but lens removal with intraocular lens implantation has become more common. Amblyopia therapy with correction of the refractive state is essential.

Juvenile cataract

Associations include:

- Hereditary
- Ocular — coloboma, ectopia lentis, aniridia, retinitis pigmentosa and posterior lenticonus
- Systemic
  - Renal disease — Alport syndrome
  - Skeletal disease — Marfan syndrome
  - Skin disease — atopic dermatitis, Marshall syndrome, Lamellar ichthyosis.
  - Chromosomal disorders — trisomy 21
  - Metabolic disease — galactokinase deficiency, Fabry disease, Refsum disease, mannosidosis, diabetes mellitus, hypocalcaemia
  - Neurological disorders — myotonic dystrophy, Wilson disease
  - Miscellaneous — chronic uveitis, drug-induced (steroids), neurofibromatosis type 2, Stickler syndrome.

Treatment comprises lens aspiration with implant. Amblyopia therapy with correction of the refractive state is essential.

15.   RETINAL ANOMALIES

15.1   Haemorrhages

May be pre-retinal, retinal and sub-retinal.

Pre-retinal haemorrhages

- Haemorrhage lies between posterior vitreous face and retina.

May be associated with Sickle cell retinopathy, trauma, subarachnoid haemorrhage (Terson syndrome), non-accidental injury but never seen in isolation; widespread retinal and sub-retinal haemorrhages also seen with or without retinal schisis (a splitting within the retina).

Retinal haemorrhages

- These may be flame-shaped, dot and blot or Roth spots (white centred superficial retinal haemorrhage).
- May be seen in retinal vein occlusions, acute papilloedema, optic disc drusen, acute hypertensive retinopathy, retinal perivasculitis (early cytomegalovirus retinitis). Roth spots are seen in severe anaemia, leukaemia, bacterial endocarditis and may also be seen in trauma. Dot and blot haemorrhages may be seen in diabetes mellitus-related retinopathy, these are full thickness in the retina. They may also be seen in shaken baby syndrome but should be associated with superficial and sub-retinal haemorrhages.

Sub-retinal haemorrhages

- Red, raised area over which the retinal blood vessels are clearly visible.
- May be seen in sickle cell anaemia, Coats disease (retinal telangiectasia), trauma including shaken baby syndrome and rarely retinal neovascularization.

15.2 Hard exudates

Yellow waxy deposits which may be retinal or sub-retinal. Focal or diffuse exudates may be seen in diabetic retinopathy (unusual to see in children), old branch retinal vein occlusion, radiation retinopathy (years later) or retinal telangiectasia.

A macular star (stellate pattern of exudates centred on the macular) may be seen in malignant hypertension, papilloedema, neuroretinitis and very rarely retinal angioma (von Hippel–Lindau syndrome or idiopathic).

Sub-retinal exudates may be seen in Coats disease (occurs in males, peaks in 8- to 10-year-olds, usually unilateral, peripheral retinal telangiectasia and aneurysmal dilatation lead to extensive areas of yellow–white retinal exudation).

15.3 Cotton wool spots

Small white lesions with fluffy edges, which are the result of localized retinal ischaemia (microvascular occlusion).

May be seen in retinal vein occlusion, acute hypertension, systemic vasculitides, human immunodeficiency virus microvasculopathy, ocular ischaemic syndromes, haematological disorders (leukaemia, dysproteinaemias), trauma to chest and long bones (Purtscher retinopathy).

15.4 Retinal neovascularization

Retinal ischaemia may result in new vessel formation, which can often lead to retinal and vitreous haemorrhage and subsequent tractional retinal detachment. New vessels may occur in the posterior pole or in the periphery.

- Posterior pole neovascularization — retinal vein or artery occlusion, retinal vasculitis, diabetic retinopathy (rare in children) or radiation retinopathy
- Peripheral neovascularization — retinopathy of prematurity, sickle cell disease, familial exudative vitreoretinopathy, incontinentia pigmenti or sarcoidosis

Mainstay of treatment, after prevention, is laser photocoagulation of the ischaemic retina.

15.5   Retinal vasculitis

Inflammation around veins (periphlebitis) or arterioles (periarteritis).

- Periphlebitis — sarcoidosis, Behçet disease, cytomegalovirus retinitis, acute retinal necrosis
- Periarteritis — systemic lupus erythematosus, dermatomyositis, polyarteritis nodosa or Wegener's granulomatosis

Examination to exclude/monitor retinal involvement during systemic treatment.

15.6   Maculopathy

Abnormality of the macula — may be the result of wrinkling, bull's eye appearance or deposition/degeneration/inflammation.

Wrinkled appearance

Striated appearance radiating out from the centre of the fovea, which causes a drop in vision. May be idiopathic (commonest), or the result of juvenile retinoschisis (X-linked) or chronic intraocular inflammation.

Bull's eye maculopathy

There is hyperpigmentation in the centre of the macula, surrounded by a hypopigmented zone around which is a final hyperpigmented zone.

Associations are long-term chloroquine use, cone-rod dystrophy, some types of cone dystrophy, juvenile neuronal ceroid lipofuscinosis and Stargardt disease (macular dystrophy starting in the teens).

15.7   Coloured macular lesions

Yellow lesions

Best's vitelliform macular dystrophy — a rare, dominantly inherited maculopathy, starting in childhood with an egg-yolk looking lesion — vision is reduced, diagnosis is made/helped by electrophysiology.

Cherry-red spots

A change in the nerve-fibre layer surrounding the fovea, such as ischaemia or deposition of abnormal metabolic by-products, results in an accentuation of the normal deep-red colour of the fovea, producing a typical cherry-red spot macula. Seen in central retinal artery occlusion, metabolic disorders such as Tay–Sachs, Sandhoff, Niemann–Pick disease, generalized gangliosidosis and sialidosis I and II.

15.8   Pale retinal lesions

Inflammatory lesions

- Single focal lesions — these may be caused by toxoplasmosis, toxocariasis, candidiasis and cryptococcus
- Multiple focal lesions — these may be cause by candidiasis, sarcoidosis, Lyme disease, choroidal pneumocystosis, presumed ocular histoplasmosis syndrome, Behçet disease, Vogt–Koyanagi–Harada syndrome (an inflammatory condition affecting the eyes, brain and skin), sympathetic ophthalmitis and tuberculous choroiditis
- Diffuse lesions — these may be seen in cytomegalovirus retinitis, acute retinal necrosis, herpes simplex retinitis and measles retinitis. Appropriate serologic and radiological investigations need to be undertaken

Non-inflammatory lesions

Focal pale lesions

- Coloboma of the retina and choroid; may be associated with a serous retinal detachment
- Retinal astrocytoma, a hamartoma seen in 50% of patients with tuberous sclerosis
- Retinoblastoma, most common childhood intra-ocular malignancy, 1 : 14,000–20,000 births. Diagnosis commonest between 1 and 1.5 years of age, 90% before 3 years. Presenting signs: leukocoria 60%, squint 22%; < 25% of cases have a positive family history
  - Treatment — uniocular enucleation (cure if no metastases)
  - Bilateral — enucleate most involved eye, local resection/focal irradiation/systemic chemotherapy/cryotherapy/laser for smaller tumours
  - Long-term follow-up and genetic counselling for patients with retinoblastoma

15.9   Diffuse pale lesions

- Non-hereditary — these include myelinated nerve fibres (myelin continues from the optic disc to include the retinal nerve-fibre layer in flame-shaped patches), large coloboma of optic disc and retina, retinal ischaemia and commotio retinae ('bruising' of the retina after blunt trauma)
- Hereditary — these include albinism and rare choroidal dystrophies, e.g. gyrate atrophy

15.10   Multiple focal/discrete lesions

- Hereditary — this includes typical and atypical retinitis pigmentosa and retinitis pigmentosa-like retinal dystrophy with systemic associations (see Section 15.14)
- Other — congenital hypertrophy of the retinal pigment epithelium (CHiRPE) also known as 'bear tracks', which has associations with familial polyposis coli

Management includes electrodiagnostic and visual field evaluation.

15.11   Retinal detachment

This is an elevation of the neurosensory retina which may be rhegmatogenous as the result of a retinal tear or hole, exudative because of inflammatory exudates, tractional most commonly secondary to retinopathy of prematurity, or solid as the result of a tumour.

In a child with high myopia and a retinal detachment the possibility of Stickler syndrome should be excluded.

15.12   Folds in the fundus

- Chorioretinal folds — fine multiple folds as a result of ocular hypotony, swollen optic discs, choroidal tumours, hypermetropia (long-sightedness), orbital pseudotumour or tumour (haemangioma or neoplasm)
- Falciform fold — large single fold seen in familial exudative vitreoretinopathy, Norrie disease, retinopathy of prematurity and persistent hyperplastic primary vitreous
- Treatment includes thorough vitreoretinal evaluation.

15.13   Retinopathy of prematurity

This is a vasoproliferative retinopathy affecting premature and very-low-birth-weight infants.

The international classification of retinopathy of prematurity (ROP) is used to describe location, extent and stage of the disease.

- Location of ROP uses the optic nerve as a reference point
  - Zone 1 is an area located around the optic nerve twice the radius of the distance from the optic nerve to the fovea
  - Zone 2 is concentric to Zone 1 extending to the nasal periphery
  - Zone 3 is the remainder of the retina
- Extent of ROP is described by how many clock-hours of the retina are involved. These may be contiguous or separate areas
- ROP is a progressive disease. It begins with mild changes at the junction of the vascularized and non-vascularized retina and may progress to, or regress from, any stage before 'Stage 3 with plus disease' at which point treatment is usually instigated

Stages of ROP

Stage 1 — Demarcation line
This is a white line, lying within the plane of the retina and separating avascular from vascular retinal regions.

Stage 2 — Ridge
The line of stage 1 has increased in volume to extend outside the plane of the retina. Isolated vascular tufts may be seen posterior to the ridge at this stage.

Stage 3 — Ridge with extraretinal fibrovascular proliferation
This may be:

- Continuous with the posterior edge of the ridge
- Posterior of, but disconnected from, the ridge
- Into the vitreous

Stage 4 — Retinal detachment – subtotal

- Extrafoveal
- Involving the fovea

Stage 5 — Retinal detachment – total
The retina is usually pulled into a funnel shape by fibrovascular scar tissue. Eyes with Stage 5 ROP usually have no useful vision, even if surgery is performed to repair the retinal detachment.

'Plus' disease
This is an indicator of activity. In order of severity 'plus' signs include:

- Engorgement and tortuosity of the posterior pole retinal vessels
- Iris vessel engorgement
- Pupil rigidity
- Vitreous haze

If ROP does develop it usually does so between 34 and 40 weeks gestational age, regardless of the gestational age at birth. Treatment (diode laser or cryotherapy) is used to destroy the avascular retina. The fundamental principle of treatment is to remove the stimulus for vessel growth, i.e. to ablate the peripheral avascular retina. Treatment is given once 'Threshold ROP' develops.

Threshold ROP is defined as:

- Stage 3 ROP:
  - Involving five or more contiguous, or eight or more cumulative, clock hours
  - In the presence of congestion of the posterior pole vessels — 'plus' disease.

Examination protocol

Which babies should be screened?

- Birth at < 32 weeks gestational age
- Birth weight ≤ 1500 g

When?

All babies must be screened at 6–7 weeks postnatal age. For the more mature baby one examination before discharge may be all that is necessary even if undertaken before 6 weeks because this gives enough information about retinal vascular development to indicate the need for further examinations.

Subsequent examinations

At least every 2 weeks until vascularization has progressed into zone 3.

- Because of the short time available for treatment, if stage 3 is imminent or present it is sometimes necessary to examine a baby more frequently

Risk factors for progression of ROP

Lower birth weight, prolonged supplemental oxygen and respiratory distress syndrome (chronic lung disease) have clearly been shown to be risk factors.

15.14 Systemic disorders associated with retinitis pigmentosa and retinal pigmentary retinopathies

- Retinitis pigmentosa — a pigmentary retinopathy characterized by night blindness (earliest symptom), progressive loss of peripheral visual field and loss of central vision (end stage). Symptoms may be present in childhood but usually do not become apparent until second or third decade of life. All forms of genetic inheritance are known.
- Early retinal changes show pigment deposition, seen in the mid-peripheral retina progressing to more diffuse patchy pigment deposition and loss.

Hearing difficulties

- Usher syndrome
  - USH 1 — retinitis pigmentosa onset by 10 years, cataract, profound congenital sensory deafness, labyrinthine defect
  - USH 2 — retinitis pigmentosa onset in late teens, childhood sensory deafness
  - USH 3 — postlingual, progressive hearing loss, variable vestibular dysfunction, retinitis pigmentosa symptoms by second decade
- Alström syndrome — retinal lesions cause nystagmus and early loss of central vision (unlike other pigmentary retinopathies where peripheral vision is lost first), dilated cardiomyopathy (infancy)/congestive heart failure, atherosclerosis, hypertension, renal failure, deafness, obesity, diabetes mellitus

- Infantile Refsum disease (peroxisomal biogenesis defect) — mental retardation, minor facial dysmorphism, retinitis pigmentosa, sensorineural hearing deficit, hepatomegaly, osteoporosis, faltering growth, hypocholesterolaemia
- Classical Refsum disease (later onset) — retinitis pigmentosa, chronic polyneuropathy and cerebellar signs
- Cockayne dwarfism — precociously senile appearance, pigmentary retinal degeneration, optic atrophy, deafness, marble epiphyses in some digits, photosensitivity, mental retardation, sub-clinical myopathy
- Mucopolysaccharidoses
- Kearns–Sayre — ophthalmoplegia, pigmentary retinal degeneration and heart block are leading features

Skin disorders

- Refsum disease
- Cockayne syndrome

Renal disorders

- Senior–Loken syndrome — renal dysplasia, retinitis pigmentosa, retinal aplasia, cerebellar ataxia, sensorineural hearing loss
- Rhyns syndrome — retinitis pigmentosa, hypopituitary, nephronophthisis, mild skeletal dysplasia
- Bardet–Biedl syndrome — obesity, rod-cone dystrophy, hypogonadism, renal anomalies, polydactyly, learning difficulties, onset by end of second decade
- Cystinosis
- Alström syndrome

Skeletal disorders

- Bardet–Biedl syndrome
- Cockayne syndrome
- Jeune syndrome — chondrodysplasia that often leads to death in infancy because of a severely constricted thoracic cage and respiratory insufficiency, retinal degeneration
- Mucopolysaccharidoses IH, IS, II and III
- Infantile Refsum disease

Hepatic disorders

- Zellweger syndrome — hypotonia, seizures, psychomotor retardation, pigmentary retinopathy and cataracts

Neurological/neuromuscular

- Kearns–Sayre syndrome
- Chronic progressive external ophthalmoplegia — retinitis pigmentosa and restrictive eye movements

- Neuronal ceroid lipofuscinosis — characterized by intralysosomal accumulations of lipopigments in either granular, curvilinear or fingerprint patterns, progressive dementia, seizures and progressive visual failure
- Hallervorden–Spatz syndrome — retinitis pigmentosa and pallidal degeneration
- Joubert syndrome — hypoplasia of cerebellar vermis, saccadic initiation failure, hyperpnoea intermixed with central apnoea in the neonatal period, retinal dystrophy
- Infantile Refsum disease
- Abetalipoproteinaemia (Bassen–Kornzweig syndrome) — steatorrhoea, pigmentary retinopathy, progressive ataxic neuropathy, acanthocytosis

16.   OPTIC NERVE DISORDERS

16.1   Optic disc swelling

Unilateral

- Association — optic nerve glioma and other compressive lesions, uveitis, posterior scleritis, papillitis, neuroretinitis, acute phase of Leber's hereditary optic neuropathy, longstanding ocular hypotony (from any cause)

Bilateral

- Association — papilloedema, malignant hypertension, cavernous sinus thrombosis, buried optic nerve drusen and bilateral papillitis. In papillitis vision is always affected whereas in papilloedema vision is only affected if chronic

16.2   Optic atrophy

Optic atrophy occurs as the result of the loss of neuronal axons. It may be primary, secondary, consecutive, primary hereditary, secondary hereditary or associated with contra-lateral disc swelling.

Primary optic atrophy

This is caused by any process affecting the visual pathways from the retrolaminar portion of the optic nerve to the lateral geniculate nucleus. Unilateral optic atrophy is caused by lesions between the globe and the chiasm while bilateral optic atrophy will be caused by lesions of the chiasm or optic tracts.

- Association — any tumour, but most commonly gliomas in children
- Treatment — neuroimaging is crucial; surveillance with colour vision, visual field analysis and electrodiagnostic testing may be necessary in cases of optic gliomas

Secondary optic atrophy

This is preceded by swelling of the optic nerve head, as a result of pressure, ischaemia or inflammation, i.e. chronic papilloedema or papillitis.

Consecutive optic atrophy

This is caused by diseases of the inner retina or its blood supply.

- Associations — include retinitis pigmentosa, cone dystrophy, diffuse retinal necrosis (e.g. cytomegalovirus retinitis, acute retinal necrosis and Behçet disease), 'cherry red spot' syndromes and mucopolysaccharidoses

Primary hereditary optic atrophy

Diffuse optic atrophy with visual loss.

- Associations
  - Simple recessive type (onset ~ 4 years)
  - Kjer juvenile dominant type (onset ~ 10 years)
  - Recessive type, DIDMOAD – **d**iabetes **i**nsipidus, **d**iabetes **m**ellitus, **o**ptic **a**trophy and **d**eafness (onset ~ 5–14 years)
  - Leber's hereditary optic neuropathy (onset ~ 16–30 years)

Secondary hereditary optic atrophy

These are hereditary neurological disorders with optic atrophy, which usually present during the first decade of life.

- Associations — Behr (recessive), Friedreich ataxia (recessive), Charcot–Marie–Tooth disease (dominant, X-linked), adrenoleukodystrophies (X-linked recessive or autosomal recessive), cerebellar ataxia type I (dominant)

16.3   Optic disc size

Small optic disc

The optic nerve may appear small (hypermetropia) or actually be smaller than expected (tilted disc or optic nerve hypoplasia).

- Treatment — exclude endocrine dysfunction in cases of hypoplasia

Large optic disc

Seen in myopia, congenital optic disc pit, optic disc coloboma and morning glory anomaly.

- Treatment — neuroimaging, especially for bilateral cases

Large optic disc cup

Most normal cups have a cup : disc ratio of 0.3 or less.

- Associations — physiological cupping (cup : disc ratio > 0.7 present in ~ 2% population) and glaucomatous cupping, where there is raised intraocular pressure with or without associated findings of: increased corneal diameter, Haab's striae (splits in the cornea caused by enlargement secondary to raised intraocular pressure), increased myopia and increased axial length of the globe

- Treatment — depends on the severity of the glaucoma and age; it can include medical treatment, laser treatment or surgery

16.4   Optic disc haemorrhages

- Associated with — acute papilloedema, papillitis, infiltrative optic neuropathy, after optic nerve sheath decompression and optic disc drusen
- Treatment — investigation to exclude early papilloedema, visual field analysis

17.   EYE MOVEMENT DISORDERS

These may be described as disorders in the primary position of gaze, anomalous eye movements and nystagmus.

- **Strabismus** (a squint) is a misalignment of the visual axes of the two eyes. Approximately 4% of children under 6 years old have strabismus. Some 25% of children with childhood-onset strabismus have either a parent or a sibling with strabismus
- **Manifest squint (-tropia)** — the eyes are misaligned
- **Latent squint (-phoria)** — a tendency for the eyes to deviate, straight eyes are maintained with effort
- **Eso-** — inward deviation
- **Exo-** — outward deviation
- **Hypo-** — downward deviation
- **Hyper-** — upward deviation

17.1   Ocular deviation in primary gaze

If a deviation between the two eyes remains the same regardless of the position of gaze it is termed **comitant**. If it does change, it is termed **in-comitant** or **non-comitant**.

Pseudo-esodeviation

- Epicanthic folds — symmetric corneal reflexes confirm the absence of true esotropia
- Narrow interpupillary distance — seen in hypotelorism

True esodeviation

Comitant esotropia

- Infantile esotropia — develops before 6 months old with a large and stable angle, cross-fixation (right eye looks left, left eye looks right) normal refractive error for age
- Non-accommodative esotropia — develops after 6 months with normal refraction
- Refractive accommodative esotropia — onset usually between 2 and 3 years associated with hypermetropia (long-sighted)
- Non-refractive accommodative esotropia — between 6 months and 3 years. No

significant refractive error but excessive convergence for near (high ratio of accommodative convergence : accommodation (AC/A ratio))

- Sensory esotropia — reduction in vision, with one eye worse than the other, which disrupts fusion, e.g. uniocular cataract
- Convergence spasm — intermittent esotropia with pseudomyopia and small pupil as a result of accommodative spasm which may be seen after trauma or as the result of a posterior fossa tumour but may be the result of a functional element

Incomitant esotropia

- VI nerve palsy — may be congenital or acquired (associated with raised intracranial pressure). Esotropia is more obvious looking into the distance
- Möbius syndrome — bilateral gaze palsies, with esotropia in 50% (as the result of superimposed VI nerve palsies). There is usually bilateral VII nerve palsies and may be associated V, IX, X nerve palsies
- Duane syndrome — caused by miswiring of the horizontal recti muscles, which leads to co-contraction of the medial and lateral recti. This leads to limited abduction with approximately normal adduction (Type I), limited adduction with approximately normal abduction (Type II), or limited abduction and adduction (Type III). The palpebral fissure narrows on adduction (as a result of globe retraction) and widens on abduction. Types I and III may have an esotropia in the primary position of gaze
- Note: if a child has a limitation of abduction but is straight in the primary position this must be Duane syndrome not a VI nerve palsy

Pseudo-exodeviation

- Hypertelorism — look for symmetry of corneal light reflexes

True exodeviation

Comitant exotropia

- Intermittent exotropia — a common condition with exotropia more often present for distance than for near. In bright sunlight the child will characteristically close the diverging eye
- Sensory exotropia — much less common in children than sensory esodeviation
- Convergence insufficiency — usually seen in older children. Convergence exercises may help but there should be a low threshold to neuroimage if there are any neurological signs or worsening despite convergence exercises

Incomitant exotropia

- Congenital III nerve palsy — exodeviation and hypodeviation of the affected eye, with ptosis and miosed pupil. There is limitation of up-gaze and adduction
- Acquired III nerve palsy — Rare; same signs as congenital condition but the pupil is dilated
- Duane syndrome Type II (see above)

17.2 Anomalous eye movements

Upshoots in adduction — on version testing

- Inferior oblique overaction — may be primary (usually bilateral and seen with esotropia but also with exotropia occurring in childhood) or secondary to a superior oblique palsy
- Duane syndrome types I, II and III — as above. Upshoots occur because of the leash effect of a tight lateral rectus muscle secondary to co-contraction of the medial rectus
- Dissociated vertical deviation — a bilateral condition most commonly seen in association with infantile esotropia. At moments of inattention/dissociation, the eye will move up and then return to its original position while the fixating eye remains still. It may occur in any position of gaze so differs from inferior oblique overaction.

Downshoots in adduction — on version testing

- Duane syndrome types I, II and III: see above
- Brown syndrome — this is not an uncommon condition where the tendon of the superior oblique muscle cannot pass freely through its pulley (the trochlear, at the superomedial orbital rim). This results in restriction of elevation in up-gaze usually just in the adducted position. There may be a coincident downshoot in adduction on vergence testing, as a consequence. It is usually idiopathic but may be acquired as the result of inflammation at the trochlear or trauma

Limitation of abduction

- VI nerve palsy — there is always an esotropia in primary position of gaze unlike Duane types I and II where there may or may not be
- Any restrictive myopathy of the medial rectus — myositis, pseudo-tumour, thyroid eye disease (very rarely in children)

Limitation of adduction

- III nerve palsy — may be congenital or acquired (see above)
- Internuclear ophthalmoplegia — a lesion in the medial longitudinal fasciculus leading to an ipsilateral adduction deficit and an abducting nystagmus of the contralateral eye
- Myasthenia gravis — very rare but may mimic an adduction deficit
- Acute myositis — restriction of movement in direction of the field of action of the affected muscle
- Duane types II and III — (see above)

Limitation of horizontal versions or gaze palsies

- Any lesion of the PPRF (paramedian pontine reticular formation) — causes ipsilateral gaze palsy
- One-and-a-half syndrome — a lesion of the PPRF/abducens nerve nucleus and adjacent medial longitudinal fasciculus causing an ipsilateral gaze palsy and ipsilateral internuclear ophthalmopleiga. A right-sided lesion would lead to an inability for either eye to look to the right, the right eye could not adduct (internuclear ophthalmopleiga) but the left eye could abduct but only with nystagmus
- Bilateral pontine lesions — result in total horizontal gaze palsies

Limitation of vertical eye movements

Can be unilateral or bilateral.

- Palsy of a muscle — superior rectus, inferior rectus, inferior oblique (up-gaze affected),superior oblique (down-gaze affected)
- Orbital floor fracture — causing entrapped inferior rectus muscle and restriction of elevation
- Orbital space-occupying lesion — capillary haemangioma, plexiform neurofibroma
- Brown syndrome — limitation of elevation in adduction, see above
- Symblepharon — attachment of the lid to the globe may cause restriction of movement, especially elevation (see above)

Vertical gaze palsy

- Parinaud syndrome — decreased up-gaze, large pupils, convergence insufficiency and convergence–retraction nystagmus. In children one of the commonest causes is a pinealoma
- Hydrocephalus — stretching of the posterior commissure results in a loss of up-gaze with or without tonic downward deviation of the eyes ('sunset' sign)
- Metabolic causes — may affect vertical eye movements. Tay–Sachs disease may cause impairment of vertical and later horizontal gaze. Niemann–Pick variants may also have vertical gaze anomalies

17.3 General limitation of ocular movements

This may be the result of multiple ocular motor palsies or it may have other causes.

Multiple ocular palsies

- Cavernous sinus lesions — very rare but may be a complication of orbital cellulitis. Tumours are very rare as are caroticocavernous fistulae
- Superior orbital fissure lesion — rare but tumours of the orbit may cause problems here (leukaemia) or infections (aspergilloma in the immunocompromised child). Tolosa–Hunt syndrome (idiopathic granulomatous inflammation), which is painful during the acute phase, may affect the superior orbital fissure and/or the cavernous sinus

- Brainstem lesions — usually encephalitis but tumours of the brainstem (glioma) may also present with ophthalmoplegia

Other causes

- Chronic progressive ophthalmoplegia — may be associated with a mitochondrial cytopathy in which case it may be isolated or part of the Kearns–Sayre syndrome
- Myotonic dystrophy — may be seen in children either as the congenital variant or the type I autosomal dominant variant which has demonstrated anticipation
- Drug toxicity — most commonly seen with phenytoin
- Acquired saccadic initiation failure (ocular motor apraxia) — may be seen in lesions of the frontoparietal cortex. Both vertical and horizontal saccades are affected. May be seen in Gaucher type III. In congenital saccadic initiation failure, vertical saccades are unaffected
- Metabolic causes — Tay–Sachs disease and occasionally other lipid-storage diseases
- Congenital fibrosis syndrome — familial, may affect all extraocular muscles. Eyes often fixed in down-gaze with bilateral ptosis and chin-up head posture

18. ABNORMAL HEAD POSITIONS

18.1 Ocular causes

- Nystagmus — a null position is a position of the eyes in the orbits where the nystagmus is most dampened; in this position the child sees better. The child adopts an abnormal head position so that the eyes are in the null position while looking straight ahead
- Unilateral ametropia (usually astigmatism) — results in a head turn but rarely a head tilt
- Strabismus — a child will usually develop an abnormal head posture to reduce the amount of diplopia. As a rule the head will turn in the direction of the action of the underacting muscle(s). To see if the head posture is the result of strabismus, patch one eye, if strabismic in origin then the head posture will improve

18.2 Types of abnormal head posture

- Chin elevation — bilateral ptosis, any elevation deficit (unilateral/bilateral – see above), nystagmus (if null position is downwards)
- Chin depression — nystagmus (null position up)
- Head tilt — may be caused by a superior oblique palsy (commonest), Brown syndrome and rarely a posterior fossa tumour.
- Head turn — lateral rectus or medial rectus palsy, Duane syndrome, nystagmus with lateral null point, manifest latent nystagmus (the nystagmus in the fixing eye dampens if that eye is adducted), homonymous hemianopia, unilateral deafness and occasionally ametropia (see above)

19. NYSTAGMUS

19.1 Character of nystagmus

- Horizontal jerk — combination of slow drift with fast corrective phase. The description is in the direction of the fast corrective phase
- Pendular — nystagmus velocity is the same in both directions but on lateral gaze this usually develops a horizontal jerk component
- Oblique — the result of a combination of horizontal and vertical directions of pendular nystagmus

19.2 Physiological nystagmus

- End-point nystagmus — fine jerk nystagmus when eyes are in extreme positions of gaze (jerk towards direction of gaze)
- Optokinetic nystagmus — jerk nystagmus induced by repetitive moving targets across the visual field. Optokinetic drum/tube train leaving station. Eyes follow target then jerk back to next target. Occipito-parietal lobe controls pursuit and frontal lobe controls saccade (jerk) back, contralateral to jerk direction
- Vestibular nystagmus — jerk nystagmus caused by altered input from vestibular nuclei to horizontal gaze centres, caloric tests

19.3 Early-onset nystagmus

- Manifest nystagmus — is usually benign but may be acquired. It is uniplanar, dampens on convergence and worsens on eccentric fixation
- Latent nystagmus — no nystagmus with both eyes open but horizontal jerk nystagmus seen when one eye is covered. Most commonly seen with infantile esotropia but may be seen with other early-onset deviations. The fast phase is towards the uncovered fixating eye
- Manifest–latent nystagmus — usually seen with infantile esotropia and dissociated vertical deviation. The nystagmus worsens with one eye occluded
- Spasmus nutans — an early onset (3–18 months) unilateral or bilateral small-amplitude high-frequency horizontal nystagmus often associated with head nodding. Most often idiopathic with resolution by 3 years of age but it may be the result of an optic pathway glioma (therefore a diagnosis of exclusion)
- Roving nystagmus — severe disruption of visual function may lead to this and the commonest causes are Leber's congenital amaurosis (severe retinal dystrophy) or optic nerve hypoplasia (bilateral)

19.4 Later-onset nystagmus

- Coarse horizontal jerk nystagmus — usually seen in cerebellar disease, with the fast phase ipsilateral to the lesion
- Torsional nystagmus — if pure, then this is usually only seen in central vestibular disease such as syringomyelia or syringobulbia associated with Arnold–Chiari malformation, demyelination and very rarely, lateral medullary syndrome in children
- Downbeat nystagmus — usually seen with lesions at the craniocervical junction (Arnold–Chiari malformation), drug toxicity (phenytoin, carbamazepine), trauma, hydrocephalus and demyeliation
- Upbeat nystagmus — usually seen in cerebellar degenerations (ataxia telangiectasia) and encephalitis; however, in babies a retinal dystrophy should be excluded (especially cone dystrophy)
- Gaze-evoked nystagmus — may be seen with lesions of the vestibulocerebellar axis, brainstem, cerebral hemispheres or after a gaze palsy or with drug toxicity (phenytoin, carbamazepine)
- Periodic alternating nystagmus — the direction of the nystagmus reverses. May be congenital idiopathic but may be seen with Arnold–Chiari malformation or cerebellar disease, trauma or demyelination
- Rebound nystagmus — attempts to maintain eccentric gaze results in gaze-evoked nystagmus which dampens and sometimes reverses direction. On returning to primary gaze a transient nystagmus develops. Usually seen in cerebellar disease
- See-saw nystagmus — pendular nystagmus in which one eye elevates and intorts while the other eye depresses and extorts and then the eyes reverse. The commonest cause is chiasmal or parasellar tumours but may also be seen in albinism as a transient finding, head trauma and syringobulbia.
- Internuclear ophthalmoplegia — the abducting eye has nystagmus (see above), lesion in the medial longitudinal fasciculus
- Monocular nystagmus — may be seen in spasmus nutans, unilateral deep amblyopia, superior oblique myokymia and optic nerve glioma
- Convergence–retraction nystagmus — seen in Parinaud syndrome (above)

19.5 Ocular causes of nystagmus

Disruption of vision will lead to nystagmus.

There may be obvious (usually bilateral) ocular disease:

- Corneal opacities
- Congenital cataract
- Microphthalmos
- Aniridia
- Oculocutaneous albinism

Less obvious ocular diseases:

- Retinal dystrophy (usually cone dystrophy or Leber's congenital amaurosis), ocular albinism
- X-liked congenital stationary night blindness
- Optic nerve hypoplasia
- Early onset optic atrophy

20. FURTHER READING

Leigh RJ. 1999. *The Neurology of Eye Movements 3rd edition.* Oxford: Oxford University Press.

Taylor DSI, Hoyt C (Eds). 2004. *Pediatric Ophthalmology and Strabismus 3rd edition.* London: Saunders.

Wright K. 1995. *Pediatric Ophthalmology and Strabismus.* London: Elsevier.

Wright K, Spiegel P (Eds). 2002. *Pediatric Ophthalmology and Strabismus 2nd edition.* New York: Springer Verlag.

Chapter 20

Orthopaedics

Vel K Sakthivel and N M P Clarke

CONTENTS

Orthopaedics

1. INTRODUCTION

This chapter aims to provide the doctor who is training to be a paediatrician with an insight into the subspecialty of Paediatric Orthopaedics. The contents of this chapter are by no means exhaustive but will offer a mode of quick revision to the paediatrician.

2. EMBRYOLOGY

- The primitive streak appears at about 12 days after conception
- Caudally, cells migrate from ectoderm and endoderm to form mesoderm. The mesoderm forms the connective tissue
- Cranially, the formation of the notochord appears in the second to third week of gestation
- Neural crest cells differentiate to form the peripheral and autonomic nervous systems
- Somites form on each other side of the notochord and develop into a specific dermatome, myotome and sclerotome
- Limb buds develop between 4 and 6 weeks
- Bone develops either in a cartilage model (endochondral ossification), or in a membrane model (intramembranous ossification)
- Primary ossification centres appear between 7 and 12 weeks. They form in the mid-portion of the bone anlage. This is responsible for the formation of the diaphysis and the metaphysis
- Secondary ossification centres develop in the chondroepiphysis. The ossification centre for the distal femur occurs at 40 weeks of gestation. This is of medico-legal importance because the presence of this centre is indicative of a complete pregnancy. All the other secondary centres occur post-natally
- There are two types of growth plates
  - Physis — which responds to compressive forces
  - Apophysis — which responds to tensile forces

3. TRAUMA

- Orthopaedic trauma accounts for 15–20% of Accident and Emergency department visits in the UK
- There are a number of anatomical and physiological variations in the paediatric skeleton which make this practice different from that of the adult practice

3.1 Anatomical and physiological differences in the paediatric skeleton

- The bony architecture in children includes a thick periosteum, a growth plate (physis), and an epiphysis (secondary ossification centre)
- The immature skeleton is much more elastic and hence absorbs more stress before actually breaking
- The ligaments are stronger than the epiphyseal plates to which they are attached so the incidence of sprains and ligamentous injuries is far less in children than of avulsion fractures of the ends of the bones
- The periosteum is thick and extremely active, producing abundant callus aiding fracture healing. Non unions are rare in paediatrics
- Remodelling helps with reshaping of a healed fracture
- The younger the patient and the closer the fracture is to a joint (metaphysis of long bones), the greater the potential to remodel
- Deformities occurring in the plane of motion of the adjacent joint will also remodel better than otherwise, i.e a dorso-volar deformity in the distal end of the radius will remodel better than a fracture which has healed with radial or ulnar deviation

3.2 Fractures unique to the immature skeleton

Growth plate (physeal) fractures

- Up to 30% of paediatric fractures involve the growth plate. Most such fractures occur through the hypertrophic zone. The commonest site of growth plate fractures is the distal radius and ulna
- A widely used and accepted classification system was designed by Salter and Harris. This classification system also has significant prognostic and treatment implications

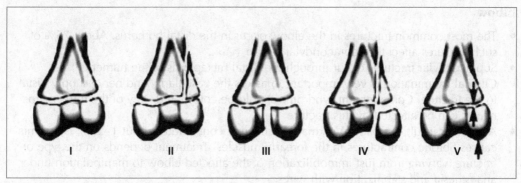

The Salter–Harris classification of growth plate injuries

Greenstick fractures

- Greenstick fractures are the most common (50%) fracture affecting the paediatric patient. They are also called **unicortical fractures** because one cortex is in continuity. There is often rotation and angulation of the fracture

Buckle fractures and plastic deformation

- Following axial loading, buckling of the metaphyseal bone occurs, leading to a buckle or Torus fracture. This is a very stable fracture and often all that is needed is a few weeks of immobilization for pain relief
- Paediatric bone is more elastic than adult bone; it absorbs more energy before fracturing. This leads to more deformation of the bone before breaking and hence there is a recognized entity called plastic deformation which is quite regularly seen in a child following injury
- There is no breach of the cortex but a deformity of the bone is seen

3.3 Fractures involving the upper limb

Shoulder

- The clavicle is the most commonly fractured long bone in a child
- Most of these fractures heal well with non-operative management methods
- **NB** The clavicle has two primary ossifying centres; the secondary centre fuses with the diaphysis at about 22–25 years of age. This can be confused with a fracture

Proximal humeral fractures

- Usually heal well with non-operative management, with good potential for remodelling
- Humeral shaft fractures should be evaluated with a good history and clinical examination. These fractures are not common without significant violence. If there is no appropriate history, there should be a high index of suspicion about child abuse, especially if the fracture is spiral

Elbow

- The most common fractures in the elbow occur in the distal humerus. About 75% of such fractures affect the supracondylar region
- Supracondylar fractures occur through the distal metaphysis of the humerus
- Clinical examination is very important to assess the vascularity and nerve supply distal to the fracture. Compartment syndrome should be considered. Any of the three major nerves can be affected by this fracture
- A vascular insult can cause Volkman's ischaemic contracture (about 1–2%). Ischaemia causes fibrotic contractures in the forearm muscles. Treatment depends on the type of fracture, varying from just immobilization of the affected elbow to manipulation under anaesthesia and stabilization with wires

Forearm, wrist and hand

- Monteggia fracture is a complex injury where there is an ulnar shaft fracture and dislocation of the radial head
- Galeazzi fracture is the association of a fracture of the shaft of the radius and disruption of the inferior radio-ulnar joint
- Treatment options range from manipulation under anaesthesia to open reduction and internal fixation
- Distal radial fractures are common, especially when the child falls on to their outstretched hand. Salter–Harris type 2 fractures are the most common fractures affecting the distal radius
- Boxer's fractures (neck of the fifth metacarpal) are common in the late teens when they suffer a punching injury

3.4 Fractures involving the lower limb

Pelvis and hip

- Uncommon
- Usually caused by high-velocity road traffic accidents
- Treatment depends on the classification and displacement. It may include:
  - Manipulation under anaesthesia
  - Hip spica
  - Closed or open reduction with internal fixation
- Complications include
  - Avascular necrosis (incidence of approximately 40%)
  - Growth arrest leading to deformities like coxa vara
  - Non-union has an incidence of about 5%

Femur fractures

- Incidence is about 1% in children under the age of 12 years
- Peak age is between 2 and 5 years
- 70% occur in the middle third, 20% in the proximal third and 10% in the distal third
- Waddell's triad — fractured femur, head injury and thoracic injury

- Consider non-accidental injury in a child with a femur fracture
- Clinical symptoms include pain and deformity. Examine for distal neurovascular deficit
- Treatment — analgesia, splinting, traction, spica, internal fixation (plates osteosynthesis, intramedullary nails)
- Complications include leg-length discrepancies

Fractures of the tibia and fibula

- Most common lower limb fractures in children
- Account for about one-fifth of paediatric long bone fractures
- Clinical symptoms — pain and deformity. Assess neurovascular status
- Fracture in toddlers — spiral fracture of the tibia in a child between 9 months and 3 years
  - Low-energy injury
  - Leads to a limp and to localized warmth and tenderness
  - Child usually crawls and prefers not to weight bear
  - X-rays may be inconclusive initially
  - Usually heal with no trouble
- Treatment generally includes analgesia, splinting. Operative treatment involves plating, nailing or external fixation

Knee

The main injuries include meniscal injuries, anterior cruciate ligament injuries and osteo-chondral defects. Others include Osgood–Schlatter disease and chondromalacia patellae.

- **Meniscal injuries**
  - Usually a twisting injury
  - Symptoms include pain, effusion, locking, giving way and snapping
  - Evaluation consists of clinical examination, diagnostic arthroscopy and magnetic resonance imaging
  - Treatment is usually arthroscopic meniscectomy
- **Anterior cruciate ligmament injury**
  - Incidence = 0.3 per 1000 per year
  - Usually a sporting injury
  - Can be associated with injury to other ligaments
  - Management involves physiotherapy and reduced activity with or without internal fixation
- **Osteochondral defects** (osteochondritis dissecans)
  - Defect involving bone and cartilage within the knee
  - Causes discontinuity of the articular cartilage
  - Aetiology unknown
  - Most commonly seen in the lateral surface of the medial femoral condyle
  - Signs and symptoms — pain, locking, effusion, may present with an acutely locked knee

- Treatment — analgesia, rest, splintage (if subchondral bone is intact)
- Arthroscopic assessment is required. If there is a 'loose body' then that should be removed
- **Osgood–Schlatter disease**.
  - Inflammation of the tibial tubercle as a result of repeated tensile forces
  - Incidence of about 2% of all growth plate injuries
  - Generally a self-limiting condition. Bilateral in about one-third of patients. Boys affected more than girls
  - Rest and analgesia are all that may be required
- **Adolescent anterior knee pain (chondromalacia patella)**
  - Pain about the knee is a common complaint. Initially hip pathology should be excluded
  - 'Chondromalacia patella' has been converted from a term meaning softening of the articular cartilage to that of an innocent condition of ill-defined anterior knee pain
  - Symptoms should be considered to be due to an unknown cause until a specific aetiology is established. If none is determined 'idiopathic anterior knee pain' is treated with physiotherapy and normally resolves

Foot and ankle

- **Ankle fractures** are classified using the Salter–Harris classification
  - Usually caused by a twisting force
  - Cause pain, deformity, swelling
  - X-rays are usually conclusive
  - Treatment includes splintage and analgesia. Can be treated by open reduction and internal fixation
- **Tarsal and metatarsal fractures** occur frequently in the adolescent patient. Diagnosis can prove difficult
  - Treatment is usually by splintage and analgesia. Internal fixation is rarely required

4. METABOLIC DISORDERS

Bone metabolism is explained in detail in Chapter 7 — Endocrinology.

4.1 Rickets and osteomalacia

- Occurs when there is a decrease in serum calcium (may be just the ionized component) or phosphorus or both
- Causes growth abnormalities and abnormal mineralization of the skeleton in children (**rickets**)
- Affects the mineralization of the skeleton alone in an adult (**osteomalacia**)

Clinical manifestations

- Apathetic and irritable
- Short attention span

- Short stature (height below the third percentile)
- Frontal bossing
- Enlargement of skull sutures (hot cross bun skull)
- Delayed dentition
- Enlargement of costal cartilages (Rachitic rosary)
- Pectus carinatum
- Delayed weight-bearing milestones
- Deformities of lower limbs (genu varum)
- Enlarged epiphyseal regions of the long bones

Radiological findings

- Cupping and widening of epiphysis
- Osteopenia of the metaphysis
- Looser's zones represent areas of weakening in the bone. Although they can predispose to fractures, they do not themselves imply that there is a fracture

Further investigation

- Bone scan may help in mild cases

4.2   Osteogenesis imperfecta

- Defect in type 1 collagen
- Four types have been identified by Sillence

Types of osteogenesis imperfecta defined by Sillence

Type	Inheritance	Sclerae	Features
I	AD	Blue	Hearing loss IA — teeth affected IB — teeth not affected
II	AR	Blue	Lethal
III	AR	Normal	Fractures at birth short stature
IV	AD	Normal	Milder, normal hearing

AD, autosomal dominant; AR, autosomal recessive.

Clinical features

- Increased fragility of bones but fracture healing process is unaffected
- Short stature
- Scoliosis
- Defective dentinogenesis
- Conductive deafness

- Ligamentous laxity
- Blue sclerae and tympanic membranes

Diagnosis

- History
- Clinical examination
- X-rays — thin cortices and osteopenia
- Histologically — wide Haversian canals, osteocyte lacunae

Management

- Aims include fracture management and rehabilitation
- May need special techniques to aid fracture management (i.e. Sofield's osteotomy)
- Ideally would have an internal fixation
- Calcitonin and calcium supplements reduce the incidence of fractures
- Bisphosphonates

4.3   Idiopathic juvenile osteoporosis

- Reduction in mineral and matrix (cf osteomalacia where there is normal matrix but reduced mineral)
- Rare
- Self-limiting
- Age of onset usually between 8 and 14 years
- Resolves spontaneously by 3–4 years after onset

Clinical features

- Bone and joint pain
- Growth arrest
- Vertebral collapse
- Metaphyseal fractures
- Diaphysis is less affected (cf osteogenesis Imperfecta in which bone is uniformally affected)

Diagnosis

- Serum calcium and phosphorus are normal
- Alkaline phosphatase is normal or slightly elevated
- Hypercalciuria may be present
- Diagnosis is usually by exclusion
- Differential diagnoses — osteogenesis Imperfecta, haematological malignancies, thyrotoxicosis, Cushing syndrome

Management

- Treatment of fractures is similar to that in the normal child
- Bracing for scoliosis

5. NEUROMUSCULAR DISORDERS

5.1 Arthrogrypotic syndromes

Arthrogryposis multiplex congenita

- Non-progressive disorder
- Congenitally rigid joints
- Sensory function is maintained but there is loss of motor function (may mimic polio)

Aetiology
- May be neuropathic, myopathic or mixed
- Decrease in anterior horn cells in the spinal cord

Possible associations
- Oligohydramnios
- Intrauterine viral infection

Clinical features
- Normal facies
- Normal intelligence
- Multiple joint contractures
- No visceral abnormalities
- Associated with teratological hip dislocations, club feet and vertical talus
- C-shaped scoliosis

Treatment
- Orthopaedically it is aimed at release of soft-tissue contractures, physiotherapy and functional bracing

Distal arthrogryposis syndrome

- Autosomal dominant disorder
- Predominantly affects the hands and feet
- Ulnar deviation of fingers, flexion contractures at the metacarpophalangeal and proximal interphalangeal joints
- Club foot and vertical talus

Larsen syndrome

- Joints less rigid than in arthrogryposis
- Multiple joint dislocations
- Flattened facies
- Scoliosis
- Cervical kyphosis

5.2   Spina bifida (myelomeningocele)

Introduction

This is a disorder of incomplete spinal cord closure or rupture of the cord secondary to hydrocephalus. It can be:

- Spina bifida occulta (defects in the bony vertebral arch but intact cord structures)
- Meningocele (sac of meninges without the neural elements)
- Myelomeningocele (sac of meninges with the protruding neural elements)
- Rachischisis (exposed neural elements with no meninges)

Antenatal diagnosis

- Raised α-fetoprotein
- Ultrasound (anomaly visible on scan)

Clinical features

- Neonatal findings such as hip dislocations, hyperextension of the knee, and club feet are common
- Fractures are common but as there are problems with sensory function, diagnosis can be difficult
- Signs and symptoms depend on the level of the spinal defect
- Increased incidence of allergic reactions, mainly latex sensitivity
- **Hips**
  - Flexion contractures with higher level involvement
  - Dislocation of the hip
  - Late hip dislocation can be a sign of tethering of the cord
- **Knees**
  - Quadriceps weakness causing difficulty in ambulation (key level is L4)
  - Flexion contractures
  - Valgus deformity
- **Ankle and foot**
  - Rigid club foot
  - Tight Achilles tendon
  - Valgus hind foot
- **Spine**
  - Scoliosis can be bony or muscular (thoracic level paraplegia) in origin
  - Rapid curve progression can denote hydrocephalus or a tethered cord

Principles of treatment

Treatment should be directed to mobilize the patient.

- Soft-tissue contracture release
- Corrective osteotomy, as required
- Functional bracing

- Surgical treatment may be required, directed at a specific problem, i.e. hip dislocation or scoliosis
- Specialized physiotherapy
- Custom-made wheelchair

5.3 Myopathies

Duchenne muscular dystrophy

- This is a sex-linked recessive myopathy
- 'Clumsy walking'
- Calf pseudohypertrophy
- Gower's sign is positive (gets up using the hands to move up the body to compensate for loss of antigravity muscles)
- Hip extensors are the muscle groups to be affected first
- Markedly elevated creatine phosphokinase
- Muscle biopsy shows absent dystrophin
- Muscle biopsy also shows foci of necrotic tissue infiltration
- Treatment is directed to keeping the patient ambulatory
- Patients are usually wheelchair-bound by the age of 15 years
- Scoliosis is a major concern in treatment

Becker dystrophy

- This is a sex-linked recessive myopathy
- Similar to Duchenne but less severe clinical picture
- Red/green colour blindness
- Patients live beyond their teens
- Dystrophin is present but abnormal

Facio-scapulo-humeral dystrophy

- This is an autosomal dominant disorder
- Facial abnormalities
- Winging of scapula
- Normal creatine phosphokinase

Myotonic myopathies

- **Myotonia congenita**
  - Defect is in chromosome 7
  - Affects chloride channels in the muscles
  - Hypertrophy seen with no weakness of muscles
  - Improves with exercise

- **Paramyotonia congenita**
  - Defect is in chromosome 17
  - Affects the sodium channels in the muscles
  - Symptoms worsen with exposure to cold
  - Worse in distal upper extremity
- **Dystrophic myotonia**
  - Defect is in chromosome 19
  - Small gonads
  - Low IQ
  - Distal involvement

6. LOWER LIMB

6.1 Developmental dysplasia of the hip

- Comprises a spectrum of abnormalities from complete dislocation of the hip to mild acetabular dysplasia
- Types of developmental hip dysplasia include dislocated hip, dislocatable hip, subluxable hip and dysplastic hip
- Incidence is 1 in 1,000 for established dislocation (15 per 1,000 for neonatal instability)
- Risk factors include being a first-born, being female, having a breech presentation and family history
- Other associated conditions include congenital torticollis, skull or facial abnormalities, hyperextension of the knee and club feet
- Clinical examination includes Ortolani test (for reducing a dislocated hip) and Barlow test (for dislocatable or subluxatable hip)
- Hip click suggests an audible or palpable noise while examining the hips, when there are no signs of instability
- Thigh skin creases may or may not be asymmetric
- Teratological dislocation means that there are other associated conditions such as arthrogryposis. These are typically stiff, high-riding and irreducible dislocations
- Screening for this diagnosis includes a neonatal physical examination and, possibly, ultrasound of the hips
- Screening can be general (all newborn babies undergo an ultrasound examination) or selective (only babies with specific risk factors undergo the ultrasound). A protocol is illustrated below.

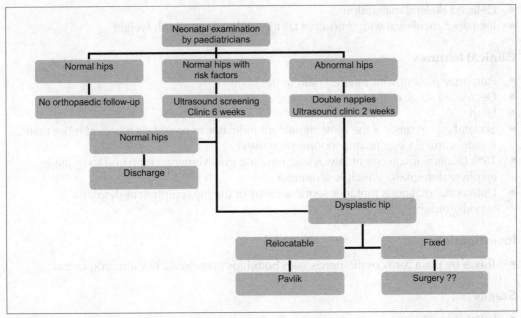

Protocol for management of developmental hip dysplasia

Treatments

- Early diagnosis — Pavlik harness has a success rate of about 85%
- Failed Pavlik harness or late presenters (> 3 months) will undergo either a closed or an open reduction augmented with a hip spica
- Late presenters, more than 2 years old, will almost certainly have, along with the above procedure, a femoral shortening osteotomy
- Even with a successful closed reduction, about 50% of patients will need a pelvic osteotomy later because there is usually a residual acetabular dysplasia

Complications

- Avascular necrosis of the proximal femoral physis
- Growth disturbances
- Coxa magna
- Residual acetabular dysplasia

6.2 Perthes disease (Legg–Calvé–Perthes disease)

This is a non-inflammatory deformity of the femoral head caused by a vascular insult leading to osteonecrosis of the capital femoral epiphysis.

- It affects more boys than girls (4 : 1)
- Usually presents between 4 and 8 years of age (can have a secondary peak between 10 and 12 years)

835

- Delayed skeletal maturation
- Increased incidence with a positive family history or low birth weight

Clinical features

- Pain (may present with referred pain in the knee)
- Decreased range of motion
- Limp
- Skeletal age at onset is the most significant indicator of prognosis (onset at more than 6 years carries a significantly poorer prognosis)
- 15% bilateral involvement (always asymmetric involvement, compared to multiple epiphyseal dysplasia which is symmetric).
- Differential diagnosis includes septic arthritis of the hip, epiphyseal dysplasia, hypothyroidism

Investigation

- This is by plain X-ray of the pelvis with both hips anteroposterior and frog lateral

Stages

- Initial stage
- Fragmentation
- Healing
- Residual

Severity

This is described in many ways but the most commonly used classification is the Herring lateral pillar classification:

- Group A — lateral pillar, lateral one-third of the femoral head shows collapse of less than 30%
- Group B — 30–50% collapse
- Group C — > 50% collapse of the lateral one-third of the capital femoral epiphysis

Treatment

- Aims to maintain the range of movement and to contain the femoral head in the acetabulum. Soft tissue release and corrective osteotomy may be required to achieve this

6.3 Slipped capital femoral epiphysis

Displacement or slipping of the proximal femoral epiphysis on the neck (this is a misnomer and it is usually the neck which slips out of alignment with the head; the head stays in the acetabulum). The defect is in the hypertrophic zone of the growth plate.

Incidence

- Two to 10 in 100,000
- Commonly seen in African-American adolescent boys
- Risk factors — obesity, positive family history
- Can be bilateral in about 25% of cases

Clinical symptoms

- Pain in the hip or knee
- Antalgic gait
- Externally rotated limb
- Decreased internal rotation of the affected limb

Classification

Classification depends on the duration of the symptoms or on ability:

- Acute — less than 3 weeks
- Acute on Chronic
- Chronic — more than 3 weeks
- Stable (can weight bear) or Unstable (unable to weight bear)

Investigations

- Plain X-ray pelvis anteroposterior and frog lateral
- Grading on the extent of slip

Treatment

- Screw fixation of the epiphysis
- Corrective osteotomy may be required in delayed presentations
- Prophylactic pinning of the contralateral hip may be considered
- Complications include avascular necrosis of the femoral head (usually occurs after treatment which includes manipulation of the head before pinning).

6.4 Congenital talipes equinovarus

- Also called 'club foot'
- Incidence is 1 in 1,000
- Ratio of male to female is 2 : 1
- No known causes but definite presence of genetic preponderance
- Various theories, such as fetal developmental arrest, myogenic and neurogenic problems, or retracting fibrosis, have been put forward
- Various associations, such as Streeter dysplasia, diastrophic dwarfism, arthrogryposis and myelomeningocele, have been documented
- Two types: positional (where the deformity is passively, fully correctable) and structural or rigid (where the deformity cannot be passively corrected)

- It is a three-dimensional deformity involving forefoot adduction and supination with hindfoot equinus and varus
- Earlier treatment improves prognosis
- Treatment can either be non-operative (serial casting, splinting) or operative (soft-tissue release with or without corrective osteotomy)

6.5 Irritable hip

- Is an idiopathic benign inflammation of the hip joint, which is one of the commonest causes of admission to a paediatric orthopaedic unit
- May be confused with septic arthritis but severe spasm, tenderness, pyrexia >30°C and ESR>20 differentiates sepsis
- Perthes disease is always diagnosed on an initial X-ray but irritable hip usually resolves spontaneously

7. UPPER LIMB

7.1 Orthopaedic brachial plexus palsy

- Paralysis of the upper limb muscles noted at birth
- Incidence is 0.4 per 1,000 live births
- Causes include pelvic dystocia, shoulder dystocia (upper cervical roots), and breech (lower cervical roots)
- There is a completely flail upper limb at birth, with full recovery in about 75% at about 4 years
- In babies for whom this does not resolve, a residual Erb's palsy is noted
- This is a C5–6 root problem manifesting with weakness in the shoulder abductors and external rotators and elbow flexion and supination
- A rarer problem involving the lower roots can sometimes ensue. This affects the C7, C8 and T1 roots and presents as loss of sensation in the hand and loss of finger flexion
- A mixed palsy (even rarer) can sometimes occur
- Electromyograms can sometimes be helpful but they are not preferred because of the baby's age and the discomfort they can cause. It is better to follow these children clinically
- Treatment involves physiotherapy to keep the joints mobile and supple
- Failure of restoration of elbow flexion by 3 months necessitates referral for consideration of surgery

8. INFECTION

8.1 Osteomyelitis

- Common in children but the incidence is decreasing
- In children it is usually acute and follows haematogenous spread (in the adult it usually follows direct inoculation)
- Pathophysiology — because the physis forms an avascular barrier there are a lot of end arteries in the metaphyseal ends of the long bones. Blood flow is very slow there and this helps bacteria to settle and multiply there, thus causing infection
- Acute (diagnosis with symptoms for less than 2 weeks), subacute (symptoms for more than 2 weeks) and chronic (missed early diagnosis) phases are noted. This depends, to an extent, on the virulence of the affecting organism and the host immune response
- Clinical features — fever, pain in the affected limb, avoidance of using the limb, limping (90% affect the lower limb), reduction of adjacent joint movement (not as severe as septic arthritis)
- Previous history of flu-like illness should be elicited and questions regarding otitis, pharyngitis and impetigo must be asked
- Investigations include full blood count, erythrocyte sedimentation rate, C-reactive protein, blood cultures, plain radiographs (may be normal in acute osteomyelitis) and bone scan (may sometimes be needed to confirm diagnosis)
- Magnetic resonance imaging and ultrasound may also be required
- Differential diagnoses include septic arthritis, fractures, neoplasms and acute infarction episodes
- Complications include chronic osteomyelitis, pathological fractures, septic arthritis and growth arrests or physeal bars
- Common causative organisms — *Staphylococcus aureus* (commonest), group B streptococcus, *Escherichia coli, Haemophilus influenzae*
- Treatment should include antibiotics to cover the respective organisms. This should usually last for 6 weeks. C-reactive protein is a good investigation with which to monitor the progress of treatment

8.2 Septic arthritis

- Most commonly affected joint is the knee, followed by the hip
- Peak age is 3 years but can affect virtually any age group
- Usually involves a single joint if it is an uncomplicated septic arthritis
- Pathophysiology — the cause is usually transient bacteraemia, direct inoculation or decompression of a juxta-articular osteomyelitis
- Clinical features
  - Fever, irritable hip and limp, refusal to use the involved extremity
  - Painful limited range of motion
  - Effusion
  - A typical attitude of the limb (as the child tends to hold the limb with the joint in a position of maximal comfort)
  - Pseudo-paralysis in the newborn should raise suspicions

- Investigations
  - Full blood count, erythrocyte sedimentation rate, C-reactive protein (normal values do not necessarily rule out infection in this age group)
  - Blood cultures
  - Microscopy, culture and sensitivity of the joint aspirate
  - Plain X-rays
  - Ultrasound
  - Magnetic resonance imaging and bone scan (can be normal if there is a tense effusion in the joint) may sometimes be required because diagnosis is often difficult
- Treatment
  - Consists of early administration of antibiotics and drainage of the purulent effusion in the joint
  - Splintage may sometimes be required
- Prognosis is good if diagnosis is early and treatment is instigated immediately. Delay in treatment can lead to early secondary arthritis with significant post-septic sequelae
- Most common organisms:
  - Neonate — *Staphylococcus aureus*, group B streptococcus
  - Child < 5 years — *S. aureus*, group A streptococcus, *Streptococcus pneumoniae*
  - Child > 5 years — *S. aureus*, group A streptococcus
  - Adolescent — *S. aureus*, *Neisseria gonorrhoeae*
- **NB** Atypical presentations — tuberculosis is on the increase in the Western world so have a high index of suspicion.

9. PAEDIATRIC SPINE

9.1 Scoliosis

- Prevalence is 0.5 to 3 per 100 (for curves between 10 and 30 degrees)
- Generally girls are affected more commonly than boys (but this may change for different age groups)
- Three-dimensional deformity (lateral curve and rotational deformity)
- Studies show both X-linked and autosomal dominant inheritance
- Recent studies have shown that certain hormonal factors, like melatonin, play an important part in the progression of this condition

Classification

- It can be idiopathic, neuromuscular, congenital, hysterical, functional and mixed with other associations (mesenchymal, traumatic, osteochondrodystophies etc.)
- It can also be classified into: Infantile (0–3 years), Juvenile (3–10 years), Adolescent (> 10 years)

Clinical features

- Asymmetry of the shoulder
- Asymmetry of the top of the pelvis
- Adams forward bend test shows a rib prominence to the side of the curve
- Lateral deviation of the head is measured (from the natal cleft) by dropping a plumb line from the C7 vertebra
- Lower limb lengths should be assessed for true and apparent limb length discrepancy
- Truncal shift should also be assessed
- Associated features, such as café-au-lait spots (neurofibromatosis), hairy patch in the lumbosacral area (spinal dysraphism), joint laxity (connective tissue disorder) should be noted
- Full neurological examination of the lower and upper limbs should be carried out

Investigations

- Plain X-rays of the whole spine posteroanterior and lateral (standing views)
- Magnetic resonance imaging and computerized tomography may be indicated depending on the neurology present and to assess for any congenital bony anomalies

Treatment

- Identify the curves that are more likely to progress (to be done by a paediatric spinal surgeon)
- Bracing (controversial in the UK but more commonly used in the USA)
- Surgery with or without spinal fusion
- Treat any intraspinal abnormalities like syringomyelia or dysraphism before attempting curve correction

9.2 Kyphosis

- Normal in the thoracic and sacral regions of the spine
- Between T5 and T12, an angle of 20–40 degrees is considered normal; 40–50 degrees is considered borderline normal; < 20 degrees is termed **hypokyphosis** and > 50 degrees is termed **hyperkyphosis**.

Causes of kyphosis

Hyperkyphosis	Hypokyphosis
Congenital	Scoliosis
Neuromuscular	Iatrogenic
Postural	
Scheuermann's disease	
Connective tissue disorders	
Metabolic	
Trauma	

10. FURTHER READING

Herring JA. 2002. *Tachdjians' Paediatric Orthopaedics 3rd edition*. Philadelphia, USA: WB Saunders.

Sillence DO, Rimoin DL. 1978. Classification of Osteogenesis Imperfecta. *Lancet* 1, 1041–2.

Staheli LT. 2003. *Orthopaedic Secrets 2nd edition*. Philadelphia, USA: Hanley & Belfuss.

Chapter 21

Respiratory

Jane C Davies

CONTENTS

Respiratory

1. ANATOMY AND PHYSIOLOGY

1.1 Embryology

In utero development is divided into four stages.

Embryonic — up to 5th week

- Lung bud grows out from the fetal foregut
- Single tube branches into two main bronchi

Pseudoglandular — 6th–16th week

- Airways grow by branching (out to terminal bronchioles)
- Cartilage and lymphatics appear from 10 weeks onwards
- Cilia appear
- Pulmonary circulation develops, arteries arising from the sixth branchial arches

Canalicular — 17th–24th week

- Conventional architecture of the lung appears
- Thinning out of distal cells in preparation for gas exchange
- Further development of arterial circulation, and appearance of venous system
- Surfactant synthesis begins
- Lung fills with fluid (lack of fluid at this and later stage (e.g. with renal agenesis) leads to pulmonary hypoplasia)

Alveolar sac — 24th–40th week

- Formation of the acinus (respiratory bronchioles, alveolar ducts and alveoli)
- Cell differentiation into type I and II pneumocytes.
- **Type I**
  - > 90% of alveolar surface
  - Major gas exchanging surface
- **Type II**
  - Thought to be the progenitor cell for type I cells
  - Produces surfactant which maintains surface tension and prevents alveolar collapse during respiration

- Surfactant-associated proteins A and D (hydrophilic) involved mainly in innate immunity
- Surfactant-associated proteins B and C (hydrophobic) important for surface tension

1.2 Fetal and postnatal lung growth

Factors affecting fetal lung growth and development include:

- Lack of amniotic fluid
- Glucocorticoids, thyroid hormones, other hormones increase maturation
- Pressure effects (e.g. compression from diaphragmatic hernia, or space-occupying lesion leads to hypoplasia)

Postnatally, lung development and growth continue for 7 years and may be adversely influenced by:

- Ventilation and oxygen toxicity
- Early infection (e.g. adenovirus, respiratory syncytial virus (RSV))
- Pressure effects of large, space-occupying lesion, e.g. lung cyst

1.3 Changes at birth and persistent fetal circulation

Vaginal delivery compresses the thorax, leading to expulsion of lung fluid and expansion of the lungs with the first breath. The increase in oxygen content leads to closure of the ductus arteriosus (which in fetal life diverts right ventricular blood away from the lungs into the systemic circulation), and the resultant increase in left atrial pressure (from increased pulmonary venous return) closes the foramen ovale. Thus, the right-sided pulmonary and left-sided systemic circulations become effectively separated. Persistent fetal circulation describes the situation where the pulmonary vasculature fails to relax, leading to ongoing right to left shunting of (deoxygenated) blood at the ductal and foramen ovale levels. Infants are severely hypoxic, mimicking the clinical picture of cyanotic congenital heart disease. Treatment includes ventilation with a high fractional inspired oxygen (FiO_2), and administration of pulmonary vasodilators such as inhaled nitric oxide or prostacyclin.

1.4 Control of respiration

Inspiration is achieved largely by diaphragmatic effort with additional expansion provided by the intercostal muscles. At rest, expiration is largely passive, although this may become active upon exercise, or in children with respiratory disease. Expiration against a partially closed glottis both prolongs this phase and raises airway pressure, leading to increased alveolar gas exchange. This is observed in the common sign of 'grunting' in infants with respiratory distress.

Respiratory drive is provided by both central (medulla) and peripheral (carotid body) chemoreceptors. In normal health, high CO_2 leads to increased respiratory drive, although in chronic lung disease sensitivity may be blunted, and there is a dependence on hypoxia for this stimulus.

1.5 Ventilation

Air passes through the trachea, major bronchi and terminal bronchioles (anatomical dead-space) before reaching the sites of active gas exchange, the alveoli. In normal health, alveolar walls are thin (one cell thick) facilitating O_2 and CO_2 exchange. In diseases affecting the alveolus, gas exchange will be impaired, leading to an increase in respiratory rate in response to both a low O_2 and a raised CO_2.

1.6 Perfusion

Perfusion is matched to ventilation via hypoxia-mediated pulmonary vasoconstriction, i.e. vascular constriction leads to diversion of blood flow away from poorly ventilated to well-ventilated areas, decreasing ventilation–perfusion (VQ) mismatch. Pulmonary arterial flow will be increased by vasodilatation in response to both high O_2 and low CO_2, whereas pulmonary vasoconstriction, and thus hypertension, is exacerbated by hypoxia and hyper-carbia.

1.7 Interpretation of oximetry and blood gases

Pulse oximetry

- Non-invasive measure of oxygen saturation based on absorption of light by oxyhaemoglobin
- Prone to movement artefact and dependent on good pulse pressure
- Widely used, but caution required in interpretation, e.g. normal saturation in a child receiving supplemental O_2 may lead to a false sense of security when there can still be significant respiratory compromise and hypercarbia
- Stable, mature values are reached by 6 months of age; normal values in awake children are 95–100% (for preterm infants) and 97–100% (for term infants and children)

Blood gas measurement

- Arterial samples are rarely indicated in children outside the intensive-care setting
- Capillary and venous samples are good surrogates for $p(CO_2)$ and pH, but not $p(O_2)$
- Transcutaneous measurements of both O_2 and CO_2 are possible, and end-tidal CO_2 is also used in the paediatric intensive-care setting
- Normal ranges
  - pH 7.35–7.45
  - $p(CO_2)$ 4.5–6.0
  - Low pH: metabolic acidosis (normal or low $p(CO_2)$, low HCO_3^-, increased base deficit) or respiratory acidosis (raised $p(CO_2)$; pH may be normalized by raised HCO_3^- if chronic)

1.8 Lung function testing

Infants

Methods for testing lung function in infancy have been developed and are in use in the research setting, although they are not yet in widespread clinical use. In general, a sedated infant is fitted with a tightly fitted face mask. After either a tidal breath or, with some methodologies, an assisted inspiration, a jacket is rapidly inflated around the infant's chest, leading to forced expiration from which flows and volumes can be measured.

Older children

From the age of between 5 and 7 years, children will usually be able to perform standard lung function tests. The following values can be obtained.

FVC — Forced vital capacity, is the total amount of air exhaled upon forced expiration.

FEV_1 — Forced expiratory volume in the first second, gives a measure of large (and medium-sized) airway obstruction.

The ratio of these two values gives an indication as to the nature of an abnormality. Restrictive lung diseases such as fibrosis lead to reduction in both parameters, with preservation of the normal ratio (approximately 80%), while obstructive diseases (asthma, cystic fibrosis) lead to a greater reduction in FEV_1 and thus a reduced FEV_1 : FVC ratio.

FEF_{25-75} — Forced expiratory flow between defined vital capacity (25% being $\frac{3}{4}$ empty) is a measure of flow at lower lung volumes, is non-effort-dependent, and is thought to be a reasonable representation of small airways function. However, the coefficient of variation, even in healthy adults, is high.

PEFR — Peak expiratory flow rate. Although useful as a home monitoring device in patients with asthma, it can be quite effort-dependent and can underestimate significant small airways obstruction.

All of the above measurements can be obtained using a simple spirometer. For more complex measurements of lung volume, patients perform plethysmography, which involves sitting inside an airtight box.

RV — Residual volume is the amount of air left in the lungs after maximal expiration. It is increased in diseases such as asthma because narrowed small airways prevent complete emptying of more distal lung and result in air-trapping.

In addition to the above, transfer factor for CO and corrected total lung CO (corrected for lung volume) give an estimate of the lung diffusion capacity. These measures are reduced in diseases where alveolae are abnormal and gas exchange is impaired, and increased in the presence of red blood cells which can absorb CO (e.g. pulmonary haemorrhage or haemosiderosis).

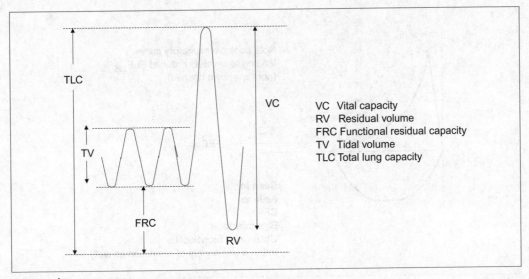

Lung volumes

VC   Vital capacity
RV   Residual volume
FRC Functional residual capacity
TV   Tidal volume
TLC Total lung capacity

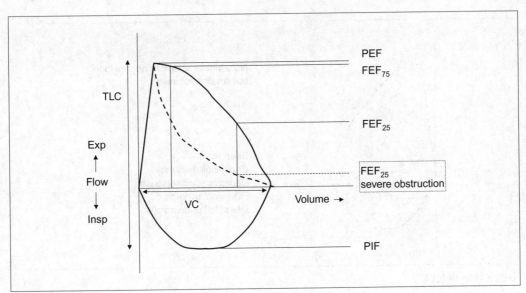

Flow volume loop

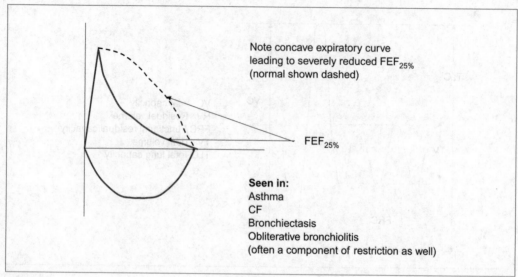

Note concave expiratory curve
leading to severely reduced FEF$_{25\%}$
(normal shown dashed)

FEF$_{25\%}$

Seen in:
Asthma
CF
Bronchiectasis
Obliterative bronchiolitis
(often a component of restriction as well)

Obstructive defect

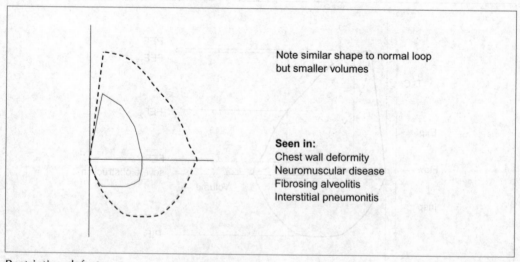

Note similar shape to normal loop
but smaller volumes

Seen in:
Chest wall deformity
Neuromuscular disease
Fibrosing alveolitis
Interstitial pneumonitis

Restrictive defect

1.9   Respiratory defence mechanisms

Pulmonary defences can be mechanical or immunological.

Mechanical defences

- **Mucociliary clearance** whereby cilia beat in a co-ordinated fashion bathed in a normal volume and composition of airway surface liquid, to bring inhaled particles to the throat where they are swallowed. Abnormal in primary ciliary dyskinesia (problem with ciliary microstructure) and cystic fibrosis (normal cilia but decreased airway surface liquid volume)
- Cough clearance

Immunological defences

- **Innate**
  - Phagocytosis by macrophages and neutrophils
  - Soluble factors including hydrophilic surfactant proteins A&D, lactoferrin, lysozyme, defensins
- **Acquired**
  - Humoral: largely immunoglobulin A (IgA) upper airway, IgG lower airways
  - Cell-mediated

1.10   Environmental influences on lung disease

- Cigarette smoke — antenatal effect on growing lung is now well established. Between 40 and 60% of British children are exposed to tobacco smoke at home. Passive smoking in children is associated with increased risk of asthma, wheeze, otitis media and sudden infant death
- Aeroallergens
- Atmospheric pollutants — ozone, particulates, lead, sulphur dioxide and CO have all been shown to increase severity of asthma

2.   EAR, NOSE, THROAT (ENT) AND UPPER AIRWAY

2.1   Nose and sinuses

Choanal atresia

Unilateral or bilateral. A congenital malformation occurring in approximately 1 per 60,000–70,000 births as a result of the failure of the breakdown of the bucconasal membrane leading to complete obstruction of the nostril(s). Bilateral choanal atresia presents immediately at birth (because the neonate is an obligate nose breather) with severe respiratory compromise and inability to pass a nasal catheter. Artificial oral airway is life-saving and surgery is required. It is associated with other congenital defects, e.g. cardiac.

Allergic rhinitis

This presents as rhinorrhoea, sniffing, altered sense of smell (and taste), +/− itchy eyes and conjunctivitis. It may be either seasonal (usually triggered by pollens, grasses, etc.) or related to environmental allergens (e.g. house dust mite, dogs, cats, horses). Often associated with an atopic family history, and there may be other features in the child, e.g. asthma, eczema. Degree of disturbance to a sufferer of severe rhinitis is probably underestimated (problems with concentration, poor sleep quality, etc.). Management should include allergen avoidance and topical (nose +/− eyes) administration of corticosteroids or cromoglycate-based agents. In severe cases, oral antihistamines may be required. Children with allergic rhinitis may also have nasal polyps.

Nasal polyps

These occur in atopic children and in cystic fibrosis (CF) (must consider CF diagnosis in any child with polyps). Children present with runny nose, nasal obstruction, decreased sense of smell and distortion of nasal shape. Polyps may respond to topical corticosteroids but are often difficult to treat, necessitating surgical removal. Recurrence post-surgery is unfortunately common.

Epistaxis

Nose bleeds are reasonably common in childhood. Usually from Little's area on the septum and often triggered by nose-picking. They are more common in inflamed/infected nose, (e.g. allergic rhinitis/polyps). If recurrent/severe must rule out a bleeding disorder, e.g. idiopathic thrombocytopenic purpura, haemophilia, leukaemia, etc. or anatomical abnormality (e.g. haemangioma, telangiectasia). Pressure under the nasal bridge is usually adequate to halt bleeding. If severe, nose may need packing. Cauterization may be undertaken for recurrent episodes.

Sinusitis

Frontal sinuses are not aerated until the age of 3–5 years, so frontal sinusitis is not seen before this age. Later, it presents with headache/facial pain (made worse by coughing/bending down), nasal congestion/discharge, concentration problems.

Sinusitis is associated with CF (almost 100% of adult patients have opaque sinuses so X-ray is not very useful). It may also be associated with humoral immunodeficiency, e.g. IgA or IgG subclass deficiency.

Treatment involves decongestants and antibiotics; surgical drainage is required in a minority.

Complications (rare but serious):

- Orbital cellulitis
- Frontal osteomyelitis
- Meningitis/cerebral abscess
- Intracranial (including cavernous sinus) thrombosis

2.2 Cleft lip and palate

This is often now diagnosed antenatally on ultrasound scanning. It can be associated with Pierre Robin sequence (micrognathia and glossoptosis), other dysmorphic syndromes (e.g. Stickler syndrome, Edward syndrome), or may occur in isolation, in which case prognosis is usually excellent. Certain antiepileptic medications are associated with increased incidence and there is some evidence of prevention with folic acid (as in spina bifida). Familial cases are not uncommon, making a genetic component very likely.

Main problems

- **Cosmetic** — Lip cleft is repaired early at approximately 2–3 months of age
- **Feeding**
  - Special teats for bottles are available for some infants
  - Feeding is facilitated by a palatal plate if cleft is severe
  - May be associated oropharyngeal inco-ordination and aspiration of feeds
  - Cleft palate surgery is usually performed by the age of 1 year
  - Speech and hearing — often associated with frequent ear infections and glue ear
  - Large cleft can cause speech difficulties
- **Airway obstruction** — If due to Pierre Robin sequence, some infants require a nasopharyngeal tube to maintain patency of the upper airway

2.3 Ears

Chronic otitis media

Chronic otitis media (glue ear) is a major cause of hearing problems and speech delay and is caused by the accumulation of thick secretions in the middle ear and recurrent acute infections. It may be associated with adenoidal hypertrophy; adenoidectomy may improve symptoms. Long-term antibiotics are not very useful.

Insertion of grommets to release the fluid and pressure is often performed. Normally they are extruded spontaneously after about 6–9 months. Studies have suggested that swimming is not harmful to a child with grommets (but they should not dive).

Deafness

Deafness can be conductive or sensorineural.

- **Conductive deafness**
  - Most common of the two types, detected in up to 3–4% of schoolchildren, often mild
  - Almost always secondary to chronic otitis media
  - Preservation of bone conductance with diminished air conductance

- **Sensorineural**:
  - Less common, 0.2–0.3% of children
  - More likely to be severe
  - Caused by either cochlear or neuronal damage (may be iatrogenic, eg. aminoglycoside toxicity)
  - Equal impairment of both bone and air conductance

Causes of sensorineural deafness

- Genetic — associated with dysmorphic syndromes
- Congenital infections (TORCH group — Toxoplasmosis, Other infections, Rubella, Cytomegalovirus, Herpes simplex)
- Birth asphyxia
- Severe jaundice
- CNS infection
  - Post-meningitis
  - Encephalitis
  - Cerebral abscess
- Aminoglycoside toxicity
- Head injury

Treatment:

- Hearing aids may be useful if there is some preservation of hearing
- Cochlear implants in selected cases
- Multidisciplinary approach

Mastoiditis

This has become rare with the use of antibiotics to treat acute otitis media. It results from the breakdown of the bony walls of mastoid air cells, secondary to ongoing bacterial middle ear infection. Presents with high fever, toxicity, irritability, marked focal tenderness over the mastoid process, discharging ear +/– deafness. If early in the process it may respond to parenteral antibiotics; in more severe cases, surgical intervention may be required.

2.4 Throat

Adenotonsillar hypertrophy and airway obstruction

Adenotonsillar hypertrophy is common in childhood, although most cases require no specific treatment and will resolve with age. More severe cases are associated with certain disease groups, for example sickle-cell anaemia and human immunodeficiency virus (HIV) infection.

Symptoms either relate to recurrent infections, or airway obstruction. Obstruction may be obvious to parents (snoring +/– apnoeic pauses, mouth-breathing), or may present with right heart failure and cor pulmonale if not recognized until late. Polysomnography may reveal obstructive episodes (increased chest excursion with diminished airflow +/− hypoxia and hypercarbia if severe), although in the majority of cases diagnosis can be made on the history.

Management is by surgical removal in selected cases.

Oropharyngeal incoordination and aspiration

Swallowing is a complex mechanism requiring intact anatomy and neuromuscular co-ordination. Diseases affecting either pathway can lead to saliva and food/drink entering the respiratory tract.

It should be considered as a cause of respiratory symptoms especially in at-risk groups such as:

- Premature babies with immature swallowing mechanisms
- Central nervous system (CNS) disease, e.g. cerebral palsy
- Anatomical abnormality, e.g. cleft palate/larynx
- Any cause of generalized hypotonia especially with bulbar involvement

Aspiration with intact swallow is also seen with severe gastro-oesophageal reflux and tracheo-oesophageal fistula.

Symptoms may be overt (choking and coughing with feeds) but are often absent. Leads to recurrent wheeze and aspiration pneumonias. It is diagnosed on video-fluoroscopy. Management depends on cause but severe cases may require surgical intervention.

2.5   Larynx

Web

Rare. If complete is obviously incompatible with life. More commonly, results in partial laryngeal obstruction, respiratory distress and stridor. Diagnosed by direct visualization and requires surgical repair.

Cleft

Very rare. Failure of closure of tracheo-oesophageal septum at 35 days of embryonic development. Presents with aspiration, choking, episodes of cyanosis +/− apnoea. May coexist with other abnormalities. Diagnosed by laryngo/bronchoscopy. Requires surgical repair.

Haemangioma

Presents with airway obstruction, cough or stridor. It may coexist with cutaneous haeman-giomata so examine the child completely. Visible as a soft mass on instrumentation of the airway and may bleed copiously if traumatized or if biopsy is attempted. Topical application of adrenaline may be life-saving in such a situation. Surgical removal often is hazardous. It may decrease in size in response to local corticosteroid injection.

Papillomatosis

Rare cause of hoarseness if affecting the larynx. It may present with stridor or barking cough. Diagnosed on upper airway examination or bronchoscopy.

Notoriously difficult to treat. There is some evidence of response to cimetidine. Initial hopes of a response to interferon appear unfounded.

2.6 Malacias

Any tubular component of the respiratory tract may be malacic (floppy).

It results in partial or complete collapse on inspiration although patency is well maintained on expiration.

- **Presentation**
  - Inspiratory stridor, respiratory distress
  - Apnoea
  - Feeding problems
  - Recurrent croupy episodes
- Diagnosis can be confirmed on laryngo/bronchoscopy (although it is usually possible clinically)
- Mild cases (the majority) become less severe with growth
- Severe cases may benefit from aortopexy or airway stenting

Causes of stridor

Common
Croup
Laryngo/tracheomalacia
Subglottic stenosis/granuloma (post-intubation)
Vascular ring
Inhaled foreign body (if large and proximally lodged)

Rarer
Epiglottitis (much less common since Hib (*Haemophilus influenzae* type B) vaccination)
External tracheal compression
Mediastinal mass, e.g. lymphoma/leukaemia
Tuberculous lymphadenopathy
Enlargement of heart/great vessels associated with congenital cardiac malformation
Laryngeal web
Haemangioma, papillomatosis
Vocal cord palsy
Vocal cord dysfunction
Hypocalcaemia

2.7   Sleep disordered breathing

A spectrum of problems, ranging from snoring through to hypoxia/hypercarbia leading to pulmonary hypertension and cor pulmonale. It may be related to local (e.g. adenotonsillar hypertrophy) or systemic (e.g. neuromuscular) disease. Take a careful history. Ask specifically about pauses in breathing signalling sleep apnoea. It may lead to disrupted sleep/ nocturnal enuresis/daytime somnolence/morning headaches (high CO_2)/underachievement at school. Definitive diagnosis on polysomnography (see Section 10.4 on management of myopathies). Treatment is tailored to cause.

2.8   Tracheo-oesophageal fistula

Failure of normal development of the primitive foregut leads to a fistula connecting the oesophagus and trachea with or without oesophageal atresia.

Oesophageal atresia presents in the immediate neonatal period with vomiting, choking (+/– an absence of gas in the abdomen, depending on the position and size of the fistula). Confirmation is obtained by attempted passage of a nasogastric tube. This may exist as part of the VACTERL constellation (**V**ertebral, **A**nal, **C**ardiac, **T**racheo-oesophageal fistula, **E**ars, **R**enal, **L**imb).

Tracheo-oesophageal fistula without oesophageal atresia will often present later. At its most obvious, the child may choke with feeds, but equally the history may be one of recurrent chest infections or wheeze. Diagnosis is made on a tube oesophagram (injection of radio-opaque dye into the oesophagus under pressure to force open a small fistula). It is often missed on bronchoscopy, particularly flexible bronchoscopy.

Treatment for both conditions is surgical.

2.9   Gastro-oesophageal reflux

There is increased risk of gastro-oesophageal reflux in premature infants, in the neurologically impaired and, probably, in severe chronic lung disease. It may also exacerbate lung problems such as asthma, which makes differentiating cause and effect difficult. Gold standard for diagnosis is the pH probe. Normal reflux index (% of time pH in lower oesophagus < 4) is 4% in older children but probably up to 10% in infants. Reflux may lead to episodes of aspiration (may be silent), which if recurrent result in irreversible lung damage. Medical treatment with combination of antacid (H_2 blocker or proton pump inhibitor) and prokinetic, e.g. domperidone. If unsuccessful, Nissen's fundoplication may be required.

2.10   Cervical lymphadenopathy

The commonest cause is upper respiratory tract infection. It usually resolves spontaneously, although small lymph nodes may persist into adult life. If chronic or severe, alternative diagnoses should be considered: e.g. infectious mononucleosis, dental disease, non-tuberculous mycobacteria, cat scratch disease (*Bartonella henselae*). If generalized, consider alternative diagnoses and look for supportive signs of malignancy (e.g. lymphoma), HIV, Kawasaki disease.

3. ASTHMA

3.1 Pathophysiology

Chronic inflammatory disease of the airways with a well-recognized genetic component in which many cells are involved, including eosinophils, lymphocytes and mast cells. Airway inflammation leads to airway oedema, and hyper-reactivity resulting in reversible broncho-constriction.

If left untreated, the inflammatory changes may eventually become chronic and irreversible, a process termed 'airway remodelling'.

From both laboratory and epidemiological studies, a protective role for infection against the subsequent development of asthma has been demonstrated, e.g. there is a decreased incidence in children with older siblings or raised on farms.

T-lymphocyte populations are biased towards a T-helper (T_{H2}) cell phenotype (interleukin (IL)-4 and IL-5 secreting, involved in IgE production), as opposed to the T_{H1} phenotype which is more commonly found in response to infection.

Symptoms

Symptoms may be classical wheeze and dyspnoea, or a cough variant. They are often worst at night or in the early morning.

Triggers

- Viruses
- Allergens (e.g. house dust mite, cats, dogs)
- Cold air
- Cigarette smoke
- Exercise
- Stress/emotional

3.2 Drug treatment

Management

Management should include:

- Identification and avoidance of precipitating factors (e.g. house dust mite, pets, cigarette smoke)
- Education — importance of long-term prophylaxis
- Recognition and management of acute attack (written plan where appropriate)

British Thoracic Society Guidelines for asthma management

Step 1 — Short-acting bronchodilators as needed (prn)

Step 2 — Low-dose inhaled steroid and prn bronchodilators

Step 3 — Increase steroid dose or add long-acting bronchodilator

Step 4 — Further increase of steroid dose or addition of leukotriene antagonist, slow release theophylline or oral bronchodilator

Step 5 — Above plus regular oral corticosteroids

Guidelines recommend stepping down treatment when control is achieved, i.e. aim for best control on lowest dose.

Treatment options beyond step 5 (very rare and needs to be under subspecialist care)

- Continuous subcutaneous terbutaline
- Intravenous immunoglobulin
- Alternative immunosuppressive drugs:
  - Methotrexate
  - Azathioprine
  - Cyclosporine A
    - gum hypertrophy
    - hypertrichosis
    - leukopenia
    - renal toxicity
    - levels required

Inhaler devices

You should know how to demonstrate each device. It is very important to choose an inhaler that is suitable for the child.

Inhaler devices

Inhaler devices

Large volume spacers	Used with metred-dose inhalers (MDIs)
	Best lung deposition
	Used with mask in young age group, and with mouthpiece when old enough to form a seal
	Static charge reduces lung delivery: leave to dry after washing — do not dry with towel
	Single puffs best administered individually
	Volumatic — salbutamol, beclomethasone, fluticasone
	Nebuhaler — terbutaline, budesonide

| Smaller spacers | (e.g. AeroChamber) more portable and versatile, although delivery with some not quite as good |
| Dry powder inhalers | Children (usually around 4–7 years) who can:
• form a seal with their lips
• hold their breath
Includes Turbohaler, Diskhaler, Acuhaler, etc. |

MDIs have poor lung deposition (most of the drug remains in the mouth and pharynx) and are not to be recommended for use alone.

Long-acting bronchodilators are useful to gain control instead of increasing steroid dose and in exercise-induced asthma. Now available in combination delivery devices with corticosteroid, which may improve compliance.

3.3 Acute attack

Signs of severity:

• Inability to talk in sentences
• Tachypnoea/tachycardia
• Inter/subcostal recession
• Use of accessory muscles of respiration
• Quiet or silent chest (poor air entry)
• Pulsus paradoxus
• Cyanosis (very late sign — beware)

In the presence of tachypnoea, a normal CO_2 level indicates a severe attack.

Management of acute severe asthma

• Oxygen
• Bronchodilator — via a spacer device has been shown to be as effective, if not more so, than via nebulizer, can be give continuously. If unsuccessful, give intravenous salbutamol with cardiovascular monitoring. Watch K^+.
• Aminophylline
  • Give loading dose slowly
• Systemic (usually intravenous) steroids
• If respiratory support is required:
  • Lowest possible inspiratory pressures
  • Short inspiratory time; long expiratory time
  • Minimal/no positive end-expiratory pressure to reduce air trapping

Causes of wheeze in childhood

Common
- Virus-associated recurrent wheeze
- Acute viral infection, e.g. RSV, adenovirus
- Asthma
- Gastro-oesophageal reflux (and aspiration syndromes)
- Cystic fibrosis
- Inhaled foreign body

Rare
- Distal bronchomalacia
- Obliterative bronchiolitis
- Bronchiectasis

4.   CYSTIC FIBROSIS

4.1   Background

Cystic fibrosis (CF) is the commonest lethal recessive disease of Caucasians, with a carrier frequency of 1 : 25, leading to disease in 1 : 2,500 Caucasian births ($>$ 6,000 patients in the UK). Previously regarded as a disease of childhood, increases in survival have swelled the adult CF population. Median survival for a child born today is estimated at 40 years.

The gene responsible encodes CF transmembrane-conductance regulator (CFTR) and is on chromosome 7. The primary function of CFTR is as a chloride-ion channel, but it also inhibits the epithelial sodium channel. CF respiratory epithelium therefore fails to secrete chloride ions (fails to absorb in the sweat gland, hence high sweat electrolytes), and hyperabsorbs sodium ions and thus H_2O, dehydrating the airway surface. Secretions are viscid, impairing mucociliary clearance and thus host defence.

CFTR is now known to have other functions (related to the transport of other substances, e.g. bicarbonate, and receptors for bacteria) but they are controversial.

Other organs affected for similar reasons include gut, pancreas, liver and reproductive tract.

Diagnosis

Sweat test
- 'Gold standard'. Values of sodium ions or chloride ions (better) $>$ 60 mEq/l are diagnostic (although a value of $>$ 40 in infants is very likely to indicate CF)
- Traditionally the test required at least 100 mg sweat, but newer methods (e.g. macroduct) require less. Conductivity (increased in CF) is also used by some laboratories.

Cases of CF with normal sweat electrolytes have been reported, so if there is a high suspicion for disease a normal sweat test does not rule out a diagnosis of CF.

- If values are in the grey area (40–60 mEq/l) a fludrocortisone suppression test is useful: 3 mg/m^2 b.d. for 2 days before the sweat test: normalizes in non-CF, no effect in CF.

Possible causes of false-positive sweat test

- Technique (evaporation leads to increased concentration and decreased volume)
- Eczema/dermatitis/ectodermal dysplasia
- Malnutrition
- Untreated hypothyroidism/panhypopituitarism
- Adrenal insufficiency
- Glycogen storage disease/mucopolysaccharidosis
- Glucose 6-phosphate dehydrogenase deficiency
- Fucosidosis
- Nephrogenic diabetes insipidus

Genetic testing
See Section 4.2

Immunoreactive trypsin
Useful in the first 6 weeks of life. Raised in CF. Often used as first test in areas with newborn screening.

Nasal potential difference
Mostly used for research purposes but useful in grey cases. Technically challenging in children.

4.2 Genetics

Over 1,000 mutations in CFTR have been identified to date. They fall into five classes. Commonest is Δ*F508*, a class II mutation which leads to defective protein folding and thus failure to reach the apical membrane. There is a relationship between pancreatic status and genotype, but correlations for lung disease have been poor to date. It should not be used to provide prognosis.

Most clinical laboratories test for up to 31 of the commonest mutations (which detects > 90% of Caucasian cases). This is useful for antenatal testing of subsequent pregnancies. Neonatal screening was approved by the government in 2001, although widespread implementation may take several years. It is universal in Australia and New Zealand.

4.3   Presentation and management

Neonatal

Commonest presentation is with meconium ileus, bowel obstruction secondary to thick inspissated gut contents. It may be antenatal and lead to meconium peritonitis. Often requires surgery, although very mild cases occasionally managed medically, e.g. with Gastrografin.

Rarer early presentations

- Pseudo-Bartter syndrome (hypochloraemic, hypokalaemic alkalosis)
- Hypoalbuminaemia, oedema, anaemia
- Bleeding from vitamin K deficiency
- Haemolytic anaemia (vitamin E deficiency)

Pulmonary

Lungs are thought to be normal at birth. Early symptoms such as cough, frequent chesty episodes and wheeze may be missed or labelled 'viral infections'. Early infection with a narrow range of organisms.

- ***Staphylococcus aureus*** — most children in UK receive long-term prophylaxis
- ***Haemophilus inflenzae***
- ***Pseudomonas aeruginosa*** — up to 80% of CF patients are chronically infected by the time they reach adolescence. Bacteria become mucoid, forming biofilms and are more difficult to eradicate when chronic. Treat with long-term nebulized antibiotics (colomycin +/− gentamicin or tobramycin). Intermittent courses of intravenous antibiotics (always at least two). Macrolide antibiotics are in more common use now. Shown to improve lung function, although mechanism of action unclear; may be anti-inflammatory
- ***Allergic bronchopulmonary aspergillosis (ABPA)*** — presents with dry cough, wheeze, variable infiltrates on chest X-ray. Diagnosed with high IgE, raised radioallergosorbent test (RAST) and precipitins. Skin-prick testing may be helpful. Treated with steroids +/− itraconazole, which may need to be prolonged.
- ***Burkholderia cepacia*** — Gram-negative, often highly resistant. Meropenem may be useful. Associated in approximately 20% with life-threatening septicaemia ('cepacia syndrome'), patient-to-patient spread is well-documented (segregation vital)
- ***Stenotrophomonas maltophilia*** — an emerging pathogen; there is accumulating evidence that it does not lead to significant deterioration.
- ***Atypical mycobacteria*** — quite common. May be an incidental finding. Treat if symptomatic, persistent, or if patient is immune-suppressed, e.g. on steroids.

Airway inflammatory response is excessive. End-result of infection/inflammation is bronch-iectasis (upper lobes common), chronic sputum production, clubbing (asthma DOES NOT cause clubbing) and hypoxia. May present with asthma-like symptoms (consider CF in cases of difficult/atypical asthma). May have haemoptysis (high bronchial arterial flow and if severe, embolization). 90% of patients die of respiratory failure.

Other treatments for lung disease

Mainstay of treatment is physiotherapy (regular — even when patient is well!). Consider bronchodilators if responsive. Many patients are on inhaled steroids (evidence lacking).

- **Recombinant human DNase**
  - Degrades viscous neutrophil-derived DNA
  - Thins sputum
  - Nebulized once daily, although treatment on alternate days is just as effective
  - Used in patients with abnormal pulmonary function tests, although some evidence that early, pre-symptomatic use is beneficial in the long term
  - Very expensive (£7,500/patient per year)

Extrapulmonary involvement

Pancreas

Exocrine insufficiency

- Presents with steatorrhoea and faltering growth
- Low stool elastase, high 3-day faecal fat
- Treat with pancreatic enzyme supplements (e.g. Creon)
- Fat-soluble vitamin supplementation
- Nutritional supplements if required
- Gastrostomy and supplemental nutrition if severe weight problems

Endocrine problems

- Diabetes is more common in older children (8–15%)
- Insidious, non-specific onset
- Ketoacidosis is extremely rare (residual pancreatic function)
- Usually require insulin. Some evidence that early use of low-dose insulin in pre-diabetic phase may protect lung function

Gastrointestinal tract

- Distal intestinal obstruction syndrome (previously called meconium ileus equivalent)
  - Rehydrate and administer Gastrografin, Golitely, etc.
  - Attention to dietary fibre and enzymes
- Hepatic cirrhosis
  - Ursodeoxycholic acid may be useful

Nose

- Polyps (up to 30%): topical steroid or surgery — often recur

Sinusitis

- Common — caused by obstruction
- Same causative organisms as lungs

Infertility

- 99% males (obstruction and abnormal development of vas deferens)
- Females subfertile, but many successful pregnancies. Pulmonary health may be severely affected during pregnancy — need careful monitoring.

Arthritis

- Probably immune-complex-mediated
- Correlates with pulmonary function tests

Vasculitis

- More common in older patients

Osteoporosis

- More common with increasing age and severity of lung disease; also long-term steroid use. Many clinics monitor using bone densitometry.

4.4 New/emerging therapies

- Ibuprofen
  - Slows reduction in lung function but has side-effects
  - Not yet in widespread use in UK
- TOBI: **tob**ramycin for **i**nhalation
  - Heavily marketed in USA where colomycin is not used
  - Very expensive, not widely used in UK
- Gene therapy
  - Still at research stage
  - Liposomes or recombinant viral vectors
  - Problems with efficiency and inflammatory response
- Dry powder antibiotics are currently in Phase III clinical trials; may improve quality of life by reducing treatment burden
  - Many others not yet in clinical arena

4.5 Transplantation

Heart–lung or bilateral lung transplants are performed, limited by the number of organs available. More recently living-related donors have been used; currently no advantage but will possibly improve with further experience.

Psychological issues are of major importance.

Possible contraindications (vary slightly with different centres)

- Long-term use of high-dose steroids
- Multiresistant organisms
- Previous thoracic surgery

- Lack of family support or psychological issues
- Severe osteoporosis

Post-transplant problems:

- Prolonged immunosuppression and infection
- Obliterative bronchiolitis is common

5.   OTHER CAUSES OF BRONCHIECTASIS

Symptoms/signs as for CF depending on severity. It may be visible on chest X-ray but computerized tomography is more sensitive. Bronchography is no longer used.

Primary ciliary dyskinesia

Previously called 'immotile cilia syndrome', this is an autosomal recessive problem (several genes probably involved). Rare, 1 per 15,000 births.

- **Presentation**
    - Neonatal respiratory distress, rhinorrhoea
    - Recurrent lower respiratory tract infections may lead to bronchiectasis
    - Sinus disease
    - Glue ear — often does not respond well to grommets
    - 50% have dextrocardia +/– abdominal situs inversus (Kartagener syndrome)
    - Male infertility (female subfertility)
- **Diagnosis**
    - Nasal brushing for ciliary beat frequency (normal > 10 Hz) and structure (electron microscopy)
    - Low exhaled/nasal nitric oxide
    - Prolonged saccharin clearance time
- **Treatment**
    - Physiotherapy
    - Antibiotics
    - ENT and hearing assessment
    - Genetic counselling

Post-infection

Classically occurs after pertussis, although may also follow measles. May occur after severe infection with any organism.

Post-airway obstruction

Highlights importance of early detection and removal of foreign bodies (see Section 8).

Tuberculosis — obstructive lymphadenopathy.

Recurrent infection

For example, immune-deficiency (see Section 7.9).

Recurrent aspiration

Idiopathic

This explains up to 60% of cases but other causes must be excluded.

Congenital

Rare.

6.   BRONCHOPULMONARY DYSPLASIA

Chronic lung disease resulting from premature delivery, surfactant deficiency and neonatal artificial ventilation.

Various definitions exist, all including the requirement for O_2 at 28 days.

Other aetiological factors include:

- Birth asphyxia
- High-concentration O_2 administration
- Fluid overload
- Infection
- Vitamin A deficiency — antioxidant effects

Of these, barotrauma from ventilation and oxygen toxicity is most important. Centres using non-invasive ventilation as the first-line therapy (e.g. nasal continuous positive-airways pressure (CPAP)), have lower incidence of bronchopulmonary dysplasia.

Incidence is reduced greatly by both antenatal steroids (increases lung maturation and surfactant production) and exogenous surfactant. (For further details see Chapter 16 — Neonatology).

Treatment

- Long-term O_2
- Corticosteroids
- Diuretics and fluid restriction may be useful
- Immunization including 'flu and Pneumovax
- Consider use of palivizumab (see Section 7.7)
- Aggressive treatment of infections
- Bronchodilators may be useful in wheezy cases
- Consider and treat coexisting gastro-oesophageal reflux (immature swallow, reduced muscle tone, prolonged intubation all increase risk)

Longer-term complications

- Reactive airways disease (e.g. risk of severe disease with RSV)
- Complications of intubation (e.g. subglottic stenosis, granulation tissue, tracheomalacia)
- Gastro-oesophageal reflux
- Pulmonary hypertension and cor pulmonale
- Growth and nutritional delay
- Neurodevelopmental disability

7. INFECTIONS

7.1 Epiglottitis

Usually caused by *Haemophilus influenzae* type b. Rare since introduction of Hib vaccine. Presents with acute-onset stridor, fever, anxiety in child.

> Do not examine throat (may precipitate fatal airway obstruction).
> Do not X-ray (although appearances may be diagnostic, wastes time and is dangerous).
> Do not upset child, e.g. taking blood, lying flat.

If suspected — urgent general anaesthesia, visualization of upper airway and intubation. Rarely need tracheostomy. Bacterial swabs at intubation. Treat with intravenous third-generation cephalosporin.

7.2 Tonsillitis

Acute tonsillitis is common and self-limiting in childhood. Presentation may be non-specific in the small child, e.g. irritability, refusal of feeds, fever, febrile convulsion. Older child usually complains of sore throat. Bacterial and viral causes (commonly adenovirus, rhinovirus, β-haemolytic streptococcus); exudate does not imply bacterial cause.

Indications for tonsillectomy

- Recurrent severe attacks of tonsillitis
- Tonsillar hypertrophy leading to airway obstruction/sleep disordered breathing
- Associated Eustachian tube obstruction with hearing impairment
- Recurrent otitis media associated with adenotonsillar infection

7.3 Croup

- Viral laryngotracheobronchitis — parainfuenza virus, influenza virus, RSV, rhinoviruses
- Common between 6 months and 5 years of age; more common in boys than girls
- Barking cough and stridor
- Child not usually toxic, may have low-grade fever
- No evidence in support of humidification

- Good evidence for a role for steroids
  - Oral single dose seems to be as good as intramuscular (dexamethasone used in most studies)
  - Some evidence for high-dose nebulized steroids, e.g. budesonide
- Nebulized adrenaline will help in acute situation but effect is short-lived
- Severe cases may require intubation and ventilation
- May be recurrent

7.4 Tracheitis

- Presentation as for croup
- Viral (same as croup) and bacterial (*Staphylococcus aureus* and *Haemophilus influenzae*) aetiologies
- Bacterial cases often more toxic
- Severe cases may require intubation

7.5 Bacterial pneumonias

Presentation

Variable depending on severity

- Cough
- Tachypnoea +/− other signs of respiratory distress (nasal flaring, grunting, use of accessory muscles)
- Fever
- Non-specific irritability/vomiting in younger infant
- Hypoxia
- Chest X-ray often patchy shadowing in infant and more commonly lobar consolidation in older child

Aetiology

- *Pneumococcus* sp. is commonest causative organism
- With increasing age, *Mycoplasma* sp. are more prevalent
- *Staphylococcus aureus* is associated with lung abscess (both staphylococci and streptococci may follow varicella virus infection)
- Rarely *H. influenzae*, streptococci, *Klebsiella* sp. (remember most pneumonias are viral in younger child)

Management

- Mild cases can be diagnosed clinically and treated with oral antibiotics out of hospital
- More severe cases — cultures (sputum if available, upper airway secretions, blood)
  - White blood cell count and differential and C-reactive protein are useful for monitoring response to treatment (but do not differentiate well between bacterial and viral infections, intravenous antibiotics)
  - Hydration (see below)
  - O_2 therapy if required
  - Rarely, severe cases will require respiratory support

Complications

Syndrome of inappropriate secretion of antidiuretic hormone (SIADH) is common. Leads to fluid retention and thus hyponatraemia, which if severe can lead to cerebral oedema and convulsions. Monitor electrolytes and osmolality (serum and urine). Management is by fluid restriction and NOT by administration of sodium.

7.6 Empyema

Collection of pus in pleural space resulting from spread of infection from lung tissue. Presents with signs of pneumonia plus unilateral decreased air entry, dull percussion note. Patient often has scoliosis toward the affected side +/− mediastinal shift. Fluid demonstrated on chest X-ray. Ultrasound may confirm presence of loculation or fibrin strands.

Management

- Requires drainage (not just aspiration)
- Some recent evidence that urokinase may assist recovery by breaking down fibrinous material
- Intravenous antibiotics
- A minority may need surgery — decortication
- Video-assisted thoracic surgery (VATS) is gaining in popularity

Complications

- Bronchopleural fistula
- Lung abscess
- SIADH

Other causes of pleural effusion

- Tuberculosis
- Chylothorax (especially post-surgery from thoracic duct ligation)
- Congestive heart failure
- Hypoalbuminaemia (with peripheral oedema, e.g. nephrotic syndrome)
- Malignancies (rare)
- Blood in pleural space will have similar chest-X-ray appearance, e.g. post-trauma

7.7 Bronchiolitis

Classically caused by RSV, common in autumn and winter (similar picture can be caused by 'flu, paraflu and adenovirus infections). Very common; > 80% children under 4 years possess neutralizing antibodies (although not very effective, hence repeated infections). Causes a range of symptoms from upper respiratory tract infections in older children and adults to bronchiolitis in the first 2 years of life. Commonest cause of pneumonia in the first year.

Presentation

- Respiratory distress and coryza
- Fever
- Hyperinflation
- Apnoea in very young infants
- Crackles widespread throughout lung fields +/− wheeze

Diagnosis

- Immunofluorescence on nasopharyngeal aspirate

Management

- Largely supportive
- Adequate hydration
- Humidified O_2 as required
- Evidence for use of bronchodilators (e.g. ipratropium bromide or salbutamol) not strong, but used frequently, often with apparent success

Groups at risk of severe disease

- Bronchopulmonary dysplasia or other chronic lung disease, e.g. CF
- Congenital heart disease (especially cyanotic or associated with pulmonary congestion/ hypertension)
- Immunocompromised children
- Disease in these children may lead to respiratory failure and requirement for ventilation

Same groups of children are at high risk for severe illness from influenza virus infection. Neuraminidase inhibitors have recently been licensed for nasal administration in high-risk patients.

Specific treatments

Ribavirin

No longer being used to any great extent because of poor efficacy, difficulties with administration (clogs up ventilator circuits) and potential teratogenicity. Used mainly in severe immunocompromise (e.g. bone marrow recipients) sometimes in conjunction with an intravenous preparation.

Vaccination

No active vaccine is currently available, and early studies with attenuated virus have led to increased severity in the subsequent infective episode. Anti-RSV immunoglobulin was useful in early studies in high-risk cases, but there were problems obtaining sufficient quantities and the usual concerns re blood products.

Humanized monoclonal anti-RSV antibody (palivizumab, Synagis) has been available in Europe since 1999 (1 year earlier in USA).

- Given as monthly intramuscular injections during the RSV season
- Shown in trials of babies with bronchopulmonary dysplasia to reduce admissions, but no effect on the severe end of the disease (paediatric intensive care, mortality)
- Recommendations for use vary (commonly chronically O_2-dependent in first 2 years of life)

7.8 Tuberculosis and atypical mycobacterial infection

See also Chapter 14 — Section 5.1.

After a fall in incidence in tuberculosis (TB) world-wide over the last two to three decades following the development of successful anti-TB chemotherapy, there is now an increase in the number of cases, both in adults and children. This largely reflects the rapid increase in numbers infected with HIV, but is also being observed in areas of extreme poverty and overcrowding in countries like the USA. A rise in cases of multi-drug resistant infection, often resulting from poor adherence to treatment in index cases.

NB. TB is a notifiable disease.

Prime example of the ability of micro-organisms either to exist within a host without causing adverse effects (TB infection) or to multiply, with or without tissue invasion and spread, and cause TB disease. Which one of these two situations evolves depends both on host (age, immune status, nutrition) and bacterial factors (numbers and virulence factors).

Pulmonary TB

The major route of infection is via the respiratory tract (more rarely via the oral route leading to gut TB — must rule out immunodeficiency).

Once organisms have been inhaled they establish themselves in the periphery of the lungs, and elicit a host inflammatory response (largely via macrophages).

Spread to regional lymph nodes may also cause hilar adenopathy.

If inflammatory response is sufficient to keep the infection in check, the lesion may calcify and form a Ghon focus, which may be identified later on chest X-ray, and may be the only evidence of previous TB in an otherwise well subject. This is much rarer in children than in adults, and the majority of TB presenting in children results from the primary infection, resulting in the period from infection to disease often being as short as weeks.

Symptoms

These vary and may be non-specific.

- Fever
- Irritability
- Weight loss and lethargy
- Cough
- Airway obstruction from lymphadenopathy; may lead to lobar collapse or less frequently to air trapping
- Dyspnoea and respiratory distress in severe cases especially if miliary
- Erythema nodosum

Radiology

- Can vary greatly from isolated focus to hilar lymphadenopathy, lobar collapse/consolidation to miliary (seed-like) shadowing throughout lung fields
- Large caseating lesions not common in children

Extrapulmonary

TB can infect most organs, in particular the brain, kidneys, gut and bone. Children are more prone than adults to extrapulmonary infection, the details of which will not be discussed further here.

Diagnosis of TB

High index of suspicion is important.

Tuberculin testing

Intradermal administration of purified tuberculin protein will lead to a T-cell-mediated reaction in sensitized individuals. Depending on the clinical situation, and whether bacillus Calmette–Guérin (BCG) has been administered, the size of reaction considered significant may differ.

Significance of reaction size

Size of reaction	Significant in:
> 15 mm	Any child
10–15 mm	High risk — birth or arrival from high-risk country
	Contact with adults in high-risk group
	Young age
> 5 mm	Contact with an open known case (if no BCG)
	Clinical or radiographic evidence
	HIV infection

Microbiology

- Sputum (rare in children)
- Gastric aspirates (morning)
- Bronchoalveolar lavage fluid
- Acid-fast bacilli may be visible on staining, otherwise culture requires up to 6–8 weeks

Some laboratories will test with polymerase chain reaction, although because this is very sensitive, false-positives can arise.

Treatment

Current guidelines state that all cases should receive at least three drugs. Quadruple therapy should be initiated where there is a risk of multiresistant TB, e.g. case or contact from a developing country.

Drug treatment is given in an initial phase of three or four drugs, followed by a maintenance phase of two drugs.

Usual first-line treatment	Potential side-effects
Isoniazid (6 months)	Peripheral neuropathy Abnormal liver function tests
Rifampicin (6 months)	Orange urine/tears Hepatic enzyme induction (drug interactions) Abnormal liver function tests
Pyrazinamide (2 months)	Liver toxicity (only active against intracellular, actively dividing forms of the bacteria. Works best early in the treatment course. Good meningeal penetration if CNS disease)

Additional therapeutic agents for high-risk/drug-resistant disease

Ethambutol

- Visual disturbance
- Perform ophthalmic examination
- Avoid in very young children

Streptomycin

- Intramuscular — rarely used in developed countries

Ciprofloxacin
Clofazimine
Kanamycin
Clarithromycin

Children are rarely open cases (i.e. smear-positive) and it is therefore unusual that they would be capable of transmitting the infection. After the first 2 weeks of treatment the child should be allowed to re-commence normal activities.

Neonatal contact

A neonate born to a mother with active TB is at serious risk of acquiring the disease. If at the time the maternal diagnosis is realized (and treatment commenced) the infant has no signs of TB, the child should receive isoniazid prophylaxis, be closely followed up, and receive a tuberculin test at approximately 3–4 months. Thereafter, the guidelines for older children should be followed.

Contact tracing is a major public health issue. Cases of paediatric TB still arise in families where a parent is known to be infected but children are not screened.

Pulmonary infection with atypical mycobacteria

Examples include *Mycobacterium avium, M. intracellulare, M. kansasii* and *M. malmoense.* Unusual except in the immunocompromised or in children with CF. Symptoms range from those seen with TB infection to much milder presentation with fever or lethargy. In some cases, diagnosis may only be suspected after new changes are seen on chest X-ray, or for example in CF when the organisms are identified in the sputum. In CF, difficulties may arise in determining whether such organisms are pathogens. Treatment of a CF child recommended if the child is unwell or if sputum is persistently positive.

Treatment
Longer than for *M. tuberculosis* (up to 2 years). Choice of agents depends on organism and sensitivities. Usually a combination of the following is used.

- Rifampicin
- Clarithromycin/azithromycin
- Amikacin
- Ciprofloxacin
- Clofazimine
- Ethambutol

Notification and contact tracing are not required.

7.9   Infections in the immunocompromised host

Pneumocystis carinii pneumonia
- **Presentation**
  - Onset may be acute or insidious (especially in the older child), with tachypnoea, respiratory distress, fever, +/– cough, bilateral crackles, hypoxia; often normocapnic in early stages
- **Chest X-ray**
  - Classically bilateral interstitial and alveolar shadowing. May be normal, unilateral, focal

- **Diagnosis**
  - Occasionally found on nasopharyngeal aspirate (NPA)
  - Usually requires bronchoalveolar lavage (BAL)
  - In rare cases, lung biopsy is required
- **Think**
  - Severe combined immune deficiency states (SCID)
  - HIV (common in 1st year of life)
  - di George syndrome
  - (CD40 ligand deficiency; previously called hyper-IgM syndrome)
- **Treatment**
  - High-dose trimethoprim/sulfamethoxazole (pancytopenia, rash, fever)
  - Pentamidine or dapsone used less frequently
  - Steroids — role established in HIV, less certain otherwise
  - If ventilated, consider surfactant
  - Prophylaxis required after treatment
- **Other**
  - Anti-*P. carinii* antibodies are common in healthy children

Cytomegalovirus

- **Presentation**
  - Usually insidious — radiological appearance and likely immunodeficiencies similar to *P. carinii* pneumonia
  - May be congenital or acquired
  - May coexist with extrapulmonary infection — ophthalmic examination required
- **Diagnosis**
  - Antigen (DEAFF, detection of early-antigen fluorescent foci) or polymerase chain reaction on NPA, BAL
  - Detection in other body fluids, e.g. urine, does not confirm cytomegalovirus as the cause of pneumonitis
- **Other**
  - Dual infection with *P. carinii* is not uncommon

Other infections

Organisms causing a similar interstitial picture in immunocompromised patients include:

- Measles
- Varicella
- Herpes simplex
- Adenovirus
- Fungi
- Mycobacteria

Lymphocytic interstitial pneumonitis

Although not related to any particular pathogen, this disorder is often confused with the opportunistic infections above, and thus is included here. Seen in children with HIV or occasionally other immunodeficiency states. Less common in adults.

- Tends to coexist with marked lymphadenopathy — parotid hyperplasia, and to decrease with falling CD4 count
- Presents either as chronic cough or hypoxia and clubbing if severe.
- May be asymptomatic and detected radiologically only.
- Treatment — nil if well, usually responds to steroids

When to suspect immune-deficiency

Normal children may have up to 10 upper respiratory tract infections per year. Suspect abnormal immune function if respiratory tract infections are:

- Unusually severe or prolonged
- Recurrent (although if same site, suspect anatomical abnormality or foreign body)
- Any case of pneumonitis/unexplained interstitial disease
- Associated with:
  - Infections in other sites, e.g. skin, liver, gastrointestinal tract, bone
  - Faltering growth
  - Persistent or generalized lymphadenopathy

8. INHALED FOREIGN BODY

This will not be diagnosed unless thought about. There are major long-term implications if not removed, e.g. lobar collapse, bronchiectasis.

Suspect signs

- Sudden-onset cough/wheeze/breathlessness
- May or may not give history of aspiration
- Ask about presence of older siblings in the case of an infant
- Unilateral signs: wheeze, absent or diminished air entry, tracheal/mediastinal deviation if severe

Chest X-ray

- Either volume loss or hyperexpansion from air trapping on affected side
- Hyperexpansion best visualized on expiratory film

Management

- Removal under rigid bronchoscopy (flexible bronchoscopy not recommended because removal is more difficult)
- Follow-up ventilation scan should be considered, especially in cases of non-inert foreign body, e.g. food. Peanuts are a particular problem because nut oil is very irritant and proinflammatory. If removal is delayed, anti-inflammatory agents, e.g. steroids, may be useful to reduce airway narrowing
- Consider post-operative antibiotics, depending on findings
- Education is important, particularly the avoidance of peanuts in young children

9. PNEUMOTHORAX

In children this is usually associated with underlying disease.

- Gas trapping (e.g. severe asthma, CF)
- Bullae (e.g. Marfan syndrome)
- Other — Langerhans cell histiocytosis (in association with fibrotic, honeycomb changes on chest X-ray)
- Iatrogenic (high-pressure ventilation), traumatic and post-operative

Symptoms and signs

- Dyspnoea, cough, chest pain
- Tracheal deviation, asymmetrical chest expansion and breath sounds
- Hyper-resonance
- +/− Subcutaneous emphysema

Management

- Depends on size on chest X-ray (all patients should have one)
- If small with minimal symptoms, can be managed conservatively and observed
- If larger with significant symptoms give O_2 (aids air absorption from pleural space) and drain. Aspiration may be sufficient, otherwise intercostal drain

Recurrent

- Consider pleurodesis
- Visceral pleura adheres to chest wall with either talc or bleomycin
- Painful. May exclude possibility of future transplantation, e.g. in CF. Consider with care

Confused with:

- Neonatal cysts, diaphragmatic hernia, severe hyperinflation, e.g. inhaled foreign body

10. NEUROMUSCULAR DISORDERS

Can impair respiratory function at any of following sites: spinal cord, peripheral nerve, neuromuscular junction and muscle.

10.1 Spinal cord

Spinal muscular atrophy

Disorder at levels of the anterior horn cells (atrophy). Autosomal recessive inheritance.

Presents as a floppy infant (Werdnig–Hoffman disease; with tongue fasciculation, preservation of eye muscles giving alert facial expression) or in less severe forms, as hypotonia and delayed motor milestones.

Respiratory involvement always seen in types I and II (diaphragm spared), common in type III. Chest may be bell-shaped. Lungs small.

Previously, severe forms would have been given a grave prognosis once diagnosed and allowed to die. More and more commonly, particularly in the USA, parents are demanding long-term ventilation. There are obvious ethical issues regarding this because there is currently no realistic chance of improvement or cure.

Myelomeningocele

Rarely affects respiration unless very high.

Cervical cord injury

Respiratory involvement depends on level.

10.2 Peripheral nerve

Guillain–Barré syndrome

- Post-viral inflammatory ascending polyneuropathy
- Respiratory involvement common and most serious manifestation (intercostals and diaphragm)
  - This will be underestimated, unless specifically monitored
  - Do not assess with peak flow (this may be normal despite respiratory muscle compromise) — use vital capacity
- Bulbar involvement may lead to aspiration. Protective intubation may be required
- Good prognosis, even in severe cases requiring mechanical ventilatory support. Usual course:
  - Evolution 2–4 weeks
  - Plateau variable
  - Resolution 2–4 weeks later

- Specific treatments
  - Intravenous immunoglobulin
  - Plasmapheresis in some cases

10.3   Neuromuscular junction

Myasthenia gravis

- Autoimmune disease with antibodies directed against the acetylcholine (ACh) receptor
- Episodic muscle weakness, often mild, e.g. ptosis
- Weakness increases with exertion
- Management strategies include a trial of anticholinesterase drugs such as pyridostigmine, thymectomy or immunosuppressive treatments

Congenital myasthenia gravis is an autosomal recessive, non-autoimmune disease in which ACh synthesis or mobilization is defective. May respond to anticholinesterase drugs, but if not, severe cases require long-term ventilatory support (see below) and assistance with feeding.

Neonatal myasthenia gravis is seen in up to 15% of babies born to affected mothers and results from transplacental passage of autoantibodies. Is transient, but affected infants may have feeding difficulties or require respiratory support. Treated with anticholinesterase drugs/exchange transfusion or plasmapheresis occasionally required.

Botulism

- Rare
- Toxins produced by *Clostridium botulinum* (usually food-borne) lead to impaired release of ACh at neuromuscular junction. Bulbar muscles involved early, with respiratory failure in most cases. Good prognosis with adequate support. Botulinum toxin is currently being used as treatment for certain diseases with muscular spasm as major component.

Tick paralysis

- Very rare

10.4   Muscle

Myotonic dystrophy

- Floppy infant in severe form
- Diaphragm involvement (eventration)
- Feeding problems +/– aspiration
- Maternal (when congenital) myotonia (muscles slow to relax eg. hard shake)
- Later problems — learning difficulties, cardiac conduction defects, baldness
- Triplet-repeat disease (others are Huntington disease, Fragile X, Friedreich ataxia) with increasing severity in subsequent generations (genetic anticipation)

Duchenne muscular dystrophy

- X-linked
- Weakness usually noted towards end of first decade
- Death is usually from respiratory failure
- Preceded by recurrent lower respiratory tract infections +/– aspiration from swallowing incoordination

Myopathies

- Respiratory involvement variable depending on type
- **Symptoms** include:
  - Respiratory infections
  - Morning headaches (CO_2 retention)
  - Daytime drowsiness
- **Management**
  - Always consider possibility of respiratory involvement
  - Lung function testing
  - Polysomnography (overnight O_2, CO_2, nasal airflow, chest wall movement, heart rate, respiratory rate +/– EEG, pH probe)
  - Non-invasive ventilation increasingly used (see below). Use once evidence of respiratory failure. Some evidence against prophylactic use in Duchenne muscular dystrophy

10.5 Respiratory failure

Inability to maintain adequate gas exchange without additional support. If chronic, pulmonary hypertension and cor pulmonale may occur. Assess severity of respiratory effort (beware if poor, exhaustion is a late and worrying sign), vital signs, evidence of cor pulmonale, oxygen saturation and blood gases. Respiratory failure may manifest with hypoxia alone or hypercarbia as well. If the latter, supplementary oxygen is not an appropriate treatment; child will need non-invasive support (see below) or intubation.

10.6 Non-invasive ventilatory support

Acute respiratory failure requiring invasive ventilation in the intensive treatment unit setting will not be dealt with in this chapter, although the systems below can also be administered long-term with the aid of a tracheostomy tube in cases where this is necessary.

Children with the neuromuscular disorders above (plus those with malacic airways and very occasionally those with chronic lung disease) may have chronic respiratory compromise and benefit from long-term ventilatory support.

This can be administered as either positive or negative pressure.

Positive pressure

Both continuous (CPAP) or bi-level (Bi-PAP) positive airway pressure can be administered through either a nose or face mask.

Both systems can be used at home with or without oxygen depending on the pathology. The devices are in general well-tolerated, the only major problem being one of pressure sores resulting from the tight-fitting mask.

Negative pressure

Devices, including the cuirass jacket, have also been used in these settings. The jacket is worn around the chest, with closely fitted seals at either end. Negative pressure applied to the jacket causes inspiration. Expiration can be passive or assisted.

The benefits of this approach include a more physiological respiratory cycle. However, movement of the child is limited by the devices, which can also be very noisy.

In the UK, negative pressure is used much less frequently than positive. It is important to remember that significant weakness of the bulbar muscles, especially with any airway malacia, can lead to airway collapse and obstruction during applied negative pressure, which can lead to failure of the device.

11. RARE DISORDERS

11.1 Congenital disorders

Cystic adenomatoid malformation

- Type 1 — single or multiple large cysts (despite shift effects, usually good post-operative prognosis)
- Type 2 — multiple small cysts
- Type 3 — solid mass (poor prognosis)

In most cases the affected lobe needs to be removed because of infection (and possible malignant transformation) risks. May be diagnosed antenatally. Cases are reported where antenatal findings appear to have been resolved by the time of birth — speculations about prognosis are therefore difficult. May be confused radiologically with congenital diaphragmatic hernia, pneumatoceles.

Congenital lobar emphysema

Over-inflation of the lobe as a result of an intrinsic deficiency of bronchial cartilage +/– elastic tissue.

- **Commonest sites**
  - Left upper lobe, right middle and upper lobes. Rare in lower lobes

- **Presentation**
  - May be asymptomatic, detected on chest X-ray
  - Neonatal respiratory distress
  - Chest asymmetry. Hyper-resonance
- **Chest X-ray**
  - Hyperlucent region. May be associated compression of other lobes
  - VQ scan may show absence of ventilation/perfusion in more severe cases
- **Management**
  - In mildest cases, manage conservatively
  - Most cases presenting in infancy are more severe and require surgical removal because of risks of infection and collapse of other areas
  - Cardiac work-up; 1 : 6 have associated cardiac abnormality

Bronchogenic cyst

- Remnant of primitive foregut derived from abnormal tracheobronchial budding
- Form up to 10% of mediastinal masses in children
- Contain normal tracheal tissue, filled with clear fluid
- May exist in various sites including paraoesophageal, with symptoms varying accordingly
- May be either symptomatic or associated with
  - Airway compression
  - Stridor
  - Lobar collapse
  - Obstructive emphysema
  - Infection
  - Haemorrhage

Barium swallow may detect filling defect. Surgical removal recommended to prevent infection, airway obstruction, or malignant transformation. Pre-operatively avoid high-pressure ventilation and air travel — cysts may expand and rupture.

Lobar sequestration

- Mass of non-functional lung; abnormal communication with airway and usually supplied by systemic circulation
- Intra- or extralobar (often associated with other congenital abnormalities and polyhydramnios). May have derived from accessory lung bud, although exact aetiology is uncertain. Lower lobes most commonly affected, more often the left. Many cases are asymptomatic. Present most commonly with recurrent pneumonia in same site
- Chest X-ray — solid or cystic (if intralobar +/− air-fluid level) mass
- Angiography required to demonstrate and delineate systemic blood supply
- Surgical removal required even in asymptomatic cases because infection will ensue if untreated

Scimitar syndrome

- Hypoplastic right lung with anomalous venous drainage (usually to inferior vena cava or right atrium) +/– systemic collateral arterial supply. 'Scimitar' sign is the vertical line caused by the right uppler lobe pulmonary vein running into the inferior vena cava
- May be asymptomatic or lead to recurrent infection
- Right lung usually functions well and surgical correction of the vascular abnormalities is usually recommended

Diaphragmatic hernia

- Incidence estimated at around 1 per 2,500–3,500 births. More common on the left. Main problems arise from the associated pulmonary hypoplasia, both on the affected side and the contralateral side when there is significant mediastinal shift. Diagnosis may be made antenatally on ultrasound
- Postnatal presentation includes respiratory distress, scaphoid abdomen and vomiting. Chest X-ray shows bowel loops inside thorax which may be confused with either cystic malformation or pneumothorax (use nasogastric tube both to confirm the diagnosis and to deflate the stomach reducing the chance of rupture)
- Often associated with other malformations, in which case prognosis is worse
- **Treatment**
  - Surgery required
  - No clear evidence, but some suggestion, that high-frequency oscillatory ventilation may help
  - Pulmonary hypertension is quite common. May respond to nitric oxide or vasodilators
- **Prognosis**
  - Even with optimal management, mortality about 50–60%
  - Survivors may have problems associated with underlying pulmonary hypoplasia

Alpha-1 antitrypsin deficiency

- Recessively inherited disorder
- Absence of liver-derived antiprotease leads to proteolytic destruction of pulmonary tissue and emphysema on exposure to oxidants, e.g. cigarette smoke and pollutants
- Rare for pulmonary problems to arise in children who are more likely to have the associated liver disease (eventual cirrhosis)
- PiMM refers to the homozygous normal state, PiZZ is homozygous deficient, PiSZ also causing disease

Alveolar proteinosis

- Aetiology is uncertain, although some cases presenting as neonates are now known to be the result of deficiency of surfactant-associated protein B and others are linked to granulocyte–macrophage colony-stimulating factor. Lipid-laden type II pneumocytes desquamate into the alveolar spaces leading to increasing hypoxia and respiratory distress

- **Chest X-ray** — resembles interstitial lung disease with widespread confluent airspace shadowing
- **Diagnosis** — made on lung biopsy
- **Prognosis** — poor
- In older child, whole lung lavages may help, but in infants, the disease is almost universally fatal. Genetic counselling required

Congenital pulmonary lymphangiectasia

- Rare dilatation of pulmonary lymphatics leading to severe neonatal respiratory distress and often pleural effusions
- Associated with congenital cardiac disorders such as obstructed venous drainage
- Prognosis very poor
- No specific treatment

11.2   Acquired disorders

Obliterative bronchiolitis

- Results from viral infection (usually adenovirus, but occasionally measles or RSV) or can follow lung or bone marrow transplant
- Severe, widespread small-airways obstruction
- Dyspnoea, wheeze and hypoxia with eventual pulmonary hypertension
- Chest X-ray — hyperinflated lungs with patchy pruning of vascular markings
- Computerized tomography — patchy areas of air trapping (honeycomb) and poor perfusion

In the early stages may have some response to bronchodilators or steroids, but often no treatment is successful. If unilateral, may go on to Swyer–James (also called Macleod) syndrome of unilateral hyperlucent lung with diminished vascularity.

Haemosiderosis

- Repeated episodes of pulmonary haemorrhage lead to accumulation of haemosiderin at the alveolar level
- Haemorrhage may be symptomatic with haemoptysis, or unrecognized, presenting with anaemia
- Aetiology is uncertain, although a subgroup of cases are associated with cows' milk protein allergy and positive antibodies and respond to dietary manipulation
- Another subgroup have Goodpasture syndrome (positive antiglomerular basement membrane antibodies)
- Similar clinical picture may occur with mitral stenosis or connective tissue diseases
- **Symptoms** — usually episodic: fever, dyspnoea, wheeze +/– haemoptysis
- **Chest X-ray** — may be normal but more commonly patchy shadowing
- **Diagnosis** — haemosiderin-laden macrophages in BAL

- **Management** — difficult
  - Acute — treat hypoxia, anaemia
  - Longer term — steroids, hydroxychloroquine or alternative immunosuppressive drugs

Sarcoid

- Extremely rare in childhood
- Multisystem granulomatous disease, may be confused with TB and chronic granulomatous disease
- **Symptoms**
  - Dry cough, dyspnoea
  - Clinical examination often unremarkable in early stages (may lead to clubbing later)
- **CXR**
  - Hilar lymphadenopathy
  - Patchy lung infiltrates
  - May be associated with extrapulmonary disease (skin, eye, kidney, gut)
- **Diagnosis**
  - Usually made on biopsy (Kveim test no longer performed)
- **Treatment**
  - May be self-limiting
  - Steroids +/– hydroxychloroquine if treatment required

Interstitial lung diseases of childhood

Group of conditions not well defined in terms of aetiology which lead to inflammation and fibrosis at the alveolar level, sometimes also termed 'cryptogenic fibrosing alveolitis' (CFA). Gradual onset dry cough, dyspnoea, hypoxia, clubbing. Widespread crackles throughout both lung fields.

- Chest X-ray/computerized tomography — ground-glass appearance
- Differential diagnosis includes pneumonitis from opportunistic pathogens, e.g. *P. carinii* pneumonitis, extrinsic allergic alveolitis. Definitive diagnosis will require an open lung biopsy
- Histological findings vary from inflammation (more likely to respond to steroids) through to severe fibrosis (steroids less likely to succeed; antifibrotics, e.g. hydroxychloroquine, may be used)
- **Prognosis** — highly variable ranging from subacute respiratory failure to a plateau phase with intermittent symptoms, or even recovery in some patients

Pulmonary hypertension

Increased pulmonary vascular pressure may be primary (rare) or more commonly occurs secondary to another disease.

These include:

- Any cause of chronic lung disease, e.g. bronchopulmonary dysplasia, CF. Chronic hypoxia leads to pulmonary vasoconstriction and arterial wall changes
- High pulmonary arterial flow from left to right shunt, e.g. large ventricular septal defect
- Obstructed pulmonary venous drainage or left heart failure (rare in childhood)

Primary pulmonary hypertension presents with hypoxia, dyspnoea and, if severe, right heart failure. May present in the neonatal period as persistent fetal circulation (see Section 1.3).

May respond to pulmonary vasodilators:

- High O_2
- Prostacyclin
- Nifedipine
- Nitric oxide
- Viagra™ (Sildenafil)

Prognosis is usually poor unless transplantation is an option

12. FURTHER READING

Beachey W. 1998. *Respiratory Care Anatomy and Physiology: Foundations for Clinical Practice.* London: Mosby.

Chernick V, Boat TF, Wilmott RW, and Bush A (Eds). 2006. *Kendig's Disorders of the Respiratory Tract in Children*, 7th edn. London: W B Saunders.

Gibson RL, Burns JL, Ramsey BW. 2003. Pathophysiology and management of pulmonary infections in cystic fibrosis. *Am J Respir Crit Care Med* 168, 918–51.

Chapter 22

Rheumatology

Nathan Hasson

CONTENTS

Rheumatology

1. JUVENILE IDIOPATHIC ARTHRITIS

This is the new classification for autoimmune arthritis in childhood and replaces 'juvenile chronic/rheumatoid arthritis'.

Definition — a chronic arthritis that persists for a minimum of 6 consecutive weeks in one or more joints, commencing before the age of 16 years and after active exclusion of other causes.

Epidemiology — 1 per 1,000 children under 16 years of age

Classification

- By mode of onset during the first 6 months
- Eight groups:
  - Systemic onset
  - Polyarticular rheumatoid factor-negative
  - Polyarticular rheumatoid factor-positive
  - Oligoarticular — persistent
  - Oligoarticular — extended
  - Enthesitis-related arthritis (enthesis = point of bony insertion of tendon)
  - Psoriatic
  - Unclassified

Systemic disease

- High remittent fever and rash with one or more of the following: hepatomegaly, splenomegaly, generalized lymphadenopathy, serositis (occasionally pericarditis)
- Arthritis may be absent at the onset, but myalgia or arthralgia are usually present

Polyarticular onset

- Five or more joints develop in the onset period, usually somewhat insidiously and symmetrically
- May be further divided by the presence of immunoglobulin M (IgM) rheumatoid factor

Oligoarticular onset

- The commonest mode with four or fewer joints involved, particularly knees and ankles
- Three clear subgroups have emerged, notably young children with positive antinuclear antibodies who are at risk from chronic iridocyclitis, older boys (aged 9 upwards) who

frequently carry the histocompatible leukocyte antigen (HLA) B27 and develop enthesitis (now classified as enthesitis-related arthritis), and those that extend past four joints (extended oligoarticular juvenile idiopathic arthritis)

- Others presenting in this way include juvenile psoriatic arthritis, the arthritis of inflammatory bowel disease and Reiter syndrome, while some are as yet unclassified

1.1 Systemic onset disease

General characteristics

- Usually begins before 5 years of age but can occur throughout childhood into adult life
- Equal in boys and girls less than 5 years old but female predominance in those over 5 years old

Clinical features

- High once-daily fever spikes for > 2 weeks
- Myalgia
- Arthralgia
- Malaise
- Rash — salmon pink or red maculopapular eruption
- Lymphadenopathy — cervical, epitrochlear, axillary and inguinal
- Hepatosplenomegaly
- Serositis — occasionally pericarditis
- Hepatitis
- Progressive anaemia
- Disseminated intravascular coagulation
- Arthritis — knees, wrists and carpi, ankles and tarsi, neck, followed by other joints

Investigations

- Erythrocyte sedimentation rate (ESR) — high
- Haemoglobin — low (normochromic, normocytic)
- White blood cell count — raised (neutrophil leukocytosis)
- Platelets — raised (> 400×10^6/l)
- IgM rheumatoid factor — negative
- Antinuclear antibodies (ANA) — negative

Course and prognosis

- Half will have recurrent episodes of systemic disease
- Progressive arthritis occurs in about one-third, irrespective of whether there are systemic exacerbations
- The younger the age of onset, the greater the risk of poor growth, both somatic and of joints
- Amyloidosis occurs in some children with persistent disease activity, predominantly among Europeans

Management

- Physiotherapy to maintain joint mobility and muscle function
- Non-steroidal anti-inflammatory drugs (NSAIDs) to control pain, inflammation and fever
- Corticosteroids in severe disease, either as pulsed intravenous, single daily dose or given on alternate days
- Methotrexate especially for arthritis
- Cyclosporin for systemic features
- Etanercept (tumour necrosis factor (TNF) receptor) or Infliximab/adalimumab (anti-tumour necrosis factor (TNF) receptor antibody) for disease that is resistant to other medical management or for patients in whom there is significant drug toxicity — very little is known of long-term toxicity, use in specialist centres only
- Anti-interleukin-1 (anti-IL-1; Anakinra) effective when other treatments failed or side-effects

1.2 Polyarticular — rheumatoid factor-negative

General characteristics

- Any age, occasionally before the first birthday
- Female predominance

Clinical features

- Polyarthritis can affect any joint; the most commonly affected are the knees, wrists, ankles and proximal and distal interphalangeal joints of the hands; metacarpophalangeal joints are often spared
- Limitation of neck and temporomandibular movement is common
- Flexor tenosynovitis
- Low-grade fever, occasionally
- Mild lymphadenopathy and hepatosplenomegaly, occasionally

Investigations

- ESR — elevated
- Haemoglobin — may be reduced
- White blood count — mild neutrophil leukocytosis
- Platelets — moderate thrombocytosis
- IgM rheumatoid factor — negative
- ANA — occasionally positive

Course and prognosis

- Variable
- May be monocyclic but prolonged over several years with good functional outcome
- Recurrent episodes tend to cause progressive deformities

Management

- Physiotherapy to maintain and improve joint and muscle function
- Splinting to prevent deformity
- NSAIDs to control pain and inflammation
- Methotrexate is very effective and can be used early on to prevent deformity
- Anti-TNF treatment if other disease-modifying anti-rheumatic drugs (DMARDs) have failed

1.3 Polyarticular — rheumatoid factor-positive

General characteristics

- Over 8 years of age at onset
- Female predominance

Clinical features

- Polyarthritis affecting any joint, but particularly the small joints of the wrists, hands, ankles, and feet; knees and hips often early, with elbows and other joints later
- Rheumatoid nodules on pressure points, particularly elbows. Vasculitis — uncommon and often late, nail-fold lesions, ulceration

Investigations

- ESR — usually elevated
- Haemoglobin — moderate anaemia
- IgM rheumatoid factor — persistently positive and in high titre
- ANA — may be positive
- HLA DR4 — frequently present
- Radiographically — early erosive changes of affected joints, particularly of hands and feet

Course and prognosis

- Persistent activity with serious joint destruction and poor functional outcome
- Additional long-term hazards include atlantoaxial subluxation, aortic incompetence and amyloidosis

Management

- Physiotherapy to maintain and improve joint and muscle function
- Splinting to preserve function
- NSAIDs
- Slow-acting drugs early
- Methotrexate
- Anti-TNF treatment if other DMARDs failed
- Surgical intervention, such as replacement arthroplasties, often required later

1.4 Oligoarticular (persistent and extended)

General characteristics

- Under 6 years of age
- Female predominance

Clinical features

- Arthritis affecting four or fewer joints: commonly knee, ankle, elbow or a single finger
- Early local growth anomalies
- Risk (2 : 3) of chronic iridocyclitis in the first 5 years of disease, ANA associated
- If four or fewer joints after 6 months then defined as persistent oligoarticular, if more than four joints are affected then it is described as extended oligoarticular

Investigations

- ESR — may be elevated or normal, initially
- Haemoglobin — normal
- White blood count — normal
- Platelets — normal
- IgM rheumatoid factor — negative
- ANA — frequently positive
- HLA A2, DR5 and DR8

Course and prognosis

- Exacerbations and remissions
- Alteration in growth of affected limb
- Long-term prognosis of joints good, except for the one in five who develop polyarthritis (five or more joints) over a period of years (extended)
- Iridocyclitis is bilateral in two-thirds, the course is independent of the joints — its prognosis depends on early detection and good management

Management

- Physiotherapy to maintain muscle and joint function
- NSAIDs
- Local corticosteroid injection — triamcinolone hexacetonide is most effective
- Frequent ophthalmological assessment (3–6-monthly)
- Methotrexate for extended oligoarticular juvenile idiopathic arthritis
- Anti-TNF treatment in extended if other DMARDs failed

1.5 Enthesitis related arthritis

General characteristics

- 9 years old and over
- Male predominance

Clinical features

- Peripheral arthritis predominantly affecting the joints of the lower limb
- Enthesopathies — plantar fascia, Achilles tendon, patella tendon
- Acute iritis
- Sacroiliac pain in some ⎫ either of these can be
- Axial disease in some ⎬ the presenting feature

Investigations

- ESR — normal to high
- Full blood count — usually normal
- IgM rheumatoid factor — negative
- HLA B27 — present 90%

Course and prognosis

- Functional outcome is good in two-thirds of cases
- Some joint extension may occur
- Over time, one-third can develop serious hip problems, cervical and other spinal involvement, impaired temporomandibular function, as well as other features of spondylitis

Management

- Physiotherapy, including hydrotherapy, to maintain mobility: particularly important if spinal involvement occurs
- NSAIDs
- Local corticosteroid injections, hip arthroplasty may be needed in a small proportion
- Sulfasalazine is the disease-modifying drug of choice, methotrexate is also effective
- Anti-TNF treatment if other DMARDs failed

1.6 Juvenile psoriatic arthritis

General characteristics

- An arthritis associated, but not necessarily coincident, with a typical psoriatic rash, or arthritis, plus at least three of four minor criteria: dactylitis, nail pitting, psoriatic-like rash or family history of psoriasis
- Female predominance
- Family history of psoriasis (common) or arthritis (but less so)

Clinical features

- Asymmetrical arthritis
- Flexor tenosynovitis
- Occasionally severe destructive disease
- Systemic features rare
- Nail pitting

- Onycholysis
- Psoriasis

Investigations

- ESR — varies with number of joints, may be high
- Haemoglobin — may fall
- White blood count — may increase (neutrophils)
- IgM rheumatoid factor — negative
- ANA — can be positive

Course and prognosis

- Young onset can be associated with iridocyclitis
- Remitting and relapsing course, even into adult life
- Occasionally severely destructive
- Occasionally spondylitis (inflammation of spinal joints) develops

Management

- Physiotherapy
- NSAIDs
- Severe destructive form may require immunosuppressants such as methotrexate
- Anti-TNF treatment if other DMARDs failed

1.7 Unclassified

All those that do not meet the criteria for the above.

2. OTHER FORMS OF CHILDHOOD AUTOIMMUNE ARTHRITIS

2.1 Inflammatory bowel disease-related arthritis

General characteristics

- Arthritis associated with either ulcerative colitis or Crohn disease
- Over 4 years of age
- Male and female predominance equal

Clinical features

- Arthritis usually occurs after the onset of bowel symptoms, but occasionally begins coincident with, or even precedes, them
- Arthritis is usually oligoarticular: knees, ankles, wrists and elbows

- Two forms:
  - Benign peripheral arthritis coinciding with active bowel disease
  - In older patients, who belong to the spondylitic group, the joint activity does not necessarily link with bowel activity

Associated features

- Erythema nodosum
- Pyoderma gangrenosum
- Mucosal ulcers
- Fever
- Weight loss
- Growth retardation
- Acute iritis — in the spondylitic group

Investigations

- Platelets — normal/elevated
- ESR — usually elevated
- Haemoglobin — usually low (normochromic, normocytic)
- White blood count — normal
- IgM rheumatoid factor — negative
- ANA — negative
- HLA B27 present in the spondylitic group

Course and prognosis

- Peripheral arthropathy involves few joints and is episodic and benign
- Prognosis for joint function is excellent
- Prognosis for the spondylitic group is similar to that of ankylosing spondylitis

Management

- Physiotherapy as appropriate
- Treatment of the underlying bowel disorder
- NSAIDs with care, because of gastrointestinal side-effects (ibuprofen may be the drug of choice and use antacids such as ranitidine
- Sulfasalazine may be helpful for both subgroups
- Infliximab (anti-TNF treatment) is effective

Causes of erythema nodosum

- Idiopathic
- Streptococcal infection
- Tuberculosis
- Leptospirosis
- Histoplasmosis

- Epstein–Barr virus infection
- Herpes simplex virus infection
- *Yersinia* sp. infection
- Sulphonamides
- Oral contraceptive pill
- Systemic lupus erythematosus
- Crohn disease
- Ulcerative colitis
- Behçet syndrome
- Sarcoidosis
- Hodgkin disease

2.2 Juvenile sarcoidosis

- Can occur at any age
- Usually presents with painless swelling of joints and marked teno-synovitis
- Can have rash
- Pan-uveitis can be severe so regular eye checks must be performed
- With musculoskeletal disease lymphadenopathy is not seen; renal disease occurs in children
- Angiotensin-converting enzyme is raised in at least 50% of paediatric patients
- Treat with steroids and methotrexate

2.3 Reactive arthritis, including Reiter syndrome

Acute arthritis occurring after an intercurrent infection, without evidence of the causative organism in the joint. Any age, but particularly male teenagers.

Clinical features

- Arthritis ⎫ Typical triad
- Urethritis/balanitis/cystitis ⎬ for Reiter
- Conjunctivitis ⎭ syndrome
- Mouth ulceration
- Fever
- Rashes, including keratoderma blennorrhagica (macules — pustular on palms, soles, toes, penis)

If only two salient features occur, it is often referred to as 'incomplete Reiter syndrome'.

Investigations

- ESR — raised
- Haemoglobin — normal
- Mild neutrophil leukocytosis

- IgM rheumatoid factor — negative
- ANA — negative
- Occasionally positive stool or urethral culture (*Shigella, Salmonella, Yersinia, Campylobacter, Chlamydia*)
- High incidence of HLA B27

Course and prognosis

- Usually self-limiting, but the arthritis can be severe and persistent
- Some may later develop ankylosing spondylitis

Management

- Antibiotics initially, if an organism is found
- Physiotherapy to maintain function of joints and muscles
- NSAIDs
- Sulfasalazine if joint problems persist

Conditions associated with HLA B27 positivity

- Ankylosing spondylitis — 95% of patients
- Reiter syndrome
- Arthritis of inflammatory bowel disease and psoriasis
- Acute iridocyclitis
- Enthesitis-related arthritis of older children
- Reactive arthritis following infection with *Salmonella, Shigella, Yersinia enterocolitica, Campylobacter*

2.4   Rheumatic fever

General characteristics

- An inflammatory reaction in joints, skin, heart and central nervous system (CNS) following a group A haemolytic streptococcal infection
- Age generally over 3 years
- Occurs in both sexes, but in girls more often than boys

Revised Jones criteria

Major manifestations	Minor manifestations
Carditis (severe pan-carditis can occur in first or subsequent attacks)	Fever
	Arthralgia
Polyarthritis (flitting)	Previous rheumatic fever and
Subcutaneous nodules	rheumatic heart disease
Chorea	Raised acute phase (ESR, C-reactive
Erythema marginatum	protein
	Prolonged PR interval on ECG

Plus supporting evidence of a preceding streptococcal infection
Throat swab positive for group A streptococcus, increased anti-streptolysin 0 and anti-DNAse B titres

Investigations

- ESR — raised if not in cardiac failure
- Haemoglobin — may fall with chronic disease
- White blood count — normal or slight rise
- IgM rheumatoid factor — negative
- ANA — negative
- ECG — may be abnormal, prolonged PR
- Echocardiogram — may show valvular or myocardial dysfunction

Course and prognosis

- Average attack lasts 6 weeks
- High risk of recurrence in patients who do not receive adequate prophylaxis against streptococcal infection

Management

- Bed rest in the acute phase
- Penicillin to eradicate residual streptococcal infection
- Salicylate therapy
- Corticosteroids in patients with significant carditis
- Prophylactic oral or intramuscular penicillin after an attack required into adult life

2.5 Infectious arthritis

Viral

- Adenovirus, parvovirus, cytomegalovirus, rubella virus, mumps virus, varicella virus

Lyme disease

- *Borrelia burgdorferi*

Bacterial

- *Haemophilus* sp. (young), staphylococcus, streptococcus, meningococcus, gonococcus
- Mycobacteria — both typical and atypical

Fungal

- Blastomycosis, coccidiomycosis, cryptococcus
- *Histoplasma capsulatum*

Other

- Mycoplasma
- Guinea worm

Differential diagnosis of childhood arthritis

- Infections
- Post-infectious arthritides
- Mechanical, including hypermobility
- Juvenile idiopathic arthritis
- Neoplasm including acute lymphoblastic leukaemia
- Other autoimmune/vasculitic diseases
- Rheumatic fever

2.6 Notes on management of arthritis

Physiotherapy, occupational therapy, podiatry, splinting

Arthritis causes contractures and the above are used to overcome this. The physiotherapist teaches active and passive joint movements aiming to maximize function and avoid contractures. Hydrotherapy is used in early disease. Splinting at night is used to prevent or help correct fixed flexion deformities. The podiatrist has a specific interest in foot care. The occupational therapist's role is to maximize the child's functioning within as normal an environment as possible using aids/adaptations as needed.

Orthoses

- Orthoses are useful in helping to prevent contractures, in maintaining a good position if contractures have been repaired and in providing joint stability
- They are particularly useful in aiding individual children with mobility
- The type of orthoses depends on the child's individual needs

For example they may be ankle–foot orthoses if there is just ankle and foot involvement, extending to the knee if the knee is involved. Should there be a scoliosis, thoracolumbar orthoses are available.

Side-effects of commonly used drugs

- NSAIDs — gastrointestinal (may need ranitidine, omeprazole), neurological (headaches, mood)
- Steroids — bone (use calcium, vitamin D), growth, cataract, weight gain
- Methotrexate — nausea (may need ondansetron) liver and bone marrow toxicity (requires monitoring of blood count and liver function)
- Anti-TNF treatment — hypersensitivity reactions, infections, particularly tuberculosis

Antinuclear antibodies

- Not diagnostic or specific for any particular disease
- React with various nuclear constituents

Causes of ANA positivity in children

- Systemic lupus erythematosus
- Juvenile idiopathic arthritis
- Chronic active hepatitis
- Scleroderma
- Mixed connective tissue disease
- Drugs, e.g. anticonvulsants, procainamide
- Epstein–Barr virus infection

3.   CONNECTIVE TISSUE DISORDERS OF CHILDHOOD

3.1   Dermatomyositis

General characteristics

- Non-suppurative myositis with characteristic skin rash and vasculitis
- Occurs in girls more often than in boys
- Peak incidence 4–10 years of age

Clinical features

- Muscle pain and occasional tenderness
- Muscle weakness — limb, girdle, neck, palate, swallowing
- Oedema
- Skin rash — periorbital heliotrope eruption and oedema
- Deep red patches over extensor surface of finger joints (Gottron's patches), elbows, knees and ankle joints
- Vasculitis and skin ulceration
- Nail-fold and eyelid dilated capillaries
- Retinitis in some
- Myocarditis with arrhythmias can occur
- Arthralgia/arthritis with contractures

- Limited joint mobility
- Gastrointestinal dysfunction
- Pulmonary involvement
- Calcinosis (after 1–2 years)

Investigations

- ESR — usually normal
- Serum muscle enzymes (creatine kinase, lactate dehydrogenase) — elevated
- Electromyogram — shows denervation/myopathy
- Muscle biopsy shows inflammation and/or fibre necrosis and small-vessel occlusive vasculitis
- ANA — positive in some

Course and prognosis

- Variable
- Prognosis usually good with adequate treatment
- A small proportion can develop extensive muscle wasting, severe contractures and widespread calcinosis

Management

- Gentle physiotherapy and splinting, followed by more active physiotherapy as muscle inflammation subsides
- Corticosteroids in sufficient dosage to restore function and normalize enzymes
- Cytotoxic drugs ciclosporin, methotrexate, azathioprine, cyclophosphamide, if required
- Anti-TNF treatment
- Careful monitoring is essential, with particular attention to palate and respiratory function, as well as to possible gastrointestinal problems

3.2 Systemic lupus erythematosus

General characteristics

- Onset usually after 5 years of age
- Before puberty, female to male incidence ratio is 3 : 1; after puberty it is 10 : 1
- Higher incidence in Blacks, Orientals, Asians, Native Americans and Latin Americans
- Can be associated with complement deficiencies C2 and C4
- Possible associations with HLA antigens HLA B8, DR2, and DR3

Clinical features

- General malaise
- Weight loss
- Arthralgia or arthritis
- Myalgia and/or myositis
- Fever

- Mucocutaneous lesions:
  - Malar rash
  - Papular, vesicular or purpuric lesions
  - Vasculitic skin lesions
  - Alopecia
  - Oral ulcers
  - Photosensitivity
- Renal disease common, even at onset
- Pulmonary — pleuritis, interstitial infiltrations
- Cardiac — pericarditis, myocarditis, Libman–Sacks endocarditis
- CNS involvement — seizures, headache, psychosis
- Cerebral dysfunction — blurred vision, chorea, transverse myelitis
- Gastrointestinal involvement — hepatosplenomegaly, mesenteric arteritis, inflammatory bowel disease
- Eye — retinitis, episcleritis, rarely, iritis
- Raynaud phenomenon, occasionally

Investigations

- ESR — raised
- Haemoglobin — low: autoimmune haemolytic anaemia in some; anaemia of chronic disease
- Leukopenia — mainly lymphopenia
- Thrombocytopenia in some
- IgM rheumatoid factor — may be positive
- ANA — strongly positive
- Antibodies to double-stranded (ds) DNA usually present in two-thirds
- Total haemolytic complement and its components low
- Anti-cardiolipin antibodies and lupus anticoagulant may be present

Course and prognosis

- Highly variable
- Relates closely to the extent and severity of systemic involvement
- Potential causes of death include infectious complications, including bacterial endocarditis
- Other problems include myocardial infarction, pulmonary fibrosis and renal failure
- Meticulous monitoring essential

Management

- Hydroxychloroquine for skin, joints, pulmonary involvement
- Corticosteroids for systemically ill patients
- Cytotoxic drugs for serious intractable disease
- Antiplatelet drugs for thrombotic episodes
- Rituximab for refractory renal, CNS and haematological disease

Revised criteria for the classification of systemic lupus erythematosus

A person shall be said to have systemic lupus erythematosus if any four or more of 11 criteria are present:

1. Malar rash
2. Discoid rash
3. Photosensitivity
4. Oral ulcers
5. Arthritis
6. Serositis:
   Pleuritis
   OR
   Pericarditis
7. Renal disorder:
   Persistent proteinuria
   ≥ 0.5g/day
   OR
   Cellular casts

8. Neurological disorder
   Seizures disorder
   OR
   Psychosis
9. Haematological disorder:
   Haemolytic anaemia
   OR
   Leukopenia
   OR
   Lymphopenia
   OR
   Thrombocytopenia

10. Immunological
    (a) Anti-phospholipid antibodies
    OR
    (b) Anti-DNA: antibody to native DNA
    OR
    (c) Anti-Sm: presence of antibody to Sm nuclear
    OR
    (d) False-positive serological test for syphilis
11. Antinuclear antibody:
    An abnormal titre of ANA

3.3 Neonatal lupus

General characteristics

- Present in neonatal period, acquired transplacentally
- Associated with maternal autoantibodies (particularly Ro/La) and with maternal lupus or Sjögren's syndrome

Clinical features

- Rash — lesions of discoid lupus or subacute cutaneous lupus
- Congenital heart block — occasional endocardial fibroelastosis
- Thrombocytopenia
- Hepatic or pulmonary disease, haemolytic anaemia — uncommon

Investigations

- ANA — particularly Ro/La
- Thrombocytopenia, anaemia, leukopenia
- Platelet antibodies — positive Coombs test
- ECG

Course and prognosis

- Cutaneous and haematological manifestations transient
- Congenital heart block permanent
- Hepatic fibrosis occasional
- Some risk of systemic lupus erythematosus in teenage or adult years

Management

- Symptomatic for transient manifestations
- Heart block may require pacemaker

3.4 Behçet syndrome

General characteristics

- A clinical triad of recurrent oral aphthous ulcers, recurrent genital ulcers and uveitis
- Male predominance
- High incidence in Japan, the Mediterranean and the Middle East

Clinical features

- Oral ulcers
- Genital ulcers
- Severe uveitis — may lead to glaucoma and blindness
- Arthritis
- Rash — skin hypersensitivity
- Bowel involvement
- Meningoencephalitis, brainstem lesions and dementia

Treatment

- Steroids, thalidomide, anti-TNF treatment are all effective

3.5 Sjögren syndrome

General characteristics

- Dry eyes (keratoconjunctivitis sicca)
- Dry mouth and carious teeth
- Parotitis
- May occur alone or in association with other rheumatic disease
- Occasional complication of renal disease or lymphoreticular malignancy

Scleroderma

Localized (majority of paediatric cases)

- Morphea:
  - Single patch
  - Multiple patches
- Linear:
  - Face, forehead and scalp (en coup de Sabre)
  - Limb (en bande)

Diffuse (systemic sclerosis/CREST (Calcinosis cutis–Raynaud phenomenon–oEsophageal hypomobility–Sclerodactyly–Telangiectasia))

- Rare in childhood; develop tightening of skin of hands, feet and face; systemic problems include respiratory and gastrointestinal problems and renal disease

3.6 Overlap syndrome including mixed connective tissue disease

General characteristics

- Overlapping features of juvenile idiopathic arthritis, systemic lupus erythematosus, systemic sclerosis and dermatomyositis
- Affects particularly older girls

Clinical features

- Arthritis
- Tenosynovitis — both flexor and extensor tendons of fingers, causing contractures
- Raynaud phenomenon — common
- Myositis
- Pleuropericardial involvement
- Dysphagia
- Parotid swelling

Investigations

- ESR — high
- Haemoglobin — often low
- White blood count — usually normal
- Platelets — can be low
- ANA — positive
- Anti-RNP antibodies in high titres indicate the designation of mixed connective tissue disease
- Anti-DNA antibodies — negative or in low titre
- IgM rheumatoid factor — occasionally positive

Course and prognosis

- Slowly develops over years
- May evolve into other recognizable conditions, such as sclerodactyly and, later, other features of systemic sclerosis or systemic lupus erythematosus may appear

Management

- Mild disease is managed with NSAIDs and/or antimalarials
- More severe disease may require corticosteroids, with or without a cytotoxic agent
- Careful monitoring is required to detect signs of potentially serious systemic disease (e.g. nephritis)

4. CHILDHOOD VASCULITIS

Childhood vasculitis encompasses a wide range of clinical syndromes that are characterized by inflammatory changes in the blood vessels. The clinical expression of the disease and its severity depend on the type of pathological change, the site of involvement and the vessel size. The two most common forms seen in children are Henoch–Schönlein purpura and Kawasaki disease.

4.1 Henoch–Schönlein purpura

General characteristics

- Inflammation of small vessels, capillaries — pre- and post-capillary vessels
- May be precipitated by infection, particularly haemolytic streptococci
- Onset generally after the age of 3 years; there is a slight male predominance

Clinical features

- Petechiae
- Rash — urticarial lesions evolving into purpuric macules, usually on the legs, feet and buttocks
- Cutaneous nodules — particularly over the elbows and knees
- Localized areas of subcutaneous oedema that affect the forehead, spine, genitalia, hands and feet
- Arthritis — transient, involving large joints
- Gastrointestinal involvement — colicky abdominal pain and/or gastrointestinal bleeding
- Renal involvement — nephritis, occasionally nephrosis

Investigations

- ESR — normal or high
- Full blood count — normal
- Haematuria and/or proteinuria and/or casts
- IgA complexes in glomeruli and involved skin

- Serum IgA is often raised

Course and prognosis

- Episodes of Henoch–Schönlein purpura are self-limiting
- Recurrences occasionally occur
- Long-term morbidity related to renal involvement

Management

- Supportive care
- Corticosteroids in severe disease

4.2   Kawasaki disease (mucocutaneous lymph node syndrome)

General characteristics

- An acute febrile disease, first described in Japan after the 1940s
- Although now seen in all racial groups throughout the world, it appears to be more common in Orientals
- Occurs in young children, even before the first birthday, and has a slight male predominance

Investigations

- ESR — high
- Haemoglobin — lowered
- White blood count — raised
- Polymorph leukocytosis
- Platelets — raised
- ANA — negative
- IgM rheumatoid factor — negative
- Echocardiography — arteriograms

Diagnostic criteria

- Fever lasting 5 days or more
- Bilateral conjunctival injection
- Changes in lips and oral cavity
- Changes in extremities — reddening and oedema of palms and soles followed by desquamation
- Polymorphous erythematous rash
- Cervical lymphadenopathy

For diagnosis a fever and four features are required.

Clinical features

As in diagnostic criteria, plus:

- Irritability
- Pericarditis
- Valvular dysfunction
- Coronary artery disease
- Arthritis and/or arthralgia
- Gastrointestinal symptoms
- Urethritis
- Central nervous system problems — aseptic meningitis
- Iritis

Course and prognosis

- Acute and convalescent stage lasts up to 10 weeks
- Coronary aneurysms or widening in some 20% of cases
- Death due to coronary vasculitis causing myocardial infarction or rupture of an aneurysm occurs in about 1% of cases

Management

- Supportive care
- Careful observation to detect and manage complications
- Salicylate therapy
- Intravenous gammaglobulin
- Steroids are used

4.3 Polyarteritis nodosa

General characteristics

- A vasculitis affecting small- to medium-sized muscular arteries in either a generalized or cutaneous form
- Age range 3–16 years with equal sex distribution

Clinical features

- Fever
- Abdominal pain
- Arthralgia/myalgia
- Rash:
  - Petechial or purpuric in the generalized form
  - Tender subcutaneous nodules and livedo reticularis in the cutaneous form
- Hypertension
- Renal involvement
- Neurological disease

Investigations

- ESR — high
- Haemoglobin — below 10 g/l
- Leukocytosis
- Urinary abnormalities
- Anti-streptolysin-O titre — elevated in some
- Histology — focal necrosis in small- and medium-sized arteries

Course and prognosis

- Cutaneous form is usually benign but relapses may occur
- Prognosis is worse in the generalized form, depending on the organ involvement

Management

- Steroids — high dose (2 mg/kg per day) in the generalized form
- Steroids and immunosuppressants for severe cases
- Penicillin prophylaxis, if streptococcal aetiology is proved

4.4 Takayasu disease (giant-cell arteritis)

General characteristics

- A panarteritis of the aorta and its large branches leading to thrombosis, stenosis or occlusion
- Primarily affects young adult women, but may occur in children
- More common in Orientals and Blacks

Clinical features

- Claudication — in the arms and also the legs, and absent pulses
- Myalgia
- Hypertension
- Malaise
- Fever

Investigations

- ESR — high
- Haemoglobin — low
- White blood count — neutrophil leukocytosis
- Using a combination of Doppler ultrasound and angiography it is possible to show occlusion, stenosis, or aneurysms

Course and prognosis

- Variable

Management

- Steroids with or without cytotoxic therapy
- Reconstructive surgery when the disease is inactive

4.5 Vasculitis with granuloma

Churg–Strauss syndrome

General characteristics

- A systemic necrotizing vasculitis of small arteries and veins, accompanying asthma and associated with eosinophilia

Clinical features

- Lung involvement — asthma, transient pulmonary infiltrates
- Rash — palpable purpuras and tender subcutaneous nodules
- Peripheral neuropathy
- Renal involvement — occasionally

Wegener granulomatosis

General characteristics

- This also is a necrotizing granulomatous vasculitis of the upper and lower respiratory tracts, accompanied by glomerulonephritis

Clinical features

- Pulmonary granulomata
- Destructive granulomata of the ears, nose and sinuses
- Rash
- Glomerulonephritis
- Eye lesions

Special investigation

- Antineutrophil cytosolic antibodies

Management

- Combined therapy with steroids and cyclophosphamide

4.6 Differential diagnosis of childhood rheumatic disorders

- Infection
- Neoplasm
- Blood dyscrasias
- Mechanical anomalies, including injury

- Biochemical abnormalities
- Genetic and/or congenital anomalies
- Oddities do occur

5. MISCELLANEOUS DISORDERS

5.1 Osteogenesis imperfecta

Osteogenesis imperfecta is a disorder of connective tissue characterized by bone fragility. The disease encompasses a phenotypically and genetically heterogeneous group of inherited disorders that result from mutations in the genes that encode for type 1 collagen. The disorder is manifest in tissues in which the principal matrix is collagen, namely bone, sclerae and ligaments. The musculoskeletal manifestations vary from perinatal lethal forms, to moderate forms with deformity and a propensity to fracture to clinically silent forms with subtle osteopenia and no deformity, as discussed below.

Osteogenesis imperfecta type 1

This is characterized by osteoporosis and excessive bone fragility, distinctly blue sclera and hearing loss. It has autosomal dominant inheritance, and occurs in 1 per 30,000 live births. Fractures may be obvious from birth. Hearing impairment is the result of otosclerosis and affects most patients from the 5th decade, but is rare in the 1st decade. Some families have dentinogenesis imperfecta — with yellow transparent teeth which are fragile. There is spontaneous improvement with puberty. X-rays show generalized osteopenia, evidence of previous fractures and callus formation at the site of new bone formation. The skull X-ray shows Wormian bones.

Osteogenesis imperfecta type II

This lethal syndrome is characterized by low birth weight and typical X-ray findings of crumpled bones and beaded ribs. Although autosomal recessive in a few cases, most cases are autosomal dominant new mutations. It affects 1 per 60,000 live births; 50% are stillborn, the remainder dying soon after birth from respiratory difficulty because of a defective thoracic cage. It is worth looking at a picture of the lethal form. X-rays show multiple fracture of the ribs, often beaded, and crumpled (accordion like) appearance of the long bones.

Osteogenesis imperfecta type III

This syndrome is characterized by severe bone fragility and multiple fractures in the newborn period which lead to progressive skeletal deformity. The sclera may be bluish at birth, but become less blue with age. It is autosomal recessive with clinical variability suggesting genetic heterogeneity. Few patients survive into adult life. X-rays show generalized osteopenia and multiple fractures, without the beading of the ribs or crumpling of the ribs seen in type II.

Osteogenesis imperfecta type IV

This syndrome is characterized by osteoporosis leading to bone fragility without the other features of type I. The sclera may be bluish at birth but become less blue as the patient matures. Inheritance is autosomal dominant. Variable age of onset and variable number of fractures, there is spontaneous improvement with puberty. X-rays show generalized osteopenia and fractures, but these are generally less than the other forms of osteogenesis imperfecta.

Management

For osteogenesis imperfecta type II no therapeutic intervention is helpful. For other forms, careful nursing of the newborn may prevent excessive fractures. Beyond the newborn period, aggressive orthopaedic treatment is the mainstay of treatment aimed at prompt splinting of fractures and correction of deformities. Genetic counselling is important. Reliable prenatal diagnosis is not available for all forms of osteogenesis imperfecta, although severely affected fetuses may be confidently recognized by X-rays, ultrasound scanning and biochemistry.

5.2   Osteopetrosis

Osteopetrosis (marble bone disease, Albers–Schönberg disease) is characterized by a generalized increase in skeletal density. There are multiple types. The most important two are listed below.

Osteopetrosis congenita

This presents in infancy (autosomal recessive) with faltering growth, hypocalcaemia, anaemia, thrombocytopenia and, rarely, fractures. Bone encroaching on the marrow cavity leads to extramedullary haemopoiesis. Optic atrophy and blindness are common, secondary to bone pressure. Diagnosis is by skeletal survey. Bone marrow transplant can be curative.

Osteopetrosis tarda

This presents in later childhood, usually with fractures, and manifestations are less severe and treatment is symptomatic.

5.3   Osteoporosis

- This can be idiopathic
- Most commonly secondary to corticosteroid use
- Seen in conditions causing decreased mobility such as cerebral palsy, neuromuscular diseases
- Dual energy X-ray absorptiometry scan for bone mineral density
- Can cause pathological fractures particularly of vertebrae
- Treat with calcium/vitamin D and bisphosphonates

5.4   Hemihypertrophy

This is often difficult to recognize. It may involve the whole of one side of the body, or be limited in extent, e.g. to just one leg. It may be congenital, in which case the tissues are structurally and functionally normal. It has been associated with mental retardation, ipsilateral paired internal organs and rarely with Wilms' tumours or adrenal carcinomas.

Hemihypertrophy can be confused with regional overgrowth secondary to neurofibromatosis type I, haemangiomas and lymphangiomas.

Beckwith–Wiedemann Syndrome (BWS)

A fetal overgrowth syndrome, mapped to gene locus 11p15.5.

Clinically the three major features are:

- Pre- and/or postnatal overgrowth (> 90th centile)
- Macroglossia
- Abdominal wall defects

The minor defects are:

- Characteristic ear signs (ear lobe creases or posterior helical pits)
- Facial naevus flammeus
- Hypoglycaemia
- Organomegaly
- Hemihypertrophy.

The diagnosis is based on

- Three major features, or
- Two major plus three or more minor features.

Infants are more likely to be delivered prematurely, 35% before 35 weeks. Exomphalos occurs in 50% of cases. Hypoglycaemia, which is usually mild and transient, occurs in 50%. Deaths from BWS can occur in infancy and are mainly caused by problems related to prematurity or congenital cardiac defects (< 10%).

During childhood, the dysmorphic features become less apparent, although the macroglossia may cause feeding problems, problems with speech and occasionally with obstructive apnoea. Surgical tongue reduction may be required in severe cases.

Overgrowth is most marked in the first few years and is associated with an advanced bone age. It tends to slow down in late childhood, and most adults are < 97th centile. Hemihypertrophy occurs in 25% of cases. Visceromegaly is common and neoplasia occurs in 5%, most commonly with Wilms' tumour followed by adrenocortical carcinoma, hepatoblastoma and neuroblastoma, those children with hemihypertrophy being the most at risk. By adolescence, the majority lead a normal life. There is controversy about abdominal tumour screening which some centres advocate should be by regular abdominal palpation and others by regular ultrasound examination or both.

5.5   Hypermobility

- Commonest cause of musculoskeletal complaints in childhood
- Causes joint pain and occasionally swelling after exercise
- Improves with age
- Differential diagnosis includes Ehlers–Danlos syndrome (skin fragility and hyperextensibility, and joint hyperextensibility), Marfan syndrome
- Management is exercise to build-up strength and reassurance

5.6   Toe walking

- Can be a normal finding up until 3 years of age, especially in hypermobile patients
- Neurological disorders include cerebral palsy, Duchenne muscular dystrophy, spinal cord problems, congenital tendo-Achilles shortening
- Leg-length discrepancy
- Habit

5.7   Foot drop

- Variety of causes
- Patient has a stepping gait and lifts the affected limb high to avoid scraping the foot on the floor
- They are unable to walk on their heel
- Possible causes
  - Lateral popliteal nerve palsy (look for signs of injury below and lateral to the affected knee)
  - Peroneal muscle atrophy
  - Poliomyelitis

5.8   Reflex sympathetic dystrophy

- Autonomic nerve dysfunction in a limb results in severe immobilization because of pain
- Osteoporosis is associated
- Physiotherapy to remobilize is the best treatment

5.9   Non-accidental injury

- Non-accidental injury can present as musculo-skeletal complaints, frequently seen with bruising
- Fractures — especially spiral or metaphyseal in the under 3-year age group more commonly
- Periosteal reactions from rotation injury
- Dislocations especially elbow

6. FURTHER READING

Ansell BM, Rudge S, Schaller JG. 1991. *A Colour Atlas of Paediatric Rheumatology.* Aylesbury: Wolfe.

Isenberg DA, Miller JJ. 1999. *Adolescent Rheumatology.* London: Martin Dunitz.

Mier RJ, Brower TJ. 1994. *Paediatric Orthopaedics.* Dordrecht, Netherlands: Kluwer Academic.

Cassidy JT, Petty RE. 2001. *Textbook of Pediatric Rheumatology,* 4th edn. New York, NY, USA: WB Saunders.

Chapter 23

Statistics

Angie Wade

CONTENTS

Statistics

1. STUDY DESIGN

1.1 Research questions

A research study should always be designed to answer a particular research question. The question usually relates to a specific population. For example:

- Does taking folic acid early in pregnancy prevent neural tube defects?
- Is a new inhaled steroid better than current treatment for improving lung function among cystic fibrosis patients?
- Is low birth weight associated with hypertension in later life?

Random samples of the relevant populations are taken. For example: pregnant women, cystic fibrosis patients, low-birth-weight and normal-birth-weight individuals.

Based on the differences found between the different groups of samples, inferences are made about the populations from which they were randomly sampled. For example:

- If the women in the sample taking folic acid have fewer neural tube defects it may be inferred that taking folic acid during pregnancy will reduce the incidence of neural tube defects in the population
- If, among our sample of cystic fibrosis patients, those taking steroids have better lung function, on average, than those on current treatment, the inference might be that steroids improve lung function among cystic fibrosis patients in general. Note that some of the patients in the sample who were on current treatment may have had better lung function than some of those using steroids, but it is the average difference that is considered
- If there is a difference in hypertensive rates between samples of individuals who were and were not of low birth weight, it may be inferred that birth weight is associated with later hypertension in the population in general

Some quantification of how the groups differ between the samples will be needed. Dependent on the nature of the data, the averages, percentages or proportions may be calculated for the samples taken. Prevalence or incidence of a disease or occurrence may be of interest.

Prevalence is the number of cases within a defined population at a specified time, **incidence** is the number of new cases arising in a given period in a specified population. For example, diabetes has high prevalence but low incidence, whereas the common cold has low prevalence and high incidence.

For the research questions given above, the suitable summaries of the outcomes may be:

- The risk of neural tube defect (number of cases divided by the number of women studied) among women taking folic acid and those who do not. The relative risk (risk in group taking folic acid divided by the risk in those that take placebo treatment) would give a measure of how effective the intervention is in preventing neural tube defects
- The difference in average lung function between those given the new steroid and those given standard therapy will provide a measure of the effectiveness of the new treatment compared to standard
- The difference in percentages of subjects developing hypertension between those who were low birth weight and normal birth weight (sometimes known as the attributable risk reduction) would provide a useful summary measure

Statistical analysis enables us to determine what inferences can be made. Studies are either experimental or observational.

1.2   Confounding

Confounding may be an important source of error. A confounding factor is a background variable (i.e. something not of direct interest) that:

- Is different between the groups being compared, and
- Affects the outcome being studied

For example:

- In a study to compare the effect of folic acid supplementation in early pregnancy on neural tube defects, age will be a confounding factor if:
  - Either the folic acid or placebo group tends to consist of older women, and
  - Older women are more, or less, likely to have a child with a neural tube defect
- When studying the effects of a new inhaled steroid against standard therapy for cystic fibrosis patients, disease severity will be a confounder if:
  - One of the groups (new steroid/standard therapy) consists of more severely affected patients, and
  - Disease severity affects the outcome measure (lung function)
- In the comparison of hypertension rates between low and not low birth weight, social class will be a confounder if:
  - The low-birth-weight babies are more likely to have lower social class, and
  - Social class is associated with the risk of hypertension

If a difference is found between the groups (folic acid/placebo, new steroid/standard therapy and low/normal birth weight) we will not know whether the differences are, respectively, the results of folic acid or age, of the potency of the new steroid or the severity of disease in the patient, or of birth weight or social class.

Confounding may be avoided by matching individuals in the groups according to potential confounders. For example, we could age-match folic acid and placebo pairs or deliberately recruit individuals of low and normal birth weight from similar social classes. We could find pairs of cystic fibrosis patients of similar disease severity and randomly allocate one of each pair to receive the new steroid while the other receives standard therapy.

1.3 Experimental studies

In experimental studies, individuals are assigned to groups by the investigator. For example, pregnant women will be assigned to take either folic acid or a placebo; cystic fibrosis patients will be assigned to either the new or current treatment. In both of these examples the second group is known as a **control group**.

Note that a control group does not necessarily consist of normal healthy individuals. In the second example the control group comprises cystic fibrosis patients on standard therapy.

Individuals should be randomized to groups to remove any potential bias. **Randomization** means that each patient has the same chance of being assigned to either of the groups, regardless of their personal characteristics. Note that random does not mean haphazard or systematic. Randomization may be adjusted to ensure that the groups are balanced with respect to potential confounders. Randomization may be stratifed or within matched pair.

Experimental studies may be:

- **Double-blind** — neither the patient, nor the researcher assessing the patients or the treating clinician, knows which treatment the patient has been randomized to receive
- **Single-blind** — either the patient or the researcher/clinician does not know (usually the patient)
- **Unblinded** (or open) — both the patient and the researcher/clinician know

It is preferable that studies are blinded because knowledge of treatment may affect the outcome and introduce a bias in the results.

Clinical trials are experimental studies.

1.4 Crossover studies

In a crossover (or within-patient) study, each patient receives treatment and placebo in a random order. Fewer patients are needed because many between-patient confounders can be removed. For example, even though pairs of cystic fibrosis patients may be chosen and randomized to groups on the basis of their disease severity, this does not ensure that the groups will be of similar age or sex.

Crossover studies are only suitable for chronic disorders that are not cured but for which treatment may give temporary relief. There should be no carryover effect of the treatment from one treatment period to the next.

1.5 Observational studies

In observational studies the groups being compared are already defined (e.g. low and normal birth weight) and the study merely observes what happens.

Case-control, cross-sectional and cohort are particular types of observational studies that, respectively, consider features of the past, the present and the future to try and identify differences between the groups.

- If we take groups of individuals with and without hypertension with the aim of identifying different features in their past that might explain a causal route for the hypertension this is a case–control study
- If we take groups of low- and normal-birth-weight babies and follow them forward in time to see whether one group is more prone to hypertension then this is a cohort study

The relative risk (RR) can be used as a measure of effect in a cohort study. A similar measure based on the odds (number of cases divided by the number of non-cases) rather than risk (number of cases divided by the number studied, i.e. cases and non-cases) in each group, known as the 'odds ratio' (OR), is appropriate for case–control studies.

2. DISTRIBUTIONS

2.1 Types of data

Data may be either categoric or numeric. If a variable is categoric then each individual lies in one of several categories. Numeric data are measured on a number scale.

Ranks give the order of increasing magnitude of numeric variables. For example:

Sample of seven readings:

| 2.3 | 5.0 | 3.9 | 1.3 | – 2.1 | 1.3 | 4.2 |

In order of magnitude:

| – 2.1 | 1.3 | 1.3 | 2.3 | 3.9 | 4.2 | 5.0 |

Ranks:

| 1 | 2.5 | 2.5 | 4 | 5 | 6 | 7 |

Note that there are seven values in the sample and the largest value has rank 7. Where there are ties (for example, the two values 1.3), the ranks are averaged between the tied values.

The mode is the value that occurs most often. In the example above:

- Mode = 1.3

The median is the middle value when the values are ranked. This is the 50th centile. In the example above:

- Median = 2.3

The **mean** is the arithmetic average. In the example above:

- Mean $= (-2.1 + 1.3 + 1.3 + 2.3 + 3.9 + 4.2 + 5.0) / 7 = 2.27$

2.2 Skewed distributions

The distribution of a set of values may be asymmetrical (skewed).

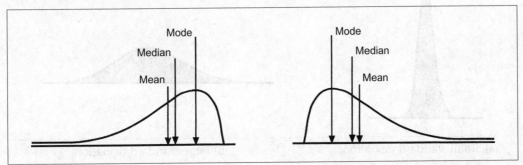

    (a) Negative or downward or left skew;   (b) positive or upward or right skew

In a sample of this type the mean is 'pulled towards' the values in the outlying tail of the distribution and is unrepresentative of the bulk of the data.

Note that the skew is named according to the direction in which the tail points. In the left-hand diagram (a), the tail points to the left, to negative values and downwards.

If the distribution is skewed then the median is preferable as a summary of the data. For example, the distribution of earnings is an upward skew, a relatively few high earners will tend to raise the mean unrepresentatively. The median (50th centile) gives a more accurate description of what most people earn — half will earn less than this figure and half above it.

2.3 Normal distribution

The normal distribution is symmetrical and bell-shaped.

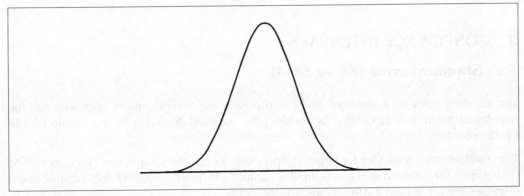

Normal distribution

2.4 Standard deviation

The standard deviation (which is equal to the square root of the variance) gives a measure of the spread of the values in the distribution. The smaller the standard deviation (or variance) the more tightly grouped the values.

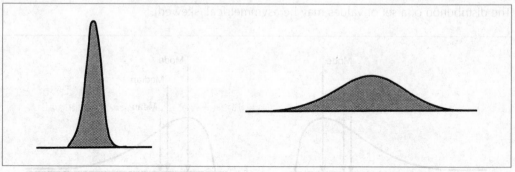

(a) Small standard deviation;   (b) large standard deviation

If the values are normally distributed, then:

- Approximately 68% of the values lie within one standard deviation either side of the mean
- Approximately 95% of the values lie within 2 standard deviations either side of the mean
- Exactly 95% of the values lie within 1.96 standard deviations either side of the mean (hence 2.5% lie in each tail, total 5% outside range)

For example, forced expiratory volume in the 1st second (FEV_1) is measured in 100 students. The mean value for this group is 4.5 litres with a standard deviation of 0.5 litres. If the values are normally distributed then:

- Approximately 68% of the values lie in the range $(4.5 \pm 1(0.5)) = (4.5 \pm 0.5) = (4, 5$ litres)
- Approximately 95% of the values lie in the range $(4.5 \pm 2(0.5)) = (4.5 \pm 1) = (3.5, 5.5$ litres)

3. CONFIDENCE INTERVALS

3.1 Standard error (SE or SEM)

The standard error is a measure of how precisely the sample mean approximates the population mean. It is calculated by dividing the standard deviation by the square root of the sample size.

The standard error is smaller for larger sample sizes (i.e. as the sample size increases, SEM decreases). The more observations in the sample the more precisely the sample mean estimates the population mean (i.e. the less the error).

The more variable the outcome (as quantified via the standard deviation) the larger the standard errors, implying less precision for a given sample size.

The SEM can be used to construct **confidence intervals** (CI).

* The interval (mean $\pm$ 1.96 SEM) is a 95% confidence interval for the population mean
* The interval (mean $\pm$ 2 SEM) is an approximate 95% confidence interval for the population mean
* The interval (mean $\pm$ 1.64 SEM) is a 90% confidence interval for the population mean

There is a 5% (or 0.05 or 1 in 20) chance that the true mean lies outside the 95% confidence interval. We are 95% confident that the true mean lies inside the interval.

There is a 10% (or 0.1, or 1 in 10) chance that the true mean lies outside the 90% confidence interval. We are 90% confident that the true mean lies inside the interval.

Note the difference between the standard deviation and the standard error:

* Standard deviation (SD) gives a measure of the spread of the data values
* Standard error (SE) is a measure of how precisely the sample mean approximates the population mean

For example, consider again the FEV_1 measurements from 100 students with mean 4.5 litres and standard deviation 0.5 litres. The standard error is calculated by combining the standard deviation and the sample size thus:

$$\text{Standard error} = (0.5/\sqrt{100}) = (0.5/10) = 0.05$$

An approximate 95% confidence interval for the population mean FEV_1 is given by:

$$(4.5 \pm 2(0.05)) = (4.5 \pm 0.1) = 4.4 - 4.6 \text{ litres}$$

i.e. we are 95% confident that the population mean FEV_1 of students lies in the range 4.4–4.6 litres.

Confidence intervals can similarly be constructed around other summary statistics, for example the difference between two means, a single proportion or percentage, the difference between two proportions. The standard error always gives a measure of the precision of the sample estimate and is smaller for larger sample sizes.

4. SIGNIFICANCE TESTS

Statistical significance tests, or hypothesis tests, use the sample data to assess how likely some specified **null hypothesis** is to be correct. The measure of 'how likely' is given by a probability known as the *p*-value. Usually, the null hypothesis is that there is 'no difference' between the groups.

4.1   Null hypotheses and *p*-values

To answer the research questions in Section 1 we test the following null hypotheses:

- There is no difference in the incidence of fetuses with neural tube defects between the groups of pregnant women who do and do not take folic acid supplements
- Lung function is similar in asthma patients who receive the new inhaled steroid when compared with the patients on current treatment
- Hypertension rates do not differ according to birth weight

Even if these null hypotheses were true we would not expect the averages or proportions in our sample groups to be identical. Because of random variation there will be some difference. The **p-value** is the probability of observing a difference of that magnitude if the null hypothesis is true.

Since the *p*-value is a probability, it takes values between 0 and 1. Values near to zero suggest that the null hypothesis is unlikely to be true. The smaller the *p*-value the more significant the result:

- $p = 0.05$, the result is significant at 5%

The sample difference had a 1 in 20 chance of occurring if the null hypothesis were true.

- $p = 0.01$, the result is significant at 1%

The sample difference had a 1 in 100 chance of occurring if the null hypothesis were true.

NB Statistical significance is not the same as clinical significance.

Although a study may show that the results from drug A are statistically significantly better than for drug B we have to consider

- The magnitude of the improvement
- The costs
- The ease of administration
- The potential side-effects of the two drugs, etc.

before deciding that the result is clinically significant and that drug A should be introduced in preference to drug B.

4.2   Significance, power and sample size

The study sample may or may not be compatible with the null hypothesis being true. If the *p*-value is small then there is a low probability of observing the samples if the null hypothesis is true and this would lead us to 'reject' the null hypothesis. A *p*-value not near to zero shows that the data are compatible with the null hypothesis.

On the basis of the study results, we may decide to disbelieve (or reject) the null hypothesis. In reality, the null hypothesis either is or is not true. This gives the fourfold situation illustrated below:

Null hypothesis:

Decision based on study results:	True	False
'Accept' null hypothesis	OK	(II)
'Reject' null hypothesis	(I)	OK

Hence the study may lead to the wrong conclusions.

- A low (significant) *p*-value (close to zero) may lead us to disbelieve (or reject) the null hypothesis when it is actually true — Box (I) above. This is known as a **type I error**.
- The *p*-value may be high (non-significant, away from zero) when the null hypothesis is false — Box (II) above. This is known as a **type II error**.

The **power** of a study is the probability (usually expressed as a percentage) of correctly rejecting the null hypothesis when it is false.

Larger differences between the groups can be detected with greater power. The power to identify correctly a difference of a certain size can be increased by increasing the sample size. Small samples often lead to type II errors (i.e. there is not sufficient power to detect differences of clinical importance).

In practice there is a grey area between accepting and rejecting the null hypothesis. The decision will be made in the light of the *p*-value obtained. We should not draw different conclusions based on a *p*-value of 0.051 compared with a value of 0.049. The *p*-value is a probability; as it gets smaller the less likely it is that the null hypothesis is true.

4.3   Parametric and non-parametric tests

Statistical hypothesis tests are either parametric or non-parametric. Choosing the appropriate statistical test depends on:

- The type of data (categoric or numeric)
- The distribution of the data (if numeric, are they normally distributed?)
- Whether the data are paired or not
- How many groups are being compared (we usually have two: diseased/healthy or treated/untreated but there may be more)

Parametric tests usually assume that the data are normally distributed. Examples are:

- *t*-test (sometimes called 'Student's *t*-test' or 'Student's paired *t*-test')
- Pearson's coefficient of linear correlation (see Section 5.1)

An unpaired (or two-sample) *t*-test is used to compare the average values of two independent groups (e.g. patients with and without disease, treated versus placebo, etc.).

A paired (or one-sample) *t*-test is used if the members of the groups are paired. For example, each individual with disease is matched with a healthy individual of the same age and sex; in a crossover trial the measurements made on two treatments are paired within individuals.

> **Non-parametric tests** are usually based on ranks (see Section 2.1). Examples are:
>
> - Wilcoxon
> - Sign
> - Spearman's Rank Correlation
> - Mann–Whitney *U*
> - Chi-squared (χ^2)

The chi-squared test is used to compare proportions (or percentages) between two groups.

5.   CORRELATION AND REGRESSION

Sometimes measurements are made on two continuous variables for each study subject. For example:

- CD4 count and age
- Blood pressure and weight
- FEV$_1$ and height.

The aim may be to quantify the relationship between the two variables. The data can be displayed in a scatterplot and this will show the main features of the data.

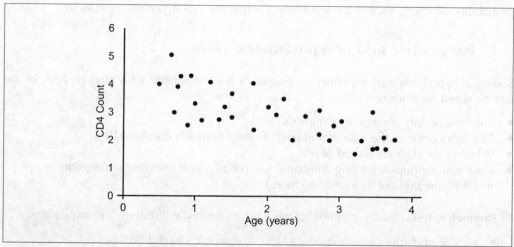

Scatterplot of CD4 count versus age

5.1 Correlation coefficients

The correlation coefficient (sometimes called Pearson's coefficient of linear correlation) is denoted by r and indicates how closely the points lie to a line.

r takes values between -1 and $+1$, the closer it is to zero the less the linear association between the two variables. (Note that the variables may be strongly associated but not linearly.)

Negative values of r indicate that one variable decreases as the other increases (for example, CD4 count falls with age).

Values of -1 or $+1$ show that the variables are perfectly linearly related, i.e. the scatterplot points lie on a straight line.

Correlation coefficients:

- Show how one variable increases or decreases as the other variable increases
- Do not give information about the size of the increase or decrease
- Do not give a measure of agreement

Pearson's r is a parametric correlation coefficient. Spearman's Rank Correlation is the most commonly used non-parametric correlation coefficient.

- Parametric correlation coefficients quantify the extent of any linear increase or decrease
- Non-parametric correlation coefficients quantify the extent of any tendency for one variable to increase or decrease as the other increases (for example, exponential increase or decline, increasing in steps, etc.)

A p-value attached to a parametric correlation coefficient shows how likely it is that there is no linear association between the two variables.

A significant correlation does not imply cause and effect.

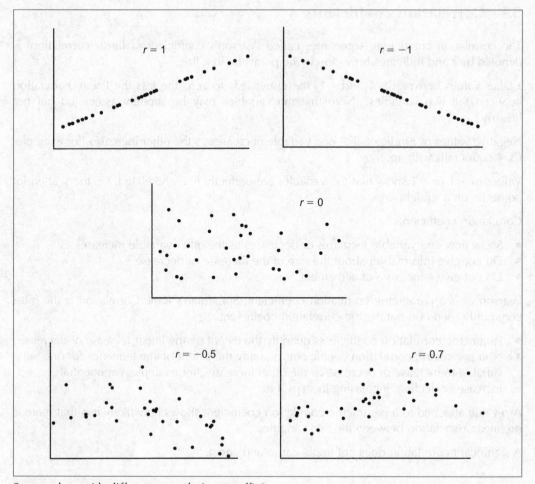

Scatterplots with different correlation coefficients

5.2 Linear regression

A regression equation ($y = a + bx$) may be used to **predict** one variable from the other.

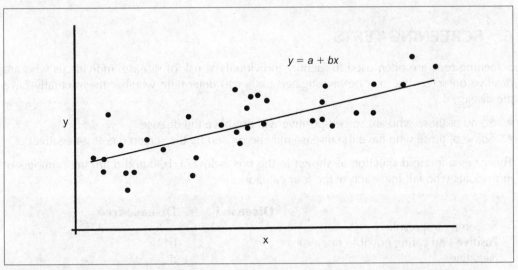

Linear regression line

- 'a' is the intercept — the value y takes when x is zero
- 'b' is the slope of the line — sometimes called the **regression coefficient**. It gives the average change in y for a unit increase in x. If 'b' is negative then y decreases as x increases

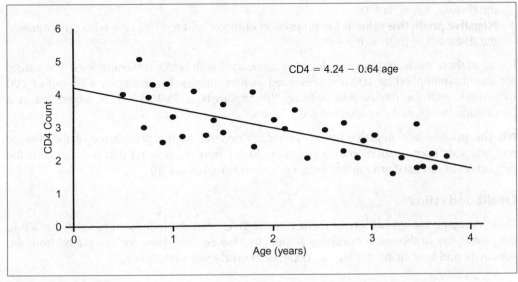

CD4 count versus age

If the units of measurement change then so will the regression equation. For example, if age is measured in months rather than years then the value of the slope (the average change in CD4 for a unit increase in age) will alter accordingly.

6. SCREENING TESTS

Screening tests are often used to identify individuals at risk of disease. Individuals who are positive on screening may be investigated further to determine whether they actually have the disease.

- Some of those who are screen-positive will not have the disease
- Some of those who have the disease may be missed by the screen (i.e. test-negative)

This gives a fourfold situation as shown in the box below (a, b, c and d are the numbers of individuals who fall into each of the four categories).

	Diseased	**Disease-free**
Screening test result:		
Positive (indicating possible disease)	a	b
Negative	c	d

There are several summary measures that are often used to quantify how good a screening test is:

- **Sensitivity** is the proportion of true positives correctly identified by the test $a / (a + c)$
- **Specificity** is the proportion of true negatives correctly identified by the test $d / (b + d)$
- **Positive predictive value** is the proportion of those who test positive who actually have the disease, i.e. $a / (a + b)$
- **Negative predictive value** is the proportion of those who test negative who do not have the disease, i.e. $d / (c + d)$

For all of these measures, larger values are associated with better screening tests. The values are usually multiplied by 100 and presented as percentages. For example, if 75 out of 100 individuals with the disease test positive, the sensitivity is $75/100 = 0.75$, expressed as a percentage this gives a sensitivity of 75%.

NB The positive and negative predictive values depend on the **prevalence** of the disease and may vary from population to population. (Recall from Section 1.1 that prevalence is the proportion of diseased among the total, i.e. $(a + c) / (a + b + c + d)$)

Likelihood ratios

These compare the probability of the test result given that the individual has the disease to the probability of the result occurring if they are disease free. They are calculated from the sensitivity and specificity and are not dependent on disease prevalence.

- **The likelihood ratio (LR) for a positive test result LR +** $= \dfrac{\text{sensitivity}}{(1 - \text{specificity})}$

- **The likelihood ratio for a negative test result, LR** $- = \dfrac{1 - \text{sensitivity}}{\text{specificity}}$

Likelihood ratios can be multiplied by pre-test odds to give post-test odds.

Example

A screening test is applied to patients with and without disease X. Of 100 who have the disease, 60 test positive; of 200 without the disease, only 20 test positive.

The following table can be constructed:

Test result	Disease X	Disease–free
Positive (indicating possible disease)	60	20
Negative	40	180

The following can, therefore, be estimated from this sample of 300 individuals:

- Sensitivity = 60/100 = 0.6 or 60%
- Specificity = 180/200 = 0.9 or 90%
- LR + = 0.6/(1 − 0.9) = 6
- LR − = (1 − 0.6)/0.9 = 0.44
- The positive predictive value is 60/(60 + 20) = 0.75 or 75% (i.e. 75% of those who test positive actually have the disease in this sample)
- The prevalence of the disease in this sample is ((60 + 40)/(100 + 200)) = 0.33 or 33%

If a particular patient had a prior odds of 1.5 of having the disease (meaning that he or she is 1.5 times more likely to have the disease than not to have it) then 1.5/2.5 (or 60%) of patients of this type will have the disease). The **posterior odds** of the patient having the disease will thus be determined by the result of the screening test:

- If the test is positive (LR +) then the odds of having the disease will be 1.5 × 6 = 9
- If the test is negative (LR −), the odds will be 1.5 × 0.44 = 0.66

Note that, as expected, the odds of having the disease rise if the test is positive and fall if the test is negative.

A posterior odds of 9 means that the patient is nine times more likely to have the disease than not, which equates to a probability of 9/10 or 0.9 (as opposed to 0.6 before testing).

A posterior odds of 0.66 equates to a probability of 0.66/1.66, or 0.4 (as opposed to 0.6 before testing).

7. FURTHER READING

Bland M. 1987. *An Introduction to Medical Research* Oxford, Oxford Medical Publications.

Kirkwood BR. 1988. *Essentials of Medical Statistics*. Cambridge, Blackwell Scientific Publications.

Altman DG. 1991. *Practical Statistics for Medical Research*. Chapman and Hall.

Armitage P, Berry G. 1987. *Statistical Methods in Medical Research*. Cambridge, Blackwell Scientific Publications.

Chapter 24

Surgery

Merrill McHoney, Vivien McNamara and Robert Wheeler

CONTENTS

Neonatal Surgery

Neonatal surgery

1. ANTENATAL DIAGNOSIS OF SURGICAL CONDITIONS

- Identify pathology and assess severity/complications
- Search for other associated anomalies
- In-utero intervention — thoracoamniotic shunt for a massive congenital cystic adenomatoid malformation with significant mediastinal shift and hydrops
- Modify pregnancy monitoring — gastroschisis (in third trimester have weekly ultrasounds and twice-weekly cardiotocographs for late intrauterine death, have an expectation of preterm labour)
- Parental counselling — opportunity for karyotyping, consideration of termination of pregnancy, information regarding early post-natal care and surgery/outcome
- Plan delivery/immediate neonatal and surgical care

2. CONGENITAL OESOPHAGEAL ANOMALIES

2.1 Oesophageal atresia and tracheo-oesophageal fistula

Oesophageal atresia (OA) and tracheo-oesophageal fistula (TOF) comprise faulty separation of the primitive embryonic trachea from the foregut (future oesophagus). Incidence is 1 in 3000 to 1 in 3500. Many are associated with pre-term labour as a result of polyhydramnios.

- 85% — blind proximal oesophageal pouch with a tracheo-oesophageal fistula to the distal pouch
- 5–10% — pure oesophageal atresia (long gap)
- 5% — H-fistula (tracheo-oesophageal) without an oesophageal atresia
- Rare — oesophageal atresia with upper pouch fistula, or upper and lower pouch fistulae

Diagnosis

- Antenatal scan — polyhydramnios, absent gastric bubble, distended upper oesophagus (interrupted foetal swallowing)
- After birth — excessive salivation, choking because of aspiration after every feed, respiratory distress with or without cyanotic episodes. Other associated anomalies are seen in 30–50%
- Confirmation — failure to pass a large-bore (10 French scale) nasogastric tube (with chest X-ray to demonstrate that the nasogastric tube is not coiled in the oesophagus) +/– bronchoscopy at surgery to confirm location of lower pouch fistula and to exclude upper pouch fistula and laryngeal cleft
- Contrast swallow is not indicated (risk of aspiration)

Management

- Stop feeds and aspirate upper pouch
- Respiratory support as required — avoid bag and mask ventilation to reduce gastric distension
- Replogle tube — sited in the proximal pouch — double-lumen gastric tube (with side holes) placed on low-pressure continuous suction preventing suction of the intestinal mucosa against the tube. Larger lumen requires flushing with 1–2 ml saline to prevent blockage with tenacious secretions
- Antibiotics if evidence of pulmonary aspiration
- Minimal handling — reduces air swallowing from crying
- Echocardiogram — ideally before surgery, especially if infant is cyanotic, there is significant cardiac murmur or infant requires cardiac support. May have duct-dependent lesion requiring prostaglandin E_1 infusion and early cardiac opinion. Repair the oesophageal atresia/tracheo-oesophageal fistula when stable
- Renal ultrasound — if urine is passed, this can be delayed until after surgery
- Spinal ultrasound — to exclude cord tethering (will be asymptomatic in the neonatal period)
- Karyotype — if infant is dysmorphic or has other system anomalies
- Parental counselling

Surgery

- Emergency ligation of fistula — seen in the premature neonate with respiratory distress syndrome
- Common anatomy (OA + TOF) — right thoracotomy, ligation of the fistula and primary end-to-end anastomosis of OA with early extubation. Trans-anastomotic tube passed for feeding. A 'tight' anastomosis may require a period of paralysis and ventilation
- Long-gap — may require complex and staged procedures

Complications

- Anastomotic leak
- Recurrent fistula
- Stricture (at anastomosis)
- Tracheomalacia
- Gastro-oesophageal reflux
- Abnormal oesophageal motility
- Missed upper pouch fistula
- Reflex bradycardia +/– respiratory arrest — vagal stimulation from a distending food bolus
- Chylothorax

2.2 Dying spells

Severe tracheomalacia exacerbated during feeding or crying, with complete airway collapse, cyanosis and cessation of stridulous breathing, followed by loss of consciousness, relaxation of the airway, and recovery.

Outcome

- Overall survival is 85–95%
- Highest risk — birth weight < 1500 g, severe associated anomalies, major congenital heart defect, ventilator dependency

3. NEONATAL INTESTINAL OBSTRUCTION

Incidence 1 in 500–1000 live births. About half will have an atresia or stenosis. After delivery, swallowed air will reach the small bowel within 30 min, the colon by 3–4 h and the rectum by 6–8 h.

Clinical presentation

- May have clinical suspicion from antenatal ultrasound — proximal bowel dilatation, 'double bubble', echogenic bowel loops (meconium ileus), polyhydramnios
- Most present shortly after birth with abdominal distension (delayed in distal obstruction), large nasogastric aspirate (> 50 ml initial volume), bilious vomiting, delayed passage of meconium (> 24 h)
- Premature neonate — delayed passage of meconium expected, bilious nasogastric aspirate may be the result of intestinal immaturity or sepsis
- Passage of flatus will exclude an atresia

Common causes

- Malrotation with volvulus
- Duodenal atresia, stenosis, extrinsic compression
- Jejunoileal atresia, or stenosis
- Meconium ileus (simple, complicated)
- Meconium plug syndrome
- Hirschsprung disease
- Ileus secondary to sepsis, paralysis/ventilation/medication
- Inguinal hernia (incarcerated)
- Anorectal malformation

Radiological diagnosis

- Abdominal X-ray
  - Proximal obstruction — a few dilated loops, mainly in the upper abdomen
  - Distal — numerous throughout most of abdomen (paucity of rectal gas suggests distal colonic or rectal obstruction)

- Partial obstruction will allow some distal gas, often mixed with meconium
- Inspect for peritoneal/scrotal calcification (meconium peritonitis/prenatal perforation)
- Water-soluble lower gastrointestinal contrast — to distinguish distal bowel obstruction (Hirschsprung disease, ileal atresia, meconium ileus/plug)
- Water-soluble upper gastrointestinal contrast — to investigate intestinal rotation abnormalities

General management

- Nasogastric tube and gastric decompression
- Replace nasogastric losses with 0.9% NaCl with KCl, ml for ml
- Intravenous fluid replacement
- Consider rectal decompression or washout after surgical consultation/review
- Broad-spectrum antibiotics if there is suspicion of intestinal ischaemia (red/shiny/oedematous abdominal wall, abdominal tenderness, absent bowel sounds, metabolic acidosis) or perforation

Megacystis-microcolon-intestinal hypoperistalsis syndrome

A rare, usually fatal, condition with degenerative smooth muscle changes in the bowel and renal tract. Abdominal distension from lax abdominal muscles and a dilated bladder. Incomplete intestinal rotation, microcolon (barium enema) with poor peristalsis. Ultrasound demonstrates hydronephrosis and megacystis (differentiate from Hirschsprung disease).

4. INTESTINAL ATRESIA

Development of the intestine is completed by 10 weeks gestation, foregut, midgut and hindgut forming with their respective blood supplies (coeliac, superior mesenteric and inferior mesenteric arteries). Liver and pancreas arise from the developing duodenum.

- Duodenal — failed vacuolization and recanalization of the developing duodenum during weeks 8 to10 of gestation. Greater association with other major anomalies and development anomalies of the pancreas/biliary tree
- Jejunoileal/colonic — follows a late intrauterine mesenteric vascular event with sterile ischaemia of the bowel (resorbed). Associated with abdominal/mechanical abnormalities (gastroschisis, mucoviscidosis in meconium ileus, with volvulus +/– cystic fibrosis, volvulus secondary to malrotation)
- Relative frequency — jejunal > duodenal > ileal > colonic > pyloric
- More proximal atresia — earlier vomiting, less abdominal distension
- Distal atresia — delayed presentation of vomiting, more abdominal distension, greater fluid and electrolyte abnormality
- Abdominal X-ray — number of dilated bowel loops suggests the approximate level of atresia
- A neonate with an intestinal atresia (as opposed to other causes of intestinal obstruction) will fail to pass any flatus, even after rectal examination

Note: The presence of a few dilated bowel loops is suggestive of a proximal small bowel atresia. It may however represent an infant with little distal midgut following a major intrauterine mesenteric vascular event which may be incompatible with life and only identified at surgery.

4.1 Duodenal obstruction

- Incidence is 1 in 2500 live births
- Intrinsic obstruction — atresia, stenosis, web
- Extrinsic obstruction — annular pancreas, malrotation, pre-duodenal portal vein
- 50% are associated with other anomalies — cardiac, genitourinary, anorectal, OA +/– TOF, malrotation, congenital diaphragmatic hernia, vertebral
- 30–40% are associated with trisomy 21
- 80% are periampullary (bilious vomiting), 20% pre-ampullary (non-bilious vomiting)

Prenatal diagnosis

- Polyhydramnios in up to 75%
- Intrauterine growth restriction, premature delivery in up to 50%
- Dilated stomach and proximal duodenum ('double bubble') on antenatal ultrasound
- Features suggesting trisomy 21 (nuchal translucency)

Post-natal diagnosis

- Index of suspicion — trisomy 21, oesophageal atresia
- Vomiting — especially bilious, initial nasogastric aspirate > 20 ml with no other obvious cause
- Abdominal X-ray — 'double bubble'

Caution — suggestive 'double bubble' with some distal gas may be duodenal stenosis or bifid biliary duct but must exclude malrotation +/– volvulus (see below).

Medical management

- Nasogastric insertion for gastric decompression, intravenous volume replacement
- Assess for other anomalies +/– karyotype if dysmorphic

Surgical care

- Laparotomy — primary repair (duodenoduodenostomy +/– duodenal tapering)
- Post-operative nasogastric replacement — initial aspirate volume may be high (100–150 ml/day), until duodenal stasis is resolved. Replace ml for ml with 0.9% NaCl (with added KCl)

Complications

- Related to co-morbid pathology — cardiac, chromosomal
- Prolonged bilious aspirates because of poor motility from delayed duodenal peristalsis

- Blind loop syndrome — chronic duodenal dilatation and secondary bacterial overgrowth

4.2 Jejunoileal atresia

- Incidence — up to 1 in 1000 to 1500 live births
- Multiple small bowel atresias — jejunal (67%), ileal (25%)
- Few associations with chromosomal abnormalities or other system anomalies
- Bowel length variable — may be foreshortened, risk of short bowel

Post-natal presentation

- Persistent bilious vomiting
- Abdominal distension — most marked with distal atresia, visible bowel loops, fluid and electrolyte disturbance
- Meconium — varies from normal colour to grey plugs of mucus

Radiology

- Dilated bowel loops — number of loops suggests level of atresia (proximal versus distal)
  - Note: In the neonate, large and small bowel are indistinguishable on X-ray because of the poor development of the haustral folds and valvulae conniventes
- Abdominal calcification — meconium peritonitis secondary to an intrauterine perforation

Medical management

- Nasogastric tube insertion for gastric decompression, volume replacement
- Cardiorespiratory support as required

Surgery

- Laparotomy — assessment of bowel length and viability, identification of all atresias, and other pathology, primary anastomosis (more than one may be required) +/– proximal stoma

Complications

- Anastomotic leak
- Stricture formation
- Nutritional — vitamin B_{12} and bile salt absorption affected from loss of terminal ileum
- Short bowel syndrome — following catastrophic small bowel loss, the survival prognosis depends partly on the presence of the ileocaecal valve (30 cm with, 50 cm without). The premature neonate has a greater capacity for functional adaptation

4.3 Colonic atresia

Rare (5% of all atresias), with an incidence of 1 in 1500 to 20,000 live births. Right colon is most commonly affected. Associated with anorectal malformation, Hirschsprung disease, small bowel atresia, renal/cardiac/limb/cerebral abnormalities.

4.4 Pyloric atresia

Rare (< 1% of all atresias), 50% are associated with polyhydramnios, non-bilious vomiting from birth, epigastric distension, single gastric bubble on X-ray, respiratory symptoms are common. Associated with epidermolysis bullosa.

5. MALROTATION

Interference with the normal return of the fetal intestine into the abdominal cavity.

- Present within the first week (55%), or by one month (80%) with only sporadic cases thereafter
- May exist with other abnormalities — exomphalos, gastroschisis, diaphragmatic hernia, cardiac anomalies associated with visceral heterotaxy
- Small bowel predominantly in the right abdomen
- The narrow mesentery is prone to kinking, and in the event of a volvulus, the entire midgut blood supply may be compromised, bowel infarction may occur in 6 h and that gut will be lost

Radiology

- Gas pattern on plain abdominal X-ray may be normal
- Signs of proximal intestinal obstruction +/– asymmetric and/or sparse distal gas pattern
- Failure of the duodenojejunal junction to cross the midline on upper gastrointestinal contrast and lie to the left of the spine
- 'Corkscrew' sign if small bowel volvulus is present
- Barium enema may show caecum/appendix in the right hypochondrium — an unreliable sign alone as the normal neonatal colon is mobile

Caution — bilious vomiting mandates an urgent water-soluble upper gastrointestinal contrast study at any time of the day/night (even if the infant is well, without abdominal distension or tenderness, with a 'normal' plain abdominal X-ray and with normal biochemistry/haematology profiles). Clinical deterioration with abdominal tenderness, cardiorespiratory collapse, metabolic and lactic acidosis, upper/lower gastrointestinal bleeding is a late sign of compromised bowel and impending death. This is a life-threatening emergency.

Surgery

- Adequate resuscitation
- Nasogastric decompression, fluid, broad-spectrum antibiotics

- Laparotomy — confirm diagnosis, untwist volvulus, assess bowel viability/length, resect necrotic bowel, proximal stoma/second-look laparotomy for uncertain viability

6. MECONIUM ILEUS

- Incidence of 1 in 1000 to 2000 live births
- 80–90% will have cystic fibrosis but only 15% of infants with cystic fibrosis will present with meconium ileus
- Thick mucus and viscid meconium, lower lactase/sucrase levels, more albumin and less pancreatic enzyme
- Obstruction of the distended meconium-filled terminal ileum. Small, unused colon, inspissated pellets of colourless mucus
- Complications occur in 50% — antenatal volvulus of the distended ileum with atresia, meconium peritonitis or pseudocyst formation
- Antenatal perforation is sterile, post-natal perforation is complicated by bacterial contamination and systemic sepsis

Diagnosis

- Uncomplicated — abdominal distension, bilious vomiting, failure to pass meconium, 'doughy' mass on palpation within 24–48 h of birth
- Complicated — abdominal wall erythema, oedema, meconium staining – suggests prenatal perforation
- Cystic fibrosis screen

Radiology

- Simple — proximal bowel dilatation, few air-filled loops, meconium mottling ('soap bubble', 'ground glass') often in the right lower quadrant
- Complicated — calcification (extravasation of meconium into the peritoneal cavity), massive bowel dilatation (atresia), displaced bowel loops (pseudocyst), ascites
- Water-soluble contrast enema — barium is contraindicated in case of existing perforation
- Alternative — N-acetylcysteine (Mucomyst) by nasogastric tube or per rectum (breaks down disulphide bridges in tenacious meconium)

Caution — gastrograffin is hyperosmolar and draws fluid into the terminal ileum from the intravascular space, softening the meconium. Adequate fluid resuscitation is vital before and during use to prevent potentially catastrophic cardiovascular collapse.

Surgery

- Simple meconium ileus, following unsuccessful therapeutic enema, laparotomy, instillation of N-acetylcysteine, or enterostomy and irrigation
- Complicated meconium ileus will require operative correction of an atresia, volvulus, pseudocyst, perforation
- Primary anastomosis +/– temporary proximal stoma

Complications

- With cystic fibrosis, 1-year survival is 75–90%
- Late complications — distal intestinal obstruction syndrome (10%), appendicitis (5%), intussusception (2%), rectal prolapse (10–30%)

Meconium plug syndrome

Failure to pass meconium or only a small inspissated plug, passed after per rectum examination, and followed by normal meconium. Usually require therapeutic enema. Exclude cystic fibrosis and Hirschsprung disease, and investigate for underlying cause.

7. HIRSCHSPRUNG DISEASE

Absence of ganglion cells in the myenteric plexus of the most distal bowel; male incidence greater than female. Occurs in 1 in 5000 births.

- Gene on chromosome 10, *RET* proto-oncogene
- Long-segment Hirschsprung disease is familial (4–7%) with equal sex incidence
- Associated with trisomy 21 (5–15% reports vary between 2–15% have Downs), high frequency of other congenital abnormalities, including multiple endocrine neoplasia
- Transition zone in the rectosigmoid junction is most common (> 75%)
- Total colonic/small bowel involvement (5–10%) — poor prognosis

Presentation

- Usually presents in infancy — poor feeding, abdominal distension, delayed passage of meconium, bilious vomiting
- Radiological evidence of distal intestinal obstruction with absence of rectal gas
- Explosive decompression following rectal examination (passage of gas excludes atresia)
- First presentation may be with acute enterocolitis (red, tender, shiny abdomen) +/– severe systemic collapse. Diarrhoea is offensive +/– blood or ischaemic mucosa. May require emergency defunctioning colostomy
- Enterocolotis can occur pre- or post-surgery, associated with *Clostridium difficile* enterotoxin

Initial management

- Nil-by-mouth, intravenous fluids, correction of electrolyte abnormalities, high colonic washouts to decompress the bowel (feeding tube, not balloon catheter)
- Fluid resuscitation + broad-spectrum antibiotics if presenting with enterocolitis
- Poor result — usually technical but may suggest long segment disease

Diagnosis

- Contrast enema — identify transition zone, exclude other pathology
- Definitive test is suction rectal biopsy for histology

Surgery

- Duhamel pull-through — excision of the involved colon, anastomosis with innervated proximal bowel (propulsion), small part of involved rectum remains (sensation and sphincter innervation). Other options are available
- Still have risk of enterocolitis following surgery (treated as above)

Outcome

- Incidence of from enterocolitis: 5–25%, increased in trisomy 21 (29–54%), associated cardiac defects, total colonic involvement (15–25%). Overall mortality from enterocolitis: 5–25%
- Surgical management for anastomotic leak, pelvic abscess, intestinal obstruction
- Medical management of soiling, constipation, frequent loose stools

8. ANORECTAL MALFORMATIONS

8.1 Imperforate anus

- Incidence of 1 in 4000 to 5000 live births
- Association with maternal diabetes
- Male (60%) — most commonly imperforate anus with rectourethral fistula
- Female (40%) — most commonly imperforate anus with rectovestibular fistula
- Imperforate anus without a fistula is uncommon (5%)
- Associated defects are common

Presentation

- Clinical examination
- Failure to pass meconium, abdominal distension, bilious vomiting (late sign)
- Passage of meconium or bubbles per urethra/vagina or meconium staining beneath perineal skin
- Neuropathic bladder if anorectal malformation is not suspected
- Following identification of other VACTERL anomalies (vertebral, anal, cardiac, tracheal, oeophageal, renal and limb)

Initial management

- Nil-by-mouth, intravenous, nasogastric decompression (passage of tube will exclude OA/TOF).
- Systematic examination, chest/abdomen/sacral X-ray, echocardiogram, renal ultrasound, spinal ultrasound (exclude cord tethering), +/– karyotype
- Prophylactic antibiotics until communication with renal tract is excluded (trimethoprim)
- Invertogram to assess level of rectal atresia (lateral shoot through, infant prone over a foam wedge, buttock elevated with a radio-opaque marker at the anal position). Thick meconium within distal bowel or straining (crying) will provide inaccurate results

Surgery

- Sigmoid loop colostomy usually within 48 h
- Distal loopagram and micturating cystourethrogram to identify anatomy of rectum and communication with urinary tract (position of fistula) +/– vesicoureteric reflux
- Posterior sagittal anorectoplasty most commonly indicated
- Various surgical options — may require complex staged procedures, urogenital surgery, dilatation of new anus, medical management of bowel control (including enema)
- Aim for colostomy closure. May be refashioned for protracted soiling (patient request)

Outcome

- Dependent on level of lesion, sacral development (S3, 4 and 5 required for urinary continence) and associated anomalies
- Low lesion — constipation (40%), soiling (15%), diarrhoea (5%)
- High lesion — constipation (35%), soiling (55%), diarrhoea (12%)

9. NECROTIZING ENTEROCOLITIS

Pathological response of the immature gastrointestinal tract to perinatal or post-natal injury. Usually seen in the first 2–3 weeks of life. Rapid and early introduction of non-breast-milk feeds, hyperosmolar feeds and bacterial infection are important aetiological factors. Progressive intestinal mucosal ischaemia, most commonly affecting the caecum, ascending colon and terminal ileum but can affect the entire intestinal tract.

Risk factors

- Prematurity
- Intrauterine growth restriction
- Antepartum haemorrhage
- Perinatal asphyxia (absent or reversed end-diastolic umbilical wave from)
- Respiratory distress syndrome
- Umbilical artery catheterization
- Polycythaemia
- Patent ductus arteriosus
- Premature rupture of membranes
- Sepsis

Radiological signs of gastrointestinal perforation

- 'Football sign' (central, oval abdominal lucency)
- Visible falciform ligament +/– an umbilical venous line in situ
- 'Wrigler's sign' (visualization of both sides of the bowel wall)
- Gas outlining the liver (left lateral decubitus view with horizontal beam projection)
- Scrotal gas (via a patent processus vaginalis)
- 'Triangles' of gas between bowel loops

- Upper abdominal lucency, especially over the liver (anteroposterior supine film, vertical beam projection)

Medical management

- Neonatal intensive care unit–continuous positive airway pressure is avoided in cases of pneumatosis and/or perforation
- Stop enteral feeds for 7–14 days (depending on severity of illness)
- Intravenous antibiotics (broad-spectrum, including metronidazole; consult local unit policy)
- Adequate intravenous analgesia
- Total parenteral nutrition
- Nasogastric tube, on free drainage with hourly aspiration and volume replacement
- Remove umbilical lines
- Regular abdominal X-rays to exclude perforation or the development of a fixed loop
- Consideration of contrast studies — assessment of possible strictures (intolerance of increasing feed volume, intestinal obstruction, or recurrent bacterial translocation following clinical recovery)

Complications

- Recurrence (10% of cases consider Hirschsprung disease)
- Perforation in 20–30%
- Overwhelming sepsis
- Disseminated intravascular coagulation
- Stricture formation — up to 20%
- Short-bowel syndrome (following extensive surgical resection)
- Lactulose intolerance — > 0.5% faecal reducing substances significant

Surgical management

- Indications — pneumoperitoneum, failure of maximal medical management, stricture formation, fixed loop +/– palpable mass
- Insertion of a peritoneal drain — may be life-saving for a tense pneumoperitoneum compromising ventilation
- Laparotomy — allows diagnosis to be confirmed, extent of disease to be assessed and peritoneal toilet to be performed and abscess cavities drained
- Localized resection with primary anastomosis
- Proximal diversion stoma +/– bowel resection
- Stoma formation — ileostomy or colostomy depending on extent/location of necrotizing enterocolitis
- May require more than one procedure, including stoma closure and stricture resection

10. BILIARY ATRESIA

Incidence is 1 in 8000 to 20,000 live births. It is the commonest indication for liver transplantation in childhood.

- **Extrahepatic biliary atresia** — progressive obliteration of part or all of the extrahepatic ducts. Aetiology uncertain
- **Intrahepatic biliary atresia** — this is less common and can be either syndromic (Alagille syndrome) or non-syndromic

Investigations

- Liver function tests (often normal enzymes with conjugated hyperbilirubinaemia), clotting
- Ultrasound (may be normal, gall bladder may be absent)
- Radionuclide Tc-99m iminodiacetic acid (^{99}Tc-HDA) scan (unimpaired hepatic uptake of isotope but failure of excretion into the duodenum after 24 h)
- Liver biopsy
- Laparotomy — operative cholangiography.

Treatment

- Hepatoportoenterostomy (Kasai procedure)
- Aim for surgery before the infant is 60 days old
- Ursodeoxycholic acid to promote bile secretion, fat-soluble vitamin supplementation
- Post-operatively — high risk of cholecystitis (prompt treatment with intravenous antibiotics)
- Fat malabsorption, cirrhosis, liver failure
- Liver transplantation may be indicated

Caroli's disease

- Autosomal recessive, congenital cystic dilatation of the intrahepatic ducts
- Recurrent acute cholangitis, biliary lithiasis, risk of cholangiocarcinoma

11. ANTERIOR WALL DEFECTS

11.1 Gastroschisis

There is controversy regarding the aetiology but it is probably the result of the intrauterine rupture of the right vitelline artery and breakdown of the abdominal wall adjacent to the umbilicus.

- Incidence of 1 in 3000 to 6000 live births, trend increasing
- Typical infant — premature, small for gestational age, lower maternal age, oligohydramnios, antenatal ingestion of aspirin, illegal drugs (vasoconstrictor side-effects), alcohol
- Risk of late intrauterine deaths, monitor fetal movements, increased ultrasound and cardiotocogram in third trimester
- Vaginal delivery is not contraindicated
- Defect is lateral (usually the right, 95%) to the intact umbilical cord

- Herniation of bowel without a covering sac, stomach, occasionally bladder, but never the liver
- Intestinal atresia is common, occurring in approximately 20% of cases. Short bowel may complicate outcome
- Rarely associated with lethal chromosomal or major structural abnormalities
- Can be confused with a ruptured exomphalos

Management at delivery

- Wrap cling-film around entire trunk, covering exposed bowel and ensure infant is well supported in the midline to reduce temperature and fluid evaporative losses
- Large-bore nasogastric tube, intravenous fluids above normal rate
- Regular visual assessment of bowel viability if closure is delayed, and during neonatal transfer

Surgical management

- Undertaken promptly after delivery. May require staged surgical repair
- Total parenteral nutrition and trophic milk via nasogastric tube
- Delay in establishing feeds is related to poor intestinal motility – bilious NG aspirates, abdominal distension, failure to pass changed stool
- Repair of atresia is present when possible

Outcome

- Morbidity is related to short bowel
- 10% risk of necrotizing enterocolitis
- Prognosis is usually good

11.2 Abdominal Compartment Syndrome

Pain/irritability, tense abdomen, poor lower limb perfusion, oliguria, increasing bilious NG aspirates, absent bowel sounds, metabolic/lactic acidosis, decreased venous return, diaphragm splinting, cardiorespiratory compromise

11.3 Exomphalos

- Failure of closure of the abdomen at the umbilical ring
- Incidence is 1 in 5000 to 1 in 10,000 live births, trend is decreasing (partly related to termination of pregnancy following identification of other lethal structural or chromosomal abnormalities)
- 40–70% have associated abnormalities — chromosomal (trisomies 13, 18 and 21), cardiac (25%), genitourinary, gastrointestinal, craniofacial, pulmonary hypoplasia
- Syndromic associations — Beckwith–Wiedemann, prune belly syndrome and pentalogy of Cantrell
- Antenatal karyotype analysis should be advocated, along with a more detailed anomaly

scan. Parental counselling in cases with severe associated abnormalities may include elective termination

Management at delivery

- Leave cord length long
- Cover exomphalos with cling-film, as per gastroschisis (reduce temperature/fluid evaporative loss)
- Support contents in the midline (vertically tie the umbilical cord to the overhead heater or incubator)
- Assess bowel colour through sac (initially transparent), look for blood (hepatic trauma), avoid sac rupture
- Nasogastric decompression, intravenous fluid/electrolyte resuscitation, temperature as per gastroschisis
- Clinical assessment — dysmorphic features (especially midline defects), karyotype, chest X-ray, echocardiacogram, renal ultrasound
- Early and regular blood glucose measurements (Beckwith–Wiedemann syndrome)
- Early surgical involvement

Surgery

- Aim for reduction of abdominal contents and complete closure
- May require staged procedures
- Massive exomphalos (especially with small abdominal cavity) or infants with multiple abnormalities may be managed conservatively. Topical application of saline, to allow eschar formation and skin overgrowth. Delayed surgical management of massive ventral hernia some years later
- Meticulous fluid management

Outcome

- Associated defects or chromosomal abnormalities have a major influence on survival
- 35% mortality, three times that of gastroschisis

12. CONGENITAL DIAPHRAGMATIC HERNIA

- Incidence is 1 in 2500 to 1 in 3500 live births
- Chromosomal abnormalities found in 5–30% of cases (trisomy 18 and 13 are most common)
- Serious associated anomalies in 40% live-born babies (cardiac and neural tube defects)
- Frequent association with intestinal fixation abnormalities including malrotation
- Resulting diaphragmatic defect and associated lung hypoplasia
- Both lungs are structurally abnormal (ipsilateral > contralateral). This is the major determining factor in the outcome of babies born alive with congenital diaphragmatic hernia
- Left-sided is more common than the right (6 : 1)
- 90% are a posterolateral defect (Bochdalek hernia)

- Poor prognostic factors — gestational age < 25 weeks at diagnosis, structural cardiac abnormality, chromosomal abnormality, polyhydramnios, contralateral lung-to-thoracic transverse area ratio < 0.5, contralateral lung-to-head circumference ratio < 0.62, left ventricular hypoplasia

Pentalogy of Cantrell

- A rare defect resulting from a severe mesodermal fusion failure
- Comprises — diaphragmatic hernia (retrosternal defect), lower sternal defect, pericardial defect, major cardiac anomaly and epigastric exomphalos

Differential diagnosis

- Congenital cystic adenomatoid malformation
- Lung sequestration
- Cystic lesions (bronchogenic, thymic, neuroenteric, duplication)
- Diaphragm eventration

Post-natal diagnosis

- Absence of visible diaphragm
- Bowel loops seen in the chest
- Tip of nasogastric tube in the chest (only if stomach herniated)
- Absence of bowel loops within abdomen
- Contralateral mediastinal shift
- Small contralateral lung

Resuscitation at birth

- Avoid bag and mask positive-pressure ventilation (minimize visceral distension)
- Prompt endotracheal intubation in the delivery room for respiratory distress
- Replogle or wide-bore nasogastric tube insertion (will need to be passed beyond the usual distance)
- Chest X-ray to confirm diagnosis, nasogastric tube position and exclude other diagnoses (congenital cystic adenomatoid malformation, pulmonary sequestration)

Medical management

- Minimal stimulation with consideration of paralysis
- Abnormal pulmonary vascular reactivity produces reduced lung perfusion, pulmonary
- hypertension, right-to-left shunting through the foramen ovale, ductus arteriosus and intrapulmonary vessels
- Surfactant used in some centres
- Maintain preductal oxygen saturations at 85–90%

Minimal ventilation pressures to reduce barotrauma. Iatrogenic injury from ventilation strategies may be significant and should be minimized

- Volume resuscitation and vasopressors (dopamine and dobutamine) often required
- Pulmonary vasodilatation with inhaled nitric oxide

- High-frequency oscillatory ventilation may be considered when conventional ventilation fails to correct hypoxia and hypercarbia, or when peak airway pressures remain high ($> 30 \, \mathrm{cmH_2O}$)
- Extracorporeal membrane oxygenation has not offered consistent results
- Persistent pulmonary hypertension of the newborn is a major determinant of survival and consideration of the timing of surgery

Surgical management

- Stabilization with medical treatment takes priority
- Operative repair includes reduction of the herniated viscera into the abdominal cavity
- Closure of the diaphragmatic defect: direct suture +/− a prosthetic patch
- Diaphragm agenesis may require more extensive surgical intervention

Complications

- Continued medical management of pulmonary hypoplasia
- Thoracic wall deformities with growth
- Detachment of prosthetic patch: may require further surgery

13. MALFORMATIONS OF THE AIRWAY AND LUNGS

13.1 Choanal atresia

- Obstruction at the level of the posterior border of the nasal septum — 90% bony, 10% membranous
- Incidence of 1 in 10,000
- Symptoms from birth (if bilateral) as neonates are obligate nose breathers
- Failure to pass a catheter beyond the posterior nares
- Transnasal surgical correction with post-operative temporary stenting

Macroglossia

- Localized — haemangioma, lymphangioma
- Generalized — hypothyroidism, Beckwith–Wiedemann syndrome (check blood glucose)
- May require surgical reduction

13.2 Laryngeal cleft

- Incomplete separation of foregut into trachea and oesophagus
- Rare condition, may occur in isolation, involves larynx +/− trachea
- Associated with — OA/TOF, cardiac, palate, genitourinary anomalies
- Feeding aspiration, recurrent pneumonia, stridor, weak cry
- May require intubation +/− tracheostomy
- Endoscopic assessment
- Surgical repair may be complex

13.3 Congenital lobar emphysema

- Overexpansion of alveolar spaces — segment or lobe (normal lung histology)
- Cartilaginous deficiency/abnormality (35–50%)
- Post-infective alveolar septal fibrosis (30%)
- Extrinsic compression — cardiomegaly from congenital cardiac anomalies in 15% (ventricular septal defect, patent ductus arteriosus, tetralogy of Fallot), aneurysmal dilatation of major vessels, bronchogenic cyst
- Acquired — preterm or small for gestational age neonates after long-term ventilation
- Inspiratory airflow — producing a 'ball-valve' defect, air-trapping and compression of adjacent lung

Presentation

- Some diagnosed antenatally on ultrasound
- Usually within a few hours of birth (50%) with severe respiratory distress
- Chest asymmetry, hyperresonant
- May be asymptomatic at birth, with symptoms by 6 months

Radiology

- Left upper lobe (42%), right upper lobe (21%), right mid-lobe (35%), rare in lower lobes
- Hyperlucent overexpanded lung
- Herniation of emphysematous segment/lung across midline (anterior to mediastinum)
- Mediastinal shift
- Compression/atelectasis of adjacent lung/lobes
- Depression of ipsilateral diaphragm
- Ventilation–perfusion scan may confirm absent perfusion/ventilation in severe cases

Management

- Mild cases — conservative, regular review with chest X-ray
- Echocardiogram
- Most require lobectomy — may be required urgently for life-threatening respiratory insufficiency. Emphysematous lobe may bulge out of the operative field

Follow-up

- After lobectomy, no significant functional impairment
- Asymptomatic overdistended lobes do not impair development of normal lung

13.4 Congenital cystic adenomatoid malformation

- May be identified on antenatal ultrasound — echogenic fetal chest mass +/– hydrops
- Some demonstrate resolution after birth (uncertainty regarding pathology/prognosis)
- 20–25% are stillborn or die rapidly from severe respiratory insufficiency
- Neonatal period — progressive respiratory distress (enlarging lesion with air-trapping)
- May require emergency surgery

- Symptoms are also related to degree of pulmonary hypoplasia (ipsilateral and contralateral), from compression
- Single lobe in 80%
- Displacement of cardiac apex
- Hyperresonant hemithorax

Radiology

- Chest and abdominal X-ray will help to distinguish between a congenital cystic adenomatoid malformation and diaphragmatic hernia (demonstrate normal intestinal gas pattern in the former but not the latter)
- Early plain films may be radio-opaque (delayed clearance of lung fluid)
- Air-filled cystic spaces, adjacent lung compression, subtle changes (appear normal)
- Computed tomography (CT) scan — precise anatomical location and extent of disease (see below)

Management

- Most will be sufficiently stable for complete pre-operative assessment (X-rays and CT)
- Symptomatic — elective lobectomy
- Asymptomatic — controversial

13.5 Pulmonary sequestration

- Congenitally abnormal non-functioning lung tissue
- No communication with the tracheo-bronchial tree
- Systemic blood supply from the aorta

Intralobar pulmonary sequestration

Sequestered lobe is contained within normal lobe. Asymptomatic or recurrent pulmonary sepsis, often in older children. Venous drainage to the pulmonary system, occasionally to the azygous/hemiazygous.

Extralobar pulmonary sequestration

Sequestered lobe has a separate pleural covering. Most common in left lower lobe, often seen on antenatal ultrasound. Associated with left-sided congenital diaphragmatic hernia (60%). Also seen with cardiac anomalies, pericardial defect, pectus excavatum, broncho-genic cysts, vertebral anomalies. May occur below the diaphragm.

Radiology

- Require CT or magnetic resonance imaging (MRI) to identify/locate abnormal arterial supply

Management

- Thoracotomy and resection, taking care with identification of blood supply (which is often large)
- Surgery advocated for risk — infection, malignancy
- Outcome is related to associated anomalies

13.6 Bronchogenic cyst

Abnormal bronchial budding. Rarely have any communication with the tracheobronchial tree. Some show early respiratory distress, recurrent pneumonia; confirm diagnosis on CT. Treatment is by surgical resection (there is a late risk of sarcomatous change).

14. NEONATAL TUMOURS

- 50% are diagnosed at delivery; a further 30% are diagnosed within a week of birth
- A palpable mass is the most common presentation
- Malignant tumours are rare, occurring 1 in 27,000 births
- Most solid tumours are benign
- Teratoma is the most common neoplasm (45% of all tumours)
- Neuroblastoma is the most common malignant tumour (15–25%)

14.1 Teratoma

- Embryonal neoplasm derived from the germ layers (ectoderm, mesoderm, endoderm)
- Most common in paraxial or midline location — sacrococcygeal (45–64%), mediastinal (10%), gonadal (10–35%), retroperitoneal (5%), cervical (5%), presacral (5%)
- Solid, cystic or mixed
- 80% benign, 20% malignant

14.2 Sacrococcygeal teratoma

- Incidence of 1 in 20,000 to 40,000 live births
- 75% female, 25% male
- Associated anomalies (18%)

Diagnosis

- Antenatal — ultrasound imaging, elevated serum α-fetoprotein/human β-chorionic gonadotrophin (see below)
- Poor prognosis — polyhydramnios, placentomegaly, gestational age < 30 weeks
- Late presentation – features of urinary or intestinal obstruction, lower limb neurology or malignancy
- Imaging — plain X-ray, MRI, CT

α-fetoprotein

Normally produced by the fetal liver, also by yolk sac tumour elements. Plot serum levels against a nomogram (levels fall rapidly following birth). Levels should fall to normal following successful resection. Elevated levels may suggest malignancy. Rising levels indicate recurrence.

β-subunit human chorionic gonadotrophin

From chorionic syncytiotrophoblastic cells (malignant teratoma). Rising levels after surgery suggest persistent or recurrent tumour.

Complications

- Placentomegaly
- Hydrops
- Cardiac failure
- Malpresentation, premature rupture of membranes, cord prolapse, placental abruption, shoulder dystocia
- Massive bleeding

Surgery

- Resection (< 2 months at latest) — may require combined abdominal and perineal approach. Technically difficult. Requires excision of coccyx
- Follow-up with 3-monthly tumour markers, clinical assessment (PR (rectal examination)) +/- further imaging
- Greatest risk of malignant change — surgery after 2 months, incomplete excision, immature elements on histology

15. SPINA BIFIDA

- Defects in the fusion of the neural tube, incidence of 1 in 500 to 1 in 2,000 live births
- Defects of increasing severity – spina bifida occulta, meningocele, myelomeningocele, myelocele

Presentation

- Less severe defects may not be apparent at birth, cutaneous stigmata (pigmentation anomalies, excess hair, lipoma, dermal sinus)
- Obvious open lesion — skin defect, cord may be protected by pia arachnoid, or there may be an open neural tube defect (exposed neural plate)
- Many are associated with central nervous system abnormalities (hydrocephalus)

Assessment

- Level of lesion (cervical, thoracic, lumbar, sacral — most will be lumbosacral), and size
- Neurological deficit — motor and sensory level, spontaneous limb movement, posture. Always begin sensory assessment from 'abnormal to normal' area
- Bladder/bowel function — appearance and sensation of perineum; rectal prolapse, absent natal cleft (paralysis of pelvic floor/sphincters)
- Hydrocephalus — bulging anterior fontanelle, persistent metopic suture, suture diastasis, setting-sun eyes, frontal bossing, enlarging head circumference (crossing percentile curves), +/− Arnold–Chiari malformation (see below)
- Orthopaedic deformities — spine (kyphoscoliosis), hips (congenital dislocation), feet (talipes)
- Other abnormalities — sacral agenesis (partial/complete), cord tethering, renal tract anomalies (hypospadias, horseshoe kidney, exstrophy), congenital heart disease, anorectal malformation, craniofacial anomalies

Neurology level

- **L3** — legs totally paralysed
- **L4/L5** — flexed hip, extended knee, no other movement
- **S1** — movement of the hip and knee, foot can dorsiflex but not plantarflex
- **S2/S3** — normal leg movements, still doubly incontinent

Immediate management

- Prone positioning (with attention to prevent faecal soiling of exposed neural tissue)
- Cover exposed neural tissue with cling-film (wrapped around trunk)
- Broad-spectrum antibiotics
- Intermittent urinary catheterization

Surgery

- Formal closure of defect with reconstruction of anatomical layers
- Ventricular shunt for hydrocephalus
- Delayed orthopaedic procedures may be required
- Clean intermittent catheterization +/− bladder augmentation procedures

Outcome

Poor prognosis with severe hydrocephalus, severe kyphosis, thoracolumbar lesions, associated malformations, poor social support

- Meningitis and ventriculitis (10–15%) requires prompt treatment
- Hydrocephalus — thoracolumbar lesion (95%), lumbosacral (60%)
- Ambulation — dependent on level of lesion, orthopaedic abnormalities, intellect. Thoracic and lumbar (few achieve independence), sacral (most), lumbosacral (many can walk with calipers but may choose a wheelchair for ease)
- Lumbosacral: with clean intermittent catheterization, nearly 90% remain continent
- Intellectual development: dependent on level, up to 40% have IQ impairment

16. MISCELLANEOUS CONDITIONS

16.1 Antenatal torsion

Presentation

- Non-tender, discoloured scrotal swelling, usually unilateral
- Differential diagnosis — hydrocoele, traumatic haematoma (breech delivery), incarcerated inguinal hernia (associated with a thickened cord), lesion secondary to patent processus vaginalis (meconium, intraperitoneal bleeding) infection, gonadal neoplasm

Investigations

- Abdominal X-ray may be helpful — identification of scrotal contents via patent processus vaginalis (air within a herniated bowel loop), meconium (antenatal intestinal perforation)
- Ultrasound — distinguish solid from cystic masses. Useful if concerned about a possible tumour

Management

- Testis is considered non-viable at the time of presentation
- Most will not remove ischaemic testis but will elect for early fixation of the contralateral side

16.2 Accessory digit

- Extra digits (polydactyly) may be simple or complex
- Tags or digit remnants — most common, near metacarpophalangeal joint of little finger
- No palpable bone in base, attached by a soft tissue stalk (containing digital nerve and vessels)
- Requires surgical excision to prevent formation of a painful neuroma
- More complex anatomy requires orthopaedic referral for formal amputation

General Paediatric Surgery

17. HEAD AND NECK SURGERY

17.1 Ranula

- A mucous retention cyst of the sublingual salivary gland caused by partial obstruction of the duct
- Presents clinically as soft, occasionally tense, clear swelling on the floor of the mouth
- Can increase in size after first appearing
- Usually symptomless, although they can be painful
- Treatment consists of marsupialization of the cyst by incising the cyst wall and suturing the edges open; thereby draining the obstructed gland. Only very occasionally is excision required

17.2 Cystic hygroma (lymphangioma)

- A lymphangioma in the head and neck
- Location is the only distinguishing feature from lymphangiomas in other sites
- A congenital anomaly caused by the failure of connection of part of the lymphatic system during embryological development
- Do not always present in the neonatal period, and the presentation is often precipitated by an unrelated infection (e.g. viral upper respiratory tact infection).
- Commonest sites of occurrence in order of frequency are:
  - Neck
  - Axilla
  - Chest
  - Abdominal
- Can be identified antenatally
- Present clinically as a brilliantly trans-illuminable multi-cystic swelling
- Usually soft
- If infected they can become tense, red and painful; occasionally progressing to abscess formation
- Can also cause symptoms by exerting pressure on adjacent structures (e.g. dysphagia, stridor, respiratory compromise)

Differential diagnosis

- Includes haemangiomas, lipomas, dermoid cysts and mixed lesions. Lymphangiomas are rarely of a 'pure' pathology; commonly they are combined with vascular or fatty elements
- Ultrasound used to confirm the diagnosis and assist with identification of macrocystic and microcystic varieties
- Occasionally CT scan is required to define extent large lesion and anatomic relationships

Treatment options

- Conservative management has become the aim — commonly after initial presentation and increase in size these lesions undergo involution; this is also common after infection
- Sclerotherapy — the most common agent is OK-432, which is a streptococcus-derived antigen. It is more successful in predominantly macrocystic lesions. Causes an acute inflammatory reaction (with acute swelling and symptoms) that causes involution but may have an adverse, temporary effect on contiguous structures (e.g. stridor).
- Surgical excision is occasionally required for larger lesions or those that do not respond to other modalities of treatment.

17.3 Thyroglossal cyst

- Thyroid gland develops as a diverticulum at the foramen caecum and descends to its cervical location in fetal life. Path is marked by the thyroglossal tract. Persistence of part or the entire tract leads to thyroglossal duct and cyst
- Presents as a midline swelling between the tongue and infra-hyoid region. Moves with swallowing and protrusion of the tongue, although this sign is relatively insensitive
- Ultrasound is indicated to identify a normal thyroid gland, and to confirm the diagnosis
- Surgical excision includes excision of the cyst, along with the tract (and central portion of the hyoid bone), all the way to the base of the tongue

17.4 Preauricular pits

- Ectodermal inclusions that occur during formation of the auricles of the ear
- Shallow, blind-ending pits which end in the subcutaneous tissues
- Present at birth and often bilateral
- Can become infected and surgical excision is sometimes recommended

17.5 Branchial arch remnants

- In weeks 4–8 of fetal life the cervicofacial region is occupied by four branchial arches with corresponding pharyngeal pouches with intervening clefts. Persistence or abnormal development leads to branchial fistulas, sinuses and cysts (least common)
- First, third and fourth branchial anomalies are all rare

- Second branchial arch fistulas and sinuses are common and are found along the anterior border of the sternocleidomastoid, usually at the junction of the middle and lower thirds. The tract ascends between the bifurcation of the carotid artery to the tonsillar fossa

17.6 Cervical lymphadenopathy

- Most common cause of neck swelling over 2 years of age
- Usually ascribed to viral infection but can also be secondary to bacterial infections in and around the head and neck
- Nodes of the anterior cervical chain are more commonly affected
- Enlargement is usually self limiting
- In toxic children, intravenous antibiotics may be required. Penicillin and flucloxacillin are used to cover staphylococcal and streptococcal infections
- If the infection is not well contained, suppuration and abscess formation supervene. The node is then tender and fluctuant with overlying redness of the skin. Ultrasound is useful in identifying pus in the centre if there is uncertainty. Incision and drainage are required
- Enlarged lymph nodes may be the result of tuberculous or atypical mycobacterial infection
- Cat scratch disease can also present with chronic enlargement. There may not be a memory of the implicating scratch, which precedes the lymphadenopathy by 3–4 weeks
- Lymphoma may present with enlarged lymph nodes. Abnormal nodes and those that persist for more than 3 months (without an obvious cause) should be biopsied

17.7 Haemangioma and arteriovenous malformations

- A congenital benign tumour affecting veins, arteries or a combination of both
- Present in 2% of newborns; the incidence increases to 10% at 5 years
- Several growth factors are thought to be involved in pathogenesis; lead to proliferation of the vascular tissues in the first months of life, with an increase in the size of the lesion
- Many subsequently regress spontaneously
- Arteriovenous malformations are always present at birth but may not be evident. Unlike haemangioma they have no propensity for regression
- A bruit may be evident
- Visible lesions may be disfiguring
- Complications — ulceration, infection, necrosis, bleeding
- Haemolysis and activation of the coagulative system may occur with large lesions
- Symptoms particular to location may occur (gastrointestinal/pulmonary bleeding, obstruction)
- Cardiac failure may occur with large arteriovenous malformations which cause a significant steal

Investigations

- Usually include an ultrasound to confirm the diagnosis and extent of the lesion
- MRI or CT scans may be required for lesions in some sites
- Angiography may assist in the anatomical definition of arteriovenous malformations

Treatment

- Conservative management — sufficient for most haemangiomas as they resolve, arteriovenous malformations that cause no symptoms can be treated conservatively
- Compression therapy — can be used for accessible lesions and may accelerate involution of haemangiomas
- Sclerotherapy — used for symptomatic lesions; multiple treatments may be required
- Interferon-α — shown by some series to be of benefit in haemangiomas that are resistant to other modalities of treatment. Treatment is required over a few months
- Surgical excision — used for lesions that give rise to complications and do not respond to conservative or other modalities of treatment
- Laser therapy — used for some superficial lesions that are disfiguring
- Embolization — used in cases in which a large feeding vessel can be identified and accessed. Particularly useful in cases with cardiac failure

18. THORACIC SURGERY

18.1 Congenital malformations

- Some congenital lesions that are not detected in the antenatal period, and that do not cause symptoms in the neonatal period, can present in childhood. They often present with recurrent chest infections and coughing
- **Congenital diaphragmatic hernia** (see section 12 above) — may remain undetected until a chest infection supervenes and is detected on chest X-ray. This is especially true for anterior hernias (of Morgagni)
- **Eventration of the diaphragm** — defined as elevation of the hemidiaphragm that results from paucity of muscle in the absence of a defect. The differential diagnosis is a phrenic nerve palsy. Eventration can sometimes present in infancy and childhood as repeated chest infections or failure to recover from a relatively minor chest infection
- **Pulmonary sequestrations, congenital cystic adenomatoid malformation and congenital lobar cysts** — may present outside the neonatal period, although they are increasingly being diagnosed antenatally. Symptomatic lesions are surgically treated after resolution of any acute complications

18.2 Chest wall deformities

Pectus excavatum and pectus carinatum

- Pectus excavatum (funnel chest) is more common than pectus carinatum (pigeon chest). Both are three times more common in males compared to females

- Aetiology of these conditions is unknown. Some form of growth disturbance in the costo-chondral junction is thought to exist, giving rise to depression (excavatum) or protrusion (carinatum) of the sternum
- Can by asymmetrical or unilateral
- Family history in some index cases
- Pectus excavatum can be seen in connective tissue diseases such as Marfan and Ehlers–Danlos syndromes; a thorough physical examination for the stigmata of these should be carried out
- Majority of patients with pectus excavatum have some deformity from birth; only 30% of patients with pectus carinatum have any abnormality at birth
- Can be a worsening of the deformity during growth spurts such as puberty.
- Most children present because they or their parents are concerned about their appearance. Sometimes this is severe enough to prevent older children and teenagers from participating in sports and other activities that cause embarrassment
- No significant effect of either condition on cardiorespiratory function. Although there was much speculation of decreased cardiorespiratory reserve in severely affected children, this has not been substantiated in studies
- Treatment
  - Most cases can be managed by reassurance. Muscle and breast development mitigate the appearance
  - Indication for surgical intervention should be critically scrutinized
  - Surgical correction has involved highly invasive procedures that resect the costal cartilages, invert the sternum with placement of metal rods or bars to correct the deformity
  - Minimally invasive procedure (the NUSS operation) has now made surgeons reconsider the indications for surgery

Poland's syndrome

- Unknown aetiology
- Characterized by hypoplasia or aplasia of the pectoralis major muscle and one or more of the following: hypoplasia or aplasia of the breast or nipple, aplasia of ribs, or syndactyly/bradydactyly

Sternal clefts

- Occur in isolation or associated with other syndromes, the most common being Cantrell's pentalogy (sternal cleft, omphalocele, pericardial and cardiac defects, and diaphragmatic hernia)

18.3   Oesophageal foreign bodies

- Children swallow a multitude of foreign bodies. Coins are the most common but the list includes pins, needles, hairclips, and small toys. Most of these items traverse the gastrointestinal tract without any difficulties. Unwitnessed ingestion can come to light because of symptoms, including choking, coughing, vomiting or regurgitation

- If the object fails to get into the duodenum the likeliest site of impaction is at the level of the cricopharyngeus, followed by the aortic and left main bronchus impressions on the oesophagus, the gastro-oesophageal junction and the pylorus
- If the development of symptoms prompts investigation, radio-opaque objects can be seen on X-ray
- Most are managed conservatively as they progress easily
- Disc batteries cause chemical injury and should be removed promptly if stuck
- Chronic hair or fibre (e.g. carpet) ingestion has occasionally lead to trichobezoars that require laparotomy

18.4 Caustic ingestion

- Caustic damage can occur through ingestion of common household products by exploring toddlers
- Alkali ingestion more commonly affects the oesophagus, whereas acid ingestion more often affects the stomach
- Oesophagus can be severely affected without any obvious oral injury
- Emergency management (National Poisons Unit)
    - ABCs (i.e. airway, breathing, circulation)
    - Steroid have been shown to have no benefit in trials
    - Endoscopy within the first 24 h to assess injury
- Patients can then be observed for symptoms of stricture formation and other complications which include:
    - Perforation
    - Mediastinitis
    - Fistulae formation
- Caustic ingestion can therefore have devastating consequences. Major palliation or reconstructive surgery may be necessary

18.5 Parapneumonic effusions

- An exudate into the pleural space during the course of a pneumonic infection
- Empyema is defined as pus in the pleural space
- Sometimes clinically difficult to distinguish between these two entities in the child who does not recover from pneumonia and has signs of an effusion. Continued pyrexia can be caused by the original disease in the former, or pleural pus in the latter. In either case culture of the fluid is usually negative
- Pressure effects of the fluid, pulmonary consolidation and thickening of the pleura can all limit chest expansion and deter recovery
- Ultrasound is helpful in defining the depth of the effusion, in identifying the presence of loculations and any pleural thickening, and in visualizing the presence of debris in the fluid to suggest pus
- Drainage is indicated by failure to resolve with adequate (albeit presumptive) antibiotic therapy. Tube thoracoscopy is usually coupled with suction (3–5 kPa)

- Fibrinolytic therapy with urokinase is used if ultrasound shows marked debris or loculations
- All patients require aggressive physiotherapy
- Chest tube is removed when drainage is ≤ 50 ml/day (usually on the 3rd to 5th day)
- Video-assisted thoracoscopic surgery is an alternative to, or adjunct to, tube drainage alone. It allows drainage of the pleural space and breaking down of any loculations and decortication in advanced cases
- Surgery (including thoracotomy for decortication) is also required when the lung fails to re-expand after tube therapy, but has had a much diminished role since the advance of fibrinolytics
- Post-operative recovery can be assessed by the return of normal flow patterns on respiratory function tests in the outpatients

19. GASTROINTESTINAL SURGERY

19.1 Abdominal wall herniae

Umbilical herniae

- Umbilicus develops by closure of the cicatrix after the cord thromboses. The cicatrix closes by fibrosis, probably aided by abdominal wall muscle contraction. Complete closure can be delayed until the 5th year of age
- Herniae present as a bulge through a circular defect in the centre of the cicatrix
- Usually symptomless, but rarely a cause of abdominal pain
- Cosmetic concerns (or teasing) are the main indications for surgery
- Surgical correction consists of repair of the defect with strong mattress sutures. This is delayed until after the 5th birthday

Supraumbilical hernia

- Less common than umbilical hernia
- Defect is sited above the cicatrix, therefore elliptical and points downwards
- Do not resolve and therefore require operative closure

Epigastric hernia

- Present as intermittent swellings usually midway between the umbilicus and the xiphisternum
- Although present from birth, usually present in school-age children, often with symptoms of abdominal pain (sometimes caused by strangulation of fat in the defect)
- The defect is often difficult to define
- Surgical correction is advised

Inguinal hernia

- A congenital abnormality caused by persistence of the patent processus vaginalis, a peritoneal tube along the path of testicular descent into the scrotum

- Incidence in general population is 1–2%; ten times more common in boys and in premature infants
- Rare association of inguinal hernia in girls with complete androgen insensitivity syndrome; girls presenting with inguinal hernia should have their chromosomes checked
- Present as intermittent swellings in groin which may reach the scrotum
- Irreducibility for prolonged periods can lead to obstruction (abdominal pain, distension and vomiting) and eventually strangulation (hard, tender swelling)
- Elective repair advised
- Patients who present with an irreducible hernia require hernia reduction and delayed repair after the resultant oedema has settled, this generally involves a 24- to 48-h hospitalization and repair before discharge
- Repair consists of reduction of the contents of the hernia, and ligation of the patent processus through a groin incision

Hydroceles

- Identical to inguinal hernia in aetiology
- Usually present as symptomless fluid-filled swellings of the scrotum that are transilluminable, and are variably reducible
- Occasionally present as tense swellings during an acute illness
- Unusual variety is a hydrocele confined to a portion of the cord only (encysted hydrocele)
- Most hydroceles (unlike hernias) resolve without surgery in the first few years of life. Surgery is indicated if they fail to resolve

19.2 Pyloric stenosis

- A condition of unknown aetiology characterized by hypertrophy of the pyloric muscle, resulting in gastric outlet obstruction
- Occurs in 1 in 500 to 1000 live births; with a male to female ratio of 4 : 1
- Strong family history in some cases
- Presentation is that of repeated, progressive, non-bilious, often forceful (typically projectile) vomiting; most commonly in weeks 4–6 after birth
  - Weight loss and dehydration common at presentation
  - Pathognomonic sign is a palpable tumour (olive) in the right upper quadrant
  - May be visible peristalsis
- Ultrasound to confirm the diagnosis only if a mass is not palpable
  - Dimensions positive for pyloric stenosis — wall thickness > 4 mm, length > 17 mm and diameter > 15 mm (younger or premature infants may have smaller measurements)
- Vomiting of stomach contents with gastric acid leads to a hypokalaemic, hypochloraemic, metabolic alkalosis
- Paradoxical aciduria in late stages

- Preoperative preparation is aimed at correcting these abnormalities
  - Acute administration of normal saline (10–20 ml/kg) is used for resuscitation
  - Fluid is prescribed at 150 ml/kg per day of 0.45% saline with KCl
  - When plasma bicarbonate is < 25 mmol/l, correction is adequate, and anaesthesia is safe
- Operative correction can be performed through a right upper quadrant incision, a paraumbilical incision or laparoscopically
- The thickened muscle is divided along its entire length down to, but not breaching, the mucosa
- Postoperative feeds are generally given after 6–12 h and most patients are discharged within 24 to 48 h after surgery

19.3   Intussusception

- Telescoping of one part of the intestine into the other
- Peak incidence between 4 months and 1 year
- Most cases are 'idiopathic' ileocolic intussusception; enlarged Peyer's patches are believed to be causative in most of these cases
- In 5–10% there is a pathological lead point — Meckel's diverticulum, duplication cyst, polyp, haemangioma, or a bleeding point in Henoch–Schönlein purpura; may present with recurrent intussusception
- Classical triad of symptoms (but not present in all patients):
  - Abdominal pain (and drawing up of legs)
  - Bleeding per rectum (red currant jelly stools)
  - Palpable mass
- Vomiting, constipation or diarrhoea may be present and may predate the occurrence of intussusception
- Complete obstruction may be present; but is usually late in the presentation
- Patients can present in extremis, with signs of shock and sepsis
- Management — careful attention to primary resuscitation and fluid management
  - Children can need up to 40 ml/kg fluid resuscitation
  - Triple antibiotics should be started when the diagnosis is suspected
  - Nasogastric decompression required if there are signs of obstruction
- Ultrasound scan confirms diagnosis, with the appearance of the typical target lesion of the telescoping bowel
- Doppler assessment can identify blood flow, or lack of it, in the bowel wall
- Plain abdominal X-ray may reveal signs of obstruction and a soft tissue mass may be seen
- Air enema under radiological control used to reduce the intussusception — with a success rate of around 85%; contraindicated if there are signs of perforation
- Laparotomy indicated for signs of peritonitis, perforation or a failed air enema

19.4   Appendicitis

- Acute appendicitis is one of the most common paediatric surgical emergencies
- Incidence increases with increasing age, but sometimes seen in children as young as 2
- Presentation in the younger child can be atypical and the diagnosis difficult
- Typical history is of colicky central abdominal pain shifting to right iliac fossa, followed by vomiting that is usually non-bilious
- Characterized by low-grade fever and mild tachycardia; may be fetor
- Localized tenderness in the right iliac fossa; localized percussion tenderness may also be present
- Advanced cases may be septic, with hypovolaemia and marked fever
- May be overt peritonitis to suggest perforation
- History in atypical cases may mimic urinary tract infection, with dysuria, frequency and fever
- Diarrhoea may be the prominent symptom, especially with a pelvic appendix

Differential diagnoses

- Urinary tract infection
- Gastroenteritis
- Mesenteric adenitis
- Pancreatitis
- Meckel's diverticulitis
- Viral illness
- Respiratory tract infection
- Diabetic ketoacidosis

Investigations

- Urinalysis to rule out urinary tract infection — urgent microscopy if urinalysis is positive, as a pelvic appendix can give rise to white cells in the urine
- In obvious cases no investigation required. Raised white blood cells and elevated C-reactive protein are often present, but are not specific
- Ultrasound scan can confirm the diagnosis in some cases that are not clear cut. The typical finding is a dilated, non-compressible appendix. There may be some free fluid in the right iliac fossa. However, a negative ultrasound does not rule out appendicitis
- Repeated examination and careful observation are the most useful tools in doubtful cases

Management

- Appendicectomy should be performed as soon as possible — by traditional right iliac fossa incision or laparoscopically
- One dose of preoperative antibiotics is given; the postoperative antibiotic regimen will be dictated by the operative findings

19.5   Meckel's diverticulum

- A congenital remnant of the vitello-intestinal duct, which is a connection between the embryonic gastrointestinal tract and the yolk sac; persistence of part of this tract results in a vitello-intestinal band, cyst, tract or a Meckel's diverticulum
- Contains all layers of the abdominal wall, and often contains ectopic gastric mucosa.
- Classically found 60 cm from the ileocaecal valve, is 5 cm long and has an incidence of 2% in the general population
- Clinical presentation depends on resulting complications
  - Intussusception can occur with the diverticulum acting as the lead point
  - Bleeding can occur as a result of ulceration secondary to acid secretion in the ectopic gastric mucosa. Melena results, with fresh blood per rectum in cases with massive bleeding. Haematemesis is sometimes present
  - Meckel's diverticulitis with/without perforation results from inflammation of the mucosa. Signs and symptoms can often mimic appendicitis
  - Intestinal obstruction can result from volvulus around the vitello-intestinal band, herniation of small bowel beneath the band or intussusception
  - May be an incidental finding
- Investigations are dictated by the clinical presentation, and can include full blood count, clotting screen and an abdominal ultrasound which can sometimes identify a Meckel's diverticulum or cysts. A Meckel's scan (using 99m-technetium) relies on the uptake in ectopic gastric mucosa, but gives a false-negative result in up to 25% of patients
- Treatment consists of resection of the diverticulum
- Treatment of incidentally found lesions is debated; some advocate excision

19.6   Undescended testis

- Defined as undescended if it is not able to be brought down into the scrotum; divided into palpable and non-palpable
- **Ectopic testis** — one that is palpable but located outside the line of normal descent (superficial inguinal pouch, perineum)
- **Retractile testis** — one that can be manipulated into the scrotum and remains there, albeit briefly; these require no surgical intervention
- Incidence of retractile testis at birth varies with gestational age
  - At term the incidence is 2–5%; at 30 weeks gestation it is 20–50%
  - Testicular descent can occur after birth
  - Overall incidence is 1% at 1 year of age. Thereafter descent is unlikely to occur. Because of the inherent risks (torsion, trauma, tumour and impaired spermatogenesis) undescended testes are fixed in the scrotum
- If testis is palpable, the inguinal canal is explored and the testis placed in the scrotum
- Boys with non-palpable testis undergo laparoscopy in an attempt to locate the testis. Occasionally the operation is performed in two stages

19.7   Testicular torsion

- Testicular torsion is a surgical emergency
- Presentation is with acute testicular pain — may be referred to the groin or abdomen.
- There is usually some swelling at presentation, a secondary hydrocele may be present. The hemi-scrotum may be erythematous in advanced cases. On examination the testis is swollen and tender
- Differential diagnosis and key points
  - Epidydimo-orchitis — difficult to differentiate, may have positive urinalysis
  - Torsion of hydatid of Morgagni — may be difficult to differentiate; localized tenderness with blue dot sign superior pole
  - Acute enlargement of a hydrocele — unable to feel testis through fluid, may have an intercurrent viral illness
  - Idiopathic scrotal oedema — erythema and oedema affecting the skin of the scrotum (often bilateral), that extends onto the perineum and inguinal region; testes are non-tender, otherwise the diagnosis is not entertained
- Investigations
  - Urinalysis and/or midstream urine should be performed to rule out infection
  - Ultrasound Doppler of the testis is sometimes entertained, but is seldom helpful in doubtful cases; the torsion may also be intermittent
- Urgent surgical exploration is required to confirm the diagnosis and save the testis

19.8   Phimosis

- Defined as narrowing of the preputial ring that prevents retraction of the foreskin. At birth the foreskin is usually non-retractile (physiological), this regresses with age
- Percentage of boys with retractile foreskin by age — newborn infants, 4%; 1-year-old boys, 50%; 4-year-old boys, 90%
- Physiological phimosis is not an indication for circumcision
- Pathological phimosis may rarely be a primary and congenital anomaly but is much more commonly secondary to repeated attacks of infection that cause scarring
- Difficulty with voiding and ballooning of the prepuce are commonest reasons for referrals, though recurrent bacterial infections (balanoposthitis) may also occur
- Usual infecting organism is *Staphylococcus* sp. — flucloxacillin or co-amoxiclav is usually therapeutic
- Chronic inflammation may lead to a rigid, fibrous foreskin
- Can also be the result of balanitis xerotica obliterans. In this condition, equivalent to lichen sclerosis atrophicus, the foreskin is thickened, inflamed, scarred and unyielding. Circumcision is perfomed in these cases
- Underlying urethral meatal stenosis is an underlying abnormality, and must be looked for in these boys

19.9   Hypospadias

- Hypospadias is an abnormality in which the urethral meatus is situated proximal to the tip of the penis on its ventral aspect
- Anatomically it is described by the position on the meatus as either:
  - Glanular
  - Coronal
  - Penile
  - Peno-scrotal
  - Perineal
- Along with the abnormality of the position of the meatus there is often a degree of deficient ventral development resulting in curvature of the penis (chordee)
- A hooded foreskin is also evidence of a ventral deficiency in penile development
- Incidence is around 1 : 300 live births
- Aetiology unknown in most cases — seen in conditions associated with deficient testosterone secretion or responsiveness (intersex disorders)
- Hypospadias with undescended testis should be investigated as potential cases of ambiguous genitalia
- Severe forms of hypospadias (e.g. peno-scrotal and perineal) are associated with renal tract (and occasionally other systems) anomalies
- Surgical correction includes correction of any chordee, tubularization of appropriate tissue to create a new urethra and skin cover. Tissues used to create the urethra include:
  - Native urethral plate
  - Prepucial skin (hence circumcision is contraindicated in patients with hypospadias)
  - Buccal or bladder mucosa
- Postoperative complications include infection, wound dehiscence, meatal stenosis and fistula formation

20.   FURTHER READING

Arensman RM et al. 2000. *Pediatric Surgery (Vademecum)*. Georgetown, USA: Landes Bioscience.

Ashcraft KW. 2000. *Pediatric Surgery*, 3rd edn. Philadelphia: W.B. Saunders Company.

Burge DM, Griffiths DM, Steinbrecher HA, Wheeler RA. 2005. *Paediatric Surgery*, 2nd edn. London: Edward Arnold (Publishers) Ltd.

Hutson JM. 1988. *The Surgical Examination of Children*. Oxford: Butterworth-Heinemann Ltd.

Nakayama DK *et al.* 1997. *Critical Care of the Surgical Newborn*. Oxford: Blackwell.

Stringer M, Oldham K, Moriquand P and Edward H. 1998. *Paediatric surgery and urology: Long term outcomes*. London: WB Saunders.

Picture permissions

The publisher would like to acknowledge the following image sources:

Emergency Paediatrics
The following figures are reproduced from the BMJ Books publication *Advanced Paediatric Life Support: The Practical Approach 4th Edition,* The Advanced Life Support Group, 2004.

Infant choking protocol, page 205
Pathophysiology of drowning, page 226

Hepatology
The following figures are reproduced from the BC Decker publication *Paediatric Gastrointestinal Disease 4th edition,* Walker, W. Allen *et al.,* 2004.

The two models of hepatic organization, page 429
The three variants of biliary atresia, page 438

Nephrology
The following figures are reproduced from the Blackwell publication *The British Journal of Urology,* Vol 81, supplement 2, April 1998. pp 33–38.

Creatinine clearance in the human fetus and newborn infant, page 663
Factional sodium excretion in the human fetus and newborn infant, page 664

The following figure is reproduced from the Blackwell publication *Clinical Paediatric Physiology,* Godfrey, S. and Baum, J.D., 1979.

Tubular function, page 668

The following figure is reproduced from the Lippincott Williams and Wilkins publication *Pediatric Nephrology 3rd edition,* Holliday, MA, Barrat, TM, Avner DE., 1994.

Renal tubular acidosis, page 684

The following figure is reproduced from the American Society of Peditrics publication *Pediatrics,* Vol 67, page 396, 1981.

Grading of vesicoureteric reflux, page 700

Index